A synopsis of
SURGICAL ANATOMY

A synopsis of
SURGICAL ANATOMY

D. J. DU PLESSIS
CHM (RAND), FRCS (ENG)
*Head of the Department of Surgery,
University of the Witwatersrand, Johannesburg;
Chief Surgeon, Johannesburg General Hospital*

Eleventh edition

**BRISTOL
JOHN WRIGHT & SONS LTD**

© **John Wright & Sons Ltd. 1975**

All Rights Reserved. No part of this publication may be reproduced, stored in a retrieval system, or transmitted, in any form or by any means, electronic, mechanical, photocopying, recording, or otherwise, without the prior permission of John Wright & Sons Ltd.

First Edition 1932
Second Edition 1934
Third Edition 1936
Reprinted 1937
Fourth Edition 1939
Reprinted 1940, 1942
Fifth Edition 1943
Reprinted 1943, 1944, 1945
Sixth Edition 1946
Reprinted 1947, 1948
Seventh Edition 1950
Reprinted 1952
Eighth Edition 1957
Reprinted 1959, 1961
Ninth Edition 1963
Reprinted 1966
Tenth Edition 1969
Eleventh Edition 1975
Reprinted 1984.

ISBN 0 7236 0384 7

Printed in Singapore
by Continental Press

PREFACE TO THE ELEVENTH EDITION

IT IS SAD to report that shortly after the appearance of the tenth edition, Mr. A. Lee McGregor died suddenly and unexpectedly. This is a severe loss to all those associated with this book and tribute must be paid to the outstanding contribution made by this remarkable man. This edition has therefore been undertaken without his help and guidance, but long discussions before his death have ensured that the basic approach has not been altered.

A general revision has been undertaken to bring the whole book up-to-date and also to eliminate those sections which were not absolutely essential because it is important to prevent a book of this type from becoming too large.

The author is indebted to Messrs. John Wright & Sons Ltd. for their unfailing help and advice.

D. J. DU PLESSIS

Department of Surgery,
 Medical School, Hospital Street,
  Johannesburg, South Africa

PREFACE TO THE FIRST EDITION

THE BOOK has been written with the object of presenting anatomical facts of practical value to the senior student and practitioner; no attempt has been made to deal exhaustively with the anatomy of the whole body; the classical textbooks are intended for that purpose. The contents of this book are presented as separate essays, any one of which is complete in itself. It is unnecessary, therefore, to read from the beginning of the book to understand any of the subsequent chapters. In the section on development no dates of the various stages have been mentioned; they are of academic value only, and it is my experience that in the effort to remember dates the student forgets the developmental facts which are of value in practice.

I must express my deep indebtedness to my teachers, the late Dr. Ryland ('Daddie') Whitaker, Dr. E. B. Jamieson, Professor Wm Wright, and many others. I must make especial mention of Sir Harold J. Stiles, who taught me the value of a knowledge of anatomy, and I must thank him for the honour he has done me in writing a Foreword for this volume.

PREFACE TO THE FIRST EDITION

To Professor Raymond Dart I am grateful for the Introduction, for advice, and for constant encouragement. I have endeavoured throughout to mention the authorities whose work I have made use of, but I should like to express here my appreciation of the fact that it is the work of others which gives this book any value it may have.

The illustrations, which form so essential a feature of the work, have been done for me by one of my students, now Dr. E. A. Thomas. I cannot thank him sufficiently for his care and patience with the drawings.

My sincere thanks are due to the publishers, Messrs. John Wright & Sons Ltd., for the great trouble they have taken in the arrangement of the text, and for the remarkable success they have achieved in the reproduction of the drawings.

A. LEE McGREGOR

62 *Muller Street,*
Yeoville,
Johannesburg, South Africa

CONTENTS

	Preface to the eleventh edition	*page* v
	Preface to the first edition	v

Part I: Anatomy of the Normal

I	The scalp	1
II	The meninges and cerebrospinal fluid	5
III	The anatomy of the normal and the enlarged pituitary body	11
IV	The thyroid and the parathyroid glands	17
V	The tonsil	26
VI	The breast	30
VII	Chest, lungs, and bronchi	41
VIII	The umbilicus	52
IX	The gut	55
X	The peritoneal fossae	67
XI	Accessory peritoneal bands	73
XII	The biliary passages	78
XIII	The kidneys and adrenals	89
XIV	The inguinal region	96
XV	The prostate	102
XVI	The ischiorectal fossa	106
XVII	The anal region	109
XVIII	The vertebral column	123
XIX	The anatomy of the child	129
XX	Nerves	136
XXI	Muscles	179
XXII	Fasciae	206
XXIII	Bones	224
XXIV	Joints, tendon-sheaths, and bursae	250
XXV	Ligaments	270
XXVI	Veins	296
XXVII	Lymphatics	324
XXVIII	Important relations	347

Part II: Anatomy of the Abnormal

XXIX	The anatomy of congenital errors	353
XXX	The anatomy of nerve injuries	448
XXXI	Bodily habitus	472
XXXII	Anatomical angles. Stiff joints	475

XXXIII	Sphincters	490
XXXIV	The relationships of the vascular pattern to surgery	499
XXXV	The teeth	572
XXXVI	The limps of infantile paralysis. 'Snapping' joints	576
XXXVII	The pathology of bone in terms of anatomy	580
XXXVIII	Rectal and vaginal examination	584
XXXIX	Anatomical bases of clinical tests	587
XL	The anatomy governing the surgery of the lymphatics	597
XLI	The anatomy governing the surgery of the sympathetic	610
XLII	The anatomy of certain diseases	651
XLIII	The anatomy of surgical procedures	733
XLIV	The anatomy of surgical approach	786
	Index	821

Part I
ANATOMY OF THE NORMAL

Chapter I

THE SCALP

TROTTER points out that the arrangement of the integuments of the scalp is similar to that on the palms of the hand and the soles of the feet, i.e., the skin is firmly bound to a subjacent aponeurosis by a densely fibrous tissue. On the other hand, the main vessels and nerves of the scalp run between the skin and the aponeurosis, whereas in the hands and feet the palmar and plantar vessels lie deep to the aponeurosis (i.e., palmar and plantar fasciae).

LAYERS OF THE SCALP

The scalp consists of five layers (*Fig.* 1):
 S   Skin.
 C   Connective tissue—dense.
 A   Aponeurosis of the occipitofrontalis or epicranius muscle.
 L   Loose connective tissue.
 P   Pericranium or periosteum.

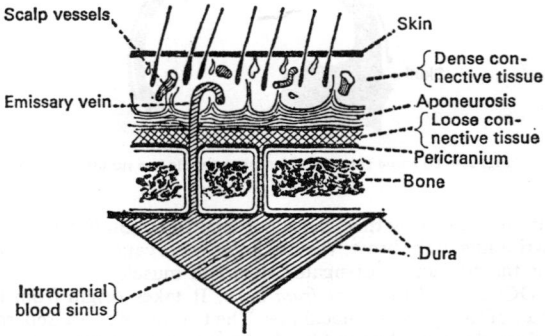

Fig. 1.—Diagrammatic representation of the anatomy of the scalp.
Note particularly the emissary vein.

Skin: This is denser here than anywhere else in the body. It contains great numbers of hairs and sebaceous glands. Therefore the scalp is the commonest site for the occurrence of sebaceous cysts.

Dense Connective Tissue: This layer acts as a very firm bond of union between the skin above it and the epicranius muscle and its aponeurosis (galea aponeurotica) beneath it. It is very dense and fibrous and contains the nerves and blood-vessels of the scalp. The vessel walls are firmly anchored by this connective tissue. For this reason wounds of the scalp bleed profusely as the torn vessels are prevented from retracting. The bleeding, on the other hand, can always be arrested by pressure against the underlying bone. Subcutaneous haemorrhage into this layer is never extensive, as expansion is limited. Inflammation here also occasions little swelling but much pain, because of the unyielding nature of the stratum. The blood-supply of the scalp is very profuse. It is therefore hardly ever necessary to cut away partly avulsed portions of scalp, as sufficient blood will enter the flap through the remaining connexions to ensure its vitality.

Aponeurotic Layer: This is muscular in front and behind. The muscles are connected by the galea aponeurotica or aponeurosis of the occipitofrontalis.

> THE FRONTALIS *has no bony origin*. It arises from the skin and subcutaneous tissue in the region of the eyebrow and root of the nose, and blends with the orbicularis oculi (*Fig*. 2). It is inserted into the galea. Its fibres run vertically and the right and left muscles

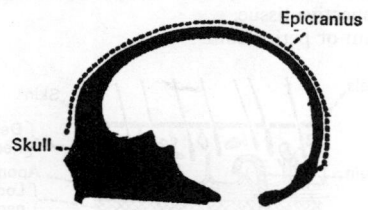

Fig. 2.—To show that the epicranius muscle has no attachment to bone in front.

> are in contact by their inner borders. In action it causes transverse wrinkling of the brow. Vertical furrows are caused by the contraction of the subjacent corrugator supercilii muscles.

> THE OCCIPITALIS *arises from bone*. It takes origin from the outer half of the superior nuchal line. The two muscles are separated by a triangular gap which is filled by an extension of the galea on its way to be attached to the same line.

> THE GALEA APONEUROTICA is a very dense strong membrane. Over the temporal region it becomes much thinner and is attached to the zygomatic arch. Wounds of the scalp do not gape unless the epicranius or galea be divided transversely, as the skin is so firmly united to this structure that only a knife can separate them.

Loose Connective Tissue: This is very tenuous and delicate. Emissary veins connecting the venous sinuses in the skull with the veins of the scalp traverse this area. It is usually overlooked that the vessels and nerves which reach the scalp from the orbit must lie in this layer for a short distance. The first three layers of the scalp can readily be separated from the pericranium through this plane. This layer forms a potential space where blood or pus may collect. Such a collection can extend over the whole dome of the skull, being limited only by the attachments of the epicranius and the galea. It may extend therefore—

Posteriorly—to the superior nuchal line.

Laterally—to the zygomatic arch.

Anteriorly—it may track into the root of the nose and the eyelids because the frontalis has no attachment to bone.

A 'black eye' can be caused in different ways:

1. It is usually due to local violence causing subcutaneous extravasation of blood into the lids. It appears within an hour or so after the receipt of the violence, and the haemorrhage occurs simultaneously in both lids.

2. A black eye may also, however, be due to a blow on the skull causing bleeding into the layer of loose connective tissue. The blood, gravitating slowly downwards under the origin of the frontalis, appears in the eyelids, taking usually a day or two to do so, and being first seen in the upper lid and only later in the lower one.

3. Fracture of the orbital plate of the frontal bone causes haemorrhage into the orbit. The blood tracks forwards under the conjunctiva, appearing in a triangular shape, the apex being at the margin of the cornea. This so-called 'flame-shaped' haemorrhage is to be distinguished from subconjunctival haemorrhage due to local violence to the eye, by the fact that in the former the posterior limit of the haemorrhage cannot be seen.

Because of its potential great extent and the presence in it of certain emissary veins, the subaponeurotic space is often called 'the dangerous area of the scalp'. An old surgical axiom states that 'if it were not for emissary veins, wounds of the scalp would lose half their significance'.

In children the dura and pericranium are more intimately attached to the skull bones than in the adult. It follows that fractures of the vault may result in tearing of the dura and pericranium so that intracranial haemorrhage may make its way through the line of fracture and collect in the subaponeurotic compartment of the scalp. No signs of compression of the brain develop until the subaponeurotic space is full of blood. When this happens signs of cerebral compression develop rapidly. Such a collection of blood has been aptly termed a 'safety-valve' haematoma.

Traumatic cephalhydrocele is a rare condition sometimes seen in young children, consisting of a swelling under the scalp made by a collection of cerebrospinal fluid which has escaped via a fracture of the vault associated with tearing of the membranes of the brain. It may become tense when the child cries.

The Pericranium or periosteum of the scalp is but loosely attached to the surface of the skull bones except at the suture lines and over the temporal fossae. At the suture lines it dips in between the adjacent bones as the sutural membrane, which is blended with the periosteum of the interior of the skull, which latter is merely the outer layer of the dura. Over the temporal fossae the pericranium is firmly fixed to the whole floor of the fossae. Collections of fluid beneath the pericranium can therefore strip it easily but cannot transgress the suture lines. For this reason such a swelling (cephalhaematoma, traumatic cephalhydrocele) will take the shape of the bone to which it is related. The features which distinguish haemorrhages in the different layers of the scalp are of great diagnostic value to the surgeon. The surgeon does not hesitate to reflect the pericranium if necessary, as the skull bones are nourished not only by the periosteum on their inner surface, but also, if not mainly, by the vessels which enter at the attachments of muscles to the bones (H. S. Souttar[1]). The big osteoplastic flaps of modern surgery rarely necrose, although frequently the only structure left attached to the bone is the insertion of muscles.

TEMPORAL REGION

In this region the scalp consists of the following layers: (1) Skin; (2) Dense connective tissue; (3) Thinned-out aponeurosis of the occipitofrontalis and the origin of two of the extrinsic muscles of the ear; (4) Temporal fascia; (5) Temporal muscle; (6) Pericranium.

Temporal Fascia: This is the only structure to which it is necessary to allude. It is attached to the superior temporal line or crest, while below it splits into two laminae which are attached to the zygomatic arch. It is exceedingly dense, which is understandable if it be remembered that it is morphologically analogous to bone. In the tortoise the temporal fossa is a bony tunnel. The practical significance is that wounds of this fascia may be mistaken for wounds of the skull, because of the firmness of the wound edges to the examining finger.

---

[1] *Br. med. J.*, 1928, **1**, 295.

Chapter II

THE MENINGES AND CEREBROSPINAL FLUID

THE meninges are: *dura mater*, *arachnoid mater*, and *pia mater*, from without in.

Dura Mater: Consists over the brain of two layers, named 'periosteal' and 'investing', which are firmly adherent excepting where they split to enclose venous sinuses (*Fig.* 3). These latter are formed in two ways: (1) By a separation of the two layers; (2) By a reduplication of the inner layer.

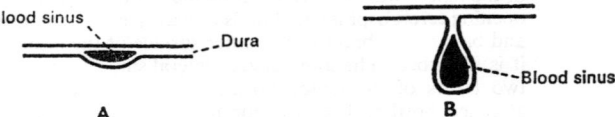

Fig. 3.—Showing the methods of formation of the intracranial blood sinuses: A, A split between the two layers of the dura; B, A reduplication of the inner layer.

THE OUTER PERIOSTEAL LAYER is the periosteum of the inner surface of the skull bones. It ends at the foramen magnum. It is firmly adherent over the base, less so over the vault, except at the sutures, where it is attached to the pericranium by the sutural membrane. It is continuous with the pericranium at the foramina.

Note that owing to the firm fixation of this layer of dura to the base, it is usually torn in fractures of the base of the skull, and as it forms part of the walls of the basal venous sinuses such as the petrosals, fractured base is frequently associated with severe bleeding from ear or nose, or into the pharynx.

In children the outer layer of dura is firmly attached to the vault. For this reason fractures of the vault in children are more apt to result in tearing of the dura and its sinuses than are similar conditions in the adult.

INVESTING OR INNER LAYER:
1. Gives sheaths to the nerves which leave the skull.
2. Becomes continuous with the dura mater spinalis at the foramen magnum.
3. Sends four processes inwards:
   a. FALX CEREBRI: A sickle-shaped reduplication which intervenes

between the medial surfaces of the two hemispheres. It contains three venous sinuses: (i) The superior sagittal along its upper border; (ii) The inferior sagittal along its lower (free) border; (iii) The straight sinus along its line of attachment to the tentorium cerebelli.

b. TENTORIUM: This is a semilunar reduplication of the dura which intervenes between the cerebellum and the occipital lobes of the brain. It therefore roofs in the posterior fossa of the skull. Its outer convex attached border is attached to the lips of the transverse sinus on the occipital bone, the mastoid angle of the parietal bone, and the superior border of the petrous temporal; it ends by being attached to the posterior clinoid process. Its inner concave free border extends forward over the attached border to become attached to the anterior clinoid process. This border bounds an oval space—'the door of the tent'—which is occupied by the midbrain. Through this opening cerebrospinal fluid finds its way from the spinal region and base of the brain to the outer surface of the brain, where it is absorbed. The transverse or lateral sinus lies between the two layers of the tentorium along the posterior half of its attached border. The superior petrosal sinus lies along the anterior half of this border.

c. FALX CEREBELLI: A small sickle-shaped fold intervening posteriorly between the two halves of the cerebellum. It contains the occipital sinus.

d. DIAPHRAGMA SELLAE: A fold of dura roofing over the pituitary fossa. It has a central aperture for emergence of the infundibulum (stalk) of the pituitary. It encloses the intercavernous sinuses.

The importance of the dura to the surgeon can hardly be over-estimated. In wounds of the head it is a barrier to infection; moreover, damaged brain tissue does not readily adhere to it. The prognosis in open injuries of the brain is largely dependent on whether or not the dura can be closed.

SPINAL DURA: A single layer continuous with the inner layer of the dura mater of the brain. It is a long tube enclosing the spinal cord but extending five vertebrae lower. Its existence as a tube ends at the 2nd sacral vertebra, but a prolongation of the membrane invests the filum terminale, ending on the back of the coccyx.

METHOD OF FIXATION: The dural tube of the spinal cord is anchored as follows:

1. It is firmly adherent to the margins of the foramen magnum, and to the 2nd and 3rd cervical vertebrae.
2. It is loosely attached at the upper and lower parts of the vertebral canal to the posterior longitudinal ligament.

THE MENINGES AND CEREBROSPINAL FLUID

3. The anterior and posterior nerve-roots which pierce it carry tubular dural prolongations which are attached to the periosteum of the bones at the intervertebral foramina.
4. The attachment to the coccyx of the investment to the filum terminale.

EPIDURAL SPACE: Between the dura and the walls of the vertebral canal lie delicate veins and fat.

SUBDURAL SPACE: This is a capillary space between the dura and arachnoid over both brain and cord. It contains no cerebrospinal fluid.

Arachnoid Mater: A delicate avascular membrane which dips into the longitudinal and lateral fissures of the brain. It ends at the 2nd sacral vertebra.

ARACHNOIDAL PROCESSES:
1. THE ARACHNOIDAL VILLI: These are fine tortuous processes described by Weed and his co-workers. They arise from the anterior surface of the arachnoid, push the dura before them, eventually perforating it and projecting into the venous sinuses and large veins. They are covered by specialized mesothelial cells which convey the cerebrospinal fluid to the blood-stream. The exact process involved is obscure, but may be filtration and dialysation.
2. THE ARACHNOIDAL GRANULATIONS (PACCHIONIAN BODIES): These are merely aggregations of arachnoidal villi clumped together. They have the same functions and relations as the villi, but are found only in adults, not in children.

Pia Mater: Very thin and delicate. All the blood-vessels to the brain and cord run on it before entering the brain or cord, yet the pia itself is avascular.

PROCESSES GIVEN OFF BY THE PIA:
1. The perivascular spaces (*Fig.* 4): The blood-vessels going to the brain lie in the subarachnoid space before piercing the pia.

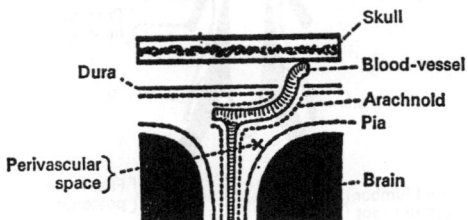

Fig. 4.—The structure of the perivascular space. (*After Cushing.*)

They carry with them into the brain a double 'sleeve' of the leptomeninges. The outer wall of the double sleeve is derived from the pia, the inner from the arachnoid. This was clearly shown by Weed.[1] This is the structure of all the perivascular spaces of the brain. The so-called Virchow-Robin space, by which is meant an adventitial lymph space within the wall of the blood-vessel itself, has, according to Weed, no existence in fact.

2. Septa dip into all the sulci and fissures of the brain.
3. Sheaths to all cranial and spinal nerves.
4. *Tela choroidea* of the fourth ventricle is the name given to the pia over the lower part of the roof of the fourth ventricle. The choroid plexuses of the fourth ventricle lie in it.
5. *Tela choroidea* of the third ventricle is the pia which lies above the roof of the third ventricle. The choroid plexus of the third ventricle and the choroid plexus of each lateral ventricle are invested by this pial process.
6. A septum into the anterior median fissure of the spinal cord is given off by the pia. Where this process is given off the pia presents a thickening—linea splendens.
7. *Ligamenta denticulata:* Twenty toothed processes extend from the pia to the dura, pushing the archnoid before them. They leave

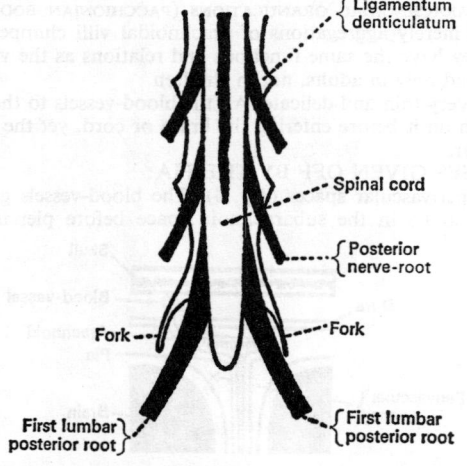

Fig. 5.—'Fork' made by lowest process of ligamentum denticulatum.

[1] 'The Absorption of Cerebrospinal Fluid into the Venous System', *Am. J. Anat.*, 1923, Jan., 191–224.

the pia midway between the anterior and posterior nerve-roots and serve to suspend the cord in the midline. The lowest ligamentum denticulatum is forked, and the posterior root of the first lumbar nerve lies on the outer prong of the fork (*Fig. 5*). In the lower region of the cord it is the surgeon's guide to the first lumbar nerve and gives him a nerve-root of known number from which he may determine the position of whatever nerve-roots he is in search of.

Subarachnoid Space: This contains the cerebrospinal fluid. It is traversed by septa lined with flat arachnoidal cells. It is also traversed by the vessels going to the brain and cord. It presents certain dilatations (cisterns) which act as a water bed to the brain:

1. *Cisterna magna*—situated posteriorly between the cerebellum and medulla.
2. *Cisterna pontis*—in front of the pons.
3. *Cisterna interpeduncularis* at the base of the brain. It contains the circulus arteriosus (circle of Willis).
4. Smaller less important cisterns.

Communications between the Cavities of the Brain and the Subarachnoid Space:

1. MEDIAN APERTURE OF FOURTH VENTRICLE (Foramen of Magendie): The median aperture in the roof of the fourth ventricle.
2. LATERAL APERTURES OF FOURTH VENTRICLE (Foramina of Luschka): Two lateral apertures, one in each lateral recess of the fourth ventricle.

Cerebrospinal Fluid:

SOURCE: It is derived (whether by secretion, filtration, or dialysation is uncertain) from the choroid plexuses of the lateral ventricles. A small amount may be derived from the perivascular spaces (which are *not* lymphatics).

REMOVAL: The fluid is passed into the venous sinuses by the arachnoidal villi, granulations, and mesothelial cells. This absorption takes place on the outer surface of the hemispheres, the fluid passing through the opening in the tentorium cerebelli to attain this situation.

LOCULATION SYNDROME (FROIN'S): If a block occurs anywhere in the vertebral canal preventing fluid passing the obstruction, the fluid below has special properties: (1) It may coagulate spontaneously as the percentage of protein in it is greatly increased; (2) It may be yellow (xanthochromia) like plasma.

Sudden increase of the intracranial venous pressure is not transmitted to the fluid below the block. Queckenstedt's test is based on this fact. (*See* p. 591.)

HYDROCEPHALUS: This is a condition due to the accumulation of cerebrospinal fluid within the skull. It may be due to: (1) Excessive production of fluid; (2) Obstruction in some part of the route along which the fluid circulates; (3) Interference with the absorption of the fluid.

OBSTRUCTION IN SOME PART OF THE ROUTE: This is the common cause. The obstruction may be in one of two places:

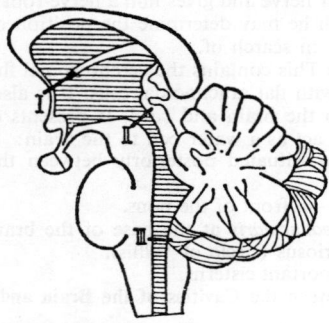

Fig. 6.—Showing the possible sites of an obstruction causing ventricular hydrocephalus. I, Blockage of the interventricular foramen (Monro); II, Obstruction in the aqueductus cerebri; III, Blockage of the median aperture of the fourth ventricle. (*After Fraser, 'Surgery of Childhood'.*)

a. Inside the Ventricular System (Fig. 6):
   i. At the opening of the lateral ventricle into the third ventricle (interventricular or foramen of Monro). This would cause distension of one lateral ventricle.
   ii. In the aqueductus cerebri (Sylvius). This would cause distension of both lateral and the third ventricles.
   iii. At the openings in the fourth ventricle (Magendie and Luschka). This would cause distension of all the ventricles. By ventriculography, i.e., injection of oxygen into the ventricles after removal of the cerebrospinal fluid, and then radiography in different positions, the site of the block may be located.

b. At the Opening in the Tentorium Cerebelli: If the 'door of the tent' is blocked by adhesions, fluid below the tentorium cannot ascend to the outer surface of the brain to be absorbed.

When surgery is necessary much may be done to relieve the condition. A local obstruction may be by-passed as in the operation of ventriculocisternostomy (Torkildsen). Excessive cerebrospinal fluid production is dealt with by draining the fluid into the blood-stream—ventriculocaval anastomosis: or into the right auricle—ventriculo-auriculostomy.

Chapter III

THE ANATOMY OF THE NORMAL AND THE ENLARGED PITUITARY BODY

NORMAL PITUITARY BODY

THE pituitary body is suspended from the base of the brain in the region of the floor of the third ventricle by a projecting stalk—the infundibulum. The organ lies in the pituitary fossa of the sella turcica of the sphenoid bone in the middle fossa of the skull. It is completely covered by a fold of dura mater, the diaphragma sellae, which is perforated by a tiny orifice for the passage of the infundibulum.

Dimensions: 13 × 8 mm.

Structure: The organ consists of two lobes, anterior and posterior (*Fig.* 7).

THE ANTERIOR LOBE is developed from a diverticulum of the epithelium of the primitive pharynx. This lobe consists of a *pars anterior* and a *pars intermedia*, which are separated from each other by a narrow cleft which is the remnant of the diverticulum from which the lobe develops. The pars anterior is kidney-shaped with the concavity posterior, partly embracing the posterior lobe. The pars anterior is very vascular, the blood-vessels reaching the gland along the infundibulum from the circulus arteriosus.

THE POSTERIOR LOBE is developed as a downgrowth from the floor of the third ventricle.

Histology:

ANTERIOR LOBE: Consists of granular epithelial cells which are arranged in cord-like alveoli separated by large thin-walled blood-vessels.

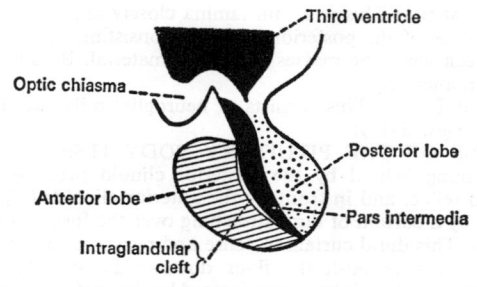

Fig. 7.—The gross structure of the pituitary body. (*After Herring.*)

12 A SYNOPSIS OF SURGICAL ANATOMY

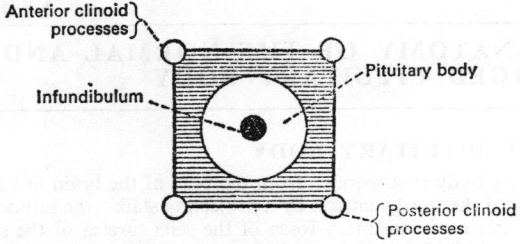

Fig. 8.—The 'four-poster bedstead' in which the pituitary body reposes. The cross-hatching represents blood sinuses.

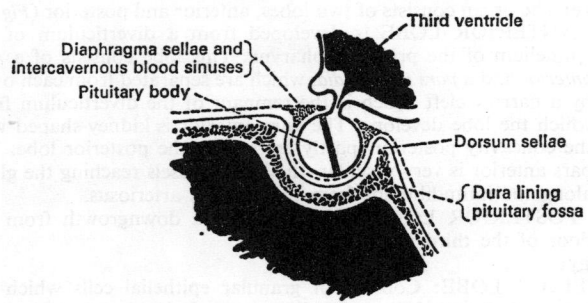

Fig. 9.—Sagittal section of the pituitary gland showing the dural relations. Notice the dura between the gland and its fossa.

PARS INTERMEDIA: This is a thin lamina closely applied to the front and sides of the posterior lobe and consisting of granular cells between which lie masses of colloid material. Blood-vessels are not numerous.

POSTERIOR LOBE: This consists of neuroglial cells and fibres.

Relationships (*Figs.* 8–13):

RELATIONS OF THE PITUITARY BODY ITSELF: The gland is overhung behind by the posterior clinoid processes and the dorsum sellae, and in front by the anterior clinoids (*Fig.* 8). It is roofed by a curtain of dura stretching over the fossa for the gland (*Fig.* 9). This dural curtain is dense and resistant. When the gland enlarges it may push the floor downwards or bulge the roof upwards. The floor is bony and formed by the roof of the sphenoidal air sinus.

THE NORMAL AND THE ENLARGED PITUITARY BODY

Four blood sinuses form a square which encloses the gland (*Fig.* 8): the cavernous sinus on each side and the anterior and posterior intercavernous sinuses in front and behind. In the outer wall of the cavernous sinus lie the third, fourth, ophthalmic branch of the fifth, and the sixth cranial nerves, and also the internal carotid artery, which is rather beneath the sinus (*Fig.* 10). Above the gland is the hypothalamus, i.e., corpora mammillaria, tuber cinereum, infundibulum, and optic chiasma.

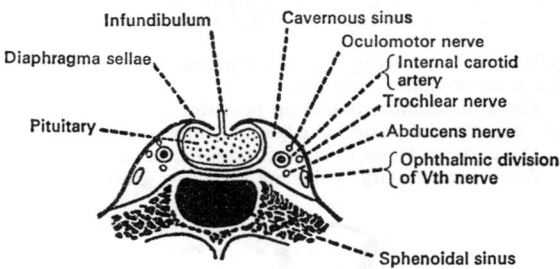

Fig. 10.—Coronal section through the pituitary body.

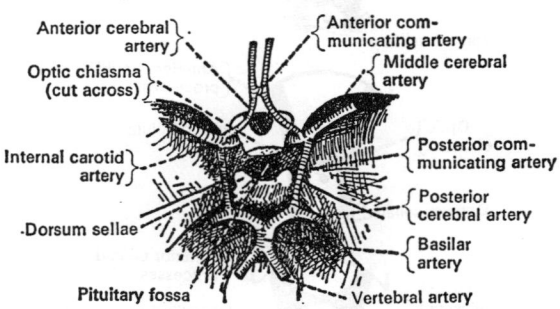

Fig. 11.—A figure to show the vascular relations (circulus arteriosus) of the pituitary fossa. The hypophysis has been removed. (*After Cope.*)

VASCULAR RELATIONS: These are shown in *Fig.* 11.
RELATIONSHIP OF THE INFUNDIBULUM TO THE OPTIC CHIASMA: The optic chiasma lies superior to the pituitary gland. It does *not* occupy the chiasmatic sulcus, but lies posterior to it (*Fig.* 12). It usually lies nearer the posterior part of the diaphragma

14 A SYNOPSIS OF SURGICAL ANATOMY

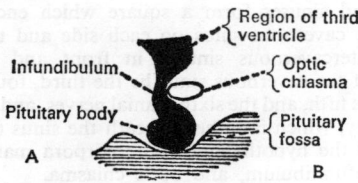

Fig. 12.—Sagittal section of the pituitary region showing the relation of the infundibulum to the chiasma. A, Posterior. B, Anterior.

sellae than the anterior. In a small percentage of cases it lies nearer the anterior clinoid (*Fig.* 13).

The infundibulum passes up posterior to the chiasma and is in contact with its posterior edge and under-surface.

The chiasma is *not* in contact with the bone.

When the pituitary is the site of a new growth it often bulges

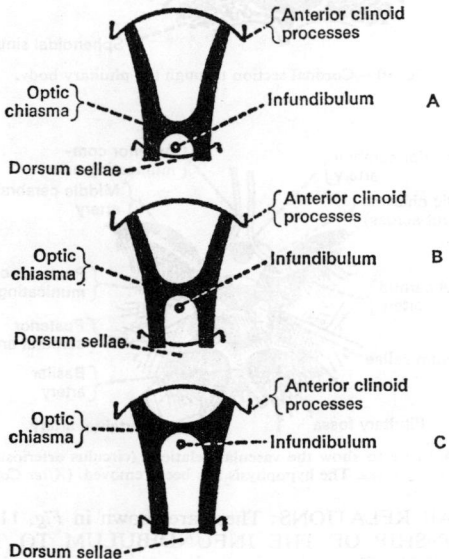

Fig. 13.—Demonstrating the variations in the situation of the optic chiasma. A, Posterior position. B, Intermediate position. C, Anterior position.

THE NORMAL AND THE ENLARGED PITUITARY BODY

or perforates the diaphragma sellae and comes to press on the optic chiasma, producing interference with the fibres conveying sight impressions from the retina. This interference produces typical defects of vision, and these give valuable information in diagnosis of the site of the lesion inside the skull. A knowledge of the method in which the visual fibres are disposed of in the chiasma is essential in effecting such diagnosis.

ARRANGEMENT OF THE RETINAL FIBRES IN THE CHIASMA: The fibres from the outer half of the retina pass back in the optic tract of the same side as that on which they arise. Those from the nasal half of the retina decussate and pass on in the opposite optic tract. Half of each macular bundle (distinct vision) goes to each side.

SUPERIOR RELATION OF THE OPTIC CHIASMA: The immediate superior relation of the chiasma is the anterior communicating artery which connects the two anterior cerebral arteries. Pituitary tumours which grow upwards, particularly the congenital cysts of Rathke's pouch (craniopharyngiomas), push the chiasma up.

ENLARGEMENTS OF THE PITUITARY

Symptoms of Pituitary Tumours: These are divisible into two great classes: (1) Constitutional symptoms due to disordered activity of the gland itself; (2) 'Neighbourhood symptoms', which are produced by the pressure of the enlarged gland on adjacent parts, especially the optic chiasma.

'NEIGHBOURHOOD SYMPTOMS': These arise from pressure on the surrounding parts, especially on the optic chiasma.

Foster Brown states that only 50 per cent of pituitary tumours give rise to visual signs. These signs are affections of the visual fields and disk changes. Whether a pituitary tumour produces visual symptoms or not depends to a large degree on the foramen

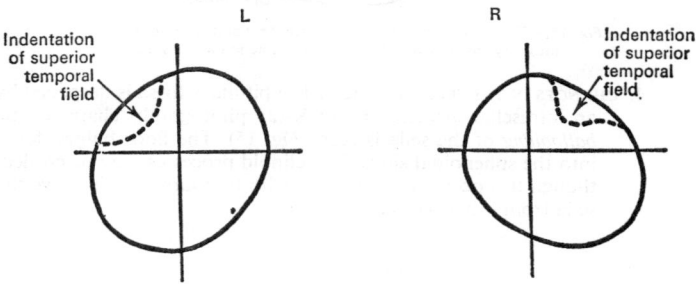

Fig. 14.—Changes in the visual fields resulting from a pituitary tumour causing bitemporal hemianopia. The solid line represents the normal field.

in the diaphragma sellae for the infundibulum. If this is large, the tumour gets through easily. If it is small, the tumour may be unable to grow upwards, and then tends to bulge through the floor of the pituitary fossa, which is the roof of the sphenoidal sinus.

1. VISUAL CHANGES: The commonest is bitemporal hemianopia which consists of a flattening of the superior temporal fields and is rarely of the same degree in the two eyes (*Fig.* 14).
2. OTHER EYE SIGNS PRODUCED BY PITUITARY TUMOURS:
   a. The third nerve, being near the pituitary, may be pressed on, diplopia and third nerve palsy resulting.
   b. Palsies of the fourth or sixth nerves are very rare.
   c. Pressure on the cavernous sinus may cause proptosis with engorgement of the lids.
3. PRESSURE ON OTHER PARTS OF THE BRAIN: With a large growth pressure may be exerted on the anterior part of the temporal lobe, causing uncinate fits, which produce sensations of smell. Pressure upwards may close the foramen of Monro and produce symptoms of hydrocephalus. Pressure up and backwards by a large tumour may cause interference with the pyramidal tract in the crus, resulting in symptoms referred to the opposite half of the body, e.g., paresis or paralysis. Pressure upwards on the floor of the third ventricle may cause persistent drowsiness. Pressure on the frontal lobes may cause mental dullness.

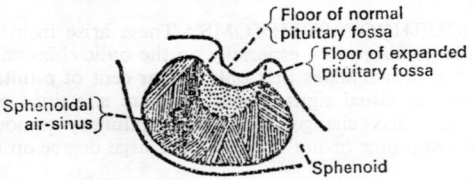

Fig. 15.—To show how a pituitary tumour expands the floor of the pituitary fossa downwards into the sphenoidal air sinus.

4. CHANGES IN THE SELLA TURCICA: The pituitary fossa is deepened by an intrasellar growth, and in X-ray photographs characteristic *ballooning* of the sella is seen (*Fig.* 15). The floor bulges down into the sphenoidal sinus. The clinoid processes may be eroded, though this occurs more usually with tumours arising above the sella from other parts of the brain.

Chapter IV

THE THYROID AND THE PARATHYROID GLANDS

THE THYROID GLAND

THE gland is composed of two lateral lobes connected by an isthmus. The lobes measure $5 \times 2.5 \times 2.5$ cm. The isthmus measures 3.7×1.2 cm.

Each lateral lobe extends vertically from the middle of the side of the thyroid cartilage to the sixth ring of the trachea. The isthmus covers the second, third, and fourth rings of the trachea. A triangular projection of gland tissue called the pyramidal lobe extends upwards from the left side of the upper border of the isthmus, and is connected to the hyoid bone above by a fibrous band or a muscle slip (levator glandulae thyroideae).

Each *lateral lobe* is roughly triangular on section.

The *superficial surface* is covered by the infrahyoid or ribbon muscles, the sternomastoid overlapping.

The *medial surface* is related to two tubes—oesophagus and trachea; two nerves—recurrent and external laryngeal; two muscles—inferior constrictor and cricothyroid.

The *posterior surface* overlaps the common carotid artery and covers the terminal part of the inferior thyroid artery.

Blood-vessels of the Gland: There are on each side two arteries (which carry many sympathetic nerves with them) and four veins.

ARTERIES:

SUPERIOR THYROID ARTERY: This, the first branch given off from the anterior surface of the external carotid, enters the gland *superficially* (*Fig.* 16). It runs downwards to the upper pole of the lateral lobe, where it breaks up into branches to the front of the gland, branches to the back of the gland, and a branch to anastomose with its fellow of the opposite side along the upper border of the isthmus. This vessel also gives off a branch to the pyramidal lobe which enters near its base where it can easily be ligated. There is no arterial supply at the apex of the pyramidal lobe which can be dissected out without fear of haemorrhage.

INFERIOR THYROID ARTERY: This is a branch of the thyrocervical trunk (which arises from the first part of the subclavian), and is a posterior relation of the gland entering it from its *deep* or *posterior* surface. It is absent in 3.5 per cent of patients.[1]

It is necessary to tie these vessels in some operations on the gland. It is obvious in *Fig.* 16 that the superior, being comparatively superficial, is easily exposed for this purpose. The inferior,

[1] Hunt, P. S., Poole, M., and Reeve, T. S., *Br. J. Surg.*, 1968, **55**, 63.

18 A SYNOPSIS OF SURGICAL ANATOMY

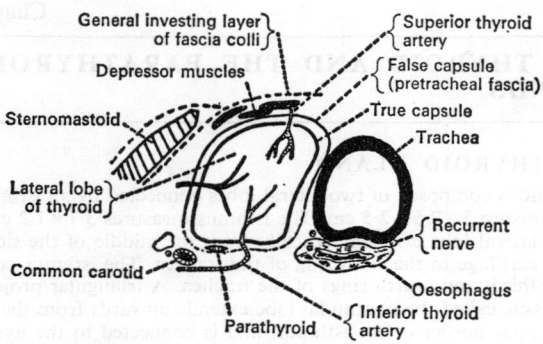

Fig. 16.—The relations of the thyroid arteries to the gland and to the capsules. Observe that, whereas the superior thyroid artery enters the superficial aspect of the gland, the inferior thyroid enters its deep aspect.

however, lies directly posterior to the gland and its exposure is much more difficult. The recurrent nerve lies behind or in front of the vessel just before the latter enters the gland, and must be protected from injury when the artery is being dealt with.

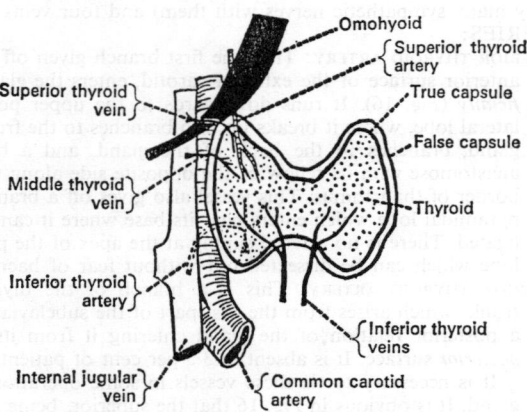

Fig. 17.—The blood-vessels of the thyroid. The veins do not accompany the arteries.

THE THYROID AND THE PARATHYROID GLANDS

THYROIDEA IMA ARTERY: An occasional vessel arising from the arch of the aorta or the innominate. When present it enters the lower part of the isthmus.

ACCESSORY THYROID ARTERIES: Small vessels to oesophagus and trachea send branches to the thyroid gland. All large arteries to the gland may be tied off and yet the blood-supply to the gland be surprisingly good because of these accessory vessels.

VEINS: The veins of the thyroid gland do not accompany their arteries (*Fig.* 17).

THE SUPERIOR THYROID VEIN, leaving the upper part of the gland, and taking as its guide the outer border of the omohyoid, crosses the common carotid artery to terminate in the internal jugular vein.

THE MIDDLE THYROID VEIN, leaving the gland about its middle, follows the inner border of the omohyoid across the carotid, ending in the internal jugular. It is a short vessel of much importance in thyroid surgery. It bleeds furiously if torn, and must be doubly ligated and cut before passing the finger between the capsules of the gland in the process of delivering an intrathoracic extension of a goitre.

THE INFERIOR THYROID VEIN, leaving the isthmus at its lower border, runs down in front of the trachea to end in the innominate of the same side. Both inferior thyroid veins may join the left innominate. They are large vessels and in thyroidectomy they are divided towards the end of the operation after the arteries have been dealt with. The reason for this is that a reversal of the procedure would cause great venous congestion in the gland.

4TH THYROID VEIN: Kocher drew attention to the frequent existence of a vein passing outwards between middle and inferior thyroid veins.

NERVES RELATED TO THE GLAND: The nerve to the cricothyroid muscle—external laryngeal—and the recurrent laryngeal nerve come into intimate relationship with the gland. One of the surgeon's main concerns, therefore, in operations on the thyroid gland is the protection of these nerves.

EXTERNAL LARYNGEAL NERVE: It is a branch of the superior laryngeal nerve and descends on the fascia of the inferior pharyngeal constrictor to supply the cricothyroid muscle which is a tensor of the vocal cord. The nerve lies close to the superior thyroid vessels at the superior pole of the thyroid (*Fig.* 18) with the nerve medial, the superior thyroid vein lateral and the superior thyroid artery between them. Usually the nerve lies outside the false capsule of the thyroid gland and can therefore be separated from the vessels by blunt dissection while operating inside this capsule. However, in some instances this cannot be accomplished because the nerve is very adherent to the artery (15 per cent) or

20 A SYNOPSIS OF SURGICAL ANATOMY

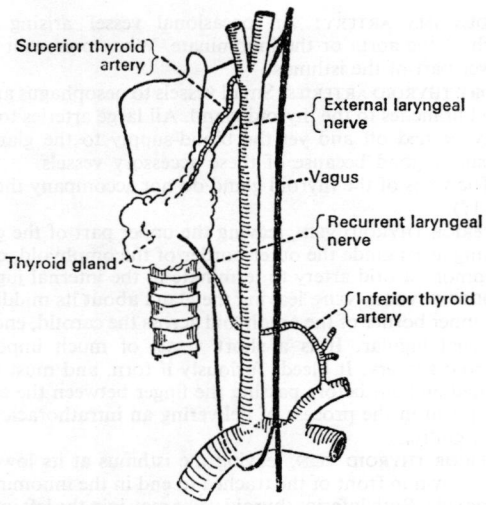

Fig. 18.—Shows the intimate relationship of the external laryngeal branch of the vagus to the superior thyroid artery. (*After Lennox Gordon.*)[1]

may even run between the branches of the artery (6 per cent)[2] and may then be injured during ligation of the vessels. This can be avoided by ligation of the branches of the superior thyroid artery and vein on the thyroid gland below the superior pole.

Injury to the nerve results in hoarseness, a decreased range of pitch and fatigue in speaking. Laryngoscopy reveals normal abduction and adduction of the cord, but the cord is irregular and wavy, lies at a lower level and has lack of tone resulting in bulging on expiration and retraction on inspiration.

RECURRENT LARYNGEAL NERVE: In the majority of cases this nerve lies in the tracheo-oesophageal groove and posterior to the inferior thyroid artery. It may, however, be further anterior where it is more vulnerable to injury during thyroidectomy (*Fig.* 19).

The nerve may be lateral (28 per cent) or anterolateral (10 per cent) to the trachea and in 30 per cent of instances it passes anterior to the inferior thyroid artery or may even be entwined with its branches. In about 50 per cent of cases the nerve is

[1] *J. Med. Ass. S. Afr.*, 1929, Oct. 12, 555.
[2] Moosman D. A., and De Weese, M. S., *Surgery, Gynec. Obstet.*, 127, 1011.

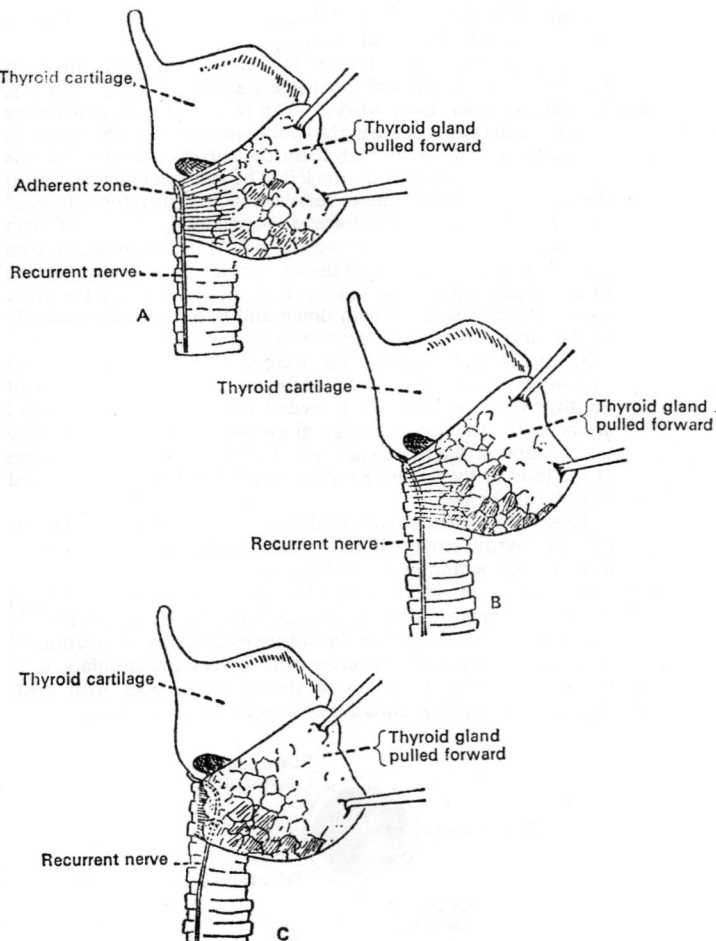

Fig. 19.—Showing the varying relationship of the recurrent nerve to the thyroid gland. In A the nerve is well posterior to the gland, lying in the tracheo-oesophageal sulcus. In B the nerve passes through the adherent zone. In C the nerve lies actually amongst the gland tissue. (*After Berlin.*[1])

[1] Berlin, D. D., *Surgery Gynec. Obstet.*, 1935, **60**, 19.

embedded in the ligament of Berry (*see* p. 24) and will thus be drawn forward with gland traction.

Injury to this nerve results in partial (abductor) or total paralysis of the cord, with hoarseness and respiratory difficulty.

NON-RECURRENT LARYNGEAL NERVE:[1] The recurrent laryngeal nerves arise from the vagus nerve in the neck in proximity to the primitive 4th aortic arch vessels which form the subclavian artery on the right and the aortic arch on the left. The recurrent nerves pass to the larynx caudal to these vessels and are therefore dragged caudally when the vessels descend. Occasionally the right fourth arch vessel fails to develop and the right subclavian artery then arises from the aorta beyond the left subclavian artery and passes to the right behind the oesophagus. In these cases the right recurrent nerve is not drawn down and passes directly medially to the larynx as a non-recurrent laryngeal nerve.

Six of 1776 nerves on the right were found to be non-recurrent.[1] In 2 instances the nerve arose at the level of the inferior pole of the thyroid gland and passed medially with the inferior thyroid artery to the tracheo-oesophageal groove and then followed the usual course of the recurrent nerve. In 4 instances the nerve arose at the level of the superior pole of the thyroid gland and passed directly to the larynx.

These non-recurrent laryngeal nerves may be mistaken for the inferior thyroid artery or the middle thyroid vein and may be ligated in error during thyroidectomy.

INTERNAL LARYNGEAL NERVE: It is a branch of the superior laryngeal nerve and penetrates the larynx through the thyrohyoid membrane. Injury to this nerve during thyroidectomy is exceptional and occurs only if the superior pole is very much enlarged. It results in loss of sensation of the laryngeal inlet with post-deglutition coughing, choking or aspiration pneumonia.

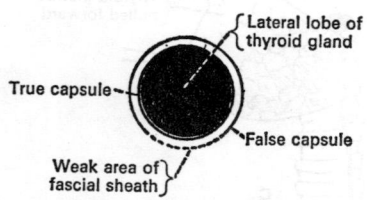

Fig. 20.—A diagram showing the weakness of the false capsule over the posterior surface of the lateral lobe of the thyroid gland.

[1] Stewart, G. R., Mountain, J. C., and Colcock, B. P., *Br. J. Surg.*, 1972, **59**, 379.

THE THYROID AND THE PARATHYROID GLANDS

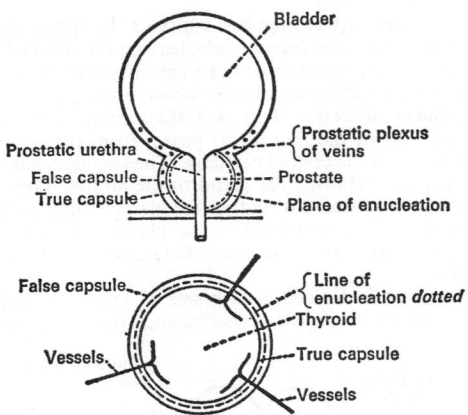

Fig. 21.—To show the plane of operative cleavage in prostatectomy and thyroidectomy. The upper figure shows that the prostate is enucleated from *both* its sheaths along the dotted line. The lower figure shows that the thyroid gland is removed *with* its true capsule, being shelled out along the dotted line, the vessels having been ligated.

Capsules: Like the prostate, the thyroid has two fibrous capsules—a true and a false. In both instances the true capsule is made up from a peripheral condensation of the connective tissue of the gland, while the false capsule is supplied by a fibrous sheet derived from a neighbouring fascia. The false capsule of the thyroid is supplied by the pretracheal fascia, that of the prostate by the visceral layer of pelvic fascia. *Fig.* 20 shows the true and the false capsules of the thyroid, and it is important to notice that the false capsule is represented by a dotted line over the back of the gland, implying that this sheath is weakest here. Compare this with the prostate (*Fig.* 21).

The false capsule of the prostate (visceral pelvic fascia) covers the whole of the gland excepting the upper surface which is in contact with the bladder. Prostatic tumours, therefore, usually grow upwards into the bladder, this being the line of least resistance. The numerous blood-vessels of the thyroid pierce both its capsules and then ramify to form a dense plexus of thin-walled vessels immediately beneath the inner or true capsule. The space between the two capsules is traversed only by the arterial and venous trunks. The surgeon, in dealing with the thyroid, secures these main trunks *between* the capsules, exercising the utmost care not to wound the true capsule because of the numerous fragile vessels which lie just under it. Contrast with this the principle underlying the enucleation of an enlarged prostate. The prostatic plexus of veins lies between the two capsules. The prostate, therefore, is *enucleated from its own true capsule*, leaving the plexus intact. Thus in the removal of the prostate both its capsules are left behind. When the thyroid is removed the removal *includes the true capsule of the organ*.

Suspensory Ligament of Berry: This is a thickening of the pretracheal fascial investment of the thyroid. It passes from the inner and back part of the gland to the cricoid cartilage. The two ligaments, right and left, form a sling anchoring the gland to the larynx. They increase in size in large goitres, thus preventing the gland falling away from the larynx, and must be severed before the gland can be removed. The recurrent laryngeal nerve is in immediate contact with the back of the ligament.

Lymphatics: The gland is drained by two sets of lymph-vessels; ascending and descending. Each consists of medial and lateral channels (*Fig.* 22).

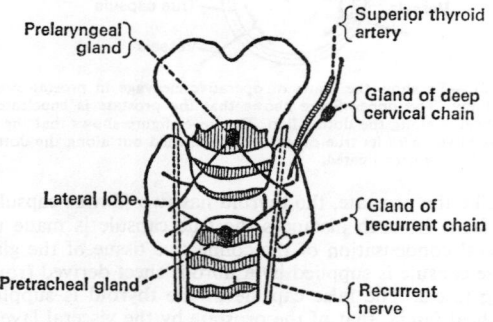

Fig. 22.—The lymphatic drainage of the thyroid gland. (*After Poirier.*)

ASCENDING VESSELS:
MEDIAL: Leave the upper border of the isthmus and go to the gland situated on the cricothyroid membrane—the prelaryngeal gland.

LATERAL: Leave the upper pole of the gland and run with the superior thyroid artery to the deep cervical glands situated at the bifurcation of the common carotid.

DESCENDING VESSELS:
MEDIAL: Pass to the gland on the trachea—the pretracheal gland.

LATERAL: Pass from the deep surface of the thyroid to small glands placed on the recurrent nerve—the glands of the recurrent chain (Poirier and Charpy).

Ectopic Thyroid Tissue: Benign thyroid follicles may be seen on histological examination in the lateral cervical lymph-nodes as an incidental finding in block dissections of the nodes in the neck for malignant tumours of other than thyroid origin. These inclusions are *not* palpable, *not* papillary in character, and are thought to reach the nodes as benign metastases along lymphatics.[1] If papillary thyroid tissue is encountered in a lymph-node it must be regarded as a malignant metastasis from the thyroid.

Occasionally palpable nodules of thyroid tissue are encountered in the area of the lateral cervical lymph-nodes. If there is lymph-node tissue in this lateral mass, or a carcinoma of the thyroid or a papillary histological appearance then this mass should be regarded as a metastasis from a carcinoma of the thyroid. In the absence of these features, however, it may be a sequestered nodule of a nodular goitre separated off from the main gland by muscular action.[2]

THE PARATHYROID GLANDS

The number of parathyroids vary from 2 to 6, but in 80 per cent of cases there are ·, 2 on each side. The total weight of 4 normal glands is about 140 mg.

Embryology: The upper parathyroids arise from the 4th branchial pouch and come to lie in close association with the upper part of the lateral lobes of the thyroid. This position is constant.

The lower parathyroids arise from the 3rd branchial pouch in association with the thymus, and descend with the thymus. Because of this embryological migration they may be found anywhere from the upper pole of the thyroid to the anterior mediastinum.

Anatomy: The glands are the size of a split pea. They are pink or brown in colour, but are frequently covered by fat, making them difficult to recognize.

The superior glands lie on the posterior surface of the middle third of the thyroid, usually above the inferior thyroid artery, but well posterior to this plane. If enlarged they may descend into the posterior mediastinum.

The inferior glands are mostly found on the posterior surface of the lower pole of the thyroid or within 1 cm. below the lower pole. They may be higher or lower, occasionally as far down as in the thymus in the anterior mediastinum. They lie in a more anterior plane than the upper glands.

Sometimes the parathyroids may be embedded in the thyroid gland.

Blood-supply: A special small parathyroid artery supplies each gland. The lower parathyroid artery comes from the inferior thyroid artery and is a guide to the gland if it lies below the lower margin of the thyroid.

The upper parathyroid artery arises from the inferior artery or from an anastomosing artery joining the superior and inferior thyroid arteries and only very occasionally from the superior thyroid artery.

There is a good collateral arterial supply from the tracheal vessels

---

[1] Nicastri, A. D., Foote, F. W., and Frazell, E. L., *J. Am. med. Ass.*, 1965, **194**, 113.
[2] Sisson, J. C., Schmidt, R. W., and Beierwaltes, W. H., *New Engl. J. Med.*, 1964, **270**, 927.

and adequate parathyroid function persists even if all 4 major thyroid arteries are ligated.

Surgical Significance: During thyroidectomy the parathyroids may be damaged or removed, resulting in post-thyroidectomy hypoparathyroidism. This must be avoided by exposing and protecting the glands.

Hyperparathyroidism may result from tumours or hyperplasia of the parathyroids. This is treated by excision of the affected glands. It can almost always be achieved through a cervical incision, but in about 1 per cent of cases a mediastinotomy is required.

Chapter V

THE TONSIL

By the tonsil is meant the faucial or palatine tonsil.

Development: The tonsil lies in a fossa, the tonsillar fossa, which is the inner extremity of the second branchial cleft. Persistence of this cleft is normal in some animals. In the human it occasionally persists as a lateral pharyngeal diverticulum, the inner opening of which is then behind the tonsil. From the epithelium in the neighbourhood of the inner end of the cleft epithelial outgrowths invade the future tonsillar fossa. These become canalized later, forming the crypts of the tonsil. Around these epithelial evaginations lymphoid tissue collects to form the lymphoid follicles of the organ. The organs are formed at the anterior end of the alimentary canal.

Situation: The tonsils are situated one on each side in the oropharynx, lying in the fossa tonsillaris, between the palatoglossal and the palatopharyngeal folds (anterior and posterior pillars of the fauces). They are visible through the mouth when the tongue is depressed. Their position corresponds on the surface of the body to a point 1·25 cm. above and anterior to the angle of the mandible. The tonsil is shaped like an almond, being also about the size of a large almond, though there is necessarily great variation. The *capsule* of the tonsil is a thin but strong fibrous structure, continuous with the pharyngeal aponeurosis. Within the capsule there are, in addition to lymphoid tissue, many mucous glands.

Relations: These are of great surgical interest. The organ has: two surfaces—medial and lateral; two borders—anterior and posterior; two poles—superior and inferior; two developmental folds related to it—the plica triangularis and plica semilunaris.

SURFACES:

MEDIAL SURFACE: This faces inwards, bounding the passage from mouth to pharynx on each side. It is covered with squamous epithelium. On the surface are seen the openings of the 12 to 20 crypts of the organ. Plugs of pus or debris are often seen filling these openings.

LATERAL SURFACE: This is separated by lax connective tissue from the superior constrictor muscle of the pharynx. The superior constrictor separates the tonsil from the following arteries: (1) External maxillary, and two of its branches—namely, (2) Ascending palatine; (3) Tonsillar.

Relation of the Tonsil to the Internal Carotid: This vessel lies 2·5 cm. behind and lateral to the tonsil, separated from the pharynx by lax alveolar tissue and fat, so that when the organ is pulled inwards by a forceps prior to its removal, *it is separated still further from the carotid*. This fact confirms the statement of W. F. Campbell[1] that it is impossible to wound the carotid during removal of the tonsil.

BORDERS:

THE ANTERIOR BORDER is in contact with the palatoglossus muscle.
THE POSTERIOR BORDER is in contact with the palatopharyngeus.

Developmental Folds:

PLICA TRIANGULARIS: This is a fold of mucous membrane passing from the lower part of the tonsil to the palatoglossal fold. It is constant in the fetus, but often disappears in the adult.

PLICA SEMILUNARIS: This is an occasional fold crossing the upper part of the tonsillar fossa.

Intratonsillar Cleft: The internal opening of the second pharyngeal pouch or fistula is not situated in the tonsil but is behind it. The cleft is present in 40 per cent of cases (Killian). It may act as a trap for particles of food, etc., lodging in it. Sir St. Clair Thomson remarks on the pity that this important depression should be called 'the supratonsillar recess', as it lies *within* the capsule of the tonsil surrounded by lymphoid tissue and is never extratonsillar. It is a convenient site for bacteria to set up inflammation and is the location of the commencement of the majority of quinsies.

Blood-supply of the Tonsil: This is very profuse, being obtained through the following arteries[2] (*Fig.* 23):

1. Anterior tonsillar—from dorsalis linguae.
2. Posterior tonsillar—from ascending pharyngeal.
3. Superior tonsillar—from descending palatine.
4. Inferior tonsillar—from external maxillary.

---

[1] *Diseases of the Nose and Throat*, 1919, 364. London.
[2] Fetterolf, *Am. J. med. Sci.,* 1912.

The veins form a plexus around the capsule, draining into the pharyngeal plexus.

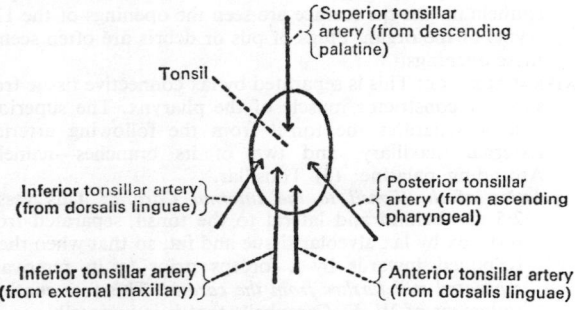

Fig. 23.—The posterolateral surface of the left tonsil to show the blood-supply. (*After Morris.*)

Nerves: The glossopharyngeal, having reached the base of the tongue, sends twigs upwards to supply the tonsil.

Lymphatics: Several vessels leave the gland, pierce the superior constrictor, and end in the superior deep cervical glands, particularly one situated just below the posterior belly of the digastric and the angle of the jaw. This gland lies on the carotid in the angle formed by the union of the common facial with the internal jugular vein. It is the tonsillar gland, also called the jugulodigastric gland.

Special Features of Practical Importance:
1. The tonsil capsule is separated by lax connective tissue from the superior constrictor, so that when the tonsil is pulled forward by a vulsellum the pharynx is not pulled with it. While this fact is true for the normal or merely enlarged tonsil it is noteworthy that—
2. Quinsy is a *peri*tonsillar collection of pus, though, as stated, the infection begins within the gland. After repeated attacks of quinsy the gland capsule is so densely adherent to the constrictor that only considerable force can separate the two. Under these circumstances the pulling forward of the tonsil displaces the pharyngeal wall inward also. It is obvious therefore from the foregoing that, having divided the attachments of the mucous membrane of the surroundings to that of the tonsil, the organ will, in the absence of previous inflammatory attacks, separate easily from the constrictor; should previous attacks of quinsy have occurred, *no plane of cleavage exists* and separation is difficult, i.e., the so-called 'adherent tonsil'.
3. When the tonsil and its capsule are removed the constrictor is exposed, and not the aponeurosis of the pharynx, which, though internal to

THE TONSIL

the muscle, is blended with and is removed with the capsule of the organ.

4. Bleeding from the tonsillar fossa after removal of the tonsil presents an important similarity to bleeding from the uterus after labour. It is an axiom in surgery that clots round the ends of blood-vessels are not disturbed for fear of re-starting the haemorrhage (*Fig.* 24). There are *two* exceptions, i.e., in the uterus and the tonsillar fossa, in both of which situations clots interfere with the *retraction* of the vessel walls by preventing the *contraction* of the surrounding muscles, i.e., the muscles bounding the tonsillar fossa in the one instance and those forming the walls of the uterus in the other. After operation for removal of the tonsils many surgeons make a practice of clearing out any clot which may be present in the tonsillar fossa.

5. Bone or cartilage may very rarely be found in the tonsil. There are two possible sources for the origin of such tissue:

   a. The late Professor S. G. Shattock[1] thought that isolated spicules of bone or cartilage in the tonsil were derived from embryonic 'rests' of the branchial arches.

   b. Ossification in the stylohyoid ligament may cause a very long styloid process to project into the tonsil, so that a bone-cutting forceps may be needed in a tonsil operation. Watt[2] has drawn attention to the fact that ossification in the stylohyoid ligament may lengthen the styloid process from the normal 2·5 cm. up to

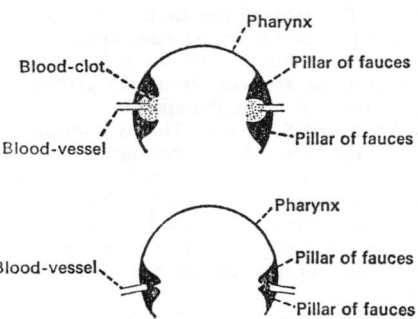

Fig. 24.—To show how clots in the tonsillar fossa, after tonsillectomy, may encourage hemorrhage. In the upper figure the vessels are prevented from closure by the clot in the tonsil beds. In the lower figure the vessels are occluded by the contraction of the muscles forming the tonsillar fossa.

---

[1] Quoted by Herbert Tilley in an address to the Clinical Congress of the American College of Surgeons, Chicago, Oct. 14, 1929.
[2] Watt, W. E., *Am. Surg.*, 1962, **28**, 1.

7·5 cm. About 4 per cent of adults may have the condition which causes symptoms in 3 per cent of cases.

These may produce pain after tonsillectomy radiating to one or both ears and intensified by swallowing. It is due to irritation of the 5th, 7th, 9th, or 10th cranial nerves when the pharyngeal mucosa rubs over the tip of the bone, post-operative cicatrization rendering the mucosa taut. Pressure by the bone on one of the carotid arteries may cause headache or pain in the face due to radiation along the appropriate artery.

Chapter VI

THE BREAST

THE breast is formed from modified sebaceous glands. It lies therefore in the superficial fascia.

Extent:

VERTICAL: 2nd to 6th ribs inclusive (the scapula covers 2nd to 7th ribs).

HORIZONTAL: The side of the sternum to the mid-axillary line. About two-thirds of the breast rests upon the pectoralis major, one-third on the serratus anterior. At its lower medial quadrant the gland rests on the aponeurosis of the external oblique, which separates it from the rectus abdominis.

AXILLARY TAIL OF SPENCE: This is a prolongation from the outer part of the gland which passes up to the level of the 3rd rib in the axilla, where it is in direct contact with the main lymph-glands of the breast (anterior axillary glands). This process of breast tissue gets into the axilla through an opening in the axillary fascia, known as the foramen of Langer. It follows that the axillary tail is *under* the deep fascia, and not, like the rest of the breast, *superficial* to this layer.

Architecture of the Gland: The breast is composed of acini which make up lobules, aggregations of which form the lobes of the gland. The lobes are arranged in a radiating fashion like the spokes of a wheel and converge on the nipple, where each lobe is drained by a duct. Eighteen to twenty ducts open on the nipple. The roundness of the organ is due to fat which fills the gaps between the portions of the parenchyma. The breast is separated from the great pectoral by fascia, *which is the deep fascia.*

THE BREAST 31

LIGAMENTS OF COOPER: The organ is anchored to the overlying skin and underlying pectoral fascia by bands of fibrous tissue called ligaments of Cooper (*Fig.* 25). In cancer of the breast the malignant cells invade these ligaments. Subsequently contraction occurs along these strands, which may cause either actual dimpling of the skin or merely attachment of the skin to the underlying growth so that the skin cannot be pinched up from the lump. If cancer cells grow along the fibrous processes binding the breast to the pectoral fascia, the mamma becomes fixed to the pectoralis major. It cannot then (as normally) be moved in the long axis of the muscle. [Cooper's name is also given to the extension which the lacunar ligament (Gimbernat's) gives to the periosteum over the iliopectineal line at the pelvic brim.]

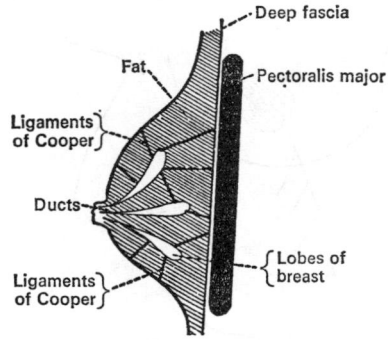

Fig. 25.—Vertical section of the breast showing the ligaments of Cooper.

THE NIPPLE lies in the 4th intercostal space 10 cm. from the mid line. The apex beat of the heart is in the 5th space 8·7 cm. from the mid line.

Arterial Blood-supply of the Breast: This is derived from:
1. The lateral thoracic artery, from the 2nd part of the axillary.
2. The perforating cutaneous branches of the internal mammary to the 2nd, 3rd, and 4th spaces.
3. The lateral branches of the 2nd, 3rd, and 4th intercostal arteries.

Venous Drainage: The superficial veins radiate from the breast and are characterized by their proximity to the skin. They are accompanied by lymphatics. The deep veins drain to axillary, internal mammary, and intercostal vessels.

Comment: Because the superficial venous and lymphatic vessels draining the breast are near the skin:

1. Skin-flaps in operations for cancer must be thin.
2. Phlebitis of one of these veins feels exactly like a thick piece of catgut immediately beneath the skin. The condition produces no discoloration and may be tensed like a bow-string by putting traction on it. The entity was first described by Favre (1922). It is called Mondor's disease (1939). The cord may take months to disappear and has no relationship whatsoever to cancer (*Fig.* 26).

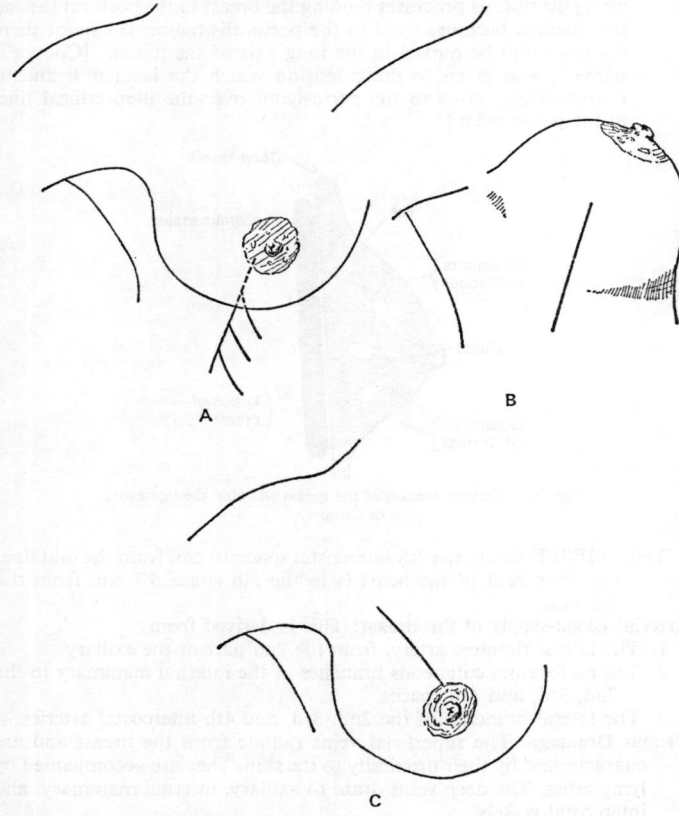

Fig. 26.—Various manifestations of Mondor's disease—the cord-like thrombosed veins are shown in three cases.

THE BREAST

Nerve-supply: The secreting tissue is supplied by sympathetic nerves which reach it via the 2nd to the 6th intercostal nerves. The overlying skin is supplied by the anterior and lateral branches of the 4th, 5th, and 6th intercostal nerves.

Lymphatic Drainage:

GLANDS: The breast itself drains mainly to the axillary glands, of which there are five sets (*Fig.* 27):

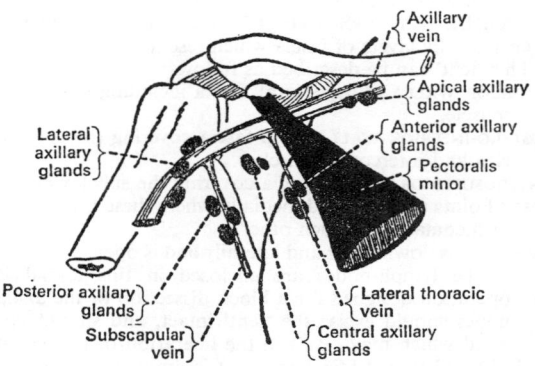

Fig. 27.—Lymph-glands of the axilla.

ANTERIOR SET (Sojius' glands or the main lymph-glands of the breast): Large glands situated along the lateral thoracic vein under the anterior axillary fold. They lie mainly on the 3rd rib. The axillary tail of Spence is in actual contact with these glands. Therefore in cancer of this process:

a. The growth appears to be separate from the breast and presents the appearance of an enlarged gland with an apparently healthy breast.

b. The anterior axillary glands may be infected, not merely by lymphatic extension, but by direct contiguity of tissue.

POSTERIOR SET: These lie along the posterior axillary fold in relation to the subscapular vessels.

LATERAL SET: Along the upper part of the humerus in relation to the axillary vein.

CENTRAL SET: Situated in the fat of the upper part of the axilla. The intercostobrachial nerve passes outwards amongst these glands. Enlargement of these glands, such as occurs in cancer, may, by pressure on the nerve, cause intense pain in the distribution of the nerve along the inner border of the arm.

APICAL SET: These are also called the infraclavicular glands. They are very important and constant in position being bounded below by the 1st intercostal space, behind by the axillary vein, in front by the costocoracoid membrane. It is noticeable that these glands lie very deeply and are not easily felt. Sir Harold Stiles taught that they might be palpated by pushing the fingers of one hand into the axillary apex from below, and those of the other behind the clavicle from above.

THE AXILLARY FASCIAL 'TENT': The axillary lymph-nodes are enclosed by layers of fascia which resemble a tent lying on its side. This 'tent' can be described as follows:

ANTERIOR WALL: Clavipectoral fascia including the pectoralis minor muscle.

POSTERO-INFERIOR WALL: Deep fascia covering the chest wall (upper ribs and intercostal muscles).

ANTEROSUPERIOR WALL: Fascia covering the subclavian vessels.

APEX: Points upwards and medially where these layers of fascia come into contact with each other.

BASE: Points downwards and laterally and is open.

The lymph-nodes are enclosed in this fascial 'tent'. Any operation designed for a block dissection of the axillary lymph-nodes should excise the 'tent' intact, and should not enter the 'tent' which may result in the liberation of malignant cells.

LYMPHATIC VESSELS: The breast is drained by two sets of lymphatics: (1) The lymphatics of the skin over the breast; (2) The lymphatics of the parenchyma of the breast.

LYMPHATICS OF THE OVERLYING SKIN. These drain the integuments over the breast, but not the skin of the areola and nipple. They pass in a radial direction and end in the surrounding gland groups. Those from the outer side go to the axillary glands. The skin of the upper part drains by vessels which go to the supraclavicular glands (members of the lower deep cervical glands). Certain of these vessels may end in the cephalic gland which lies in relation to the vein of the same name in the deltopectoral triangle. The vessels from the skin over the inner part of the gland go to the internal mammary glands which lie in relation to the veins of that name. These glands lie in the upper four or five intercostal spaces or behind the related costal cartilages. It is of great surgical moment to observe that the lymphatics of the skin over the breast communicate across the middle line, and that a unilateral disease may become bilateral by this route. In mammary cancer secondary invasion of the skin appears in the form of discrete nodules (*Fig.* 28). This has been explained by Sampson Handley: the lymphatic trunks from the skin drain each a separate portion, and there is no communication between adjacent territories. When cancer cells grow along these vessels the process results in nodules separated from each other by apparently healthy intervening skin.

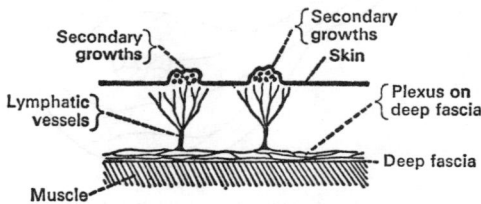

Fig. 28.—Showing the discrete nature of secondary cancerous nodules in the skin, owing to the fact that the lymphatics draining adjacent territories of the skin do not communicate with each other. (*After Sampson Handley*.)

LYMPHATICS OF THE PARENCHYMA OF THE BREAST: The subareolar lymph plexus of Sappey is a collection of large lymph-vessels situated under the areola (*Fig.* 29). The hitherto accepted view that most of the lymph draining the breast tissue passes to the subareolar plexus of Sappey is no longer tenable. Haagensen[1] expressed doubts on clinical grounds that the main direction of lymphatic drainage in the breast is centripetally to the subareolar plexus.

Turner-Warwick,[2] using intravital techniques such as the flow of radio-active gold after an injection into the breast, makes important observations:

a. The axillary glands receive about 75 per cent of lymph draining the breast tissue. These vessels, arising in the lobules, pass directly outwards in the substance of the breast, receive tributaries on the way, and pass through the axillary tail to the axilla. Most go to the anterior gland group, a few pass to the posterior group. From there they run to central and apical groups, coming to lie on the inferomedial and anterior aspects of the axillary vein (*Fig.* 30).

At no time do these vessels run on the deep fascia. Though the subareolar plexus does communicate with the lymphatics of the breast tissue, it is not a collecting zone for the breast lymph.

b. Lymphatics from the deep surface of the breast pass through the great pectoral muscle on their way to the axillary or internal mammary glands (*Fig.* 30).

[1] Haagensen, C. D., *Diseases of the Breast*, 1956, 28. Philadelphia and London: Saunders.
[2] Turner-Warwick, R. T., *Br. J. Surg.*, 1959, 46, 574.

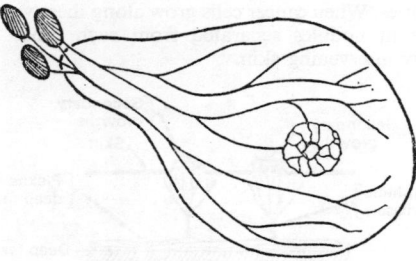

Fig. 29.—The main lymphatic pathways from the breast passing through the axillary tail to the anterior gland group.

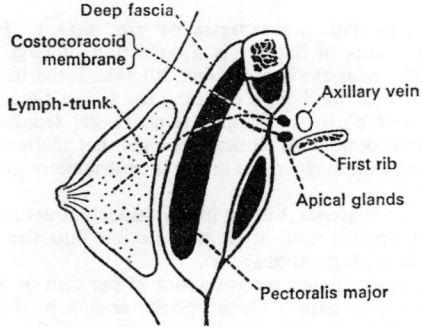

Fig. 30.—Showing the direct pathway of deep lymphatics of the breast through the great pectoral muscle to the axillary glands.

    c. The plexus of the deep fascia consists of fine lymphatic vessels. They do not act as a normal pathway for lymph from the breast to the regional glands.

    d. The internal mammary gland group is an important lymph pathway from both the medial and lateral halves of the breast. Lymph enters the thorax along the anterior perforating branches of the internal mammary artery and along the lateral perforating branches of the intercostal vessels. Most of this lymph goes to the internal mammary chain, but a small amount may pass to the posterior intercostal glands lying near the heads of the ribs (*Fig.* 31).

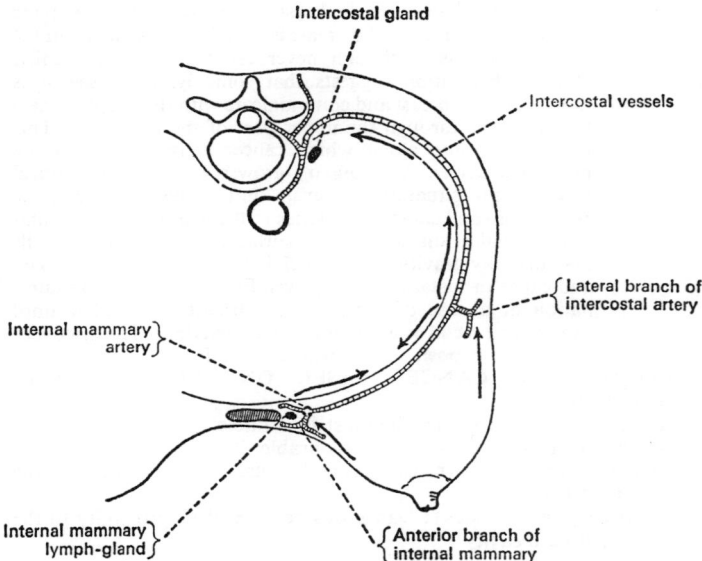

Fig. 31.—The routes into the chest of lymph from the breast. The arrows show the direction of lymph flow. (*After Thorek.*)

At the level of the first interspace fine lymphatics connect the right and left internal mammary chains behind the manubrium sterni, and small glands may be found there (Rouvière).[1]

Handley and Thackray[2] investigated 150 cases of early breast cancer and reported that half of the tumours in the inner half, and one-fifth of those in the outer half of the breast had metastasized to the internal mammary glands. In 10 per cent of each group the axillary glands were not involved.

This work focuses attention on the importance of the internal mammary gland pathway in the spread of breast cancer. It is necessary to remember that when lymph channels are blocked, tumour cells may spread in a retrograde direction, and that the accepted principles underlying the surgery of

---

[1] Rouvière, H., *Anatomie des Lymphatiques de l'Homme*, 1932. Paris: Masson et Cie.
[2] Handley, R. S., and Thackray, A. C., *Br. med. J.*, 1954, 1, 61. Quoted by Turner-Warwick.

cancer of the breast are the keystone of treatment. The lower and inner quadrant of the breast is only 2·5 cm. away from the xiphoid process. Although never established anatomically, clinical observation suggests that some lymph-vessels pass down from the breast and communicate with the subperitoneal lymph-plexus through the upper part of the linea alba. This is a short route along which cancer cells may reach the peritoneal cavity. A secondary growth in the subperitoneal plexus in this situation may erupt on the inner surface of the peritoneum and cause secondaries in the liver by the implantation of malignant cells on its surface. Further, cancer cells may drop by gravity into the pelvis from the upper abdomen and cause metastases in the pelvis. For this reason no examination of a case of cancer of the breast is complete until vaginal and rectal examinations have been done. The discovery of a pelvic deposit would negate operation.

PROGNOSIS IN CANCER BASED ON THE LYMPHATIC DRAINAGE:

UPPER OUTER QUADRANT: The most favourable.

LOWER OUTER QUADRANT: Less favourable.

UPPER INNER QUADRANT: Dangerous because of its proximity to the mediastinum.

LOWER INNER QUADRANT: Dangerous because of its proximity to the peritoneal cavity.

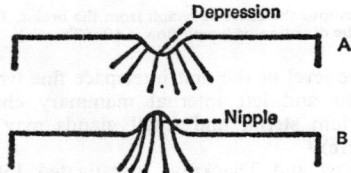

Fig. 32.—Showing the evolution of the nipple. A, The early invagination stage. B, The evagination stage.

'Retraction' in Breast Pathology: It is perhaps unnecessary to stress the importance of retraction as a physical sign in pathological conditions affecting the breast, but it would appear essential to particularize as to the pathological anatomy of the sign, as some confusion undoubtedly exists. Three forms of retraction need consideration:

1. CONGENITAL RETRACTION OF THE NIPPLE: In the development of the breast there is first a downgrowth of epithelium from the future site of the nipple, forming a pocket or invagination of the skin. Only shortly before birth is this depression pushed up to

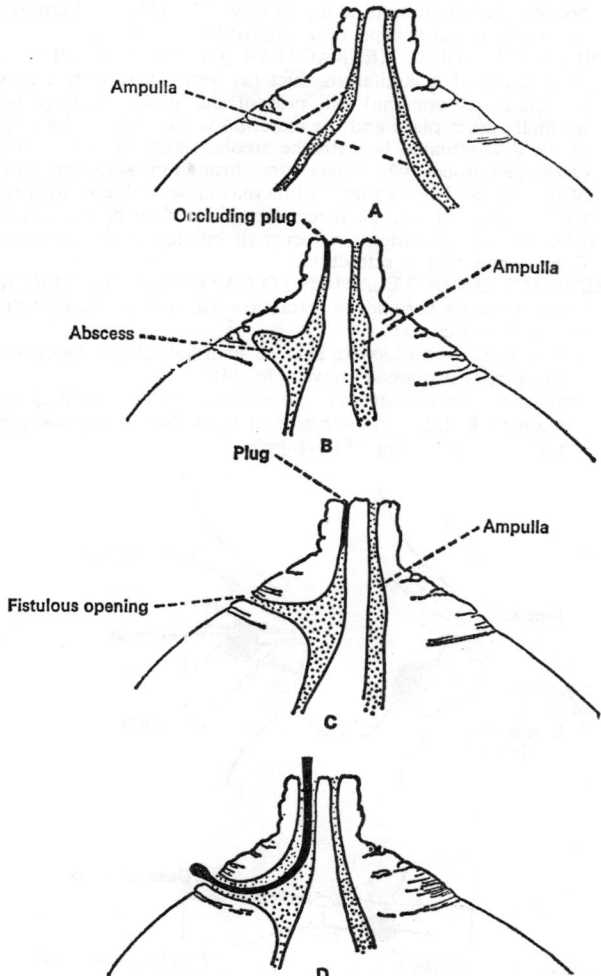

Fig. 33.—A, Normal anatomy of lactiferous ducts. B, Lactiferous duct abscess. C, The abscess has ruptured. Note relation of fistulous opening to areola. D, Probe in fistulous track.

40 A SYNOPSIS OF SURGICAL ANATOMY

become an evagination or nipple (*Fig.* 32). This evagination may never occur and a depression exist throughout life.

2. INFLAMMATORY RETRACTION OF THE NIPPLE: Any obstruction of a lactiferous duct (as may occur with a plug of keratin at its opening) will prevent the slight discharge which normally takes place and the secretion will collect in the ampulla of the duct situated beneath the areola. Infection usually results, causing an abscess which may burst through the skin near the edge of the areola. The resultant fistula may close and later the process will be repeated or a persistent lactiferous duct fistula may form (*Fig.* 33). The persistent or recurrent inflammation will result in fibrosis and nipple retraction.

3. RETRACTION IN RELATION TO CANCER OF THE BREAST: There are three varieties of retraction which may occur, each due to a different cause:

    a. RETRACTION OF THE SKIN: Due to invasion of the ligaments of Cooper, as explained above (*Fig.* 34).

    b. RETRACTION OF THE NIPPLE: Due to extension of growth along the main milk ducts and subsequent retraction as fibrosis occurs, leading to indrawing of the nipple.

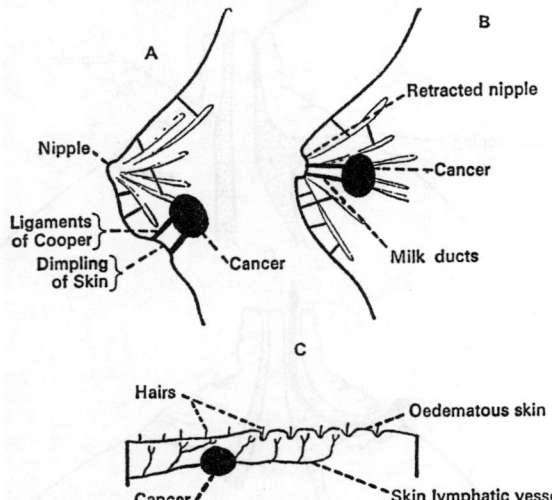

Fig. 34.—Illustrating the pathology of breast retraction. A, Dimpling of the skin due to the pull exerted by the ligaments of Cooper. B, Retraction of the nipple due to retraction of the milk ducts. C, Peau d'orange due to lymphatic obstruction.

c. PEAU D'ORANGE: In this condition the pits of the hair-follicles appear to be retracted beneath the level of the surrounding skin. The condition is due to blockage of the lymphatics draining the skin, leading to a stagnation of lymph and oedema of the skin.

Chapter VII

CHEST, LUNGS, AND BRONCHI

1. THE CHEST WALL

PARTS of the sternum are used to determine the situations of deeper structures. The upper border corresponds to the lower border of the 2nd thoracic vertebra. A pin pushed back at the middle of its upper border would transfix the inner border of the innominate artery just below its division. In the child the top of the aortic arch may reach the upper border of the manubrium, whereas in the adult it is about the level of the centre of this bone.

The Angle of Louis—a slight transverse prominence formed by the junction of the manubrium with the body of the sternum—is an important landmark. Here the 2nd costal cartilage articulates with both these bones. Although the 1st rib is mainly concealed by the collar bone, the 1st costal cartilage can be felt below it. The 2nd rib is the one most easily identified in counting the ribs. The angle of Louis corresponds to:—

The lower border of the 4th thoracic vertebra.

The bifurcation of the trachea. This is one vertebra higher in the infant.

The site where the pleural sacs meet.

The arch of the aorta begins at this level. It ends at the same level posteriorly as it arches back. The highest point of the arch reaches the centre of the manubrium.

The xiphisternal junction is at the level of the disk between the 9th and 10th thoracic vertebrae.

The roots of the lungs lie opposite the 4th, 5th, and 6th thoracic spines midway between them and the inner border of the scapulae.

The intercostal spaces are widest between the inner ends of the 2nd and 3rd costal cartilages. They become narrower between lower ones. Therefore the internal mammary vessels are best ligated in the 2nd or 3rd space where they lie behind the intercostal muscles half an inch from the side of the sternum. The vessels lie on the pleura above the 3rd costal cartilage. Below this level they are separated from it by slips of the transversus thoracis muscle. The 3rd space would therefore be the site of choice for internal mammary ligation.

The internal mammary artery gives two small anterior intercostal arteries to each of the upper five or six spaces, and perforating branches which come through the same spaces and pass through the great pectoral muscle, supplying it and the breast. Those emerging from the 2nd, 3rd, and 4th spaces are of considerable size and should be secured before division in radical mastectomy, to prevent bleeding and retraction through the anterior intercostal membrane.

Barrett[1] points out that the ribs and costal cartilages, by virtue of their attachments to sternum and vertebrae, form a series of hoops. Thus conditions which affect one part of the circle alter the shape of the other, so that any prominence or depression must be considered in relationship to the thoracic cage as a whole. A notable example is the prominence sometimes seen at a costochondral junction and often mistaken for a tumour. It is in fact a buckling due to unequal rib growth.

II. THE LUNGS AND BRONCHIAL TREE

In preparing this chapter the author wishes to express his indebtedness to the writings of Doctor Richard H. Sweet of Boston, Mass., and Sir Russell C. Brock of London.

The significance of the segmental structure of the lungs is apparent when it is realized that:

   a. The segmental architecture of the lungs is fairly uniform.
   b. Infections and neoplastic processes are often localized to one or more adjacent segments.
   c. Conservation of lung tissue is thus often possible in removal of diseased areas.

A detailed knowledge of the anatomy of the lungs and bronchi is essential not only in localizing but also in the surgical handling of diseases of the lungs. Each lung consists of ten segments which, though they appear to be in continuity, are yet separate entities. The parenchymal substance of adjacent segments is distinct. They fill with air proximodistally like the opening of a fan. Each has its own bronchus, artery, and veins. There is little anastomosis between adjacent segments, and thus individual segments can be excised with little loss of blood or leak of air, if intersegmental planes can be adhered to.

Fissures of the Lungs: Each lung is divided into lobes by the oblique or horizontal fissure. The surface marking begins at the 6th costochondral junction and follows the line of the 6th rib to meet the tip of the 3rd thoracic spinous process. The upper end of the fissure is a little higher on the left than on the right, and Brock emphasizes that it is lower than usually given, being at the 5th rib or interspace or even the 6th rib. This knowledge is essential in locating and operating on lung abscesses.

---

[1] Barrett, N. R., *Ann. R. Coll. Surg.*, 1958, 23, 372.

The horizontal fissure occurs on the right side only. It is marked out by a line extending out from the 4th costal cartilage to strike the oblique fissure in the mid-axillary line at the level of the 5th rib. This fissure is frequently absent or incomplete.

Both fissures are subject to developmental variability and their situations may be considerably distorted by pathological processes such as bronchiectasis and other conditions causing fibrosis.

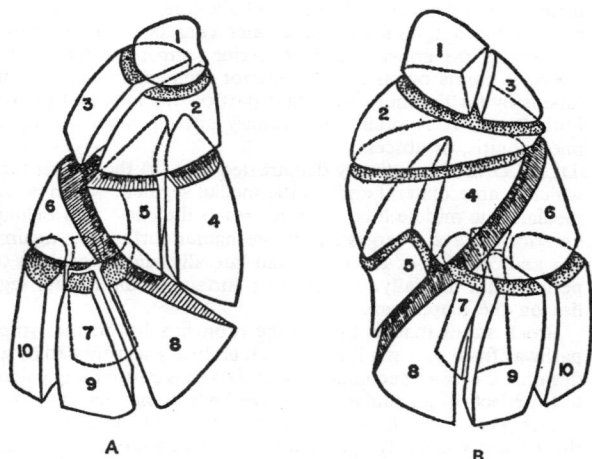

Fig. 35.—A, The segments of the right lung. Upper lobe: 1, Apical; 2, Anterior; 3, Posterior. Middle lobe: 4, Medial; 5, Lateral. Lower lobe: 6, Superior; 7, Medial basal; 8, Anterior basal; 9, Lateral basal; 10, Posterior basal. B, The segments of the left lung. Upper lobe: 1, Apical; 2, Anterior; 3, Posterior; 4, Superior lingular; 5, Inferior lingular. Lower lobe: 6, Superior; 7, Medial basal; 8, Anterior basal; 9, Lateral basal; 10, Posterior basal. (*By courtesy of Sweet—modified by Thomas.*)

Segments of the Lungs: Each lung consists of ten segments which have a somewhat constant disposition and relationship to the overlying ribs. Each extends to the pleural surface. Sweet states that, but for the fact that the lingular bronchus on the left usually comes from the upper lobe bronchus, the arrangements on the two sides would be essentially the same. On both sides the superior segment of the lower lobe is often anatomically fused with the upper lobe, especially behind.

The apparent complexity of the segmental anatomy is simplified by reference to the diagrams (*Fig. 35*).

44 A SYNOPSIS OF SURGICAL ANATOMY

Right Lung:

UPPER LOBE: Comprises three segments: (*a*) apical, (*b*) anterior, and (*c*) posterior. The dome of the lung is formed by the apical segment which has anterior, posterior, medial, and lateral surfaces. The anterior segment has anterior and medial surfaces, whilst the posterior segment presents laterally and posteriorly. The inferior surfaces of anterior and posterior segments form the base of the upper lobe. The inferior aspect of the anterior segment is separated from the middle lobe by the horizontal fissure, whereas the posterior part of the longitudinal fissure intervenes between the posterior segment of the upper and the superior segment of the lower one.

Brock points out that the posterior segment of the right upper lobe is by far the most important part of this lobe and perhaps of both lungs. It is often the primary site of tuberculosis, septic pneumonitis, or abscess.

MIDDLE LOBE: Is vertically demarcated into (*a*) the lateral segment which is anterolateral and (*b*) the medial segment which is anteromedial. The middle lobe does not reach the chest wall behind. Its anterior surface is largest, while triangular surfaces lie against the 4th and 5th ribs of the chest wall laterally and in relation to the pericardium medially. The inferior surface of the medial segment lies on the diaphragm.

Brock states that as the middle bronchus lies in the lymphatic pathway from the right lower lobe, it is closely surrounded by glands draining the lower and middle lobes. It is thus particularly vulnerable to the effects of glandular enlargement which may result in bronchiectasis, etc. Near the acute angles formed by branching bronchi there usually lies a lymph-gland. The presence of calcified glands, so often seen near the lung hilum at operation or in X-ray pictures, is a monument to the severe lymphadenitis which must have existed at some stage in the patient's history.

LOWER LOBE: This lobe, the largest of the three, is made up of a superior and an inferior portion.

THE SUPERIOR SEGMENT is related by its posterior surface to the 4th to the 8th ribs. On the medial and lateral aspects it extends round to the fissure and comes into contact with the posterior segment of the upper lobe. This segment therefore has a surface abutting on the mediastinum and another against the lateral chest wall. The inferior portion of the lower lobe, the longest part of it, comprises four segments. It lies on the diaphragm and is made up of the following parts to all of which the term 'basal' should be added.

The posterior segment contributes to the mediastinal surface of the lobe.

The lateral segment is also partly posterior.

The anterior segment is lateral also.

CHEST, LUNGS, AND BRONCHI

The medial segment (cardiac) is entirely medial and diaphragmatic.

AZYGOS LOBES OF THE LUNG: There is much confusion in the terminology of accessory lobes of the lung, the term 'azygos' being applied to all without further distinction. 'Azygos' means a median unpaired structure. Such lobes may occur in three situations. E. P. Stibbe,[1] to put the nomenclature on a sound basis, suggests the following classification:

There are three varieties of supernumerary lobes of the lung.
1. The lobe of the azygos vein—due to abnormality of the azygos vein.
2. The upper azygos lobe—not associated with abnormality of the azygos vein.
3. The lower azygos lobe—previously called azygos lobe. The second and third types are of no practical importance. They are accessory lobules of lung tissue. One or other is rarely found, and is 'upper' or 'lower' according as its situation is above or below the hilum of the lung.

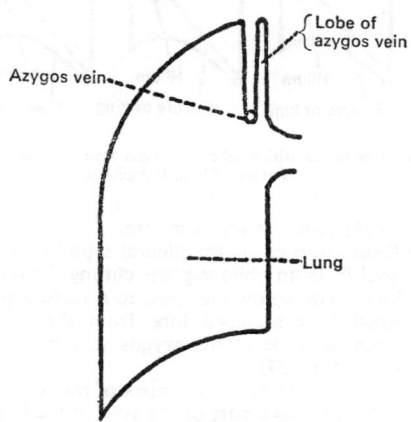

Fig. 36.—The lobe of the azygos vein.

LOBE OF THE AZYGOS VEIN: This accessory lobe is important because:
1. Its existence may cause unusual appearances in a radiograph of the chest.
2. It may be the site of disease of the lung.
3. It is necessary to realize its significance if it is discovered in operations on the lung or at post-mortem examination.

[1] *J. Anat.*, 1929, 53, July, 303–13. The account given here is largely taken from this lucid article.

Definition: A part of the upper inner surface of the right lung is cut off from the rest of the lung by a double pleural septum—the 'meso-azygos' (cf. mesocolon)—which contains at its apex the upper part of the azygos vein (*Fig.* 36). The meso-azygos, therefore, divides the pleural cavity into an upper compartment containing the accessory lobe, and a lower one for the rest of the lung.

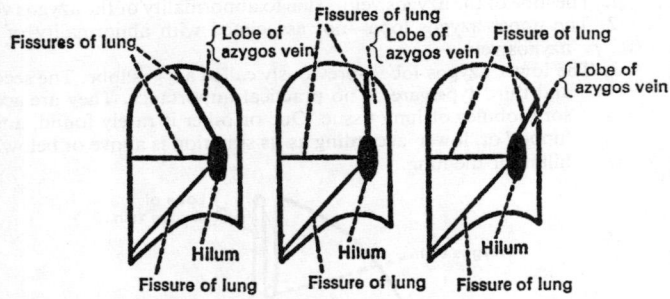

Fig. 37.—Various forms which lobe of azygos vein may assume. Mediastinal surface of lung is depicted.

Extent of the Lobe: It varies in size.

The fissure formed by the pleural septum cuts the lung at any level from an oblique plane cutting the outer surface of the lung 5 cm. below the apex, to a vertical plane cutting off a small tongue-shaped lobe from the mediastinal surface. Thus the lobe of the azygos vein may take one of three forms (*Fig.* 37).
 1. It forms the whole apex of the lung.
 2. It forms a part of the apex of the lung.
 3. It takes no part in the formation of the lung apex.

The fissure containing the meso-azygos and vein extends nearly to the root of the lung, resembling a normal lung-fissure.

Aetiology of the Condition: The developing bud of the right lung has to pass outwards under an arch formed by the anterior end of the right posterior cardinal vein (the future azygos vein). If the long bud does not quite clear the arch, so that part of the lung is lateral to and part medial to the vein, the vein becomes embedded in the developing lung, and the part medial to the vein is the lobe of the azygos vein. The condition is of distinct rarity. It was first described by Worsberg in 1777.

X-ray Appearance: The lobe itself is not seen, but its outer boundary, i.e., the meso-azygos and azygos vein, demarcates the lobe (*Fig.* 38). The meso-azygos is seen as a fine line coursing from the apex of the lung downward with a convexity outward, and then inward so as to approach the mediastinum at about the level of the angle of Louis (2nd costal cartilage). The line ends in a small dense shadow about the size of a pea. The line itself is the meso-azygos, the dense shadow is the azygos vein.[1]

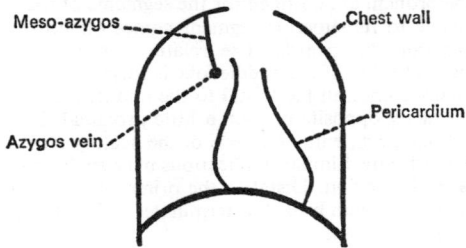

Fig. 38.—Diagrammatic representation of radiograph of thorax showing azygos vein and meso-azygos.

Left Lung:

UPPER LOBE: Consists of five segments. The lower two comprise the superior and inferior lingular segments which both have anterior, lateral, and medial surfaces. The lower part of the inferior segment lies on the diaphragm, adjacent to the pericardium.

The upper part of this lobe is arranged very much as on the right, having anterior, apical, and posterior segments. Owing to the manner of bronchial division, the two latter segments are sometimes described as a single apico-posterior segment. As each receives an independent bronchus, artery, and vein, they are fittingly classified separately.

LOWER LOBE: Is smaller than its fellow on the right. It comprises five segments and their arrangement is very similar to that on the right. Thus there is a superior segment and four basal ones, lateral, anterior, medial, and posterior. The latter presents partly on the medial surface of the lobe. The anterior and medial basal segments are grouped by some authors as a single anteromedial segment because of the manner of bronchial supply. Each ultimately has its own bronchus, etc.

Bronchial Tree:

RIGHT LUNG: The right main bronchus is more vertical than the left and is wider and shorter. The bronchus to the upper lobe passes

[1] Stoloff, E. Gordon, *Am. J. Roentg.*, 1929, Nov., 466.

48 A SYNOPSIS OF SURGICAL ANATOMY

laterally and a little upwards for just over a centimetre and then branches rapidly into the three divisions of the lobe—apical, anterior, and posterior.

On the front of the main bronchus, just beyond the origin of the upper lobe bronchus, is a groove in which the pulmonary artery lies. Just distal to this the middle lobe bronchus arises from the anterolateral aspect. It soon divides into its medial and lateral segmental branches. Distal to the origin of the middle lobe bronchus, all the bronchi are destined for the segments of the lower lobe. The bronchus to its superior segment comes off posteriorly and runs horizontally backwards. The relationship of the origin of this bronchus to that of the middle lobe is surgically important. Though it usually comes off just distal to the middle lobe bronchus, it may arise exactly opposite or even a little proximal. Should this be the case it may, e.g., entail removal of the healthy middle lobe in lower lobe lobectomy. Similar implications may apply to segmental resections in this region. Distal to the origin of the superior segmental bronchus the main bronchus terminates in four bronchi to the basal segments (*Fig.* 39).

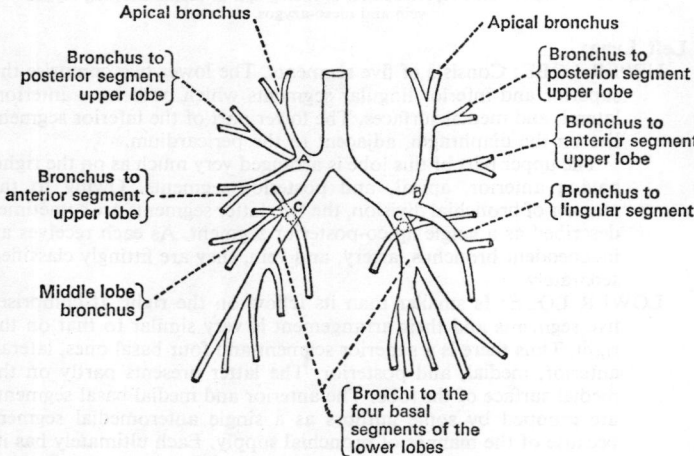

Fig. 39.—The anatomy of the bronchial tree. A, Right upper lobe stem bronchus. B, Left upper lobe stem bronchus. C, The dotted circle shows the origin of the bronchus to the superior segment of the lower lobe. It arises from the posterior aspect of the stem bronchus. (*Re-drawn from Shanks and Kerley*).

LEFT LUNG: The left main bronchus is longer than the right and less vertical. About 5 cm. from the trachea it divides into the left upper lobe stem bronchus and that to the left lower lobe. After this bifurcation the upper stem bronchus curves laterally. The bronchus to the lingular segment occurs as a bifurcation of this tube a little more than a centimetre from its origin. This bronchus to the lingular segment divides into a branch to each of the two lingular segments. The stem bronchus to the upper lobe having divided to form the lingular bronchus soon subdivides into a branch to the anterior segment and another to the apical and posterior segments which soon divides into a bronchus for each of these two segments.

The left lower lobe bronchus gives off first the bronchus to the superior segment which comes from its posterior aspect. There are usually three bronchi to the basal segments; one for the posterior, one for the lateral, and one for the anterior and medial basal segments which soon divides to supply them.

This description of the bronchial tree is the common one but anomalies are frequent. Sweet describes a supernumerary bronchus which is found in about 50 per cent of cases. It arises just distal to the origin of the superior segment bronchus to the lower lobe. It may occur in either lung and is sometimes called the subsuperior bronchus.

Brock points out that the main practical importance of the lingula is its liability to be involved with the left lower lobe in bronchiectasis. It may be small or large. Each bronchopulmonary segment is a unit in the architecture of the lungs. Its parenchyma is distinct from that of its neighbours. It is supplied by one or more branches of the pulmonary artery and is drained by its own veins. In general the bronchus and its main branches to the segment are central in position. The arteries tend to occupy a position nearer the centre of the segment than the veins, which tend to lie mainly along the intersegmental planes, and are thus useful guides in delineating the segments.

Brock[1] states that though lung abscesses may result from embolic infection carried by the blood-stream, they are much more commonly due to inhalation of infected, usually particulate, material into the bronchi. The site of the resulting abscess or suppurative pneumonitis is dependent on posture and bronchial anatomy. The right lung is more commonly affected than the left. After operations on the upper respiratory areas the upper lobes are more commonly affected than the lower, whereas after abdominal operations the opposite obtains. A pre-exising bronchial infection is the main source of lung infection after laparotomy, the infected material flowing directly to those parts of the lung in which suppuration commonly occurs.

---

[1] Brock, Sir R. C., *The Anatomy of the Bronchial Tree*, 1947, Ch. 2. London: Oxford University Press.

50 A SYNOPSIS OF SURGICAL ANATOMY

Pulmonary Vessels:

RIGHT PULMONARY ARTERY: Runs transversely for a short distance in front of the right main bronchus until it reaches the anterior aspect of the upper lobe bronchus where it supplies its first branch to the upper lobe. This vessel soon divides into a branch for its apical and another for its anterior segment. Having given off this branch the artery bends downwards, lying in a groove on the anterior surface of the bronchus below its upper lobe branch. It is in this situation that the artery to the posterior segment of the upper lobe arises. This vessel can only be found by dissection in the depths of the fissures as it enters the lobe beneath the fissure. The middle lobe is supplied as a rule by two branches of the pulmonary artery which arise at the base of the confluence of the fissures distal to its posterior segmental branch to the upper lobe. They enter the lobe in close relation to the middle lobe bronchus. Having supplied the middle lobe, the pulmonary artery ends by supplying the lower lobe segments. The vessel to its superior segment arises first passing downwards and backwards to this segment. A spray of vessels then supplies the basal segments (*Fig.* 40, A).

LEFT PULMONARY ARTERY: The main trunk is longer than on the right. It trends upwards, outwards, and backwards above the main bronchus where it gives off the first branch which supplies the

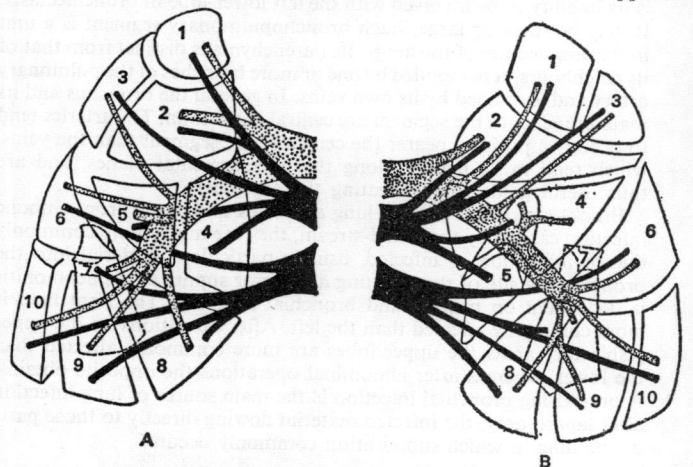

Fig. 40.—Diagrams of the blood-supply to A, the right lung, B, the left lung; arteries, stippled; veins, black. (*By courtesy of Richard Sweet.*) See *Fig.* 35 for segment names.

apical and posterior segments. The vessel then arches over behind the upper lobe bronchus giving off branches to the upper three segments of the lobe. In the interlobar fissure the main vessel gives off a single lingular artery which divides into a vessel to each segment of the lingula.

The left lower lobe arteries come from the interlobar part of the main vessel much as on the right. They come off more distally arising close to the bronchi of their segments of supply (*Fig.* 40, B).

VENOUS ARRANGEMENTS: Are much the same on the two sides. The veins draining the segments converge to form larger trunks and end as the superior and inferior pulmonary veins at the hilum of the lung. The superior pulmonary vein receives the apical, posterior, and anterior segmental veins and two or more veins from the middle lobe. The inferior pulmonary vein receives the veins from the lower lobe segments. At the hilum of the lung the veins are the most anterior structures.

Bronchial Vessels: The bronchial arteries are small vessels which supply nutrition to the lungs. There is usually one main artery to each lung. It arises from the aorta just beyond the origin of the left subclavian or it may come from one of the upper aortic intercostals. One or more smaller arteries may arise from the thoracic aorta.

The bronchial and pulmonary circulations intercommunicate freely on both the arterial and venous sides. These are not therefore closed circuits as was at one time believed. Marchand et al.[1] point out that the bronchial circulation is unique in that the artery arises from the systemic circulation, whereas its venous component enters the pulmonary system. The numerous anastomoses between the systems are of great significance in many forms of lung disease. Virchow[2] (1851) pointed out that ligation of the pulmonary artery did not cause gangrene of the lung. Cases of complete stenosis of the pulmonary artery may survive for many years.

These authors show that the arterial and venous arrangements are such that the arterial supply to the hilar and subpleural structures is separate from the bronchial artery; they call these the pleurohilar arteries. The intrapulmonary bronchi and bronchioles drain via the deep or true bronchial veins and empty into the pulmonary venous system including the left atrium, whereas the pleurohilar veins drain into systemic veins (azygos on the right and left superior intercostal or accessory hemi-azygos on the left) by a separate system of vessels which communicate freely with the pulmonary veins.

Pulmonary Agenesis: A lung is completely absent. The cause is unknown. There are often coexistent congenital defects. About 150 cases are recorded. The condition is compatible with good health and old age.

---

[1] Marchand, P., Gilroy, J. C. and Wilson, V. H., *Thorax*, 1950, 5, 207.
[2] Virchow, R., *Virchows Arch.*, 1851, 3, 171. (Quoted by Marchand et al.)

Chapter VIII
THE UMBILICUS

Level: Typically it is on the same level as the highest points of the iliac crests, i.e., the disc between the 3rd and 4th lumbar vertebrae. It is, however, variable in position, and is therefore unreliable as a landmark.

Its level has some significance as a test in another connexion: it is normally above the midpoint between the top of the head and the soles of the feet. In the condition known as achondroplasia (a type of dwarfism) it is below this midpoint.

Congenital Abnormalities at the Umbilicus:
1. PERSISTENCE OF VITELLO-INTESTINAL CANAL:
    a. IN ITS WHOLE LENGTH: Faeces are discharged at the umbilicus when the cord drops off, as the vitello-intestinal canal is then in direct communication with the small intestine at one extremity and with the skin surface at the other.
    b. IN ITS DISTAL PART ONLY: A raspberry-red tumour is seen at the umbilicus when the cord falls off.
    c. IN ITS CENTRAL PART: The umbilicus itself is normal, but at some later time in life a cystic tumour develops deep to it.
2. PERSISTENCE OF CONNEXION BETWEEN URACHUS AND BLADDER: Urine is discharged at the umbilicus.
3. HERNIA: Owing to persistence of the one-time communication between the peritoneal cavity and the extra-embryonic coelom of the umbilical cord through the umbilicus, a congenital umbilical hernia develops. Umbilical herniae may be classified as follows: (*a*) Hernia of the umbilical cord; (*b*) Umbilical hernia, (i) of children, (ii) of adults.
    a. HERNIA OF THE UMBILICAL CORD: Such a hernia may contain a considerable proportion of the abdominal viscera, being known as a hernia of the umbilical cord or congenital umbilical hernia. The coverings of the hernia are amnion, Wharton's jelly, and peritoneum, and are so thin that the contents of the hernia may be seen through the coverings. There is no skin over the protrusion except at its edges. This condition is also known as *exomphalos*, and according to its degree is defined as being *complete* or *partial*.
    b. UMBILICAL HERNIA:
        i. *Of Children:* This is due *primarily* to one of two causes: (α) Persistence of a small peritoneal process in the root of the cord: (β) Imperfect closure on the part of the linea alba immediately above the umbilicus. *Secondary* factors such as straining at

THE UMBILICUS

stool or coughing may determine the onset of a hernia at one of these weak areas, such herniae being small, with a strong tendency to natural cure. That such a cure does not by any means always occur (as is frequently taught) is amply borne out by statistics.

  ii. *Umbilical Hernia of Adults* is dealt with below.

4. WEEPING UMBILICUS: A condition where the umbilicus fails to heal after the cord falls off. It is seen to be bright red and to discharge watery fluid. This is due to implantation of gut epithelium (columnar) at the umbilicus during the recession of the vitello-intestinal duct (Keith). To cure the condition it is necessary to scrape away this epithelium.

5. ECTOPIA VESICAE: In this condition the lower part of the anterior abdominal wall is absent and the gap is occupied by the posterior wall of the bladder. The umbilicus is malformed and exists as a crescent limiting the deficiency above.

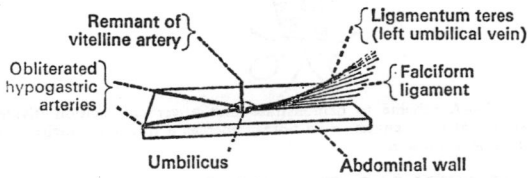

Fig. 41.—Scheme to show the remains of blood-vessels connected with the umbilicus.

VASCULAR REMNANTS: The remains of three blood-vessels end at the umbilicus (*Fig.* 41):

  a. The left umbilical vein, which becomes the ligamentum teres of the liver, ends at the umbilicus.

  b. and *c.* The hypogastric arteries of the fetus are found after birth as the obliterated hypogastric arteries, which pass up over the lower abdominal wall to the umbilicus. They may, very exceptionally, remain patent.

  d. Exceptionally a fibrous cord may connect the umbilicus to the gut or mesentery. This is a remnant of the artery of the vitello-intestinal duct.

Acquired Abnormalities:

1. ACQUIRED UMBILICAL HERNIA (umbilical hernia of adults): The umbilical cicatrix becomes greatly stretched, allowing a process of peritoneum and coils of gut to escape through it. It is usually large and must be cured by operation. In operations for umbilical herniae it is of the first importance to realize that the fibres of the rectus sheath run transversely into the linea alba and umbilicus.

54 A SYNOPSIS OF SURGICAL ANATOMY

Mayo devised an incision, running transversely across the abdomen, to deal with umbilical hernia, as the fibres of the rectus sheath are then simply separated and the abdominal wall is not further weakened (*Fig.* 42). If a vertical incision is used, the fibres of the sheath are divided, thus adding to the already existent weakness of the abdominal wall.

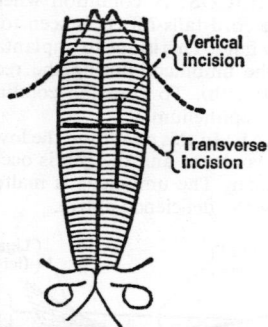

Fig. 42.—A scheme to demonstrate that a vertical incision divides the rectus sheath at right angles to its fibres, whereas a transverse incision merely separates adjacent fibres.

2. **CAPUT MEDUSAE**: The umbilical area is one of the sites of communication between the portal and systemic circulations. The ligamentum teres carries small veins to the liver (portal) which communicate at the umbilicus with the veins of the anterior abdominal wall, which are systemic. Should obstruction occur to the flow of portal blood through the liver, some of that blood is shunted along the veins of the ligamentum teres to the umbilicus and so to the systemic veins here. These latter are radially arranged at the umbilicus, and when dilated give an appearance suggestive of the spokes of a wheel, which is called the 'caput Medusae'.

3. **DISCHARGES AT THE UMBILICUS**: There is a tendency for pathological collections inside the abdomen, such as abscesses and collections of bile, to discharge at the umbilicus. Much the commonest cause of a discharge from the umbilicus is an area of inflammation in the depth of the depression which is due to neglect or inability to cleanse properly. Concretions or umbilical stones may form under similar circumstances due to the accumulation of skin secretions. Such conditions are readily cured by packing with ribbon gauze which allows proper drainage.

4. **NEW GROWTHS**: The umbilicus is an occasional site for the occurrence of warts or papillomata. These require very careful

investigation. It may happen that a cancer in the liver extends along the round ligament to the umbilicus and is seen on the surface as what appears to be a papilloma. If a portion of this is examined microscopically and found to be cancer of some intra-abdominal organ (columnar or adenocarcinoma), it is of the first importance both diagnostically and also from the point of view of treatment, because in addition to denoting the presence of a primary growth elsewhere, it indicates the uselessness of trying to remove the primary growth, as at least one secondary growth (that at the umbilicus) already exists.

Chapter IX

THE GUT

Duodenum:
SIZE: The duodenum is 25 cm. long. It makes a C-shaped bend which embraces the head of the pancreas. It consists of three parts:
FIRST PART: Extends up, backwards, and to the right to the level of the upper border of the 1st lumbar vertebra. It is 5 cm. long.
SECOND PART: Extends downwards to the level of the lower border of the 3rd lumbar vertebra. It is 7·5 cm. long.
THIRD PART: Extends to the left, then upwards to the level of the left side of the 2nd lumbar vertebra. It is 12·5 cm. long.
RELATIONS:
FIRST PART:
Anterior: Quadrate lobe of the liver.
Posterior: Portal vein, gastroduodenal artery, and bile-duct.
The vena cava is behind these.
Superior: Epiploic foramen and hepatic artery (horizontal part).
Inferior: Head of the pancreas.
SECOND PART:
Anterior: Gall-bladder, transverse colon, and small gut.
Posterior: Renal vessels, the pelvis of the kidney, and the kidney.
Right: Hepatic flexure of the colon.
Left: Head of the pancreas. It is pierced about the middle by the bile and pancreatic ducts.
THIRD PART:
Anterior: Superior mesenteric vessels, the root of the mesentery, the transverse colon and mesocolon.
Posterior: Inferior vena cava, aorta, spermatic vessels of both sides, the left sympathetic trunk, and the left psoas.

Superior: Head of the pancreas.
Inferior: Small gut.

PERITONEAL RELATIONS: In general the C which this part of the gut makes is covered anteriorly and on its convexity by the peritoneum except where the transverse colon crosses the second part and holds the peritoneum away (*Fig.* 43). The posterior surface and concavity of the C are devoid of peritoneum. The first 2·5 cm. of the first part is entirely covered by peritoneum except for a small part above and behind (cf. caecum).

In the region where the bile-duct enters the second part, a diverticulum of the duodenum may occur. It owes its existence to the fact that at a very early developmental stage more than one outgrowth from the gut takes place to form the liver. Usually all except one (the permanent bile-duct) disappear. Parts of a second outgrowth may remain, forming a blind protrusion from the bowel. Such a diverticulum is devoid of peritoneal covering. This is of surgical importance, as its removal would be attended by grave risks of peritonitis because the retroperitoneal tissues have little resistance to infection.

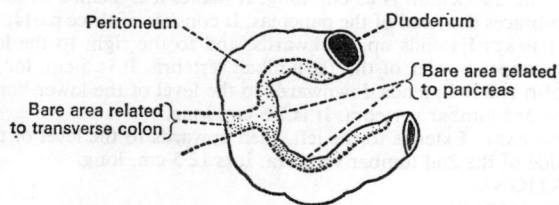

Fig. 43.—Peritoneal relations of the duodenum. The stippled area is uncovered by peritoneum and is in relation to the pancreas in the concavity of the gut and in relation to the transverse colon where this crosses the descending portion of duodenum.

Duodenojejunal Flexure: The duodenojejunal flexure is at the left side of the 2nd lumbar vertebra just below the pancreas. It is a fixed part of the gut and easily found. It is supported by a ligament containing unstriped muscle which passes to it from the region of the left crus of the diaphragm and the tissue about the coeliac plexus. This is the suspensory ligament of the duodenum (ligament of Treitz).

Small Intestine (Jejunum and Ileum): The average length of this part of the intestine is 7 m. The upper two-fifths are jejunum, the lower three-fifths are ileum. It is entirely surrounded by peritoneum. It is important to note that the length of the small gut is variable, the extremes being 4 and 9 m.

THE GUT 57

THE PART OF THE SMALL GUT WHICH LIES IN THE PELVIS:
1. The terminal ileum, except the last 5 cm. which are fixed in the right iliac fossa.
2. The 1·5 m. of small gut beginning at a point 1·8 m. from the duodenojejunal flexure to a point 3·4 m. from the flexure. This is due to the fact that the mesentery to this part of the small gut is longer than that to other parts. These are the parts of the small gut which are likely to be affected in pelvic peritonitis.

The small gut is suspended by its mesentery. This extends from the left side of the 2nd lumbar vertebra to the right iliac fossa, crossing the third part of the duodenum, aorta, vena cava, and right ureter in its course. It is 15 cm. in length along this line of attachment. Along its free border it is necessarily as long as the small gut—7 m. Its depth is 15 cm., except in relation to the part of the small gut which occupies the pelvis, where it is 20 cm. broad.

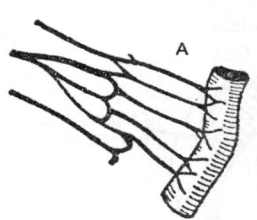 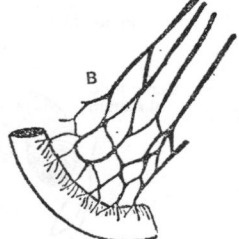

Fig. 44.—Arrangement of the arteries to the small intestine.
A, Jejunum. B, Ileum.

DIFFERENCES BETWEEN THE ILEUM AND JEJUNUM:
These are well known. The least well-known distinction is the only one of use to the operating surgeon who wants to be sure at a glance if a part of the gut is upper or lower small gut. This distinction depends on the blood-supply (*Fig.* 44). *Jejunum:* One or two arterial arcades in the mesentery with parallel vessels 3·7 cm. long going to the gut. *Ileum:* Two or three arterial arcades in the mesentery with parallel vessels 1·2 cm. long going to the gut.

A diverticulum—Meckel's—may be found on the antimesenteric border of the ileum in cases where the vitello-intestinal duct partly persists. It occurs 61 cm. from the ileocaecal valve, is found in 2 per cent of persons, and is 5 cm. or more in length. It has the calibre of the ileum.

Large Intestine: The large intestine is 1·8 m. long. Its longitudinal muscle coat is arranged round it in three bands, the taeniae coli. These bands

58 A SYNOPSIS OF SURGICAL ANATOMY

are 1·2 m. long. It is therefore 'gathered' by the muscle to form characteristic sacculations. Its two terminations, rectum and appendix, are completely surrounded by muscle. These two portions are therefore not sacculated.

PERITONEAL RELATIONS: Those parts with mesenteries—transverse colon, pelvic colon, and appendix—are completely surrounded by peritoneum except for a narrow band between the two layers of the mesenteric attachment. The other parts are devoid of peritoneum posteriorly. The caecum and the rectum have special relations.

CAECUM: Is completely surrounded by peritoneum, except a small part posteriorly and superiorly (cf. first 2·5 cm. of duodenum).

RECTUM (*Fig.* 45):
The first third is covered anteriorly and at the sides by peritoneum.
The second third is covered anteriorly only by peritoneum.
The third third has no relation to peritoneum.

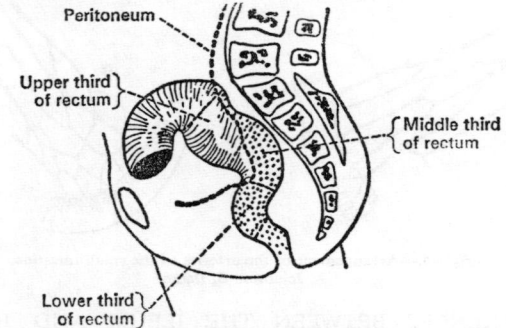

Fig. 45.—Peritoneal relations of the rectum.

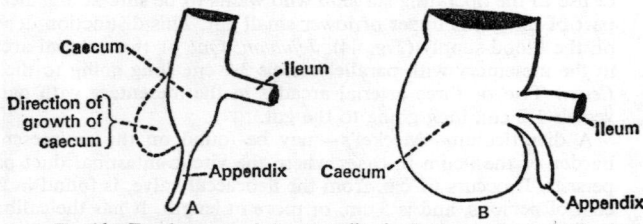

Fig. 46.—Development of the appendix. A, Caecum at an early developmental stage showing the future appendix below. The dotted line shows how the appendix is pushed medially by the outgrowth of the right wall of the caecum. B, The adult condition.

The peritoneum is firmly attached to the upper third and loosely to the middle third.

Appendix: The appendix is the commencement of the large gut. At an early embryonic stage it has the same calibre as the caecum and is in line with it. It is formed by excessive growth of the right wall of the caecum which pushes the appendix to the inner side (*Fig.* 46). It may persist in its early and infantile form and is then most liable to catch foreign bodies. It varies in length from 2·5 to 23 cm. The average length is 9 cm. Congenital absence of the appendix is extremely rare—0·0009 per cent (Collins[1]).

It has the same coats as the large gut, but the muscular coat may be deficient in parts so that the peritoneum and mucous membrane are separated only by connective tissue through which infection may readily spread from the mucous membrane to the peritoneum. Its wall contains much lymphoid tissue. Much lymphoid tissue is collected at the entrance to the alimentary canal in the pharynx (tonsils, adenoids). Much lymphoid tissue is collected at the entrance to the large gut in the terminal ileum and appendix.

POSITIONS: These were explained by Sir Frederick Treves in the form of a clock (*Fig.* 47).

11 o'clock: Paracolic. 3 o'clock: Promontoric.
12 o'clock: Retrocolic. 4 o'clock: Pelvic.
2 o'clock: Splenic.   6 o'clock: Mid-Poupart
                                  or mid-inguinal.

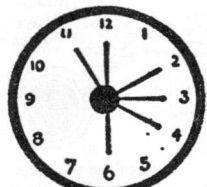

Fig. 47.—Positions of the appendix. 11 o'clock, Paracolic; 12, Retrocolic; 2, Splenic; 3, Promontoric; 4, Pelvic; 6, Mid-inguinal. (*After Treves.*)

11 AND 12 O'CLOCK POSITIONS: The appendix passes upwards, and may be to the outer side—paracolic (11)—or directly behind the caecum—retrocolic (12). The organ may be partly or entirely behind the peritoneum. It is sometimes in front of the kidney.

2 O'CLOCK OR SPLENIC POSITION: The organ passes in a direction towards the spleen. It is entirely intraperitoneal and goes in front of or behind the terminal ileum. If inflamed it may affect this

[1] Collins, D. C., *Am. J. Surg.*, 1951, **82**, 689.

part of the ileum and cause *much* vomiting (an unusual thing in appendicitis) and even obstruction of the small gut; it is particularly liable to result in a general peritonitis, and is the most dangerous position which the appendix may occupy.

3 O'CLOCK OR PROMONTORIC POSITION: Its relations are much as in the last type. It is directed transversely inwards towards the promontory of the sacrum.

4 O'CLOCK OR PELVIC POSITION: The appendix hangs over the pelvic brim into the true pelvis.

6 O'CLOCK POSITION: Appendix passes down towards the middle of the inguinal ligament.

Mesenteries of the Large Gut:

MESENTERY OF THE APPENDIX: May be complete or incomplete. The appendicular artery reaches the appendix along this mesentery. If the mesentery is incomplete, the artery lies on the wall of the appendix in its distal part and the wall of the vessel may be eroded in suppurative appendicitis, or early thrombosis of the appendicular blood-vessels may occur.

TRANSVERSE MESOCOLON: Is a double fold of peritoneum which suspends the transverse colon from the anterior border of the pancreas. The middle colic artery runs in the mesocolon (*Fig.* 48). This artery runs downwards and not up—as students often say,

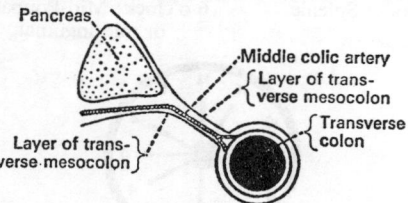

Fig. 48.—The attachment of the transverse mesocolon to the anterior border of the pancreas.

the reason being that they visualize the artery as seen in illustrations where the transverse colon has been pulled up in order to show the vessel, which then appears to run upwards.

Large Mesenteries and their Attachments (*Fig.* 49):

PELVIC MESOCOLON: Has a ∧-shaped attachment. The left limb of the ∧ is attached to the brim of the left side of the pelvis. The right limb of the ∧ passes from the apex down to the third piece of the sacrum. The apex of the ∧ is situated exactly over the left ureter where it crosses the pelvic brim. This is the surgeon's guide to the left ureter. The mesocolon carries the superior haemorrhoidal vessels.

THE GUT 61

1. The mesentery of the small gut—the attachment to the posterior abdominal wall is oblique.
2. The mesentery of the transverse colon—the attachment to the posterior abdominal wall is transverse.
3. The mesentery of the pelvic colon—the attachment to the posterior abdominal wall is of an inverted V shape.

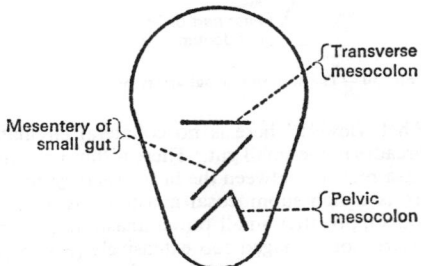

Fig. 49.—The manner of the attachments of the mesenteries to the posterior abdominal wall.

Blood-supply of the Gut: The primitive gut is divisible into fore-, mid-, and hind-gut. The foregut ends and the midgut begins where the bile-duct enters the second part of the duodenum. The midgut ends and the hindgut begins at the junction of the left with the middle third of the transverse colon. Each portion of the gut has its own artery.

The artery of the foregut is the coeliac.
The artery of the midgut is the superior mesenteric.
The artery of the hindgut is the inferior mesenteric.
The first part of the duodenum up to the entrance of the bile-ducts has therefore the same blood-supply as the stomach.
The blood-supply of the stomach is so profuse that any one of the large vessels supplying the organ is sufficient to maintain its vitality providing the marginal anastomotic vessels are patent. It is this fact which enables the organ to be so freely mobilized in oesophago-gastric anastomosis. The small bowel has a generous vascular supply. The colon is less adequately supplied than other parts of the bowel. The rectal supply is better than that of the colon.

SUPRADUODENAL ARTERY OF WILKIE (*Fig.* 50): The right gastric or hepatic artery gives off a small vessel which runs on the first part of the duodenum. This is the supraduodenal artery. It was suggested as a factor in the aetiology of duodenal ulcer by Wilkie, who considered the vessel to be an end artery.

62 A SYNOPSIS OF SURGICAL ANATOMY

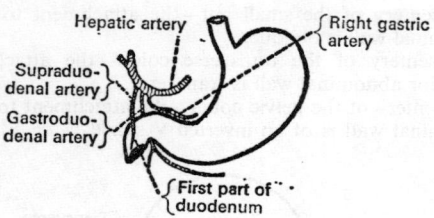

Fig. 50.—The supraduodenal artery of Wilkie.

Blood-supply of Small Bowel: There is no collateral circulation beyond the terminal arcades in the small gut.[1] There is thus no communication between the vasa recta or between the branches they give off to bowel wall, but there is a rich submucosal anastomosis which ensures an adequate blood-supply after small bowel anastomosis, provided that the vasa recta are not damaged too extensively (Fig. 51).

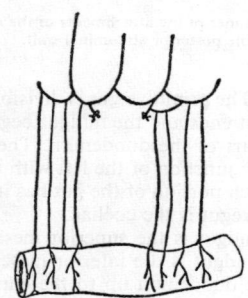

Fig. 51.—Small intestinal anastomosis. Preparing for the junction.

Blood-supply of Large Bowel:
  APPENDICULAR ARTERY: A branch of the ileocolic which runs *behind* the terminal ileum to reach the appendix, and is accompanied in this course by the lymphatics of the appendix.
  MARGINAL ARTERY: Along the concavity of the three-sided square made by the large gut, there courses an artery made up by anastomotic vessels from the different main vessels going to the large

[1] Akkinis, A. J., *J. Anat. Paris.* 1930, 64, 200.

THE GUT   63

intestine (*Fig.* 52). It is the marginal artery and is capable of supplying the gut through these anastomoses even though one of the large feeding trunks be severed. This artery can maintain the vitality of the left colon even after the inferior mesenteric has been ligatured at its origin (Archibald). It is, however, never wise to assume this during operations on the colon. It has been shown for example by Singleton[1] that the anastomosis between the left and middle colic arteries is absent in 5 per cent of cases. Ligature of one of these vessels would thus jeopardize the blood-supply of the splenic flexure region of the colon. The only safe procedure is to inspect the colonic blood-supply in planning resections. After mobilization the vessels can usually be seen through the peritoneal attachment if the bowel is held up to display them.

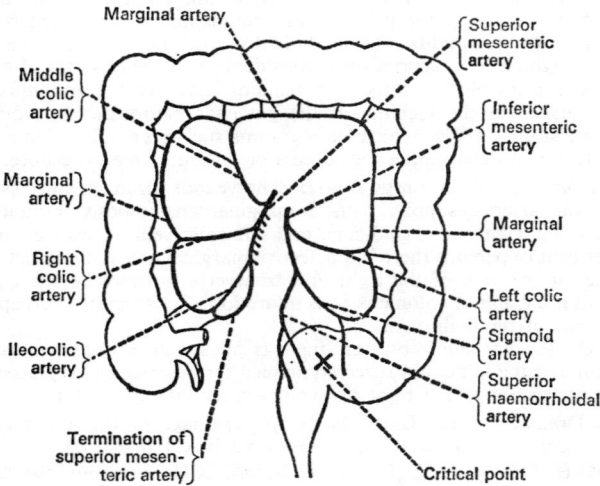

Fig. 52.—Blood-supply of the colon, showing the marginal artery and the so-called 'critical point' of Sudeck.

It is also sound procedure to delay bowel section until a late stage in operations on the gut, as by that time colour changes may indicate vascular inadequacies and indicate the site of safe section. Arthur Allen of Boston stresses that fat should not be trimmed off bowel ends in preparation for anastomosis as by this means the blood-supply to the gut is impaired. O. Wangensteen,

[1] *Surgery*, 1943, **14**, 328.

on the other hand, clears bowel ends of fat for almost a centimetre (*see also* section on Anatomical Principles underlying the Surgery of Colon Cancer, p. 598).

'CRITICAL POINT' OF SUDECK: There is a satisfactory anastomosis between the lowest sigmoid branch of the inferior mesenteric artery and the superior haemorrhoidal branch of the same vessel. The opposing view expressed by Sudeck (1907) and other investigators and taught until recently is incorrect.

In resection of the pelvic colon for cancer it is mandatory to remove the paths of lymphatic spread, and therefore the inferior mesenteric artery below the origin of the left colic or even at its origin from the aorta should the gland spread warrant this. The marginal artery will in at least 70 per cent of cases (Goligher[1]) ensure the blood-supply of the left colon. The rectum and lower 5 to 7·5 cm. of the pelvic colon are adequately nourished by the inferior and middle haemorrhoidal arteries and no single case of sloughing has occurred in a considerable personal series of cases. The principle none the less remains that the surgeon must be satisfied of the viability of the gut ends before deciding on the anastomosis. The avoidance of trauma such as crushing clamps is a factor in determining the success or failure of the procedure.

Venous Drainage of the Large Bowel:[2] The venous drainage corresponds to the arterial supply, with a marginal anastomosis joining the ileocolic, right colic, mid-colic and left colic veins. However, in 20 per cent of persons there is a defective marginal anastomosis between the major veins of the right and transverse portions of the colon. This is a cause of colonic venous infarction after surgical interruption of one of the main veins.

On the left side, however, there is always an excellent marginal vein and the left colon is recommended for oesophageal replacement in preference to the right to avoid venous infarction of the bowel.

Lymph Drainage of the Gut: The lymph drainage of the gut may be considered under two heads: (1) Stomach; (2) Intestines.

LYMPH DRAINAGE OF THE STOMACH: Each of the three branches of the coeliac axis takes a share in the arterial supply of the stomach. The organ may be divided into three lymphatic areas corresponding fairly closely to the arterial territories. The lymph-glands concerned in the drainage of the stomach are:

1. Hepatic group
   - *a.* Hepatic
   - *b.* Cystic
   - *c.* Subpyloric

   Lie on the hepatic artery or its branches.

---

[1] Goligher, J. C., *Br. J. Surg.*, 1954, 41, 351.
[2] Nicks, R., *Ibid.*, 1967, 54, 124.

THE GUT 65

2. Gastric group { *a.* Superior / *b.* Inferior } { The superior group lie on the left gastric artery.

3. Pancreatico-lienal group { Lie on the splenic artery or its branches.

HEPATIC GLANDS: These lie in the lesser omentum along the bile-ducts; an outlying member is in relation to the neck of the gall-bladder along the cystic artery. This is the cystic gland. They receive lymph from the liver and gall-bladder.

SUBPYLORIC GLANDS: These are in the angle between the first and second parts of the duodenum on the head of the pancreas in relation to the bifurcation of the gastroduodenal artery. They receive the lymph from the right two-thirds of the greater curvature of the stomach which comes through the inferior gastric glands.

GASTRIC GROUP: This consists of (*a*) superior, and (*b*) inferior sets.

a. Superior Glands: The superior glands are divisible into:
  i. Upper—on the upper part of the left gastric artery.
  ii. Lower—on the lower part of the left gastric artery (i.e., along the left half of the lesser curvature of the stomach between the layers of the lesser omentum).
  iii. The paracardial are grouped around the neck of the stomach.

b. Inferior Glands: The inferior glands lie along the pyloric half of the greater curvature of the stomach between the layers of the greater omentum.

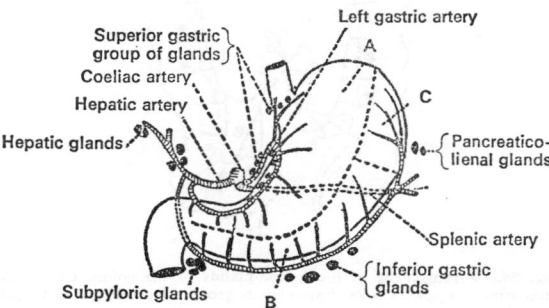

Fig. 53.—The lymph territories of the stomach are indicated by the letters A, B, C. Area A represents the upper two-thirds of the organ; Area B, the right two-thirds of the lower third; Area C, the left third of the lower third. A drains to superior gastric glands; B drains to inferior gastric glands; C drains to pancreatico-lienal glands.

PANCREATICO-LIENAL GLANDS: These lie along the splenic artery in relation to the upper border of the pancreas. Some occur in the gastrosplenic ligament in relation to the short gastric branches of the splenic.

THE EFFERENTS FROM ALL THESE GLANDS go to the lymph-glands around the coeliac axis in front of the aorta, i.e., the coeliac group of pre-aortic glands.

Divide the stomach by a line in its long axis, two-thirds of the stomach being to the right of this line, one-third to the left. Divide the left third into two by a line at the junction of its upper third and lower two-thirds. This marks out the three lymph territories of the organ (*Fig.* 53).

LYMPH DRAINAGE OF THE INTESTINE: The glands are arranged on a plan common to all parts of the large and small intestine. They are very numerous and arranged in three groups: (1) Proximal; (2) Intermediate; (3) Distal. (*Fig.* 54.)

THE PROXIMAL GLANDS are situated on the main blood-vessels to the gut, i.e., superior mesenteric, ileocolic, right colic, left colic, middle colic, inferior mesenteric, superior haemorrhoidal, sigmoid.

THE INTERMEDIATE GLANDS are situated along the larger branches of the above-named vessels.

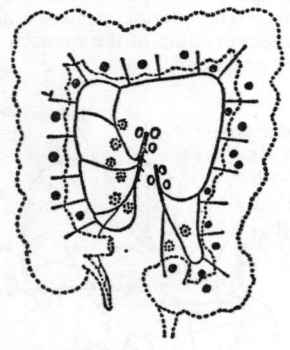

Fig. 54.—Arrangement of the lymph-glands of the colon. Clear circles: proximal group. Stippled circles: intermediate group. Black circles: distal group.

THE DISTAL GLANDS are situated near the gut between the numerous small vessels entering the gut. Some of these glands lie on the gut. The lymph goes for the most part from the gut to the distal glands and thence to the intermediate glands. It is, however, of the first importance to realize that lymph from the gut may miss the distal set and go direct to the intermediate or even the proximal set.

This plan is the same throughout the large and small intestines. The lymphatics from the territory of any one of the large arteries converge on the main trunk of the vessel so that the lymph drainage is divided up fairly accurately into areas corresponding to the main arteries.

This fact governs the operative treatment of cancer of the gut, so that if a cancer occurs at the caecum for instance, the whole of the gut supplied by the ileocolic and right colic arteries, together with these arteries and their branches and the related peritoneum, is removed to ensure the removal of the whole lymph territory which converges on these vessels.

Chapter X

THE PERITONEAL FOSSAE

THESE are of great surgical importance, as owing to the possibility of portions of gut entering the fossae and becoming strangulated there, such fossae may serve as sites of internal herniae. The fossae are:
1. The lesser sac of the peritoneum—always present.
2. The duodenal fossae:
   a. Left duodenal:
      i. Paraduodenal—occasionally present (in 20 per cent of persons).
      ii. Superior duodenojejenal—often present (in 50 per cent of persons).
      iii. Inferior duodenojejunal—often present (in 25 per cent of persons).
   b. Inferior duodenal—often present.
   c. Mesenterico-parietal fossa of Waldeyer.
3. The caecal fossae:
   a. Ileocolic—often present.
   b. Ileocaecal—often present.
   c. Retrocaecal or subcaecal—often present.
4. The intersigmoid.

1. **Lesser Sac of the Peritoneum:** Occasionally part or the whole of the small gut may enter this space through the foramen epiploicum (Winslow).[1]

[1] According to some authors this condition is not acquired, but is a congenital error of rotation of the gut.

68 A SYNOPSIS OF SURGICAL ANATOMY

THE FORAMEN OF WINSLOW is the communication between the greater and lesser sacs of the peritoneum (*Fig. 55*).

LEVEL: 12th thoracic vertebra.

SIZE: Up to 3 cm.

RELATIONS:

Anterior: The right free border of the lesser omentum containing the bile-duct, hepatic artery, and portal vein.

Posterior: The right adrenal gland and inferior vena cava.

Superior: The caudate process of the liver.

Inferior: The first part of the duodenum and hepatic artery (its transverse part).

It is apparent that this orifice is surrounded by such important structures that should it be the cause of gut strangulation it does not admit of surgical enlargement in any direction. Usually the gut is easily delivered from the fossa. If it cannot be delivered, the lesser sac is opened through the great omentum and the gut aspirated. After this it reduces more readily.

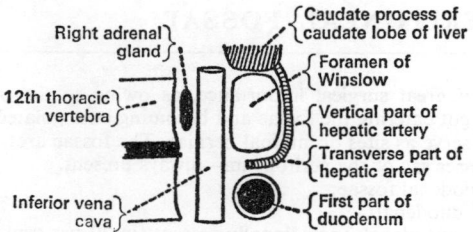

Fig. 55.—Boundaries of the foramen epiploicum (Winslow).

2. Duodenal Fossae:

PARADUODENAL FOSSA (*Fig. 56*): This fossa lies to the left of the duodenojejunal flexure and is open to the right and upwards.

It occurs in 20 per cent of persons. It never exists together with other types of duodenal fossae.

BOUNDARIES:

Above: Pancreas and renal vessels.

Right: Aorta.

Left: Kidney.

Anterior: The inferior mesenteric vein runs in the anterior wall of the fossa.

Treves advised that should the fossa be the site of strangulated gut, its surgical enlargement be effected in a *downward* direction, to avoid injury to the inferior mesenteric vein.

THE PERITONEAL FOSSAE 69

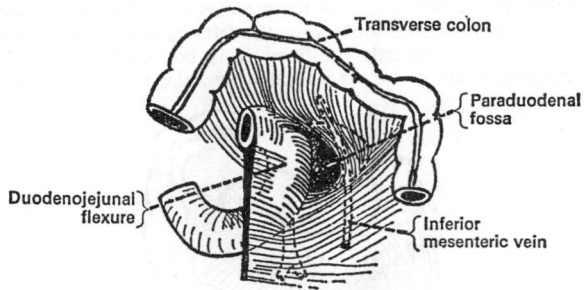

Fig. 56.—The paraduodenal fossa.

SUPERIOR AND INFERIOR DUODENOJEJUNAL FOSSAE
(*Fig.* 57): These often exist. They are formed, when present, by
two peritoneal folds running to the left from the region of the
termination of the duodenum.

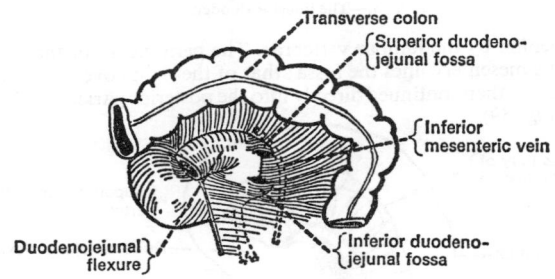

Fig. 57.—The superior and inferior duodenojejunal fossae.

SUPERIOR DUODENOJEJUNAL FOSSA: Looks downwards. It is about
2·5 cm. in depth and is in front of the 2nd lumbar vertebra.

INFERIOR DUODENOJEJUNAL FOSSA: Looks upwards. It is in front of the
3rd lumbar vertebra.

INFERIOR DUODENAL FOSSA (*Fig.* 58): This is an occasional
opening which extends behind the third part of the duodenum.

MESENTERICO-PARIETAL FOSSA OF WALDEYER: The classic
description of the fossa is that of Moynihan:[1] 'The most usual
position of this fossa is in the first part of the mesojejunum,
immediately behind the superior mesenteric artery, and immediately

[1] Lord Moynihan, *Retroperitoneal Hernia*, 2nd ed., 1906.

below the duodenum. The fossa varies considerably in size. The fossa has its orifice looking to the left, its blind extremity to the right and downwards. In front it is bounded by the superior mesenteric artery (or its continuation, the ileocolic artery), and

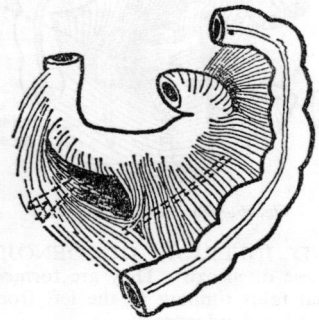

Fig. 58.—The inferior duodenal fossa.

behind by the lumbar vertebrae. The peritoneum of the left leaf of the mesentery lines the fossa; that of the right covers the blind end, and is then continued directly into the posterior parietal peritoneum.' (*Fig. 59*).

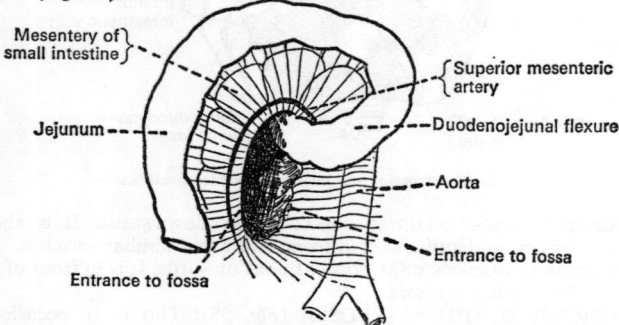

Fig. 59.—The mesenterico-parietal fossa of Waldeyer.

Herniae into this fossa are rare—eight times less common than herniae into the left duodenal fossae. Observe that:[1]

[1] For many of the facts given here I am indebted to Francis R. Brown, *Br. J. Surg.*, 1925, **13**, 367.

THE PERITONEAL FOSSAE

1. A swelling produced by a hernia into this fossa would occupy the right half of the abdominal cavity.
2. The contents are small intestine.
3. The symptoms will be those either of an internal strangulation, or of duodenal ileus (due to obstruction of the afferent bowel).
4. The orifice of the fossa is so large that it is very unlikely to be the cause of strangulation. If such exists it is caused by adhesions about the orifice or the sac or by axial twisting of the intestine at the neck of the sac.
5. The intestine can usually be withdrawn from the sac without difficulty. Should enlargement of the fossa be necessary to effect reduction, the relationship of the superior mesenteric vessels to the fossa must be remembered. The fossa can only be incised in a *downward* direction.

3. Caecal Fossae:

ILEOCOLIC OR SUPERIOR ILEOCAECAL FOSSA: This is formed by a fold of peritoneum extending between the ascending colon and the terminal ileum—the ileocolic fold.

BOUNDARIES:

Anterior: The ileocolic fold contains the ileocolic artery and vein.
Posterior: Ileum and its mesentery.
Right: Ascending colon.

The fossa is open to the left.

ILEOCAECAL FOSSA: This is formed by the ileocaecal or bloodless fold of Treves, which extends from the terminal ileum to the caecum and the mesentery of the appendix.

BOUNDARIES:

Anterior and Inferior: Ileocaecal fold.
Superior: Posterior surface of the ileum and its mesentery.
Posterior: Mesentery of the appendix.

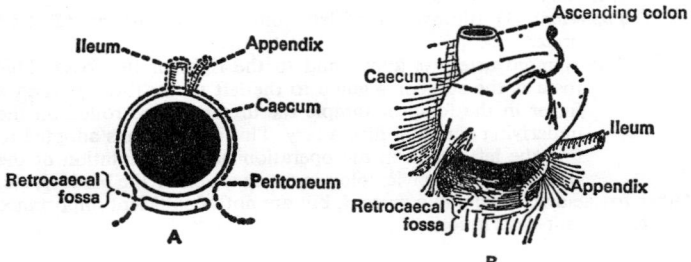

Fig. 60.—Showing the retrocaecal or subcaecal fossa. A, Represents the fossa as seen on horizontal section through the caecum. B, Shows the caecum retracted up to expose the fossa.

72 A SYNOPSIS OF SURGICAL ANATOMY

RETRO- OR SUBCAECAL FOSSA (*Fig.* 60): This is posterior to the caecum.

BOUNDARIES:
  Anterior: Posterior surface of the caecum.
  Right: Peritoneum of the right colic gutter.
  Left: Mesentery.
  Posterior: The iliac fossa covered by parietal peritoneum.
  It often contains the appendix.

4. **Fossa Intersigmoidea:** The pelvic mesocolon has a parietal attachment shaped like an inverted V. The apex of the ∧ is at the bifurcation of the left common iliac artery (*Fig.* 61). The right limb descends to the third piece of the sacrum, the left limb runs along the inner wall of the pelvis. At the apex of the ∧ is a fossa which is always present in infancy but may disappear later. It is represented in many cases merely by a dimple.

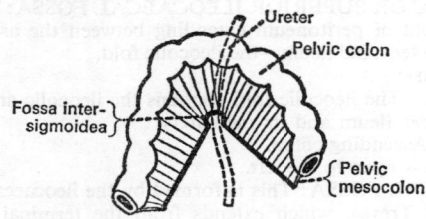

Fig. 61.—To show the fossa intersigmoidea lying at the apex of the ∧ attachment of the pelvic mesocolon. The ureter is shown passing down behind the fossa.

RELATIONS:
  Anterior: Peritoneum.
  Posterior: (1) Bifurcation of left common iliac artery; (2) Left ureter.
  The sigmoid artery is above and to the right of the fossa. This fossa is the surgeon's guide to the left ureter (Stiles). With a finger in the fossa or dimple the ureter can be rolled on the underlying common iliac artery. This is the means adopted to find the left ureter in the operation of transplantation of the ureter into the pelvic colon in extroversion of the bladder, etc.

Other fossae are occasionally present, but are not of sufficient importance to warrant description.

Chapter XI

ACCESSORY PERITONEAL BANDS[1]

THERE are frequently found in the abdominal cavity accessory peritoneal bands or membranes. They are of much interest and practical importance as they have been held to cause obstruction to the faecal current by kinking or angulating portions of gut. There are different views as to their causation, and much controversy has centred round this matter generally.

Theories of Causation:

EVOLUTIONARY THEORY: This is the view of Arbuthnot Lane, who holds that these bands are a result of the assumption of the erect posture—that is to say, that the vertical position of the body has caused the development of these peritoneal processes as 'ligaments' to hold up the gut and prevent its sagging downwards. This view is not now generally accepted, although it is agreed that these accessory membranes are most often present in that type of habitus where the viscera of the abdomen are low in position.

INFLAMMATORY THEORY: Championed by Jackson and others. The view is discarded. There are strong arguments against it; (1) The bands are very regular in situation and appearance; (2) The blood-vessels in the bands are long, tenuous, parallel vessels, quite unlike the blood-supply of inflammatory tissue.

CONGENITAL THEORY: This is the most widely accepted view. The bands are often present at birth. They are best explained by a reference to development: gut undergoes most complicated alterations in position during the developmental process of rotation. During this migration primitive ventral and dorsal mesenteries largely disappear and secondary ones develop. Failure of parts of the original membranes to disappear and minor alterations in the development of the secondary ones result in the accessory membranes found at birth. It is important to realize that, though they exist at birth, these bands rarely produce symptoms and then usually in adult life.

Accessory Peritoneal Bands or Membranes:

1. GENITO-MESENTERIC FOLD OF DOUGLAS REID:[2] Sixty or more years ago Douglas Reid described, in the fetus, a triangular fold of peitoneum which extended into the region of the brim of the pelvis, from the back of the terminal mesentery of the small intestine. It is on the right-hand side. It becomes less marked in the adult where,

---

[1] For much of the matter of this chapter I wish to acknowledge my indebtedness to the masterly article of R. B. Carslaw on 'Right-sided Visceroptosis', *Br. J. Surg.*, 1928, 15, 545.

[2] *J. Anat.*, 1911, 45, 73.

to use Reid's expression, it becomes soldered to the peritoneum of the posterior abdominal wall. It extends from the junction of the second and third parts of the duodenum to the region of the suspensory ligament of the ovary or testis. It contains lymph-glands and blood-vessels and may establish close relations or adhesions to appendix, ovary, and other structures. It may thus bury the appendix or bind down the caecum, and Reid considered that through its lymphatics and blood-vessels it might be responsible for the spread of infection between ovary and appendix, etc. Its chief surgical value to-day is that it is often the cause of binding down and kinking of the appendix. In the adult it is relatively bloodless and may thus be safely divided when, as is often the case, it prevents delivery of the appendix. It is often the cause of obstructive appendicitis when it angulates this organ.

2. **LANE'S ILEAL MEMBRANE** (*Fig.* 62): This is a thickening of the parietal peritoneum in the region of the right iliac fossa extending from the right iliac fossa to the antimesenteric border of the terminal 5 or 7 cm. of the ileum. It is held by Lane that the continued contraction (i.e., shortening) of this band may kink the small gut at this place. In opposition to this view it is held that though minor degrees of obstruction may occur, it is not a common finding, and the ileum is not hypertrophied above the band, which would be the case if obstruction existed.

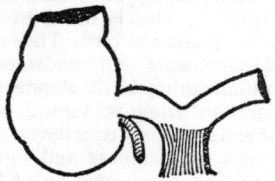

Fig. 62.—The ileal band.

3. **MESOSIGMOID MEMBRANE** (Lane's 'first and last kink') (*Fig.* 63): This corresponds on the left side to the ileal membrane on the right. It is a thickening and shortening of the peritoneum of the left iliac fossa binding the junction of the iliac and pelvic colons down to the pelvic brim. Lane called it the 'first and last kink' because it is the *first* to appear according to his evolutionary theory and the *last* in the sense that it is the last (or lowermost) part of the gut to be affected by a band. Lane holds that very commonly this band causes symptoms of partial obstruction. The view is not popular.

ACCESSORY PERITONEAL BANDS

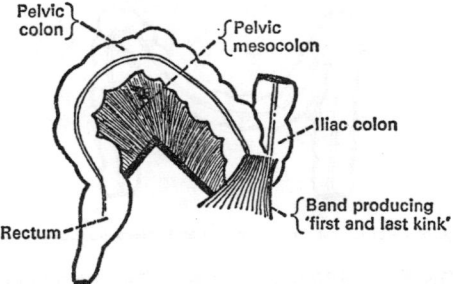

Fig. 63.—Showing Lane's 'first and last kink' and the method of its production.

4. **MESOCOLICOJEJUNAL MEMBRANE** (*Fig.* 64): This is a band of varying length extending from the under-surface of the transverse mesocolon to the antimesenteric border of the proximal part of the jejunum.

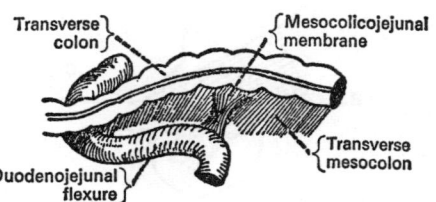

Fig. 64.—The mesocolicojejunal membrane.

5. **INTERCOLIC MEMBRANES**: These are peritoneal folds which bind together: (1) The ascending colon and proximal part of the transverse colon in the region of the hepatic flexure; (2) The descending colon and distal part of the transverse colon in the region of the splenic flexure (Payr's membrane).

Carslaw thinks that this membrane is a part of the great omentum which has become attached excessively far out. It has the effect of causing so-called 'double-barrelled' colon and is held to be an occasional cause of partial obstruction to the onflow of the contents of the gut (*Fig.* 65). There is little evidence in support of this contention.

76 A SYNOPSIS OF SURGICAL ANATOMY

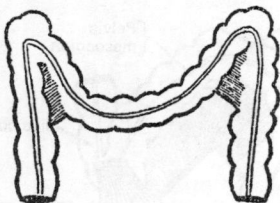

Fig. 65.—'Double-barrelled' colon and intercolic membranes.

6. **JACKSON'S MEMBRANE** (*Fig. 66*): This is a fold of peritoneum, thin and diaphanous, which extends from the posterior abdominal wall in the region to the right of the ascending colon, in a direction downwards and inwards, and is attached to the anterior longitudinal band of the ascending colon or caecum. It may even extend from the hepatic flexure to the caecum, or over only part of this segment of the gut. The blood-vessels are thin, long, and parallel, as shown in *Fig. 66*.

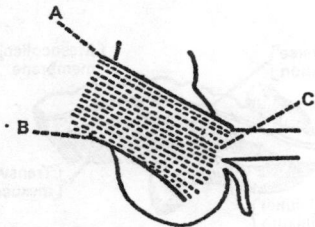

Fig. 66.—Jackson's membrane. The membrane lies between the thick lines A and B. The lines between, (C), represent the parallel, fine blood-vessels so characteristic of this membrane.

7. **CYSTOGASTROCOLIC BAND**: A fold which stretches from the gall-bladder across the duodenum to the great omentum or transverse colon. It may produce symptoms dating from birth of partial obstruction to the outlet from the stomach (*see below*).
8. **MESENTERY TO THE ASCENDING COLON**: Either the ascending or descending colon may have a mesentery. This is due to faulty fixation of the gut to the posterior abdominal wall during development. If a mesentery exists, the ascending or descending colon is not firmly fixed to the loin, but is dependent from it by a fold of peritoneum (*Fig. 67*). In the case of the

ACCESSORY PERITONEAL BANDS 77

descending colon this is not common and is of little significance. In the case of the ascending colon it is of the utmost significance. When supplied with a mesentery the ascending colon falls away

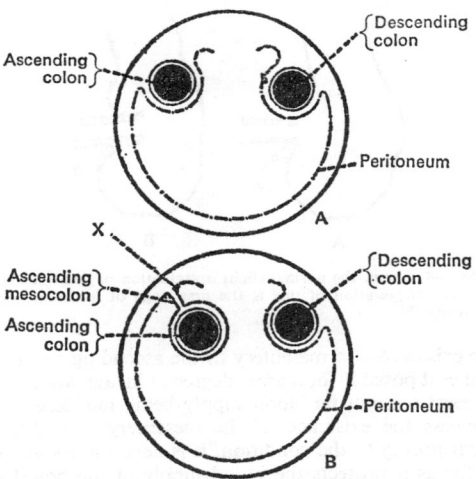

Fig. 67.—A diagrammatic transverse section through the abdomen, showing in A the normal relation of ascending and descending colons to the peritoneum; in B the ascending colon has a mesocolon. X is an exaggeration of the thickening of the peritoneum indicated in the body by a white line which marks the line of junction of the ascending mesocolon with the posterior parietal peritoneum.

from the loin and drags the caecum and hepatic flexure with it. Though the possession of such a mesentery may never render its owner uncomfortable, it plays a supremely important part in: (*a*) Duodenal ileus; (*b*) Volvulus of caecum; (*c*) Ileocaecal intussusception.

VOLVULUS OF THE CAECUM: The caecum may become twisted around its own long axis—the condition of volvulus. This cannot occur if the gut is firmly fixed to the abdominal wall. The condition is therefore predisposed to by the existence of a mesentery to the ascending colon.

INTUSSUSCEPTION: The ileum normally projects very slightly into the caecum at the ileocaecal valve. This may, under certain conditions, form the starting-point of an invagination of the gut into the caecum. When this occurs the condition is progressive and the invaginated gut travels farther and farther into the ascending colon, dragging the caecum and appendix with it (*Fig.* 68). This condition is more likely to occur if the caecum is not firmly anchored to the posterior abdominal wall. On the other hand,

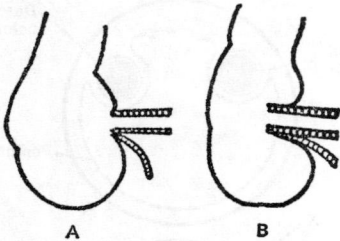

Fig. 68.—A, Shows the normal slight invagination of ileum into caecum at the valve. An exaggeration of this is the first stage of intussusception of the ileocaecal varity (B).

the existence of a mesentery to the ascending colon and caecum makes it possible for a great degree of invagination of the caecum to exist without its blood-supply being interfered with, so that whereas the existence of the mesentery is a disadvantage in predisposing to the condition, it is nevertheless an advantage in as far as it protects the blood-supply of the bowel—preventing strangulation and gangrene.

Chapter XII

THE BILIARY PASSAGES

Bile-ducts: From the porta hepatis emerge the right and left hepatic ducts, which join to form the common hepatic duct. This is in turn joined by the cystic duct (2·5–4 cm. long) from the gall-bladder to form the common bile-duct.

The cystic duct is only 0·25 cm. in diameter, like a match-stick.

THE COMMON BILE-DUCT is 7·5–10 cm. long and runs down first in the right extremity of the lesser omentum and then behind the first part of the duodenum to open into the ampulla of Vater. As a rule the main duct of the pancreas (Wirsung) enters this ampulla also. The bile and pancreatic fluids, therefore, enter this common vestibule, which opens into the duodenum on the papilla duodeni, which is situated on the postero-medial aspect of the second part of the duodenum about its middle. The orifice is less than 0·2 cm. in diameter. If a 3-mm. dilator is not readily transmitted by the sphincter it is injudicious to pass larger ones as they may inflict injury sufficient to cause later stricture formation.

The retroperitoneal portion of the bile-duct lies behind the head of the pancreas. In 85 per cent of cases part or all of the duct is covered by pancreatic tissue. In 15 per cent it is completely uncovered by pancreas, lying in a groove of that organ (Baldwin).[1] This groove is of importance to the surgeon as it can be palpated between thumb and fingers when the second part of the duodenum and head of pancreas are mobilized. Though a normal bile-duct would itself not be palpable in that situation, gall-stones would be; moreover, the groove indicates the precise position of the bile-duct.

The bile-duct varies considerably in its diameter and in cases where it contains stones it may vary still more. It has been generally held that the duct dilates after cholecystectomy in an attempt to

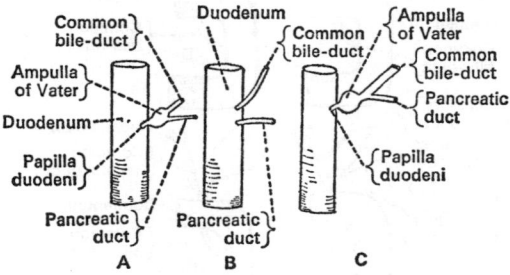

Fig. 69.—Methods of termination of the pancreatic and common bile-ducts. A, Both ducts open independently into the ampulla of Vater. B, The ducts open into the bowel independently of each other. C, The ducts join together, and open into the ampulla by a common channel. A stone lodged in the latter would block both ducts.

take over the reservoir function of the gall-bladder. Le Quesne et al.[2] have shown that there is no evidence that the bile-duct becomes dilated after cholecystectomy. Moreover after cholecystectomy and removal of stones from the duct a dilated common duct does not diminish significantly in calibre.

---

[1] Baldwin, W. M., *Anat. Rec.*, 1911, 5, 197.
[2] Le Quesne, L. P., Whiteside, C. G., and Hand, B. H., *Br. med. J.*, 1959, 1, 329.

80 A SYNOPSIS OF SURGICAL ANATOMY

VARIATIONS IN THE TERMINATIONS OF THE BILE AND THE PANCREATIC DUCTS are amply explained by *Fig.* 69. A stone blocking the papilla duodeni will in A and C prevent both

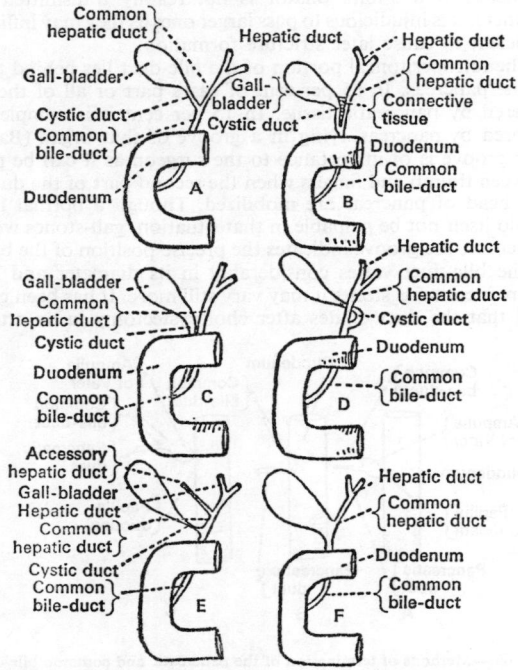

Fig. 70.—Variations in the bile-ducts. **A**, The ducts as usually described. **B**, The common hepatic and cystic ducts lie parallel, being joined by connective tissue. **C**, The common hepatic and cystic ducts join just before the duct enters the duodenum. **D**, The cystic joins the common hepatic duct on its *left*. **E**, Accessory right hepatic duct. **F**, Absence of cystic duct—the common hepatic duct enters the gall-bladder and the common bile-duct leaves it. (*After Flint*.)

bile and pancreatic fluids from reaching the duodenum. The importance of the secretions entering a common cistern is obvious when it is remembered that the governing factor in the pathology of acute haemorrhagic pancreatitis is the fact that the bile and pancreatic ducts open into the duodenum by a common orifice. (Regurgitation of bile into the pancreas along its duct is thought to be the determining factor in this disease in a large percentage of cases.)

VARIATIONS IN THE BILE-DUCTS (*Fig.* 70): E. R. Flint[1] has shown that:
1. The cystic duct usually joins the common hepatic to form the common bile-duct within 2·5 cm. of the upper border of the duodenum.
2. Frequently the common hepatic and cystic ducts lie parallel, being joined by connective tissue for some distance before becoming one duct.
3. The union of the cystic and common hepatic ducts is frequently behind the duodenum or the pancreas, and may only occur just before the duct pierces the wall of the duodenum.
4. Usually the cystic duct joins the common hepatic on its right side. It may, however, join the front, back, or even the left side of the common hepatic by taking a spiral course behind it.
5. An *accessory bile-duct* is not uncommon. It is sometimes an accessory right hepatic duct which leaves the right extremity of the porta hepatis, runs down parallel to the cystic duct and behind it, in front of the right hepatic artery, and joins the common hepatic duct anywhere between the site of its formation and the entrance of the cystic duct into the common duct. In the author's experience this duct is very rare. It is much more usual, nay common, to find ducts of varying size going directly from liver into gall-bladder.
6. The cystic duct may be absent, the common hepatic duct entering the gall-bladder and the common bile-duct leaving it. It is,

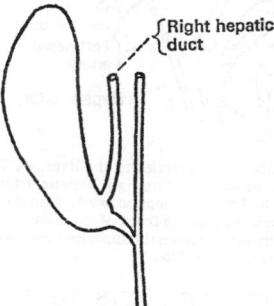

Fig. 71.—Note the important anomaly of the right hepatic duct terminating in the cystic duct. Thus there is no common hepatic duct.

[1] *Br. J. Surg.*, 1922, 9, 509.

82 A SYNOPSIS OF SURGICAL ANATOMY

perhaps, more accurate to describe the gall-bladder in these cases as being sessile. The condition is important, as gall-stones can readily enter the common duct.

7. A rare anomaly described by Milroy Paul[1] shows the right hepatic duct entering the inner end of the gall-bladder. Its surgical importance is considerable. Should it be ligatured, jaundice would result as there is little communication of bile channels between the two parts of liver drained by right and left hepatic ducts (*Fig. 71*).

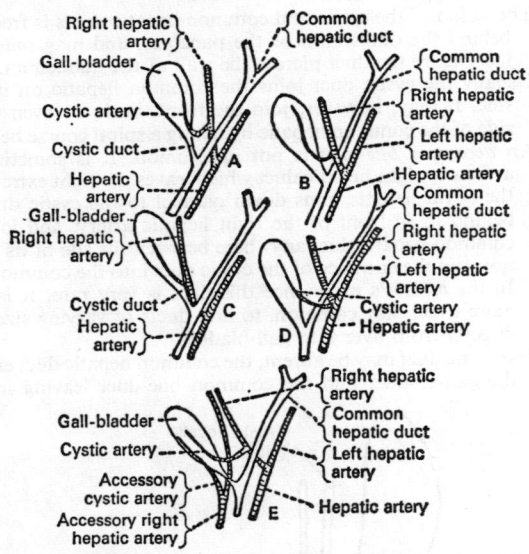

Fig. 72.—Abnormalities in the arteries to the liver. A, The blood-vessels as usually described—i.e., the normal. B, The right hepatic artery passes in front of the common hepatic duct. C, The right hepatic artery parallel to and very near the cystic duct. D, The cystic artery passes in front of the common hepatic duct. E, An accessory right hepatic artery arising from the superior mesenteric artery and giving off an accessory cystic artery. (*After Flint.*)

RELATIONS OF THE BILE-DUCTS TO THE ARTERIES TO THE LIVER: Normally the hepatic artery lies to the left of the bile-duct and divides near the liver into right and left branches, the right branch passing behind the common hepatic duct. The cystic

[1] Paul, Milroy, *Br. J. Surg.*, 1948, 35, 383.

artery is a branch of the right hepatic and lies most commonly between the cystic duct and liver, i.e., above and medial to the duct. Arterial anomalies are very common (*Figs.* 72, 73). The following facts were determined by Flint:
1. The right hepatic artery may arise from the superior mesenteric artery or elsewhere.
2. The right hepatic artery may be double.
3. The right hepatic artery may pass in front of the common hepatic duct.
4. The right hepatic artery may lie parallel to and very near the cystic duct and is often behind it.
5. The cystic artery may pass in front of the common hepatic duct.
6. An accessory cystic artery may exist, and arises from the right hepatic, the left hepatic, or some other branch of the hepatic trunk.

The cystic artery tethers the gall-bladder. It can be felt as a taut string when the proximal part of the gall-bladder is pulled laterally and can thus be identified. When the artery is divided the inner part of the gall-bladder becomes much more mobile. Lahey warned of the danger of reactionary haemorrhage due to retraction of the cystic artery, should it and the cystic duct be included in the same ligature.

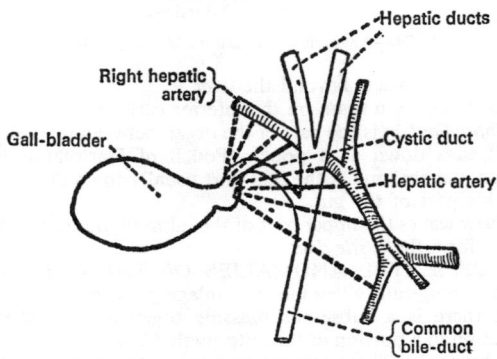

Fig. 73.—A figure to show the great variation in the origin and course of the cystic artery. The interrupted lines show the various positions other than the normal (thick black line) which the vessel may occupy. (*After Rio-Brancho.*)

It is important to bear in mind that the cystic artery has no accompanying vein. Venous drainage of the gall-bladder passes by a number of small vessels through the gall-bladder bed into the liver. These should as far as possible be secured in operations for the removal of the gall-bladder. Occasionally a vein may be found passing with the cystic artery, or independently of it, into the portal vein.

Gall-bladder: The gall-bladder holds about 45 ml. and is 7·5–10 cm. long. It consists of fundus, body, infundibulum, neck, and cystic duct (*Fig.* 74).

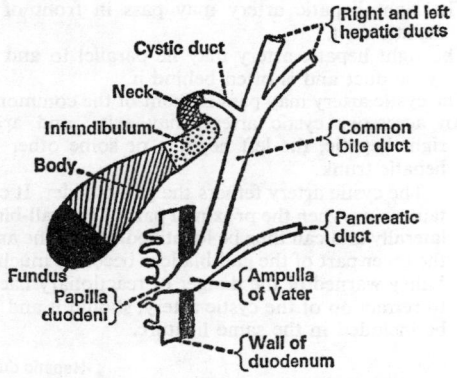

Fig. 74.—Anatomy of the gall-bladder. (*After Wilkie.*)

The *fundus* projects beyond the liver.

The *body* lies in a fossa on the inferior surface of the liver.

The *infundibulum* is the part of the organ between the body and neck; it sags down as a pouch (Pouch of Hartmann) towards the duodenum, and is the first part usually to contract adhesions to this part of the gut.

The *neck* leaves the upper part of the infundibulum and soon narrows to form the *cystic duct*.

DEVELOPMENTAL ANOMALIES OF THE GALL-BLADDER: Embryologically when the liver anlage grows out from the primitive gut there is a subserous massing together of epithelial cells in relation to a portion of the outgrowth. Cavitation occurs in relation to these cells. These cavities coalesce and form the gall-bladder and its duct. As a result of aberrations of this process several abnormalities may occur (*Fig.* 75).

1. Congenital absence of the gall-bladder is extremely rare. At the Mayo Clinic[1] it was found twice in 10,000 cases in which surgery or necropsy had been carried out.

[1] Ferris, D. O., and Glazer, I. M., *Surgery*, 1965, 91, 359.

2. The gall-bladder may be septate, transversely or longitudinally.
3. The gall-bladder may be double with a single cystic duct.
4. The gall-bladder may be double with separate ducts opening into hepatic or common or both ducts. The serosa may be separate or common.

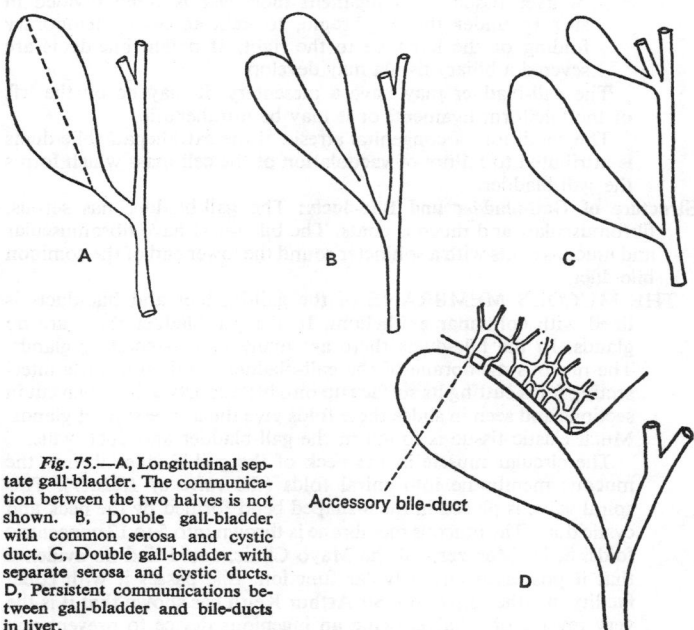

Fig. 75.—A, Longitudinal septate gall-bladder. The communication between the two halves is not shown. B, Double gall-bladder with common serosa and cystic duct. C, Double gall-bladder with separate serosa and cystic ducts. D, Persistent communications between gall-bladder and bile-ducts in liver.

5. Small ducts may connect gall-bladder with liver. Usually these become obliterated. They may persist, which is one of the reasons why drainage is mandatory after cholecystectomy. Hayes and Coller[1] have suggested and practised a search of the gall-bladder bed for the remains of such hepatocystic communications and the insertion of a small catheter to relieve jaundice due to otherwise irremediable obstruction (external biliary fistula).
6. It is of interest to compare the condition just described with persistence of bile-duct remnants in the left triangular ligament

[1] Hayes, M. A., and Coller, F. A., *Ann. Surg.*, 1952, 135, 98.

of the liver. The left lobe of the liver is originally the same size as the right. It regresses when the physiological hernia of the embryo becomes reduced. The left triangular ligament marks the site of this disappearance. Thus it may contain bile-ducts and their remnants and sometimes isolated islands of liver tissue. This ligament moreover is often divided in surgery under the diaphragm, to gain access by temporary folding of the left lobe to the right. If patent bile-ducts are severed a biliary fistula may develop.

The gall-bladder may have a mesentery, it may be on the left of the falciform ligament, or it may be intrahepatic.

The condition of congenital atresia of the extrahepatic bile-ducts is attributed to failure of vacuolation of the cell mass which forms the gall-bladder.

Structure of Gall-bladder and Bile-ducts: The gall-bladder has serous, fibromuscular, and mucous coats. The bile-ducts have fibromuscular and mucous coats with a sphincter round the lower end of the common bile-duct.

THE MUCOUS MEMBRANE of the gall-bladder and bile-ducts is lined with columnar epithelium. In the gall-bladder there are no glands. In the bile-ducts there are many mucus-secreting glands. The mucous membrane of the gall-bladder is raised in little intersecting folds cutting its surface up into little courtyards. When cut in sections and seen in slides these folds give the impression of glands. Much elastic tissue is found in the gall-bladder and duct walls.

The circular muscle in the neck of the gall-bladder throws the mucous membrane into spiral folds (the *valve of Heister*). This spiral valve is placed in the S-shaped bend formed by the neck and cystic duct. The mucous membrane is thrown into 5 to 12 concentric folds. S. H. Mentzer,[1] of the Mayo Clinic, could find no evidence that it possessed any valvular function. Bile passes it with equal facility in either direction. Sir Arthur Keith has shown that it is the very reverse of a valve, being an ingenious device to prevent any obstruction to inflow or egress resulting from kinking at the gall-bladder neck (Robinson[2]).

The mucous glands in the bile-ducts can secrete mucus at much greater pressure than that at which the liver cells can secrete bile. If the bile-duct is blocked, the liver may, because of the increase of pressure in the duct system, be unable to secrete bile, which is then absorbed into the blood. The mucous glands in the ducts, however, go on secreting mucus. A patient may therefore be green with jaundice while his ducts contain mucus (white bile).

---

[1] *Archs Surg., Lond.*, 1926, 13, 511, quoted by Robinson.
[2] Arris and Gale Lecture, 'Short-circuit Operations in the Treatment of Cholecystitis', *Lancet*, 1930, 1, 673.

THE BILIARY PASSAGES 87

Vascular Arrangements of the Gall-bladder and Common Bile-duct: The blood-supply to the extrahepatic bile-ducts is generous, the main contributor being the posterior-superior pancreatico-duodenal artery assisted by the hepatic and cystic.

THE VEINS OF THE COMMON BILE-DUCT: There is a venous plexus on the wall of the supraduodenal portion of the common duct which is of value in the recognition of the common duct at operation. This venous plexus is only visible when the overlying peritoneum has been removed. It does not extend on to the cystic duct.[1]

THE VEINS OF THE GALL-BLADDER drain into the quadrate lobe area of the liver directly or via the pericholedochal plexus and ultimately enter the hepatic veins, not communicating with the portal vessels.

THE LYMPHATICS OF THE GALL-BLADDER run in two groups to the glands in the free border of the lesser omentum and thence to the pre-aortic group. Cancer of the gall-bladder is uncommon and of very grave prognostic import, none the less the lymph drainage from the viscus is so channelled that at an early stage of the disease block dissection may embrace the entire pathological process.

Paths of Infection: To reach the gall-bladder infection must follow one of the following anatomical routes (R. P. Rowlands[2]):

1. The blood-stream per: (*a*) Cystic artery from distant sources, e.g., septic teeth; (*b*) Portal vein from the less remote source represented by the gut.
2. The lymph-stream, from the liver, pancreas, or appendix.
3. The bile-ducts, by spread downwards from the liver or upwards from the gut.
4. Duodenal ulcer or inflamed appendix when the duodenum or appendix is in direct contact with the gall-bladder.

There is no recognized pathway for lymph from the liver to reach the gall-bladder, which negatives Graham's theory of lymphatic infection reaching the gall-bladder from the liver and explains the great rarity of carcinoma of the gall-bladder in secondary carcinoma of the liver or primary carcinoma of that organ.[3]

Position of Gall-bladder in Radiographs: The gall-bladder as seen by the X-rays may normally occupy any part of the following quadrilateral (F. Davies[4]) (*Fig.* 76):

Vertical Extent: From the upper border of the 12th thoracic vertebra to the lower border of the 4th lumbar vertebra.

---

[1] Saint, J. H., *Br. J. Surg.*, 1961, 47, 489.
[2] *Br. med. J.*, 1930, 1, 185.
[3] Patey, D. H., and Whitby, L. E. H., *Br. J. Surg.*, 1933, 20, 585.
[4] *Br. med. J.*, 1927, 1, 1138.

Transverse Extent: From a point 2·5 cm. to the right of the median plane to a point 10 cm. to the right of this plane.

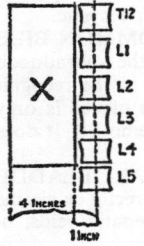

Fig. 76.—The position of the gall-bladder in cholecystography. Normally the gall-bladder may occupy any part of the quadrilateral marked X. (*After Davies.*)

The commonest situation is for the gall-bladder to lie vertically in the angle between the 12th rib and 1st lumbar vertebra (*Fig.* 77). The angle it makes with the vertical position is subject to variation of anything up to 45°, depending upon the habitus of the individual.

Shoulder-tip Pain: When the sensory terminations of the phrenic nerve are irritated pain may be referred to the sensory nerves arising from

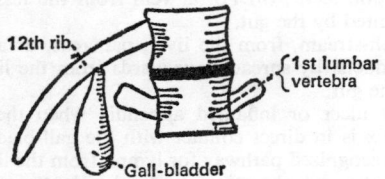

Fig. 77.—A very usual position of the gall-bladder as shown by cholecystography.

the same segments of the spinal cord (C. 3, 4, 5). Thus it comes about that in such cases pain is referred to the skin overlying the acromion process, this area being supplied by the descending supraclavicular nerve (C. 3, 4).

The phrenic nerve takes no part in the innervation of the peritoneum overlying the gall-bladder or bile-ducts. Biliary colic or lesions of the biliary duct apparatus cannot *per se* cause shoulder-tip pain. This referred pain can only arise if the peritoneum on the under-surface of the diaphragm is irritated, e.g., by inflammatory exudate. If such an exudate occurs, inflammation of the gall-bladder may produce such pain, though it is an unusual sign of acute cholecystitis. Cope and others have remarked that shoulder-tip pain is commoner in gastric or duodenal perforations than in gall-bladder lesions. Pain and possibly hyperaesthesia referred to the left shoulder —Kehr's sign—may occur in cases of ruptured spleen (effused blood irritating the peritoneum on the under-surface of the diaphragm). Cases are also encountered of intraperitoneal rupture of ectopic gestation where the patient's chief complaint is pain referred to the left acromion, for the same reason.

Shoulder pain may be caused by irritation (inflammation) of the serous membranes lining the surfaces of the diaphragm, i.e., the pleura above or the peritoneum below. Both are supplied by the phrenic nerve. If the irritation is anterior the pain is referred above the clavicle. Should the inflammation or irritation be posterior the pain is referred to the acromion. It is not, however, possible from the position of the pain to determine whether it is referred from the upper (pleural) or lower (peritoneal) surface of the diaphragm.

Chapter XIII

THE KIDNEYS AND ADRENALS

Kidneys:
POSITION: The long axis of the kidney is parallel to, but not coincident with, the long axis of the 12th rib. (The long axis of the spleen is parallel to and coincident with the long axis of the 10th rib.) Both kidneys normally lie entirely above the level of the umbilicus, the lower poles being about 2·5 cm. above the highest point of the iliac crest. The right kidney reaches the upper border of the 12th rib, the left reaches the lower border of the 11th rib. The outer border of the organ lies half an inch lateral to the outer border of the sacrospinalis muscle. The pelvis of the kidney is seen in pyelograms to lie opposite the 1st and 2nd lumbar transverse processes.

RELATIONS:
RELATIONS TO THE 12TH RIB: This rib is separated from the kidney by the pleura and the diaphragm. The diaphragm, therefore, intervenes between the kidney and the pleura. It sometimes happens that there is a small gap between the slips of the diaphragm arising from the lumbocostal arch and the 12th rib, in which case the kidney and pleura are separated by a little connective tissue only.

It is seen from *Fig.* 81 that the 12th rib is oblique while the lower border of the pleura is horizontal. The two cross like an X. The angle between the 12th rib and the outer border of the

	RIGHT KIDNEY	LEFT KIDNEY

ANTERIOR—
(*Fig.* 78)
	Below: hepatic flexure of colon.
	Medial: second part of duodenum.
	
	Above: adrenal, liver.[1]
		Below: splenic flexure.
		Crossing the middle:
		  Pancreas and splenic vessels.
		  Below pancreas is jejunum.[1]
		  Above pancreas is stomach[1] and spleen.[1]
		Above: adrenal.

MEDIAL—	Inferior vena cava, ureter.	Duodenojejunal flexure, inferior mesenteric vein, adrenal, ureter.
LATERAL—	*Below:* ascending colon.[1] *Above:* liver.[1]	*Below:* descending colon.[1] *Above:* spleen.[1]
POSTERIOR— (*Figs.* 79, 80)	Same in both kidneys. Each kidney rests upon four muscles: psoas, transversus abdominis, quadratus, diaphragm. The lumbocostal arches, last thoracic, ilio-hypogastric and ilio-inguinal nerves, and subcostal vessels are between kidney and quadratus, the anterior layer of the lumbodorsal fascia intervening.	

[1] Structures indicated thus are separated from the kidney by peritoneum.

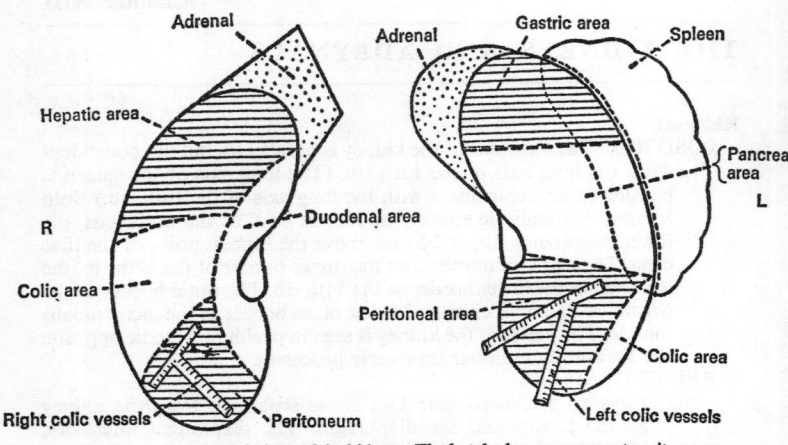

Fig. 78.—Anterior relations of the kidneys. The hatched areas represent peritoneum.

sacrospinalis is the kidney angle. Kidney pain is usually referred here, and pressure here may elicit pain in kidney lesions. The lumbar incision for exposure of the kidney commences here.

THE KIDNEYS AND ADRENALS 91

In cases where the 12th rib is very short it does not project beyond the outer border of the sacrospinalis. In such cases the pleura may be opened on exposing the kidney by this route, as the 11th rib is sometimes mistaken for the 12th.

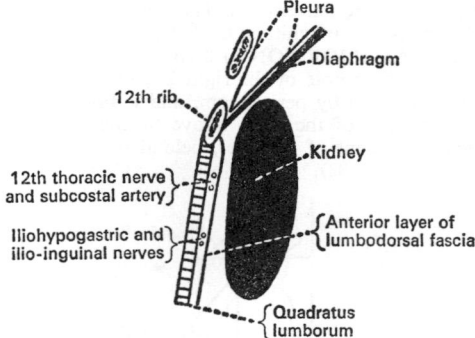

Fig. 79.—Schematic representation of the posterior relations of the kidney.

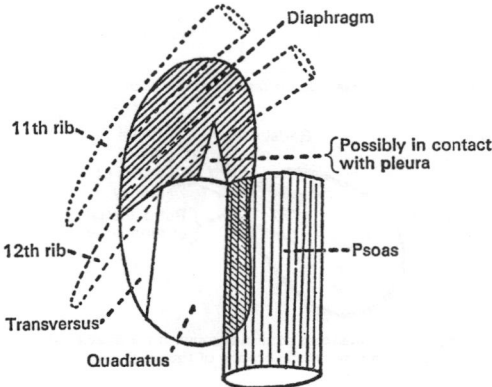

Fig. 80.—The posterior relations of the kidney, showing its relation to diaphragm and ribs, and the area where it may lie in contact with the pleura.

RELATIONS AT THE HILUM: The renal artery gives two branches which go behind the ureter on the right, and one on the left (*Fig.* 82).

92 A SYNOPSIS OF SURGICAL ANATOMY

NERVE-SUPPLY: Thoracic 10, 11, 12 through small splanchnic and splanchnicus imus nerves. The nerve-supply of the large intestine is the same. Renal lesions such as calculus, therefore, may, and often do, cause reflex interference with peristalsis. Such cases may simulate acute obstruction of the large gut.

BLOOD-SUPPLY: Renal arteries. The blood-supply to the kidneys is similar in relative magnitude to that of the lungs and thyroid.

HEPATORENAL (MORISON'S) POUCH: There is a deep recess above the upper pole of the right kidney. This is the *hepatorenal pouch*. It is lined by peritoneum, and is bounded in front by the inferior surface of the liver, above by the posterior layer of the coronary ligament of the liver, behind by the peritoneum on the diaphragm (*Fig.* 83).

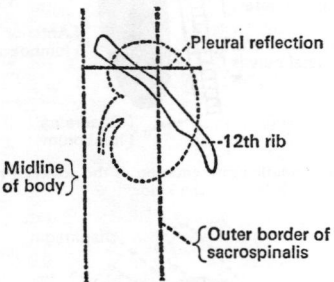

Fig. 81.—Showing certain important posterior relationships of the kidney.

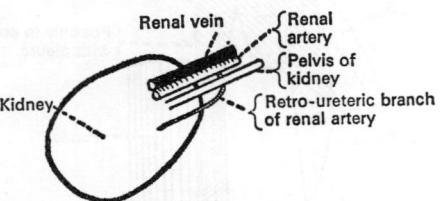

Fig. 82.—Transverse section through the kidney to show a retro-ureteric branch of the renal artery.

With the body lying horizontal this recess is the lowest level of the peritoneal cavity, excluding the pelvis. Extravasations of fluid are likely to collect there, especially after operations on the liver and bile-passages. The pouch is therefore usually drained after such operations if leakage is feared.

THE KIDNEYS AND ADRENALS

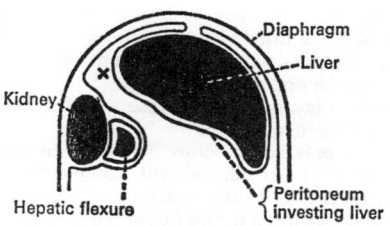

Fig. 83.—The hepatorenal or Morison's pouch (X).

FASCIAL RELATIONS: The kidney has three capsules: (1) Its proper capsule; (2) A fatty capsule; (3) The renal fascia.

PROPER CAPSULE: A fibrous membrane stripping easily from the organ. In inflammatory diseases it is frequently adherent and cannot be stripped without tearing the kidney tissue.

FATTY CAPSULE: The kidney is embedded in a peculiar type of fat. This fat is condensed at its periphery to form the renal fascia. It is likewise condensed where the kidney is in contact with it, because of the continuous impact due to the pulsation of the kidneys.

RENAL FASCIA: Is continuous with the extraperitoneal connective tissue (*Fig.* 84). It is arranged as follows:

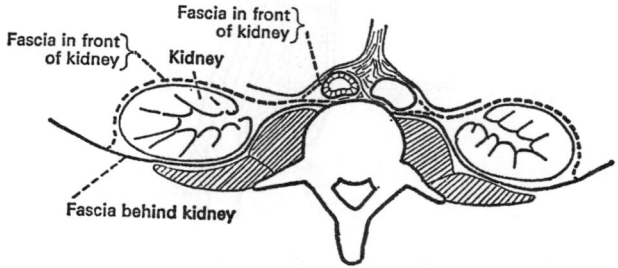

Fig. 84.—The diagram shows that the renal fascia invests each kidney completely. (*After Mitchell.*)

Laterally: At the outer border of the kidney it splits to enclose the organ: lateral to this it is fused with fascia transversalis.

Posteriorly: It blends with the fascia on the psoas and quadratus. The attachments are feeble and the kidney and its capsules are readily separated from the underlying muscles.

Medially: Mitchell[1] has shown that, contrary to current teaching, the renal fascia fuses with the connective tissue round the great vessels and does not *extend* in front of them to fuse with its fellow on the opposite side.

Above: The two layers join, and fuse with the fascia on the under aspect of the diaphragm.

Below: The fascia is closed below. Thus, as Mitchell has shown, the renal fascia is an investment completely surrounding the kidney (*Fig.* 84). Thus perinephric collections of fluid will be completely enclosed in this fascia. The compartment is weakest below and should increasing pressure of such a collection lead to rupture, this will occur inferiorly into the pelvic cellular tissue. Its line of extension will be to the opposite side and not upwards.

The adrenal is enclosed in a separate loculus of this fascia; therefore in removal of the kidney, when it is shelled out from its fatty capsule, the adrenal remains in situ; furthermore, in movable kidney the adrenal does *not* move with the kidney, for the same reason (*Fig.* 85). That the integrity of the adrenal gland is not always secured by such a fascial arrangement has

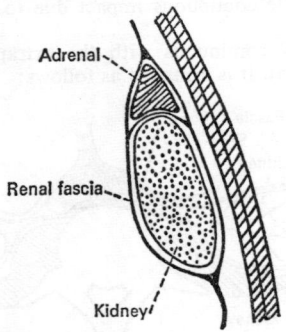

Fig. 85.—To show that the renal fascia completely invests the kidney. (*After Mitchell.*)

been made abundantly clear by Davie.[2] This observer found in 6 out of 1500 routine post-mortems that the kidney and the adrenal were so intimately fused that nephrectomy in these cases would have resulted in coincident adrenalectomy. This matter is of the first importance in the surgery of the kidney,

[1] Mitchell, G. A. G., *Br. J. Surg.*, 1950, 37, 257.
[2] Davie, T. B., *Br. J. Surg.*, 1935, 22, 428.

and it behoves the operator to make a careful examination of the kidney when exposed at operation so that measures may be taken to guard against inadvertent removal of the adrenal gland. In all these cases there is a small interspace filled with connective tissue between the inferomedial angle of the adrenal and the kidney where a separation of the two structures may be begun. A survey of the development of the organs concerned explains the occurrence. The adrenal cortex develops from the upper part of the Wolffian ridge, the testis or ovary from the lower. The kidney is developed from tissue lying some distance below these structures. When the gonads descend, the kidney and adrenal become approximated. At this age the adrenal is larger than the kidney and envelops its upper pole. As a rule development of the two organs proceeds independently and each organ develops a fibrous capsule, fatty tissue separating them. At times the organs may remain in such intimate relationship that separation can only be effected by dissection, and it is in these cases that the dangers indicated above obtain. Davie and Mitchell point out that this close developmental interrelationship is the basis on which Grawitz based his theory that hypernephromata arise from adrenal rests in the kidney.

The kidney is retained in place mainly by intra-abdominal pressure; the fatty capsule assists. Diminution of this fat is a factor which predisposes to undue mobility of the kidney. If the kidney becomes mobile, it is most likely to move downwards because of gravity and respiratory movements. The kidney has, under certain conditions, a very great mobility.

Adrenals: The right adrenal is shaped like a top hat. The left adrenal is shaped like a cocked hat. Each has an anterior and a posterior surface. Each of these surfaces has two relations (Wright).

RELATIONS (*Fig.* 86):

The left adrenal has 'slipped' down the medial border of the kidney, being arrested by the renal vessels, its lower pole being in contact with these, whilst its upper pole is in contact with the upper pole of the spleen. Thus it comes about that the right adrenal is usually higher than the left, just the reverse of the relative positions of the kidneys.

Between the two adrenals are the crura, the aorta, the coeliac artery, the coeliac plexus, and the inferior vena cava.

BLOOD-SUPPLY:

ARTERIES: Three to each: (1) Superior adrenal from the inferior phrenic; (2) Middle adrenal from the aorta; (3) Inferior adrenal from the renal.

VEINS: One only. Drains on the right into the vena cava; on the left into the left renal.

96 A SYNOPSIS OF SURGICAL ANATOMY

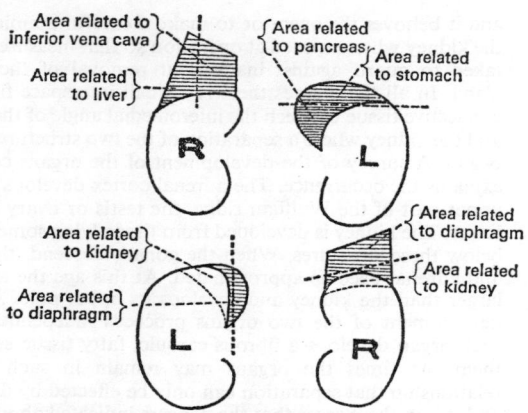

Fig. 86.—The relations of the adrenals. R, Right kidney. L, Left kidney. The anterior surfaces are shown above, the posterior below.

	RIGHT	LEFT
ANTERIOR—	*Medial:* inferior vena cava. *Lateral:* part of bare area of liver.	*Superior:* stomach. *Inferior:* pancreas.
POSTERIOR—	*Inferior:* kidney. *Superior:* crus of diaphragm.	*Medial:* crus of diaphragm. *Lateral:* kidney.
HILUM—	Near upper end.	Near lower end.
PERITONEAL RELATIONS—	Not related to peritoneum, except a tiny area below.	Separated from stomach by peritoneum.

Chapter XIV

THE INGUINAL REGION

Descent of the Testis: The testis is formed in front of the kidney. Its descent (described on p. 405) is a complicated process which depends on the gubernaculum testis, steroid hormones, and maternal gonadotrophins. Shortly before birth the testis reaches the bottom of the scrotum being invaginated into a tube of peritoneum—the processus

THE INGUINAL REGION 97

vaginalis. This process becomes occluded, first at its upper end, the internal abdominal ring, then just above the testis leaving a sequestrated sac of peritoneum, below which is the tunica vaginalis testis. The portion of the process between the two sites of occlusion is the last to become obliterated.

Anatomy of the Inguinal Region and of Inguinal and Femoral Hernia:

INGUINAL CANAL: A triangular slit 3·8 cm. long, almost horizontal in direction, which lies just above the inner half of the inguinal ligament. At its lateral end is the abdominal inguinal ring (internal inguinal ring), at the medial end is the subcutaneous or external inguinal ring.

The internal inguinal ring is an opening in the fascia transversalis midway between the anterior superior iliac spine and the symphysis pubis just lateral to the inferior epigastric artery. The ring is shaped like the letter V with the open end pointing laterally and superiorly. The arms are called the crura. The superior crus is attached to the transversus muscle by fascial slips so that when the transversus abdominis muscle contracts the internal ring is drawn laterally, thus increasing the obliquity of the exit.

The subcutaneous inguinal ring is triangular, and lies very obliquely above and lateral to the pubic crest. It is an opening in the external oblique. The spermatic cord emerges from it, lying on the inferior margin of the ring, and *lateral* (not medial) to the pubic spine (H. S. Souttar).[1] The spine is more easily felt from the outer side in inguinal hernia and from the inner side in femoral hernia.

The fascia transversalis is part of the endo-abdominal fascia, deriving its name from the overlying transversus muscle. The lower part of this fascia is thickened to form the iliopubic tract (Thomson's ligament)[2] which stretches from the anterior superior iliac spine laterally to the pubis medially. It lies posterior to and adjacent to the inguinal ligament, forms the inferior border of the internal ring, bridges across the femoral vessels, and reinforces the anterior margin of the femoral sheath. The iliopubic tract, if well developed (which it is in the majority of cases), can be used in groin hernia repair.

The aponeurosis of the transversus abdominis muscle[2] extends downwards from the arched muscle to become attached into a variable length of Cooper's ligament between the pubic tubercle and the medial edge of the femoral vein. It is intimately adherent to the underlying fascia transversalis. The strength of the posterior wall of the inguinal canal will vary with the extent of this aponeurosis.

---

[1] *Br. med. J.*, 1924, 1, 367.
[2] Condon, R. E., *Hernia*, 1964 (ed. Nyhus, L. M., and Harkins, H. N.). Philadelphia: Lippincott.

BOUNDARIES OF THE CANAL:

Anterior: External oblique in its whole length. Internal oblique in its lateral third.

Posterior: Fascia transversalis and the aponeurosis of the transversus abdominis muscle in its whole length. Falx inguinalis (conjoint tendon) in its inner half. Reflex inguinal ligament in its inner third.

Floor: The upper surface of the inguinal ligament (external oblique), which forms a furrow (Poupart's ligament).

INGUINAL HERNIA:

AN INDIRECT INGUINAL HERNIA traverses the canal. It is invested by the coverings of the spermatic cord: (1) External spermatic fascia from external oblique; (2) Cremasteric fascia from internal oblique; (3) Internal spermatic or infundibuliform fascia from fascia transversalis.

The constriction in strangulated inguinal hernia is in 50 per cent of cases at the internal ring, and in the remaining 50 per cent at the external ring (St. Bartholomew's Hospital surgeons' observations). The constriction at the internal ring must be divided in a lateral direction because the inferior epigastric artery is medial to the ring.

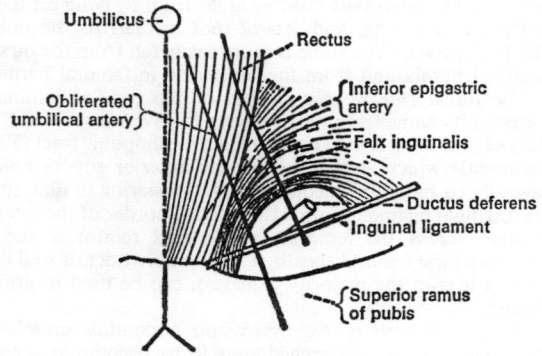

Fig. 87.—Posterior surface of lower part of anterior abdominal wall showing the triangle of Hesselbach.

DIRECT INGUINAL HERNIA is probably not congenital, though R. W. Murray[1] ascribes it to a process of peritoneum passing through a congenital opening between the fibres of the falx inguinalis. The indirect variety is invariably congenital (Hamilton Russell)

[1] Quoted by Thomson and Miles, *Manual of Surgery*, 1926, 3, 149. London.

THE INGUINAL REGION 99

because of the presence of the remains of the processus vaginalis. Direct herniae are now looked upon as being herniae through the linea semilunaris. Direct hernia leaves the abdominal cavity medial to the inferior epigastric artery through the triangle of Hesselbach (*Fig.* 87). This triangle is seen on looking at the inner surface of the anterior abdominal wall.

Triangle of Hesselbach: Lateral boundary—inferior epigastric artery; medial boundary—outer border of the rectus; lower boundary—inguinal ligament.

It is divided into medial and lateral halves by the obliterated umbilical artery (lateral umbilical ligament). Direct hernia leaves this triangle through its outer or inner part, and is therefore: (1) A lateral direct hernia; (2) a medial direct hernia.

Coverings of Direct Hernia:

Lateral direct hernia: The same coverings as the indirect type, except that the covering it receives from the fascia transversalis is not that part of the fascia prolonged from the margins of the internal ring. The inferior epigastric artery is lateral to the hernia opening.

Medial direct hernia: (1) External spermatic fascia; (2) Falx inguinalis or conjoint tendon; (3) Fascia transversalis.

Direct hernia is generally less oblique in direction than the indirect, though this is not always true. In direct hernia the opening in the fascia transversalis lies directly opposite the external ring, and the examining finger passes straight back through the openings and not in an oblique direction as in indirect hernia.

FEMORAL HERNIA: Passes through two orifices: (1) The femoral canal, which is the inner compartment of the femoral sheath; and (2) The fossa ovalis (saphenous opening)—an opening in the fascia lata of the thigh, 3·8 cm. below and 3·8 cm. lateral to the pubic tubercle.

THE FEMORAL SHEATH is a funnel-shaped fascial channel which invests the femoral vessels and passes down behind the inner half of the inguinal ligament. It is formed by two fascial layers (*Fig.* 88). Its anterior wall is formed by the fascia transversalis continued down behind the inguinal ligament in front of the femoral vessels. Its posterior wall is formed by the fascia iliaca passing down behind the vessels.

Anterior Wall: covered by fascia lata in which is the fossa ovalis.

Posterior Wall: lies on the psoas and pectineus.

Outer Wall: straight.

Inner Wall: oblique and shorter than outer wall.

Compartments: three, a lateral for the femoral artery, an intermediate for the vein, and a medial called the femoral canal (*Fig.* 89).

100 A SYNOPSIS OF SURGICAL ANATOMY

FEMORAL CANAL: Is 1·2 cm. long and 1·2 cm. wide. It lies under cover of the fascia cribrosa, which covers over the saphenous opening. It contains a lymph-gland belonging to the deep subinguinal group. The femoral ring is the mouth of the canal.

FEMORAL RING:

Boundaries:

Anterior: Inguinal ligament.
Posterior: Pectineus.
Lateral: Femoral vein.
Medial: Lateral sharp edge of the lacunar ligament. This edge gives a fascial extension backwards for half an inch along the iliopectineal line (brim of pelvis) where it blends with

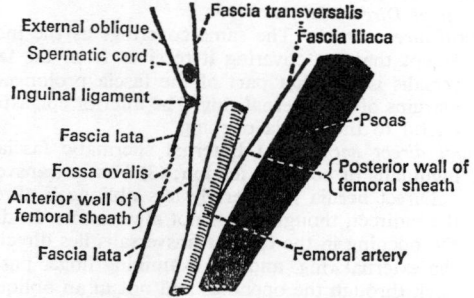

Fig. 88.—Longitudinal section of femoral sheath.

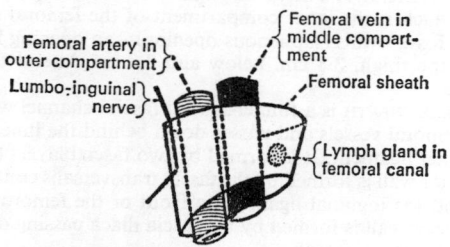

Fig. 89.—Compartments of femoral sheath.

the periosteum. This fascial extension is called *Cooper's ligament*. The surgeon closes up the femoral canal by sewing this ligament to the inguinal ligament or to the falx inguinalis (conjoint tendon), hoping thus to prevent the recurrence of hernia.

THE INGUINAL REGION

Contents: Femoral septum, which is a fat-pad plugging the ring.

ABNORMAL OBTURATOR ARTERY: Usually the obturator and inferior epigastric vessels each gives a pubic branch which is small, and these anastomose at the back of the pubis. In 30 per cent of cases the pubic branch of the inferior epigastric is very large, taking the place of the obturator artery, and being known as the abnormal obturator artery. It passes down in relation to the femoral ring to reach the obturator foramen (*Fig.* 90).

In its descent it may stick to the side of the femoral vein (the safe position). In 10 per cent of persons with such an abnormal artery, the vessel passes down along the edge of the lacunar ligament, which is the inner boundary of the femoral ring (the dangerous position). In strangulated femoral hernia the constricting agent is sometimes the outer edge of the lacunar ligament, and it must be divided to relieve the pressure. It is necessary, therefore, in cases where an abnormal artery exists, to exercise great care in dealing with this ligament, as serious haemorrhage follows division of the vessel.

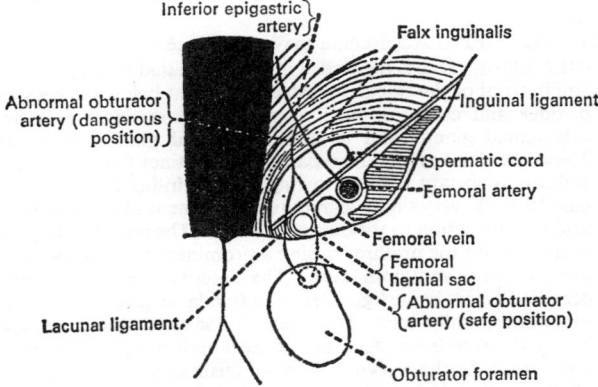

Fig. 90.—Posterior surface of lower part of anterior abdominal wall showing the course of the abnormal obturator artery.

COVERINGS OF FEMORAL HERNIA: A hernia passing down the femoral canal emerges through the saphenous opening. It has therefore as coverings: (1) Fat forming femoral septum; (2) Anterior wall of femoral sheath; (3) Fascia cribrosa.

Having become subcutaneous, the hernia, if it continues to enlarge, often takes a recurrent course across the inguinal ligament, following the line of the superficial inferior epigastric vessels.

Chapter XV

THE PROSTATE

THE organ is composed of glandular tissue in a fibromuscular stroma. It is the size and shape of a chestnut. It surrounds the first 3 cm. of the urethra. It is traversed by the ejaculatory ducts. It and the caecum are both broader than they are long: Prostate 3 cm. long, 3·8 cm. broad; caecum 5·7 cm. long, 6·4 cm. broad. The organ consists of five lobes and has five surfaces.

Lobes: The five lobes are: Anterior, posterior, two lateral, and middle.

ANTERIOR LOBE: Lies in front of the urethra and contains little or no glandular tissue. Adenomata therefore seldom, if ever, occur here (Cabot).

POSTERIOR LOBE: Lies behind the middle lobe. Adenomata never occur here—primary carcinoma of the prostate is said to begin here.

LATERAL LOBES: Adenomata may occur here.

MIDDLE LOBE: This is the wedge of tissue situated behind the urethra and in front of the ejaculatory ducts. It is just below the neck of the bladder and contains much glandular tissue. Here also lie the subtrigonal glands and all the subcervical glands of Albarran. These are mucous glands, separate and distinct from the prostate, and are important because, owing to their intimate relation to the bladder neck, very slight degrees of enlargement of these glands may lead to obstruction to the outflow of urine. The middle lobe projects normally into the urethra, raising a prominence on its floor—crista urethralis or verumontanum. The internal urethral meatus is occupied below by a slight elevation (uvula vesicae) also due to the subjacent middle lobe. This lobe is the one where adenomata begin *par excellence*. The line of least resistance is upwards into the urethra. As the growth enlarges it pushes the mucous membrane of the urethra before it, and extends into the bladder, and may entirely *block* the internal meatus. The growth may project as a large pedunculated mass into the bladder. The effort of straining to urinate squeezes it on to the internal meatus, which is thus entirely blocked (*Fig.* 91). It is obvious that the growth has insinuated itself through the grip of the internal sphincter between the mucous membrane of the floor of the urethra and the internal sphincter (sphincter vesicae). This muscle cannot therefore shut off the prostatic urethra from the bladder, the result being that urine is constantly trickling into this part of the urethra. As it should normally contain no urine, the constant desire to pass urine, which is so troublesome to those with enlarged prostates, is ascribed to this fact.

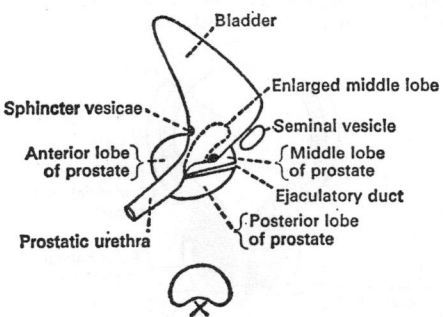

Fig. 91.—Sagittal section of bladder and prostate showing normal projection of middle lobe of prostate into prostatic urethra. Interrupted line shows the direction of growth of middle lobe when it enlarges; obviously it will render the sphincter of the bladder incompetent to prevent urine constantly entering the prostatic urethra. Lower figure shows contour of internal urinary meatus, and normal elevation caused by middle lobe of prostate (X).

Surfaces: These are: Base, or superior surface (above), apex (below), posterior surface, two inferolateral surfaces, and anterior surface.
RELATIONS:
  BASE: Continuous with neck of bladder, a groove intervening in which are veins.
  APEX: Rests on upper surface of superior layer of the urogenital diaphragm.
  POSTERIOR: Rests on anterior wall of rectum and can be felt by a finger in the rectum.
  INFEROLATERAL (2): Related to and supported by that part of the levator ani called the levator prostatae.
  ANTERIOR BORDER OR SURFACE: Behind the symphysis and connected with it by puboprostatic ligaments.

Fascial Relations:
1. CAPSULES: Two—true and false (*Fig.* 92).
  THE TRUE CAPSULE is formed by a condensation at the periphery of the gland. Cabot and others deny its existence. They say an adenomatous prostate shells out because the non-adenomatous tissue is pushed to the periphery of the gland and the adenomata are shelled out of this compressed gland tissue.

THE FALSE CAPSULE is formed by the visceral layer of pelvic fascia which gives a sheath common to bladder and prostate and is absent where the two organs are in contact. For this reason adenomata of the prostate tend to grow upwards into the bladder, this being the line of least resistance.

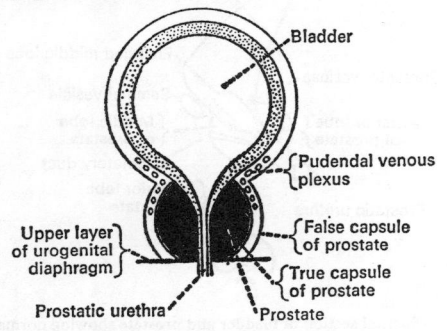

Fig. 92.—Capsules of the prostate.

The pudendal plexus of veins (prostatic) lies between the two capsules and receives in front the deep dorsal vein of the penis.

In the operation of suprapubic prostatectomy the surgeon 'enucleates' the prostate. It is enucleated from *both its capsules*, so that the pudendal plexus of veins between the sheaths is undisturbed. The prostatic urethra is removed with the gland and the ejaculatory ducts are torn across. The removal is therefore totally different to the removal of the thyroid where the gland is removed *with* its true capsule, leaving only the false capsule behind. As a result of prostatectomy the patient is sterile. This arises from the fact that the prostatic urethra with its musculature has been removed with the prostate, and though the ejaculatory ducts discharge into the prostatic cavity, this is now lined with fibrous tissue which is unable to expel its contents per urethram. Ejaculation therefore does not occur, the seminal fluid being voided at the next act of micturition. The patient is therefore not impotent though he is sterile. Many surgeons divide the ducti deferentes at the subcutaneous abdominal rings after prostatectomy with the object of preventing the spread of infection from prostatic cavity to epididymis. This procedure prevents the onset of epididymitis.

2. FASCIAE BEHIND THE PROSTATE (and in front of the rectum —*Fig.* 93): In the early fetus the peritoneum of the pelvic floor extends down as a pouch behind the prostate. This pouch is

THE PROSTATE 105

ultimately shut off from the peritoneal cavity and exists as two layers of fascia with a potential space between them. These two layers are attached to peritoneum (floor of Douglas's pouch) above, and to the urogenital diaphragm and perineal body below. This is the fascia of Denonvilliers (prostato-peritoneal fascia). The

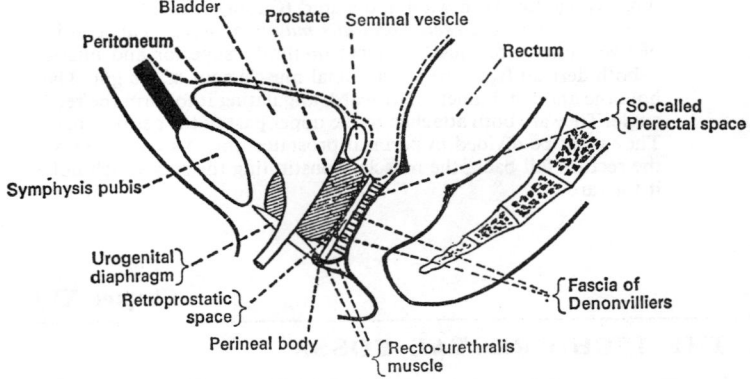

Fig. 93.—The fasciae behind the prostate.

anterior of these two fascial layers is firmly attached to the prostate. The posterior layer is not quite so firmly blended with the sheath of the rectum (derived from visceral layer of pelvic fascia). The potential space between the fascia is the space of Denonvilliers (the retroprostatic space of Proust). The so-called 'prerectal space'

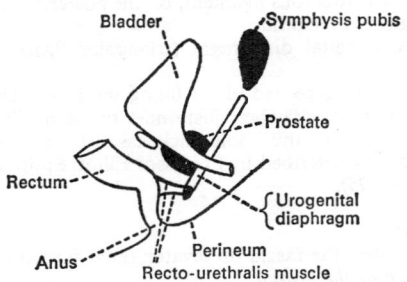

Fig. 94.—Diagram to show the recto-urethralis muscle.

between the rectum and the fascia of Denonvilliers is not a space at all, potential or actual.

In the performance of perineal prostatectomy the surgeon must find his way *between* these two fascial layers by opening the space of Denonvilliers. This is an essential step of the operation, and failure may mean damage to the rectum. It is most difficult at times to find this passage 'between wind and water' (Cabot).

Fig. 94 shows the *recto-urethralis muscle of Roux*. This consists of two bundles of muscles—recto-urethralis superior and inferior —both derived from the longitudinal muscle coat of the gut. They hold the anorectal junction forward, angulating it to form the rectal angle. They are both attached to the upper part of the perineal body. They must be divided in perineal prostatectomy, as only then will the rectum fall back, the muscles constituting the stay which holds it forward.

Chapter XVI

THE ISCHIORECTAL FOSSA

THIS cavity is pyramidal in shape. It is 5 cm. long, 5 cm. deep, and 2·5 cm. wide.

BOUNDARIES:
  LATERAL: The fascia covering the obturator internus muscle and the ischial tuberosity.
  MEDIAL: The fascia covering the levator ani muscle; the external sphincter of the anus.
  POSTERIOR: Sacrotuberous ligament, on the posterior surface of which is the gluteus maximus.
  ANTERIOR: Urogenital diaphragm (triangular ligament).
  FLOOR: Skin.

Under the skin is a large pad of fat filling the fossa. There is here no deep fascia such as exists elsewhere just under the skin. The deep fascia is separated from the skin by the whole thickness of the pad of fat filling the fossa. This fascia was described by Professor Elliott Smith and named the 'fascia lunata' (*Fig.* 95).

Fascia Lunata:
  RELATIONS:
    MEDIAL: It covers the fascia on levator (anal fascia) and *ends at the lower end of the levator*.
    LATERAL: Covers fascia on obturator internus (obturator fascia) and

THE ISCHIORECTAL FOSSA

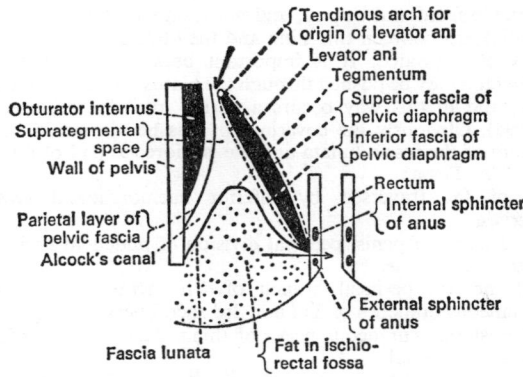

Fig. 95.—Coronal section of the ischorectal fossa. Note the fascia lunata. The upper arrow shows the hiatus of Schwalbe. The lower arrow shows the course frequently taken by ischiorectal abscesses which rupture into the rectum.

is attached to ischium. The internal pudendal vessels and nerves are between these two layers, and thus Alcock's canal is formed (and not by a splitting of the obturator fascia) (*Fig. 96*).

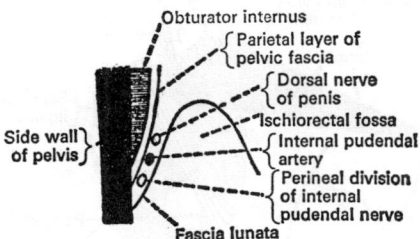

Fig. 96.—To show how Alcock's canal is formed by the pelvic fascia and the fascia lunata.

ANTERIOR: The fascia fuses with the urogenital diaphragm.

SUPERIOR: The upper arched portion of the fascia is called the *tegmentum*. There is a space between this tegmentum and the apex of the fossa, which space is the suprategmental space and contains fat.

Hiatus of Schwalbe: The levator ani arises from the pubic bone in front, the ischial spine behind, and the obturator fascia between these points. At times it arises from a tendinous sling, which is attached only to bone in front and behind, and not to fascia at all. There is then a potential gap between this sling and the obturator fascia. This is the hiatus of Schwalbe. It is important because a process of pelvic peritoneum may be pushed through the hiatus into the suprategmental space, and in this way occurs a hernia into the ischiorectal fossa (*Fig.* 95). Obviously the coverings of this hernia would be the tegmentum of the fascia lunata and the ischiorectal pad of fat.

Contents of the Fossa:
1. Pad of fat traversed by inferior haemorrhoidal vessels and nerves.
2. Dorsal nerve of penis, perineal division of pudendal nerve, internal pudendal vessels.
3. Small nerves: perineal branch of 4th sacral nerve; perforating cutaneous branches of 2nd and 3rd sacral nerves; gluteal branches of posterior cutaneous nerve of thigh. The fossa therefore has a rich nerve-supply.

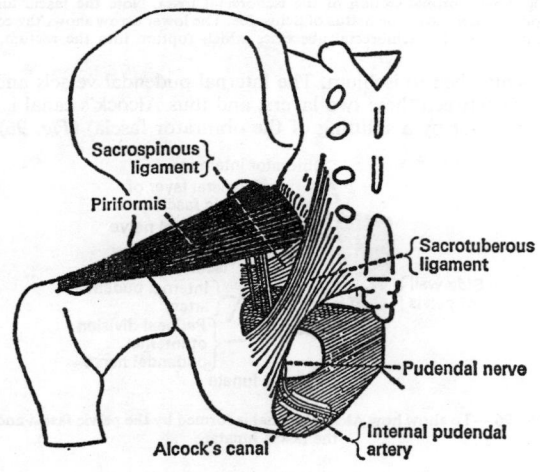

Fig. 97.—Alcock's canal.

Alcock's Canal: Runs forward on outer wall of fossa 3·8 cm. above the lower border of the ischial tuberosity (*Fig.* 97). It contains the internal pudendal vessels and nerve. The nerve divides into its two divisions, dorsal nerve of penis and perineal division, as soon as it enters the fossa; at the same point it gives off the inferior haemorrhoidal nerves.

THE ANAL REGION 109

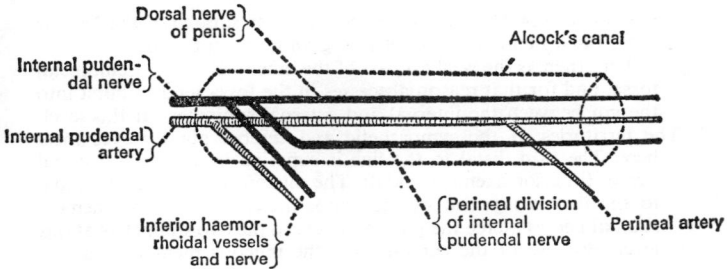

Fig. 98.—Alcock's canal (dotted) and its contents.

The artery does not divide, but gives off inferior haemorrhoidal vessels at the posterior part of the canal, and the perineal branch at the anterior extremity of the canal (*Fig.* 98).

Chapter XVII

THE ANAL REGION

I. THE PECTINATE LINE[1]

DEVELOPMENTALLY the anal canal has a twofold origin: (1) An ingrowth from the skin—the proctodeum; (2) The downgrowth of the hind-gut towards the surface.

The *anal membrane* is the partition which divides the proctodeum from the hind-gut. It disappears, as a rule, leaving only a wavy whitish line to mark its situation at the lower part of the anal canal. This is the *pectinate line*. It has considerable importance anatomically, but much more surgically. Its surgical importance may be gathered from the considered statement of Pennington[2] who said that 85 per cent of all proctological diseases occur in this area. It is an important *boundary region*.

Anatomical and Surgical Importance of the Line:
1. The squamous epithelium of the skin meets the columnar epithelium of the gut at this line. The line is said to be covered with transitional epithelium.
2. (*a*) The fascia lunata of Elliott Smith (*see* pp. 106, 107) ends at this level by fusing with the fascia over the levator ani between the

[1] The author has welcomed Professor Goligher's suggestion that the term 'Hilton's Line' be discontinued because its significance is imprecise.
[2] *Rectum, Anus, and Pelvic Colon*, 1923. Philadelphia.

two sphincters. (b) The fascia on the lower surface of the levator (anal fascia) ends here by blending with the gut wall.

This, then, is the weakest part of the inner wall of the ischiorectal fossa, and for that reason abscesses in the fossa tend to burst into the gut between the internal and external sphincters at this level.
3. The territories of the sympathetic and cerebrospinal nerves meet here. The skin distal to the line is supplied by the cerebrospinal nerves (inferior haemorrhoidal). The mucous membrane proximal to the line is supplied by the sympathetic. The inferior haemorrhoidal nerves pierce the gut wall between the two sphincters at this level. Because of the nerve-supply the mucous membrane above

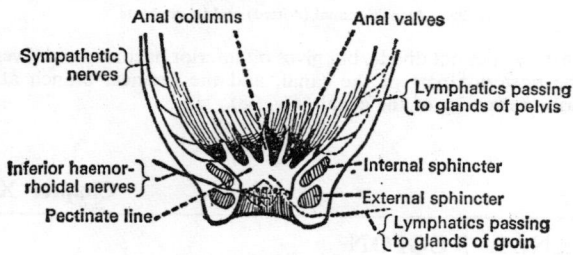

Fig. 99.—Anatomy of the pectinate line.

the line is relatively insensitive, while the skin below the line is exquisitely sensitive. As haemorrhoids are usually situated just above this line they are often covered by skin below and mucous membrane above. Therefore, when injecting piles to thrombose them, the surgeon puts his needle into the upper (mucous-membrane covered) part of the pile, and avoids the sensitive skin below. Carcinoma of the rectum is 'silent' for a long time because it causes no pain. The type, however, which occurs here is agonizingly painful because it involves cerebrospinal nerves.
4. True or internal haemorrhoids occur above this line.
5. The pectinate line is the lymphatic watershed of the region. The mucous membrane and gut above the line is drained into pelvic lymph-glands—sacral and hypogastric. The skin distal to the line is drained into the superficial subinguinal glands in the groin by lymphatics which run round the *inner* side of the root of the thigh.
6. The *anal valves* are found on this line. The anal canal has a number of longitudinal ridges of mucous membrane on its inner surface. These, the anal columns or columns of Morgagni, are connected together at the pectinate line by transverse folds covered by mucous membrane on their upper and skin on their lower surfaces.

These are the anal valves. Fissure in ano is sometimes caused by the rupture of one of these folds (usually by the passage of scybala). It is intensely painful because cerebrospinal nerve-ends are exposed in the floor of the fissure. The tag formed by the torn valve is called the 'sentinel pile'. It is not a pile. Above each anal valve is a small pocket called a rectal sinus.

7. *Anal papillae:* The anal membrane is covered by skin below and mucous membrane above. It may be found entire at birth, causing the condition of imperforate anus. It usually disappears entirely, though often there are triangular tags found on the pectinate line which are remnants of the anal membrane. They are called anal papillae, and may cause irritation and pruritus ani, though usually they are symptomless.

8. It is of use to remember that diseases peculiar to the skin occur distal to this line, whilst those peculiar to mucous membrane occur proximal to the line.

9. *Fistula in ano:* Too little attention has been paid to the existence of certain tubular structures which open into small depressions, anal sinuses, which lie just above the shelf formed by an anal valve. These tubular structures, whether glands or sinuses, have been recognized since 1880. They represent all that is left of certain complicated glands found in the anal region in some of the lower animals. These tubes penetrate the coats of the rectum partially or completely, and in the opinion of Pennington, Gordon Watson, and others, they play a part of first-rate importance in rectal pathology. Parks[1] considers that 90 per cent of fistulae in ano derive from these vestigial glands. Organisms enter these crypts, find shelter and multiply, and eventually give rise to abscesses which rupture, causing fistulae in ano or rectal sinuses.

Long since Goodsall enunciated a valuable law in regard to the position of the internal orifice of a complete fistula in ano: If the anal circumference be divided into an anterior and a posterior half by an imaginary transverse plane, the internal opening of a fistula behind this plane is in the *midline* of the rectum posteriorly; the inner opening of a fistula opening on the skin in front of this plane is at a point on the rectal wall corresponding in position to the external opening.

10. *Piles* are varicose veins of the anus, and occur in relation to the pectinate line. In the lower rectum there is an important communication between the veins of the portal and the systemic circulation. A reference to *Fig.* 100 shows how the superior haemorrhoidal vein (portal) communicates with the middle and inferior haemorrhoidal veins (systemic). The superior haemorrhoidal vein has no valves; so the veins in the anal columns (columns of Morgagni)

[1] Parks, A. G., *Br. med. J.*, 1961, 1, 463.

have to support the pressure all the way from where the portal vein enters the liver. If it be remembered, further, that these veins penetrate the muscle wall of the rectum through buttonhole openings, it can be realized how straining at stool, constipation, prolonged standing, etc., may cause dilatations of these veins— i.e., piles. It is furthermore readily understood how, in portal obstruction, the portal-systemic anastomosis in the rectum may be one of the paths of the collateral circulation of venous blood, which may be evidenced as piles.

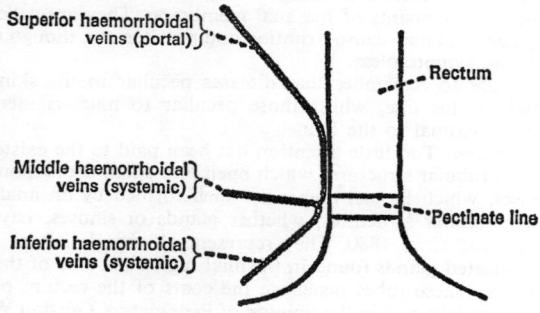

Fig. 100.—Showing the portal-systemic anastomosis in the lower rectum.

Piles may occur, therefore, above the pectinate line or below it, or may be a mixture of the two. Thus internal, external, or interoexternal piles are found. Internal piles are varicosities of the superior haemorrhoidal veins in the anal columns. External piles form a bluish cushion of veins in the skin round the anus. These two varieties may be connected by small veins crossing the pectinate line.

The arrangement of pile masses is that of the anatomy of the superior haemorrhoidal vein, which is explained by *Fig.* 101. Observe that primary piles occur at positions corresponding to the numbers 3, 7, 11 on a clock face.

There are three varieties of false external piles:

a. One type is properly styled haematoma ani (thrombotic pile), and is due to straining causing rupture of one of the small perianal veins; it appears clinically as a bluish swelling of variable size at the anal verge.

b. This type is not venous but merely a tag of skin at the anus. These tags are formed as a result of 'attacks of piles'. Thrombophlebitis of a haemorrhoidal vein causes an area

of swelling and oedema of the related segment of the anal skin; subsidence of the oedema leaves a dog-eared tag of skin.
  c. This variety is the 'sentinel' pile described on p. 111.

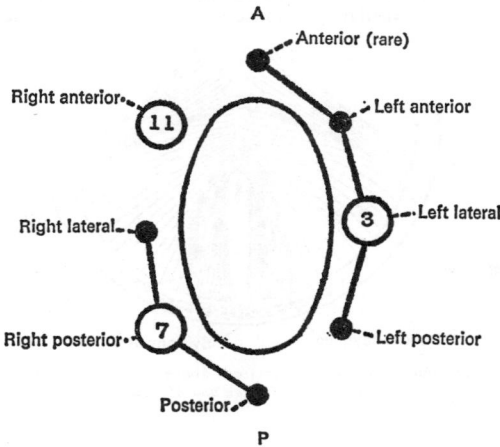

Fig. 101.—The anatomy of piles. The superior haemorrhoidal artery gives off a right and a left branch. The right branch and left branch divide as shown in the figure. The circles represent the primary branches, the black dots show the the secondary branches. The veins correspond, and piles are called primary or secondary according to their situation. A, Anterior; P, Posterior. The numbers in the circles show the clock-face positions where primary piles occur. (The anus is seen with the subject in the lithotomy position.) (*After Abel.*[1])

II. THE ANAL SPHINCTERS

In 1934 Milligan and Naunton Morgan[2] published the results of their researches on the muscle control of the anus. This paper is a classic. It served to dispel much false teaching and to establish sound surgical precept. This section summarizes the work of these authors.

Muscles: (1) Levator ani. (2) Sphincter ani externus. (3) Muscles of anal canal.

  LEVATOR ANI: The levators, originally muscles acting on the tail, now form the pelvic diaphragm. They support the viscera of the pelvis. Each muscle arises from bone in front and behind, and from parietal layer of pelvic fascia between, along a line (the white line)

---

[1] *Lancet*, 1932, April, 2.
[2] Milligan, E. T. C., and Morgan, C. Naunton, *Lancet*, 1934, 2, 1150, 1213.

extending from back of pubis to ischial spine. The nerve-supply is from the 3rd and 4th sacral (*see Fig.* 185, p. 198). The muscle is composite, being made up by iliococcygeus, pubococcygeus, and puborectalis from behind forward (*Fig.* 102).

ILIOCOCCYGEUS: Arises from posterior part of white line and ischial spine; often vestigial, it is inserted into coccyx and anococcygeal raphe.

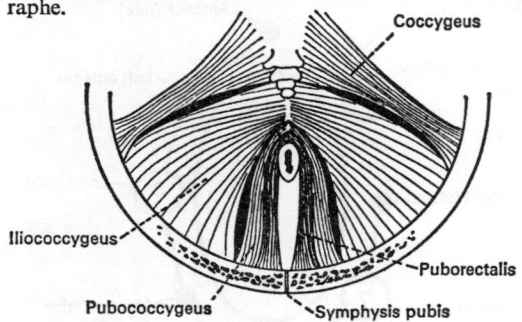

Fig. 102.—The floor of the pelvis seen from above to show the levatores ani. (*Modified from Milligan and Morgan.*)

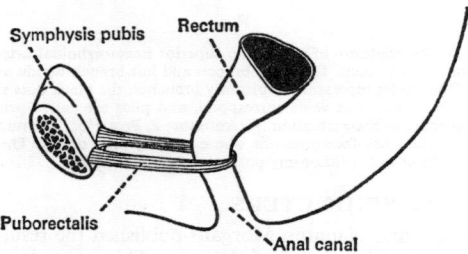

Fig. 103.—To show how the anorectal junction is angulated by the sling formed by the puborectalis muscles.

PUBOCOCCYGEUS: Arises from back of pubis and anterior part of white line. Fibres pass almost horizontally backwards beside rectum, superior to the previous muscle, and form a dense raphe behind rectum.

PUBORECTALIS: Arises from back of pubis, passes backwards and downwards at the side of the rectum, and, meeting its fellow posterior to this viscus, forms a powerful muscular sling, angulating anorectal junction and anchoring rectum to pubis (*Fig.* 103).

This muscle is an important part of the anal sphincteric apparatus. It can be felt with an examining finger along the whole length of the sling. It is an important part of the anorectal ring (*Fig.* 104). Nerve-supply: 3rd and 4th sacral.

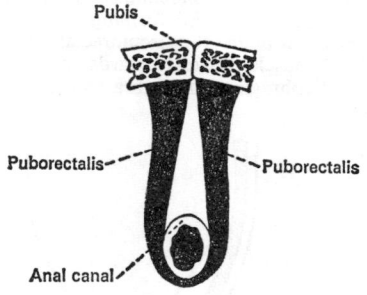

Fig. 104.—Plan of the puborectalis muscle sling.

SPHINCTER ANI EXTERNUS: Because of a better understanding of the functions of the anal sphincters this muscle has less clinical significance than has hitherto been accorded to it. It is 8 to 12 cm. long and 2·5 cm. wide at the anal level where it forms the so-called 'Umbrella Ring'. The outer or superficial portion has a tendinous posterior attachment to the anococcygeal raphe whence it passes forward as two bands encircling the anus and joining anteriorly to be inserted into the central tendinous point of the perineum, together with levator and perineal muscles. The deeper part of the muscle forms a complete sphincter to the anal canal, being closely applied to the internal sphincter. Above it blends with the puborectalis and below with the other muscles at the central perineal point. Nerve-supply: 3rd and 4th sacral (*Fig.* 105).

MUSCLES OF ANAL CANAL: As elsewhere in the bowel there are longitudinal and circular muscle layers.

LONGITUDINAL MUSCLE: Extends down between puborectalis and the deep and superficial parts of the external sphincter without and the internal sphincter within. It tends to blend with the muscles lying exteriorly and takes a share in the formation of the anorectal ring. It is reinforced by fibres of the puborectalis. As the muscle passes between internal and external sphincters it becomes fibro-elastic. Some of these fibres pass through the internal sphincter to enter the submucous space mingling with the musculus submucosae. At the pectinate line they tether the anal skin by gaining attachment to it, thus dividing the submucous space containing the internal haemorrhoidal venous plexus from the subcutaneous perianal space where the external plexus lies, and where the lower end of the internal sphincter is situated. Most of the fibres of the fibro-elastic part of the longitudinal muscle pass through the subcutaneous external sphincter to gain attachment into the true skin forming the corrugator cutis muscle. Others pass through the ischiorectal fossa. Anteriorly the longitudinal muscle passes forwards to gain attachment to the urogenital diaphragm and urethra as the recto-urethralis muscle (*Fig.* 105).

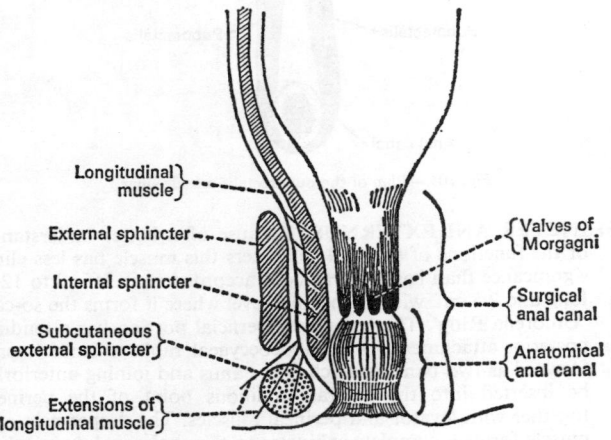

Fig. 105.—The surgical and anatomical anal canals. (*By courtesy of Morgan and Thompson.*)

CIRCULAR MUSCLE: In the region below the anorectal ring the circular muscle layer of the rectum becomes increasingly thickened to form the internal sphincter ani. A depression may be felt just within the anal margin, between the lower end of the internal sphincter and the 'umbrella ring' formed by the subcutaneous external sphincter.

It is apparent that the longitudinal muscle is an arrangement which binds the sphincters together.

Clinical Applications: Anatomically the anal canal extends from the valves of Morgagni—the dentate or pectinate line—to the anal verge. The surgical anal canal extends from the anorectal ring, i.e., the site where the rectum passes through the levator ani, to the anal margin.

Below the dentate line the skin of the anal canal is pale and smooth and contains no hair follicles or glands and is firmly attached to the deeper structures. The mucosa over the internal haemorrhoidal plexus, formed by the submucous veins above the anal valves, is lax and the skin over the external plexus under the anal skin is loosely attached. Thus submucous and subcutaneous (perianal) potential spaces exist.

When piles prolapse and become infected or strangulated, the mass—intero-external pile—which appears is divided into two portions by a deep groove due to the binding down of the skin at the white line by its attachments to the fibro-elastic extensions of the longitudinal muscle (*Fig.* 106).

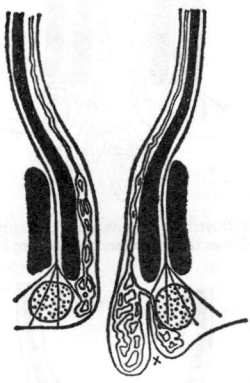

Fig. 106.—Diagrammatic representation of a strangulated pile. The X shows the deep fissure between internal and external haemorrhoidal plexuses produced by the attachment of the fibro-elastic extensions of the longitudinal muscle to the skin. (*After Milligan and Morgan.*)

Liberal communications pass between the internal and external haemorrhoidal plexuses. When the internal piles are delivered the external plexus becomes turgid and presents as a ring of veins. This is good evidence that most of the blood from this plexus drains via the internal one (*Fig.* 107).

NATURE OF THE ANAL SPHINCTER: It is apparent from the foregoing that the lower 3·7 cm. of the alimentary canal is surrounded by a complex apparatus which allows proper control of emptying. The puborectalis, external sphincter, and internal sphincter act together as a whole. The upper part of the mechanism forms the palpable anorectal ring (*Fig.* 108). The sphincteric apparatus is under somatic and autonomic control through the 3rd and 4th sacral nerves.

O. Swenson[1] of Boston states that when a faecal mass descends, the trigger area for contraction of the sphincters is the anal mucosa.

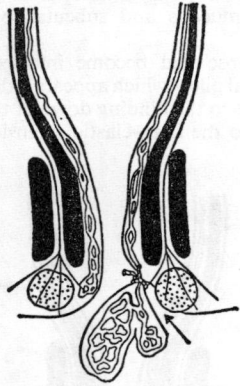

Fig. 107.—The diagram illustrates the anatomical features concerned in removing a pile. The arrow shows the line of section. (*After Milligan and Morgan.*)

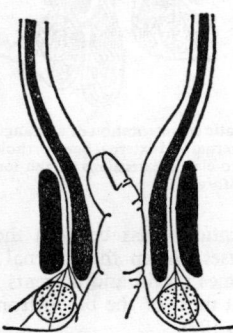

Fig. 108—Palpation of the anorectal ring. (*After Milligan and Morgan.*)

If this is removed soiling is apt to occur. Rectal continence depends on the integrity of the anorectal ring. It is necessary to have this advice constantly in mind as boldness in the surgery of the anal

[1] Personal communication.

canal is often the only way to cure sufferers of old-standing and complex rectal fistulae.

Bennett and Goligher[1] emphasize the fact that internal sphincterotomy is followed by faecal soiling in the anal region in 30 per cent of cases, and even though this is minor in nature it is disturbing. They go on to say that continence normally depends in greatest measure on the voluntary muscles of the anal region, the external sphincter and the puborectalis—the internal sphincter being concerned with the refinements of anal continence.

For effective sphincteric control the distal 5 cm. of the rectal mucosa must be preserved. This implies that in anterior resection of the rectum, where the distal bowel is preserved to avoid colostomy, the level of bowel section must be not less than approximately 10 cm. from the anal verge.

RE-ORIENTATION OF SPHINCTERS: Eisenhammer[2] drew attention to the importance of the internal sphincter ani in surgery of the anal canal. He pointed out that the ring of white fibres surrounding the lower end of the anal canal is the lower end of the internal sphincter and not the subcutaneous external sphincter as had hitherto been generally believed. Morgan and Thompson[3] investigated the matter further. As a result it is now known that:

1. The internal and external sphincters of the anus are comparable to two tubes of muscle one within the other.
2. Under certain conditions, e.g., anaesthesia or stretching of the anus, the lower end of the internal sphincter lies lower than, and internal to, the external sphincter.
3. The internal sphincteric fibres are white, those of the external are red (*Fig.* 109).
4. In operations for piles the muscle exposed is the internal sphincter.
5. In anal fissure the muscle in the floor of the fissure is the internal sphincter.
6. The division of this muscle cures the fissure by removing the cause of painful spasm.
7. There is no such thing as the pecten band.

TOTAL RECTAL BIOPSY: Providing the bowel is properly prepared and judicious use is made of antibiotics, certain apparent liberties may be taken with the anal sphincteric apparatus.

The rectum is often the site of polyps, villous and other tumours which can neither be safely nor completely removed through a sigmoidoscope. In such cases excellent access is obtained by a vertical midline incision from tip of coccyx to a point just short of the anus. The rectum is divided in the line of the incision, its edges

---

[1] Bennett, R. C., and Goligher, J. C., *Br. med. J.*, 1962, 2, 1500.
[2] Eisenhammer, S., *S. Afr. med. J.*, 1951, 25, 486.
[3] Morgan, C. Naunton, and Thompson, H. R., *Ann. R. Coll. Surg.*, 1956, 19, 88.

retracted, and the tumour can then be seen and removed *in toto* with part of the rectal wall if necessary. David[1] has gone further and advised that the skin and bowel incision should be extended to divide the anal musculature, laying open the whole anal canal. With proper suture methods, although a temporary leak may develop, neither fistula nor incontinence results.

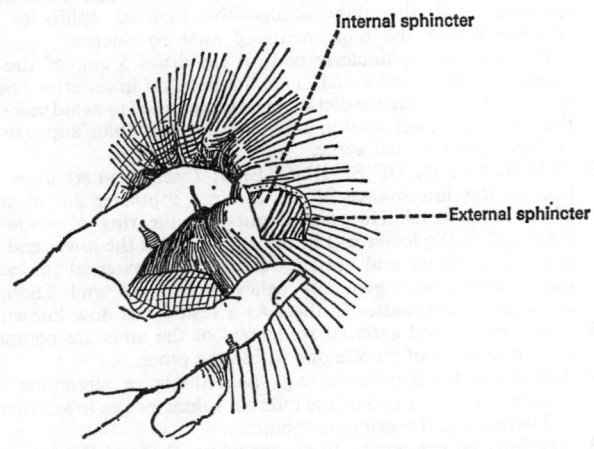

Fig. 109.—The relationship of internal and external sphincters at the lower end of the anus.

III. FISTULA IN ANO

A fistula in ano follows spontaneous rupture or surgical drainage of an anorectal abscess and the various types of fistulae therefore depend on the types of preceding anorectal abscesses.[2]

More than 90 per cent of anorectal abscesses are the results of infection in the anal intramuscular glands. These glands lie in the intermuscular space between the circular and longitudinal muscles of the anal canal and drain by narrow ducts which pierce the circular muscle to open into the crypts at the dentate (pectinate) line in the anal canal (*Fig.* 110). Infective material may be forced into these glands during defaecation (particularly with diarrhoea) and this results in abscess formation.

The abscess will track along the duct to discharge internally in the related crypt at the dentate line but eventually will also track downwards

[1] David, V. C., *Surgery*, 1954, 14, 387.
[2] Eisenhammer, S., *Dis. Colon Rectum*, 1966, 9, 91.

THE ANAL REGION 121

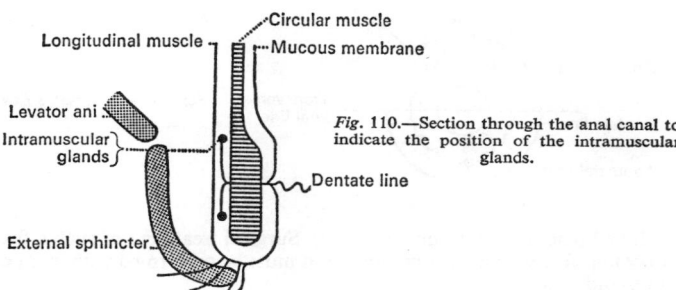

Fig. 110.—Section through the anal canal to indicate the position of the intramuscular glands.

towards the skin and discharge fairly close to the anus to produce a fistula in ano. A similar outcome may result from external surgical drainage.

The majority of these glands arise posteriorly in the midline and are situated in the lower part of the intermuscular space. Anorectal infection is therefore usually encountered in this region and the resultant fistula is a low-level anal fistula discharging at the dentate line in the midline posteriorly (*Fig*. 111).

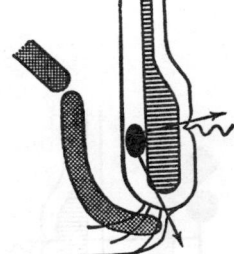

Fig. 111.—Low anal intermuscular abscess resulting in a low anal fistula.

The infection in the intermuscular space reaches the skin by tracking along the terminal fibres of the longitudinal muscle. These fibres also offer a route of spread into the ischiorectal fossa.

According to Goodsall's law, if the external opening is posterior to a transverse line drawn through the anus, the internal opening is at the midline posteriorly, but if the external opening is anterior to this line, the internal opening is at the dentate line exactly opposite the external opening (*Fig*. 112).

Occasionally the abscess forms in an intramuscular gland in the upper part of the intermuscular space and then the internal opening of the fistula

122 A SYNOPSIS OF SURGICAL ANATOMY

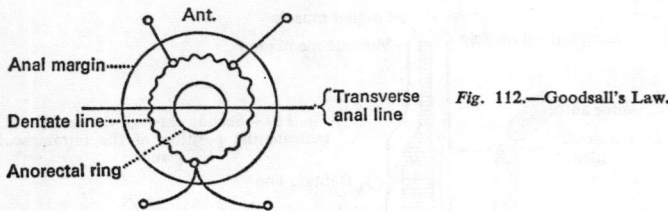

Fig. 112.—Goodsall's Law.

will be higher in the rectum (*Fig.* 113). Surgical treatment of such a fistula may interfere with anal continence and must be performed with great care to avoid this.

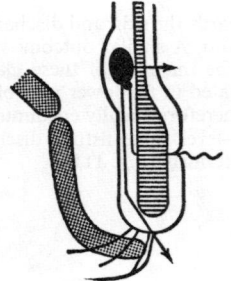

Fig. 113.—High anal intermuscular abscess resulting in a high anal fistula.

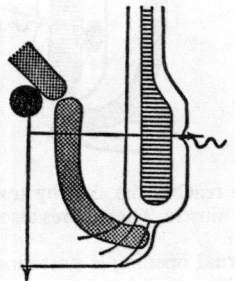

Fig. 114.—Ischiorectal abscess discharging externally but with an associated fistulous opening.

Abscesses in the ischiorectal fossa are rare but may occur either from an aberrant anal gland which has pierced the whole anal musculature or as a result of direct, lymphatic or blood spread from the anal canal. Such abscesses will rupture externally to produce an external sinus only. If the abscess formed in an aberrant anal gland, it may break through into the anal canal to produce a fistula, opening at the dentate line but with an extension of a blind sinus higher up in the ischiorectal fossa (*Fig.* 114).

The pelvirectal abscess above the levator ani muscle is actually an extraperitoneal pelvic abscess resulting from diseases such as Crohn's disease, appendicitis, ulcerative colitis or diverticulitis. It may break through into the rectum above the anorectal ring and through the levator muscle

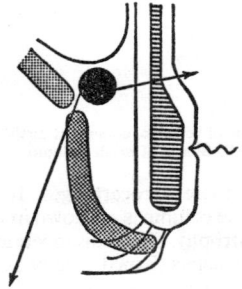

Fig. 115.—Pelvirectal abscess resulting in a supralevator fistula.

onto the skin to produce a supralevator fistula (*Fig.* 115). Surgical excision of such a fistula may produce complete anal incontinence unless special precautions are taken to avoid this.

Subcutaneous and submucous fistulae result from minor abscesses in the subcutaneous and submucous spaces. They are of little importance and are easily cured by surgical opening of the track.

Chapter XVIII

THE VERTEBRAL COLUMN

THE vertebral column consists of thirty-three bones. Five are fused to form the sacrum, four to form the coccyx.

Curves of the Column: These are: (1) Primary; (2) Secondary.
 PRIMARY: These exist at birth: *thoracic* and *sacral* (*Fig.* 116, A).
 SECONDARY: These develop after birth: *cervical* and *lumbar*. The cervical appears when the child holds its head up after the third month; the lumbar curve develops when the child sits up after the fifth month (*Fig.* 116, B).

Intervertebral Fibrocartilages: The column is lengthened by these discs, which comprise one-third to a quarter of its total length. The shape

124 A SYNOPSIS OF SURGICAL ANATOMY

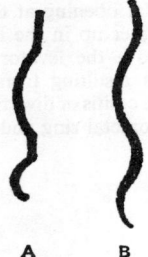

Fig. 116.—A, Diagrammatic representation of shape of vertebral column at birth, i.e., only the thoracic and sacral curves exist. B, Shape of adult column.

of the column is largely dependent on these fibrocartilages. If the bones alone are articulated, the shape of the column is as shown in *Fig.* 117, B. In later life, after 60, the discs atrophy. Their disappearance gives rise to the bowed back of old age, which is shaped exactly as the column is shaped when the bones are articulated without fibrocartilages.

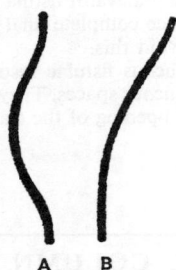

Fig. 117.—Shape of vertebral column (excluding lower lumbar and sacral portion). A, Complete with intervertebral fibrocartilages. B, Intervertebral discs removed. (*After Lovett.*)

Bearing and Transmission of Weight: The column performs the important function of weight bearing and transmission. Should one or more of the vertebrae be diseased (as in tuberculous disease of the spine), a factor comes into play which is not seen anywhere else in the body, i.e., the diseased segments are crushed by the superincumbent weight and the products of the disease in the interior are squeezed out. This accounts for the great frequency of cold abscesses in tuberculosis of the spine. As the result of this collapse the spines of the diseased bodies

THE VERTEBRAL COLUMN 125

become more prominent, and form a projection or hump, as the arches of the vertebrae are not affected by the disease and are held in position by the ligaments and muscles attaching them to adjacent bones. This weight-bearing function of the vertebral bodies may in itself be a cause of hump-back in cases where the architecture of a vertebra is damaged as the result of a blow or other injury. Kümmell described cases where after an injury to the spine a slow collapse of a vertebra occurred, producing much disability. This was ascribed to interference with the blood-supply. It is now looked upon as the result of an undetected fracture. There results insufficient immobilization with subsequent collapse of the vertebral body. Watson Jones[1] has shown how such lesions should be treated by use of the physiological splint supplied by

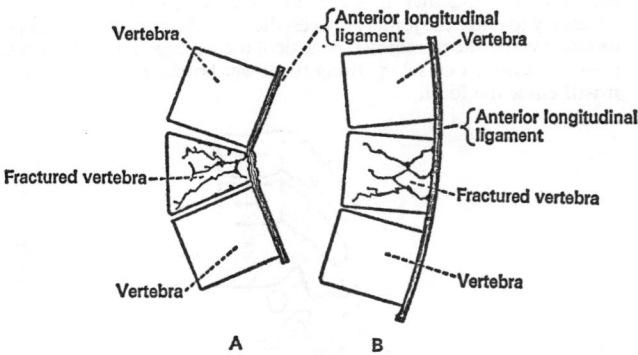

Fig. 118.—To show how extension of the spine restores the contour of a crushed vertebra. The part played by the anterior longitudinal ligament is shown. A, Column in flexion, vertebra collapsed. B, Column in extension, vertebra restored to normal shape.

the anterior longitudinal ligament of the spine. This is a powerful band uniting the vertebral bodies. The patient is transported in the prone position, which maintains extension of the vertebral column. Later a plaster case is applied to the trunk with the spine hyperextended. By this means the buckled vertebra is pulled back to its original shape by its attachments to the intervertebral fibrocartilages above and below, assisted by the resistance offered by the powerful anterior longitudinal ligament (*Fig.* 118). In 1949 Nicoll reported that in cases of stable fractures with simple wedge deformity, treatment by bed rest and immediate exercises was eminently satisfactory.

[1] *Br. med. J.*, 1931, Feb. 21, 300.

Articulations: Adjacent bones articulate with each other by their bodies through the intervention of articular discs, and through their articular processes. Each vertebra has upper and lower pairs of articular processes. For the most part these are arranged vertically, except in the cervical region, where they are more transverse. Thus dislocation of vertebrae can occur without fracture only in the neck (*Fig.* 119). Anywhere else in the column a pure dislocation cannot occur because of the direction of the articular processes, and the injury is therefore necessarily a fracture-dislocation, as the articular processes must break off before the bodies can move apart. In connexion with the articular processes, Sir Harold Stiles pointed out that the plane of the thoracic inferior articular processes continues in the line of the lower border of the lamina. In the operation devised by Hibbs for fixing the vertebrae together in cases of tuberculosis of the spine, it is necessary to enter the joints between the articular processes of adjacent thoracic vertebrae to remove the articular cartilage. This is readily done then by passing a chisel up along the lower border of the lamina when it will enter the joint.

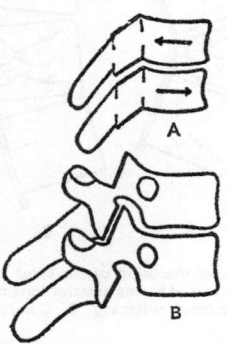

Fig. 119.—A Showing how dislocation of a cervical vertebra may occur without fracture. B, Dislocation of thoracic vertebrae must be associated with fracture because of the nature of the joints between the articular processes, and the direction of these processes.

Intervertebral Foramina: These are formed by the articulation of the bones with each other, and are usually proportionate in size to the spinal nerves emerging through the foramina. Putti has shown that in the lower lumbar region the foramina are often so small that there is just room for the emergence of the nerves, which therefore fill the foramina. The lumbar nerves *increase* in size from 1 to 5. The lumbar intervertebral foramina *decrease* in size from above down, resulting in the large lower lumbar nerves having to negotiate smaller foramina than the thin upper lumbar nerves. Should there be swelling of the nerve-sheath, or should the bony ring become narrowed by disease, the emerging nerve will be pressed upon, resulting in the condition of sciatica.

Transverse Processes: In the cervical regions these are very short. In the thoracic region they lie exactly behind the necks of the ribs, which splint them. In the lumbar region they are long and have big powerful muscles attached to them, e.g., the quadratus lumborum and psoas. It happens sometimes (more often than was thought before the introduction of radiography) that lumbar transverse processes are pulled off by the violent action of the attached muscles. This is a possible, though unusual, cause of persistent pain and weakness in the back.

Abnormalities in the Bones: Accessory vertebrae may exist in any region of the column. Accessory parts of vertebrae may exist. This may produce serious deformity. This is typically seen in cases where a vertebra is represented by only one lateral half of its body. The result is a bending of the spine to one side—the condition of *scoliosis*. From the nature of its cause it is difficult to correct the condition.

THE VERTEBRAL ARCHES may be incomplete, producing the condition known as *spina bifida* in which the cord is unprotected by bone in some part of its course.

SACRALIZATION: The 5th lumbar vertebra is frequently joined in whole or in part to the sacrum. This is known as sacralization of the 5th lumbar vertebra. It is often devoid of symptoms. In other cases the transverse process of the 5th lumbar vertebra may come into contact with the subjacent ala of the sacrum, forming what Sir Robert Jones called a 'transverse lumbosacral joint'. Such a condition may also be symptomless, but may cause persistent painful back, either directly because of friction between the two bones, or because the lumbrosacral trunk passing down in relation to the bones is irritated.

The 5th lumbar transverse process passes upwards and outwards to avoid contact with the posterior part of the iliac crest. It may: (1) Articulate with the crest; (2) Be fused with the crest owing to ossification of the iliolumbar ligament. These latter conditions may also cause painful back.

Neurenteric Canal: According to McRae[1] the neurenteric canal is a transitory communication between the primitive gut, the chordal canal, and the dorsal surface of the embryo. It exists for a few days in the third week of embryonic development. In the adult it is situated at a point corresponding roughly with the cervical spine. Defective closure of the canal may result in an adhesion, cyst, or canal, connecting part of the respiratory or gastro-intestinal tract with the spine, spinal cord, or dorsal surface of the embryo. Therefore posteriorly

[1] McRae, D. L., *Am. J. Roentg.*, 1960, **84**, 3.

situated thoracic or upper abdominal tumours or cysts, in the presence of anomalies of the cervical or upper thoracic vertebrae, should direct attention to their possible origin from the primitive neurenteric canal. The low situation of a mass of this kind is explained by the descent of the diaphragm.

Movements of the Column: These are flexion, extension, side-bending, and rotation.

FLEXION AND EXTENSION take place in the cervical, lumbar, and dorsolumbar regions.

SIDE-BENDING AND ROTATION: This is a composite movement. It has been shown conclusively by Lovett and others that in bending the spine to one side, i.e., in the coronal plane, rotation of the spine must occur for mechanical reasons. The spine has been compared in this respect to a very thin lath. If this is bent edgewise, it will rotate in so doing.

Spinal Localization: Early in fetal life the spinal cord extends the entire length of the vertebral canal. Soon the column grows much more quickly than the cord, and ultimately a great disproportion exists between the extent of the two structures. In the adult the cord ends at the 2nd lumbar vertebra. The dural sac ends at the 2nd sacral vertebra.

At birth the cord ends at the *3rd lumbar vertebra* (and not at the lower end of the column). The segment of the cord which corresponds to a given vertebra is therefore above the level of that vertebra. The only part of a vertebra which is accessible throughout the column is its spine. The spinal segments are therefore localized in terms of the spines of the vertebra.

In the cervical region a vertebral spine is one lower in number than the corresponding cord segment, i.e., the 5th spine is opposite to the 6th cervical cord segment.

In the upper thoracic region the spines are two lower in number than the corresponding cord segment, i.e., the 3rd spine corresponds to the 5th thoracic segment.

In the lower thoracic region the spines are three lower in number than the corresponding cord segment, i.e., the 7th spine corresponds to the 10th thoracic segment.

This scheme, though not strictly accurate, is a good practical method for localizing segments in terms of spines.

RELATION OF THE MOST PROMINENT SPINE IN DISEASE AND INJURIES OF THE CORD:

1. In tuberculous kyphosis the centre of the diseased area corresponds to the most prominent spine.
2. In fracture-compression of a vertebra the most prominent spine is the one above the crushed vertebra.
3. In fracture-dislocation of the spine the most prominent spine is the one below the displaced vertebra.

Chapter XIX

THE ANATOMY OF THE CHILD

Head:
DIMENSIONS: At birth the circumference of the infant's head averages 33 to 35 cm. It gains 7·6 cm. in the first six months. At the end of the first year it is 45·7 cm. At five years it is 50 cm. At ten years it is 53 cm.

FONTANELLES: The skull at birth is only partly ossified, there being gaps between the bones which are filled in by a membranous structure which consists of three layers. The inner is the outer layer of the dura, the middle is the future periosteum of the skull bones, the superficial layer is the aponeurosis joining the occipitalis and frontalis muscles. These gaps are called fontanelles. They serve two very important purposes: (1) They admit of some overlapping of the skull bones during the moulding and pressure which the skull undergoes during birth; and (2) They permit of growth of the brain.

It is of the utmost importance to note that the normal skull only develops round a normal brain. (The term 'normal' is here used as implying absence of gross anatomical defect.) There are six fontanelles at birth. One is situated at each angle of a parietal bone. Two are therefore median and four are lateral. The four lateral close within a few weeks of birth. The median fontanelles are posterior and anterior.

THE POSTERIOR FONTANELLE is situated where the two parietal bones meet the occipital bone. It closes soon after birth.

THE ANTERIOR FONTANELLE is vastly the most important. It is situated at the place where the two parietal bones and the frontal bone come close together (*Fig.* 120).

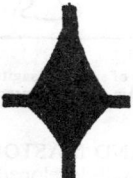

Fig. 120.—Shape of the anterior fontanelle.

Shape: It is rhomboid in shape. Each of its four angles marks the end of a suture.

Size: It measures about 3·8 cm. in length by 2·5 cm. in breadth.

Significance:

Developmental significance: There is here for two years after birth a non-rigid area which permits of increase in size of the brain.

Clinical significance: Valuable information is obtained from the fontanelle. The degree of tenseness of the membrane gives an index of the intracranial pressure. On the other hand, abnormal depression of the membrane indicates an insufficiency of body fluids. The fontanelle is of great service for further purposes: (1) Through its lateral angle a needle may be passed into the lateral ventricle of the brain; (2) The superior sagittal sinus may be approached through the membrane (*Fig.* 121). Veins are very hard to find in babies. The superior sagittal sinus is readily accessible here for either the withdrawal of blood or the giving of intravenous drugs or fluids. There are two points to remember in this connexion: (*a*) The sinus is very close to the surface, 0·32 to 0·48 cm.; (*b*) The sinus is exactly median in position.

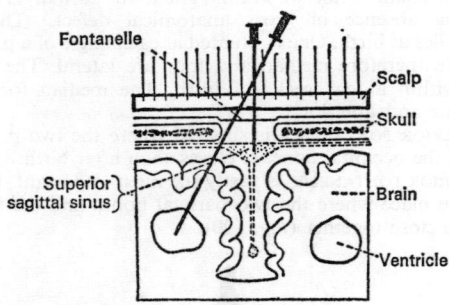

Fig. 121.—Puncture of superior sagittal sinus and lateral ventricle of brain through anterior fontanelle.

TYMPANIC ANTRUM AND MASTOID PROCESS: The tympanic (mastoid) antrum is a well-developed cavity at birth. The mastoid process does not begin to develop until the end of the 2nd year, the same age at which the mastoid air-cells begin to develop (*Fig.* 122). If it is noted that the auditory tube is relatively wide at birth and that infection easily spreads along it from the nasopharynx to the tympanic cavity, it will readily be understood that though no mastoid process exists for the first two years of life, yet mastoiditis

THE ANATOMY OF THE CHILD 131

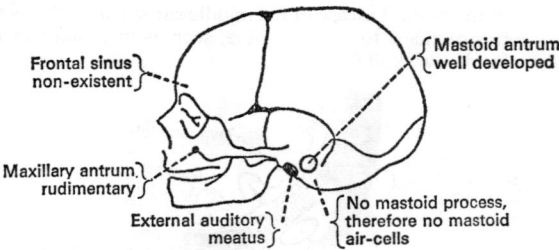

Fig. 122.—Condition of air-sinuses at birth.

is common at this period. In this connexion there are one or two anatomical points to be remembered which are of importance:

1. Before the mastoid process develops, the facial nerve is a subcutaneous structure and is in danger of being cut by an incision behind the ear which extends too far down (*Fig.* 123). In the adult the nerve is 2·54 to 3·8 cm. from the surface, being pushed to the base of the skull by the development of the mastoid process.

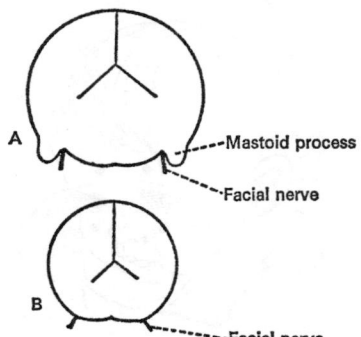

Fig. 123.—Adult skull. A, Demonstrating the protection afforded to the facial nerve in the adult by the mastoid process. B, Infant's skull; the nerve is superficial, as the mastoid process is undeveloped in the infant.

2. There is in the infant a strip of cartilage uniting the squamous and petrous parts of the temporal bone. This cartilaginous strip is very thin and lies under the dura and temporal lobe

132 A SYNOPSIS OF SURGICAL ANATOMY

of the brain. Disease of the middle ear spreads readily through this cartilage to cause trouble, such as meningitis or abscess, inside the skull (*Fig.* 124).

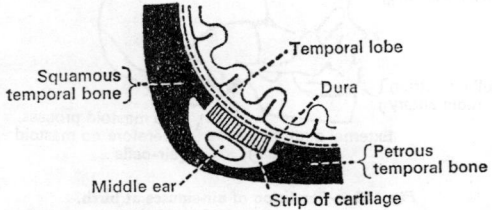

Fig. 124.—Scheme to show the readiness with which disease of the middle ear in the infant may cause intracranial complications.

FRONTAL SINUS: This does not exist at birth. It begins to develop as an outgrowth from the nose during the first year. It is rarely evident before the 7th or 8th year. It reaches full development between the 15th and 20th years.[1]

MAXILLARY ANTRUM (SINUS): At birth the maxillary antrum is rudimentary (*Fig.* 125). It reaches full development between the 15th and 20th years.

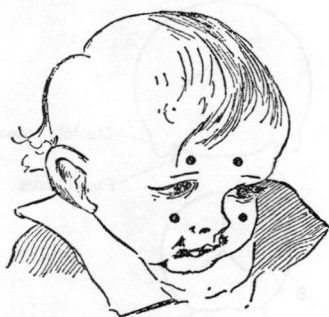

Fig. 125.—This baby is a year old. The frontal and maxillary sinuses are rudimentary and the sites of their future development are marked by black spots.

THE MANDIBLE: All traces of the cartilage uniting the two halves of the mandible at the symphysis menti have disappeared at birth. At this time they are united by fibrous tissue. Ossification is complete within the first year.

[1] Sir St. Clair Thomson *Diseases of the Nose and Throat*, 1919, 240. London.

THE ANATOMY OF THE CHILD 133

Suctorial Pad: The roundness and fullness of the infant's cheeks are due to the presence in the cheek of a large pad of fat known as the suctorial pad. This lies anterior to the masseter, on the buccinator. It is pierced by the parotid duct and is represented in adults by the buccal pad of fat which is relatively much smaller. It is of assistance in the act of sucking. It is worth noticing that the reason why the newborn child, though edentulous, does not present the unsightly appearance of the toothless adult is because the suctorial pad prevents infalling of the cheeks.

Teeth: Though the teeth only begin to appear at the sixth month of life, yet the rudiments of most of the teeth, both temporary and permanent, exist at birth. The exceptions are the second and third molars. The rudiment of the second appears at the fourth month after birth, and that of the third about the fifth year.

Larynx: (epiglottis to cricoid): In the adult lies opposite the 3rd, 4th, 5th, and 6th cervical vertebrae. In the fetus at birth it lies opposite the 3rd and 4th cervical vertebrae. It gradually descends till puberty.

Rima Glottidis: This is the same length in both sexes till puberty. After that the rima in the male grows faster, so that in the adult male the rima is 2·5 cm. long, and in the adult female only 1·8 cm. long.

Thorax: The thorax at birth and for two years after is circular on section; the adult thorax is oval (*Fig.* 126). The diameter of the adult thorax

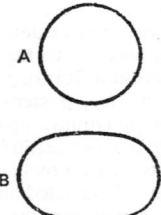

Fig. 126.—A. The circular shape of the child's thorax on section.
B, The oval shape of the adult thorax.

may therefore be increased by thoracic breathing. This is impossible in the child, as the surface area of a circle cannot be increased within a circumference the length of which remains constant. For this reason respiration in the first two years of life is almost entirely abdominal (diaphragmatic), and only in later years does intercostal (thoracic) respiration take much part in breathing. Children therefore are liable to pneumonia, etc., after abdominal operations, as there exists then an abdominal wound which is painful on respiratory movements, and the child restricts these movements as much as possible, thus interfering with the excursions of the diaphragm. The result is that the lungs are improperly ventilated and secretions tend to accumulate in them which may become infected and cause pneumonia, more particularly as expelling these secretions by coughing is intensely painful (as anyone knows who has had the unfortunate experience even in later life).

Hibernating Gland: There lies in the posterior triangle of the infant a mass of fat which extends down behind the trapezius towards the scapula. This is said to be the remains of a collection of fat which exists here in hibernating animals, acting as a storage for use during their long sleep. It is said, moreover, that this fat is histologically different from ordinary fat and may give rise to a special form of tumour.

Subcutaneous Fat: This is of a very firm feel in the healthy child, and the curves of the baby are due to the filling out of the skin by the underlying fat. In conditions of wasting from any cause the fat is absorbed and the skin becomes wrinkled and feels much thinner than in the healthy child.

Spinal Column: The child is born with two curves in its vertebral column. These are called primary curves and are thoracic and sacral in position. When the head is held up after the age of three months, its weight causes the neck to be curved with a convexity forwards. On sitting up at the age of six months, the lumbar curve develops. These two latter curves are called secondary curves (*see* p. 123).

Spinal Cord: The cord ends at a level only one vertebra lower in the newborn child than in the adult. It therefore ends at the 3rd lumbar vertebra.

Thymus Gland:

IN INFANCY: At birth the organ extends from the cricoid to the 4th costal cartilage, lying anterior to the trachea, great vessels of the thorax, and the pericardium. It is of pyramidal shape, greyish-white in colour, and has anterior, posterior, and right and left lateral surfaces. It has a definite connective-tissue sheath.

IN THE ADULT: The gland lies behind the manubrium, anterior to the great vessels of the superior mediastinum. It is noteworthy that:
1. The organ is always connected to the thyroid by a strand of tissue known as the thyrothymic ligament.
2. It receives a good blood-supply from the vessels in the neighbourhood: inferior thyroid, internal mammary, innominate, and intercostals. The venous drainage is by one or two large lobular veins going to the innominates and by superior vessels joining the thyroid veins.
3. The gland has a profuse lymphatic drainage (into internal mammary, anterior mediastinal, and paratracheal glands), noteworthy in that certain of the lymphatics open directly into veins, without first traversing lymph-glands.
4. The gland is an organ which is active during the growth period. After maturity a process of retrogression occurs in the gland, although it never entirely disappears. The old idea that the

THE ANATOMY OF THE CHILD

gland disappears at puberty is incorrect. In over 250 thymectomies for myasthenia gravis in patients between the ages of $2\frac{1}{2}$ and 60 years, Keynes[1] could always identify both lobes. The size varies at all ages between wide limits—in adults from 2·7 to 32 g.

5. Modern experimental work suggests a close physiological relationship between thyroid and thymus glands.
6. According to Holmes Sellors[2] islets of thymic tissue are occasionally found in the anterior mediastinal fatty tissue.

Abdominal Cavity:

THE LIVER is relatively very large at birth and occupies much of the abdominal cavity.

PERIRENAL FAT: There is very little perinephric fat either in infants or young children. This means that the kidney is much more intimately related to the peritoneum in young children than it is in adults. This has an important bearing in injury and disease.

In *injuries* to the kidney from external violence, the overlying peritoneum is very seldom torn in adults. In children it is much more easily torn, for no perinephric fat separates the kidney and peritoneum as is the case in adults (*Fig.* 127).

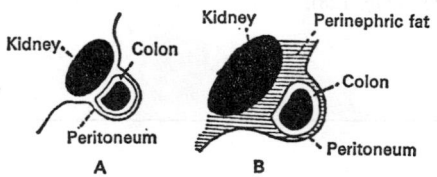

Fig. 127.—Relation of kidney to colon and overlying peritoneum. A, In the child. B, In the adult. Demonstrating the greater liability of injury to the peritoneum in the child in cases of rupture of the kidney.

With regard to *disease*, the hepatic flexure of the gut on the right and the splenic flexure on the left lie in actual contact with the kidney, no peritoneum intervening.

THE OMENTUM is small and undeveloped in infancy and childhood. The omentum, once called the 'policeman of the abdomen', is the most important factor concerned in localizing inflammatory processes in the abdominal cavity, e.g., acute appendicitis. The relative under-development of the omentum in the child is one of the factors which make inflammatory disease so serious in the abdomen of the child.

[1] Keynes, G., *Br. med. J.*, 1954, 2, 659.
[2] Holmes Sellors, T., *Report of the International Society of Surgeons*, 1961, p. 328. Imprimerie Médicale et Scientifique, 67 Rue de l'Orient, Brussels.

136   A SYNOPSIS OF SURGICAL ANATOMY

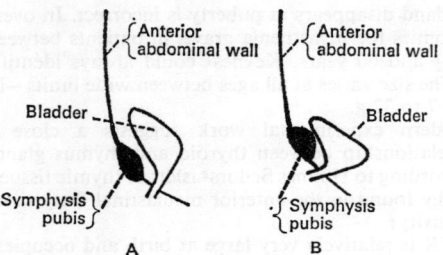

Fig. 128.—Position of the empty bladder. A, In the child, an abdominal organ. B, In the adult, a purely pelvic organ.

THE BLADDER: The cavity of the true pelvis is undeveloped at birth. There is therefore no gut in the fetal pelvis. Similarly the bladder in the child at birth and during infancy is an abdominal organ whether full or empty. In the adult it is when empty entirely pelvic in position and only rises into the cavity of the abdomen proper when distended (*Fig.* 128).

Chapter XX

NERVES

I. THE CUTANEOUS NERVE-SUPPLY OF THE HEAD AND NECK

A great number of nerves take part in supplying the skin of the head and neck (*Fig.* 129).
1. **The Fifth Cranial Nerve** is mainly responsible for the cutaneous supply of the face and scalp. All three of its divisions assist in this supply.
   THE FIRST OR OPHTHALMIC DIVISION gives:
   a. The supra-orbital nerve.
   b. The supratrochlear nerve.
   c. The infratrochlear nerve.
   d. The external nasal nerve.
   e. The lacrimal nerve.
   THE SECOND OR MAXILLARY DIVISION gives:
   a. The infra-orbital nerve, which divides into palpebral, lateral nasal, and superior labial branches.

NERVES 137

    b. The zygomatic nerve, which divides into zygomaticofacial and zygomaticotemporal.

  THE THIRD OR MANDIBULAR DIVISION gives:

    a. The auriculotemporal nerve.

    b. The mental nerve.

2. **The Tenth Cranial** or **Vagus Nerve** gives off the auricular branch of the vagus or Arnold's nerve.

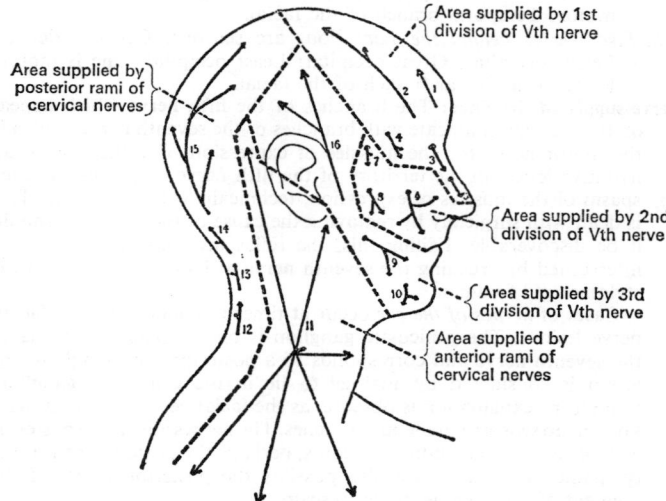

Fig. 129.—Cutaneous nerve-supply of head and neck. 1, Supratrochlear; 2, Supra-orbital; 3, Infratrochlear; 4, Lacrimal, 5, External nasal; 6, Infra-orbital; 7, Zygomaticotemporal; 8, Zygomaticofacial; 9, Buccinator; 10, Mental; 11, Anterior rami of cervical nerves; 12, 13, 14, 15, Posterior rami of cervical nerves. The broken lines demarcate the main supply areas.

3. **The Anterior Rami of the Cervical Nerves** contribute:
    a. The nervus cutaneus colli   C. 2, 3
    b. The great auricular nerve   C. 2, 3
    c. The lesser occipital nerve   C. 2
    d. The supraclavicular nerves   C. 3, 4

    These are all branches of the cervical plexus and represent all the cutaneous branches of this plexus.

4. **The Posterior Rami of the Cervical Nerves** contribute:
    a. The great occipital nerve   C. 2

b. The least or third occipital nerve   C. 3
   c. The medial branches of   C. 4, 5
   The great and least occipital nerves are the medial branches of the posterior rami of C. 2 and 3 respectively.

COMMENTS

Nerve-supply of the Scalp:
  1. *Five Nerves in Front of the Ear:* Four are sensory: Supra-orbital; Supratrochlear; Zygomaticotemporal; Auriculotemporal. One is motor: Temporal branch of the facial.
  2. *Five Nerves behind the Ear:* Four are sensory: Great auricular; Lesser occipital; Great occipital; Least occipital. One is motor: Posterior auricular branch of the facial.

Nerve-supply of the Face: The branches of the fifth nerve which appear on the face communicate with branches of the seventh nerve, which is the motor nerve for the muscles of expression. For this reason an irritative lesion in the territory of the fifth nerve may cause a reflex spasm of the muscles of expression, technically called *facial tic*. This is dealt with surgically by removing the cause of the irritation should it be discoverable. Failing this, the reflex arc may be temporarily interrupted by crushing the seventh nerve at its emergence from the stylomastoid foramen.

Cases of *herpes of the ear* occur at times in connexion with facial-nerve lesions. The geniculate ganglion is on the pars intermedia of the seventh nerve and corresponds to a posterior root ganglion; the lesion is considered by analogy to lie in the geniculate ganglion, though the explanation is obscure, as the facial nerve has, so far as is known, no sensory cutaneous branches. The herpes affects the posterior wall of the external auditory meatus, perhaps the posterior half of the tympanic membrane, and also possibly the posterior aspect of the segment of skin joining pinna to scalp.

Nerve-supply of the External Ear (*Fig.* 130):

  THE PINNA:
   THE LATERAL SURFACE is supplied by two nerves: the great auricular supplying the lower third, the auriculotemporal supplying the upper two-thirds.
   THE MEDIAL SURFACE: The lower third is supplied by the great auricular, the upper two-thirds by the lesser occipital.
  EXTERNAL AUDITORY MEATUS: If this channel be divided into two by a vertical plane in its long axis, the skin lining the anterior half is supplied by the auriculotemporal nerve, while that of the posterior half is supplied by the auricular branch of the vagus, which also supplies that narrow territory of skin which joins the pinna to the skull behind.
  TYMPANIC MEMBRANE: The outer surface of the ear-drum is covered by skin, the anterior half of which is supplied by the

NERVES 139

auriculotemporal nerve, the remaining portion by the auricular branch of the vagus.

The auricular branch of the vagus which assists in the innervation of the external auditory meatus is considered to be the remains of the nerve of the first visceral pouch. The fact, however, is not devoid of clinical significance. Leonard Williams has drawn attention to the possibility of persistent cough resulting from the

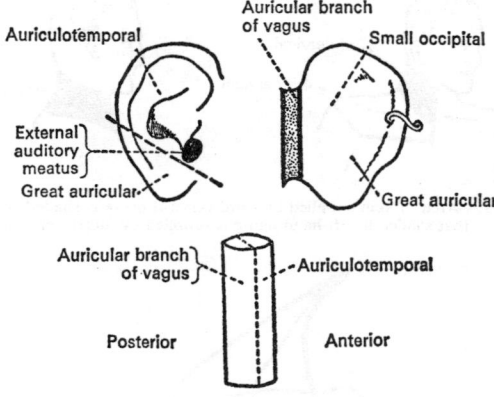

Fig. 130.—Nerve-supply of pinna and external auditory meatus. The lower figure represents the external auditory meatus.

irritation of wax in this canal; cases of intractable earache have been cured by adjusting some gastric disorder. Rarely sufferers from hiatus hernia complain of earache which disappears after the repair of the hernia. To explain these facts it is necessary to recall that the vagus supplies the lungs, bronchi, and stomach. The auricular branch of the vagus was once known as the alderman's nerve. Aldermen, those lovers of good cheer, were said, when replete at banquets, to stimulate their jaded appetites by dropping cold water behind the ear. Apparently this acted by reflexly encouraging gastric peristalsis.

The Supraclavicular Nerves arise from C. 3 and 4. It is of clinical significance that these two nerves have separate territories (*Fig.* 131). In Erb's paralysis there is often an area of anaesthesia in the territory of C. 4. Herpetic lesions may affect the territory of one only of these nerves. It is of still greater significance to observe that, in addition to the neck, these supraclavicular nerves supply the skin of the upper thorax as far down as the level of the second rib in front. The area of skin immediately below this is supplied by the second thoracic nerve. It follows, therefore, that a transverse lesion of the spinal cord anywhere between the fourth cervical and second thoracic segments will give the same level of anaesthesia or line of hyperaesthesia anteriorly. For this reason this is the only region of the body where such a line is of little assistance in determining the exact level of the cord lesion. The

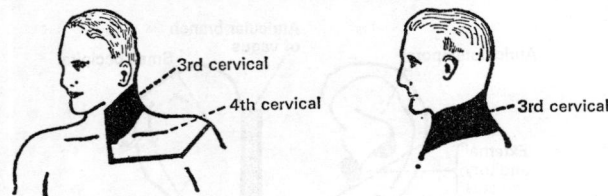

Fig. 131.—Area of skin supplied by third cervical nerve is shaded. Area below that shaded in left-hand figure is supplied by fourth cervical.

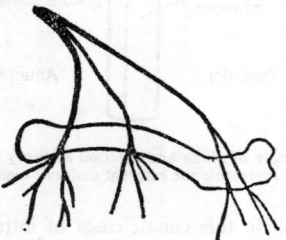

Fig. 132.—The descending supraclavicular nerves.

supraclavicular nerves cross the clavicle (*Fig.* 132). Occasionally one of the nerves may pass through a foramen in the clavicle. Excessive pain may follow if a branch of the nerve is involved in the callus following a fractured collar-bone. Apart from fracture, irritation of one of the nerves may cause severe pain. Stiles advises resection of a part of the middle supraclavicular nerve when it is exposed in incisions above the middle third of the clavicle, to avoid its inclusion in scar tissue later.

Other Points to be Noted: Observe that:
1. The area of the cheek supplied by the great auricular nerve is immediately in front of the angle of the jaw and is about 3 cm. in diameter.

NERVES 141

2. The lowest cervical nerve to give a cutaneous branch is: in front, C. 4; behind, C. 5.
3. The only cervical nerves to give cutaneous branches are: anterior rami, C. 2, 3, 4; posterior rami, C. 2, 3, 4, 5.

II. THE GANGLIA OF THE FIFTH NERVE

The fifth nerve is:
1. The sensory nerve of the face and front half of the scalp.
2. The motor nerve to the muscles of mastication, excepting the buccinator.
3. It has been regarded as the nerve of taste, but *see* p. 147.

This extraordinary nerve is characterized by the great number of communications it makes with the facial nerve (motor to the face) and by the number of ganglia situated on it. It communicates with every branch of the facial which appears on the face.

The fifth nerve has five ganglia on it: (1) The semilunar or Gasserian on the nerve-trunk; (2) The ciliary on the first or ophthalmic division; (3) The sphenopalatine on the second or maxillary division; (4) The otic on the third or mandibular division; (5) The submaxillary (Langley's) on the third or mandibular division.

All these ganglia, except the semilunar, receive motor, sensory, and sympathetic roots.

Semilunar (Gasserian) Ganglion: Corresponds to the ganglion on the posterior root of a spinal nerve. The plan of this ganglion is therefore the same as that of the cerebrospinal ganglia (*Fig.* 133). The ganglion is half-moon-shaped, with two surfaces, upper and lower, and two borders, posterosuperior and antero-inferior.

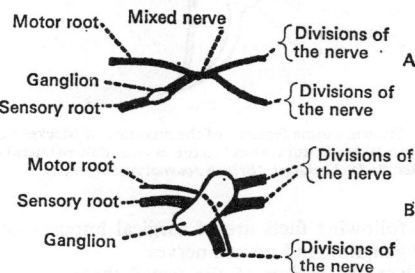

Fig. 133.—To show that the semilunar ganglion is the homologue of the ganglion on the posterior root of a spinal nerve. A, Spinal nerve. B, Fifth nerve.

RELATIONS:

THE LOWER SURFACE is in relation to the bed of the ganglion—that is, a hollow on the apex of the petrous temporal bone and the cartilage filling the foramen lacerum. The great superficial petrosal and great deep petrosal nerves join under the ganglion to form the nerve of the pterygoid canal (Vidian). The motor root of the fifth nerve (portio minor) is under the ganglion.

THE UPPER SURFACE is related to the gyrus hippocampus of the temporal lobe.

MEDIAL is the cavernous sinus and internal carotid artery.

THE POSTEROSUPERIOR BORDER gives off the sensory root.

THE ANTERO-INFERIOR BORDER: Three nerves join it: first, second, and third divisions of the fifth nerve.

The motor root makes no connexion with the ganglion, but goes through the foramen ovale to join the mandibular division outside the skull.

THE DURAL RELATIONS are of great surgical importance. At each side of the pituitary body there lies between two layers of dura mater the cavernous blood-sinus. Invaginated into the sinus through the opening through which the fifth nerve leaves the posterior fossa is a diverticulum of dura (*Fig.* 134). This is Meckel's cave, which contains: (1) The sensory and motor roots of the fifth nerve; (2) The semilunar (Gasserian) ganglion; (3) The terminations of the 1st, 2nd, and 3rd divisions of the fifth nerve.

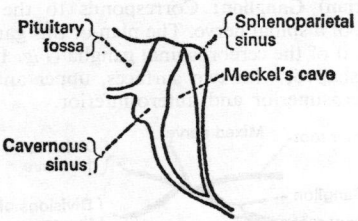

Fig. 134.—Showing some features of the anatomy of Meckel's cave. Observe that there are two layers of dura lateral to the cave, and three lateral to the cavernous sinus. (*After R. D. Lockhart, 'British Journal of Surgery'.*)

The following facts are of surgical importance in operations on the ganglion and related nerves.

1. Over the region of the 'cave' three layers of dura form the lower half of the outer wall of the cavernous sinus (*Fig.* 135).
2. The outer wall of the cave is fused with the dura bounding the sinus laterally.
3. The outer wall of the cave is not adherent to the ganglion.
4. The inner wall of the cave is adherent to the ganglion.

NERVES 143

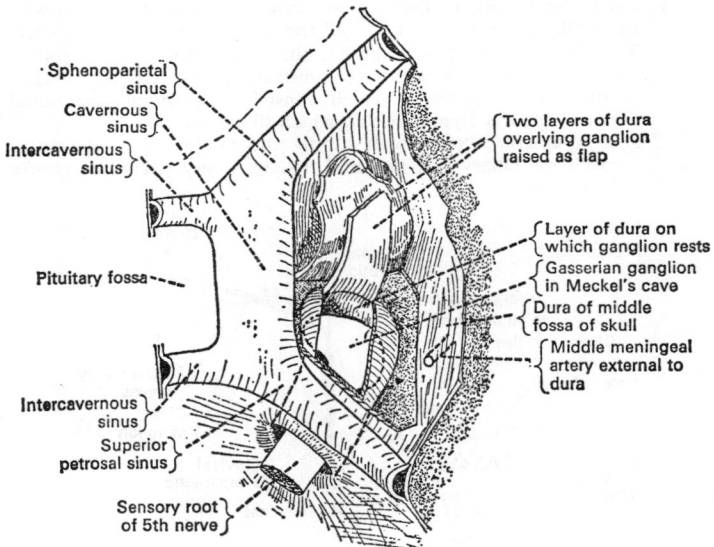

Fig. 135.—Diagrammatic representation of Meckel's cave, to show the dural relations of the semilunar ganglion and the venous sinuses in its vicinity. Notice that the middle meningeal artery is immediately lateral to the ganglion.

5. Between the outer wall of the cave and the dura bounding the sinus laterally are found: (*a*) *Posteriorly*—The superior petrosal sinus widening out to join the cavernous sinus; (*b*) *Anteriorly*—The sphenoparietal sinus joining the cavernous sinus (sometimes). Because of these vascular relationships the surgeon in approaching the ganglion goes through the middle region of the outer wall of the cave.

Ciliary Ganglion: This is the size of a pin's head.

SITUATION: Near the apex of the orbit—between the optic nerve medially and the lateral rectus on the outer side.

ROOTS:

MOTOR: From the inferior branch of the oculomotor nerve.

SENSORY: From the nasociliary branch of the first division of the fifth nerve.

SYMPATHETIC: From the plexus round the ophthalmic artery.

144 A SYNOPSIS OF SURGICAL ANATOMY

BRANCHES: Fifteen to twenty short ciliary nerves which pass with the optic nerve to the back of the eyeball, which they pierce. The short ciliary nerves supply: the ciliary body (oculomotor), which is concerned with accommodation; the circular muscle of the iris (oculomotor), which constricts the pupil; the radial fibres of the iris (sympathetic), which dilate the pupil.

The sympathetic fibres which supply the dilator pupillae muscle reach the ciliary ganglion and iris by a very circuitous course (*Fig.* 136):

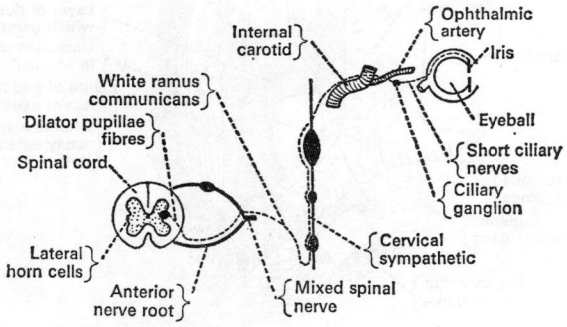

Fig. 136.—Ciliary ganglion. Dotted line represents course of sympathetic fibres which supply dilator pupillae muscle.

1. Fibres arise from a centre in the frontal lobe of the brain which go to the pupil-dilating centre in the medulla and thence to the ciliospinal centre in the lower cervical cord.
2. Fibres take origin from the cells of the lateral column of the spinal cord in the lower cervical and upper thoracic region (C. 7, 8, T. 1).
3. They leave the cord by the anterior root of the second thoracic nerve, which gives off the second white ramus to the sympathetic chain.
4. They travel up the whole length of the cervical sympathetic trunk in the neck.
5. They join the cranial sympathetic trunk, that is, the plexus which the cervical sympathetic gives off at its upper end to accompany the internal carotid into the skull.
6. They leave the internal carotid in the cavernous sinus to accompany the sympathetic plexus round the ophthalmic artery.

NERVES 145

7. They leave the ophthalmic artery as the sympathetic root to the ciliary ganglion.
8. They leave the ciliary ganglion in the short ciliary nerves to pierce the eyeball and supply the radial (dilator) fibres of the iris.[1]

ARGYLL ROBERTSON PUPIL: In locomotor ataxia and general paralysis of the insane (diseases of the cord and brain) the pupil usually becomes very small, and contracts to accommodation but not to light (observe the 'a' of Argyll and of accommodation). The lesion is thought to lie in the ciliary ganglion. Tumours of the superior corpora quadrigemina may cause a similar phenomenon.

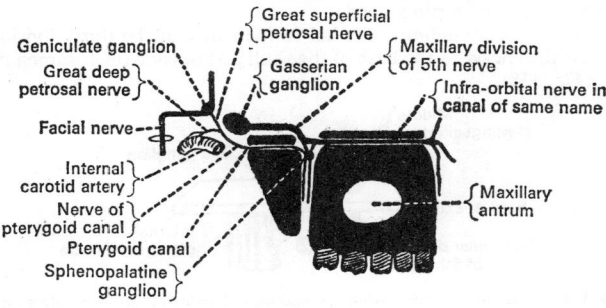

Fig. 137.—Sphenopalatine ganglion (Meckel's).

Sphenopalatine or Meckel's Ganglion: Connected with the maxillary division of the fifth nerve. It is the size of the head of a small tack (*Fig.* 137).

POSITION: In the upper part of the pterygopalatine fossa.

ROOTS:

MOTOR AND SYMPATHETIC: They reach the ganglion through the nerve of the pterygoid canal (Vidian). This nerve is formed in the skull underneath the semilunar ganglion by the union of a nerve from the geniculate ganglion of the facial (great superficial petrosal) with a branch from the plexus round the carotid (great deep petrosal). It reaches the posterior border of the ganglion through a bony canal—the Vidian or pterygoid canal.

SENSORY: From the maxillary division of the fifth nerve.

---

[1] Observe that this account of the dilator pupillae fibres is that given by anatomists. Neurologists, e.g., Purves-Stewart and Cameron, state that the fibres leave the sympathetic in the skull, go to the semilunar ganglion, thence via its ophthalmic division to the nasociliary nerve; they are conveyed to the iris by the long ciliary nerves without going through the ciliary ganglion.

BRANCHES: The ganglion and its connexions resemble a man hanging on by two arms to the rope formed by the maxillary nerve. The branches run in all directions except outward and forward:

ASCENDING: Orbital to the periosteum of the orbit.

DESCENDING: Anterior palatine to palate. This nerve gives off the middle and posterior palatine nerves and one of the nasal nerves.

INWARD: Nasopalatine and nasal—to nose and septum through the sphenopalatine foramen which is just internal to the ganglion.

BACKWARDS: The pharyngeal—through the canal of the same name to the mucous membrane of the roof of the pharynx.

Otic Ganglion: Connected to the mandibular division of the fifth nerve. It is the size of a pin's head.

POSITION: Very definite. Medial to the trunk of the third division of the fifth nerve at the base of the skull just outside the foramen ovale (*Fig.* 138).

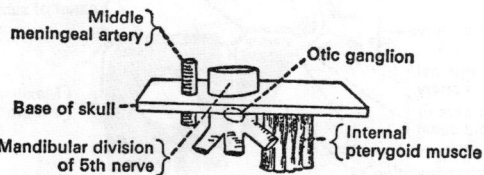

Fig. 138.—Schematic representation of mandibular division of fifth nerve showing, as a dotted circle, the otic ganglion medial to the nerve.

RELATIONS:
  LATERAL: Mandibular nerve.
  MEDIAL: Tensor palati muscle.
  POSTERIOR: Middle meningeal artery.
  ANTERIOR: Internal pterygoid muscle.

ROOTS:
  MOTOR: From the nerve to the internal pterygoid (from mandibular).
  SENSORY: The lesser superficial petrosal (fibres from the seventh and ninth cranial nerves).
  SYMPATHETIC: From the plexus on the middle meningeal artery.

BRANCHES:
  1. MOTOR to two tensors—the tensor tympani and tensor palati.
  2. SECRETORY to the auriculotemporal nerve—carrying secretory fibres for the parotid (probably derived from the glossopharyngeal through the small superficial petrosal).

COMMUNICATIONS:
  1. To the auriculotemporal nerve.
  2. To the nerve of the pterygoid canal.
  3. To the chorda tympani nerve.

NERVES 147

Submaxillary or Langley's Ganglion: It is the size of a pin's head.
POSITION: On the outer surface of the hyoglossus muscle depending from the lingual nerve (*Fig.* 139).

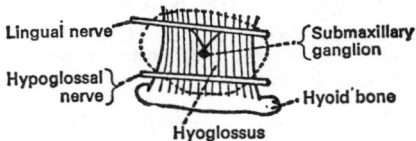

Fig. 139.—Submaxillary or Langley's ganglion. The dotted line is the submaxillary gland.

RELATIONS:
  LATERAL: Submaxillary gland.
  MEDIAL: Hyoglossus muscle.
  ABOVE: Lingual nerve.
  BELOW: Submaxillary duct.
ROOTS:
  MOTOR (secretory): From the chorda tympani (facial) through the lingual.
  SENSORY: From the lingual.
  SYMPATHETIC: From the plexus round the external maxillary artery.
BRANCHES: It hangs from the lingual nerve by two filaments, the posterior going from the lingual to the ganglion, the anterior going from the ganglion to the lingual, to be distributed through it: (1) To the submaxillary gland and duct; (2) To the sublingual gland; (3) To the mucous membrane of the mouth and tongue (through the lingual nerve).

Pathway for Taste: In early editions of this work the accepted view at that time was enunciated that the fifth nerve is the ultimate pathway for all taste sensations. Following, however, the observations of Cushing and others that removal of the Gasserian or semilunar ganglion causes no permanent loss of the sensation of taste, the view then held becomes untenable.

1. Taste sensation in the anterior two-thirds of the tongue passes via the lingual nerve to the chorda tympani, thence to the facial nerve in the canal for the facial nerve, and so to the geniculate ganglion, whence the impulses go in the nervus intermedius to the pons.

2. From the posterior third of the tongue taste sensations pass via the glossopharyngeal nerve to the brain-stem. Temporary loss of taste over the anterior two-thirds of the tongue may follow removal of the semilunar ganglion. This is due to swelling of the axons of the lingual nerve consequent on their degeneration,

148 A SYNOPSIS OF SURGICAL ANATOMY

this swelling causing pressure on the taste fibres travelling via the lingual to the chorda tympani. Taste returns when degeneration is complete.

III. THE NERVES IN THE NECK

These are: (1) Cranial nerves: 7, 9, 10, 11, and 12. (2) Cervical nerves: (*a*) 1–8, anterior divisions; (*b*) 1–8, posterior divisions. (3) Thoracic nerves: 1. (4) Cervical sympathetic.

Cranial Nerves

Seventh: Facial Nerve: Emerges from the stylomastoid foramen at a point 2·5–4 cm. deep to the middle of the anterior border of the mastoid process. Almost at once it enters the parotid gland. Before doing so it gives off three branches:

Posterior auricular: This nerve associates itself with the artery of that name, and runs back in the groove behind the pinna to supply the occipitalis muscle and the auricularis posterior.

Nerve to stylohyoid: A long thin twig.

Nerve to digastric (posterior belly): A short fat twig, which gives a communication to the glossopharyngeal nerve, which communication soon leaves this latter, as the nerve to the stylopharyngeus.

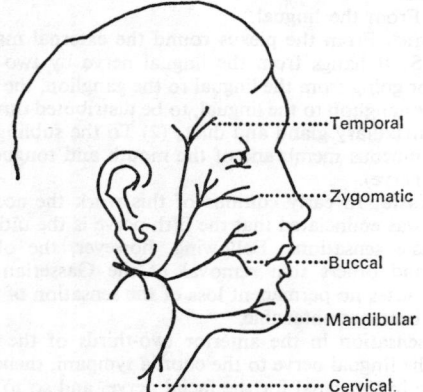

Fig. 140.—The facial nerve after its emergence from the stylomastoid foramen.

In the parotid the facial lies superficial to the posterior facial vein and external carotid artery. It soon divides into two divisions: (1) The *temporofacial* which runs sharply upward; (2) The *cervicofacial*

NERVES 149

which continues the course of the parent trunk downwards, forwards, and outwards (*Fig.* 140). These divisions in turn divide to form the goose's foot (pes anserinus), the branches of which leave the anterior border of the parotid and pass as five twigs to the temporal, zygomatic, buccal, mandibular, and cervical regions, to supply the muscles of expression, which include the buccinator, the frontalis, and the platysma. All these nerves communicate on the face with branches of the fifth cranial.

THE MANDIBULAR BRANCH OF THE FACIAL has important relations. It passes down, continuing the course of the main trunk, just *behind* the angle of the mandible. It then lies deep to the platysma between it and the deep cervical fascia, crossing the inferolateral surface of the submaxillary gland. It turns *up* and crosses the lower border of the mandible to supply the quadratus labii inferioris muscle. Incisions made behind the angle of the jaw, e.g., mastoid process to hyoid bone, will cut this branch of the facial unless the cut is made at least 2·5 cm. behind the angle. The result of division of the nerve is temporary paralysis of the muscle, so that the mouth will be asymmetrical.

The Last Four Cranial Nerves lie together at the base of the skull, where they are all anterior to the internal jugular vein and posterior to the internal carotid artery. They soon diverge from each other.

Ninth: Glossopharyngeal Nerve: Crosses the internal carotid superficially, lying deep to the external carotid, hooks round the stylopharyngeus muscle, runs deep to the hyoglossus, and so reaches the base of the tongue. Where it lies in the jugular foramen it has two ganglia on it:
(1) The superior ganglion, which is small and gives no branches;
(2) The petrous ganglion, which is larger and communicates with:
(*a*) The superior cervical sympathetic ganglion; (*b*) The auricular branch of the vagus; (*c*) The ganglion nodosum of the vagus. The petrous ganglion gives off:

THE TYMPANIC BRANCH: The tympanic branch of the glossopharyngeal nerve (Jacobson's nerve) goes to the otic ganglion on the third division of the fifth nerve. Although the fifth and ninth nerves lie near each other at the base of the skull, the tympanic nerve takes a long detour to get to its destination (*Fig.* 141). It passes through a small foramen easily found on the sharp bony ridge separating the carotid canal from the jugular foramen, and so reaches the medial wall of the tympanic cavity. Here it breaks up into a plexus—the tympanic plexus—which supplies the mucous membrane of the middle ear, the mastoid cells, and the auditory tube. It is assisted in the formation of this plexus by two twigs from the sympathetic plexus round the internal carotid artery (the superior and inferior caroticotympanic nerves). The tympanic nerve then leaves the plexus as a twig which lies in the petrous bone, and is soon joined by a nerve from the geniculate ganglion of the facial nerve. The nerve formed by this junction is the *small superficial petrosal nerve*, which lies in a groove on the upper surface of the petrous temporal bone just lateral to the groove for the great superficial petrosal nerve. The small petrosal then leaves the skull, passing either through the suture between the great wing of sphenoid and petrous temporal, or through the foramen ovale, or through

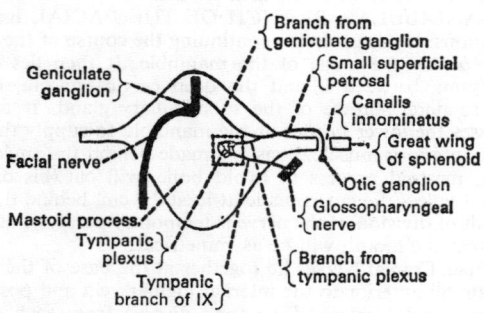

Fig. 141.—Small superficial petrosal nerve.

the canalis innominatus (a tiny foramen sometimes present which lies posterior to the foramen ovale). Having left the skull, the small petrosal enters the otic ganglion on the tensor palati muscle as its sensory and secretory roots. The secretory fibres to the parotid gland, which reach it via the auriculotemporal nerve, are brought to the otic ganglion by the small superficial petrosal, and reach the auriculotemporal in a twig sent to it from the otic ganglion.

The glossopharyngeal nerve itself gives the following branches: (1) Communicating from facial; (2) Nerve to the stylopharyngeus; (3) Pharyngeal; (4) Tonsillar; (5) Lingual. (*Fig.* 142.)

It has been shown that the communication to the glossopharyngeal from the facial arises from the nerve to the posterior belly of the digastric, and this communication is given off again incorporated in the nerve to the stylopharyngeus. This latter nerve is given off by the glossopharyngeal where the latter hooks round the stylopharyngeus. Having supplied this muscle, most of its fibres pass into the pharynx to the mucous membrane.

PHARYNGEAL NERVES:

1. Small branches to the mucous membrane of the pharynx.
2. A large branch which goes to the pharyngeal plexus.

NERVES 151

TONSILLAR NERVES: These come off at the base of the tongue and form the plexus known as the circulus tonsillaris over the tonsil, which supplies also the mucous membrane of the soft palate and isthmus faucium.

LINGUAL NERVES: The terminal branches of the glossopharyngeal supply the posterior third of the tongue with the special sense of taste and with ordinary sensation (touch, heat, cold). The anterior two-thirds of the tongue are supplied with special sense by the chorda tympani branch of the facial, and with ordinary sensation by the lingual branch of the trigeminal.

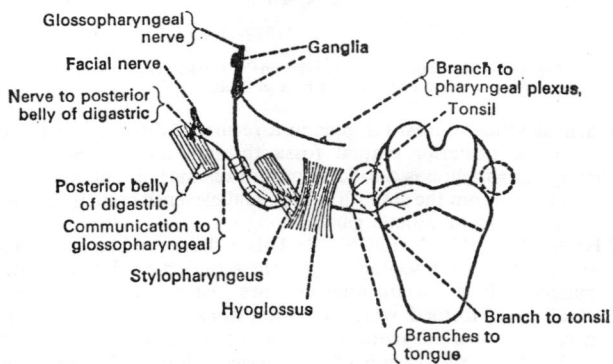

Fig. 142.—Glossopharyngeal nerve.

Tenth: Vagus Nerve: The tenth cranial nerve pursues a perfectly straight course from the jugular foramen to where it enters the thorax by crossing the first part of the subclavian artery on the right, and passing anterior to the subclavian on the left. At the base of the skull it is posterior to the internal carotid, in front of the internal jugular, and associated with the ninth, eleventh, and twelfth cranial nerves; it soon comes to lie in the groove between the jugular and carotid in the carotid sheath, and keeps this position in relation first to the internal and then to the common carotid (*Fig.* 143). It presents, therefore, very much the same relationship as the common and internal carotids lying in front of the cervical sympathetic trunk. It has two important ganglia on it: (1) The ganglion jugulare; (2) The ganglion nodosum.

1. THE JUGULAR GANGLION: This is in the jugular foramen. It gives off: (*a*) The auricular nerve; (*b*) A meningeal nerve; (*c*) Branches of communication.

   a. THE AURICULAR (ALDERMAN'S NERVE OR ARNOLD'S NERVE) passes outwards across the bulb of the internal jugular vein and enters a canal in the outer wall of the jugular foramen. It emerges between the anterior border of the mastoid process and the external acoustic meatus. It communicates three times with the facial nerve, twice in the bone, and once behind the ear. It supplies the posterior half of the skin lining the acoustic meatus and tympanic membrane.

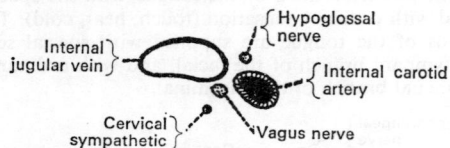

Fig. 143.—Showing immediate relations of right internal carotid a little below base of skull.

b. THE MENINGEAL BRANCH goes in a recurrent direction to the dura of the posterior cranial fossa through the jugular foramen. The jugular ganglion is a kind of nerve-exchange, as communications reach it from the seventh, ninth, and eleventh cranial nerves and superior sympathetic ganglion.

2. THE GANGLION NODOSUM: This is the second largest ganglion in the neck, being second only to the superior cervical sympathetic ganglion. It is 1·8 cm. long and lies just below the base of the skull. It is formed where the accessory portion of the spinal accessory joins the vagus, and is connected by big *communications* with: (1) The first loop of the cervical plexus; (2) The superior cervical sympathetic ganglion; and (3) The hypoglossal nerve.

It gives off two important nerves: (1) The pharyngeal; (2) The superior laryngeal.

THE PHARYNGEAL BRANCH OF THE VAGUS passes as one or two nerves between the internal and external carotids to the pharyngeal plexus on the middle constrictor.

THE SUPERIOR LARYNGEAL NERVE passes deep to both the internal and external carotids. It divides deep to the internal carotid into the internal and external laryngeal nerves.

The Internal Laryngeal Nerve passes under the posterior border of the thyrohyoid muscle, pierces the membrane of the same name together with the superior laryngeal vessels, and supplies the mucous membrane of the larynx (superior laryngeal—sensory to the larynx).

The External Laryngeal Nerve passes downwards on the inferior constrictor deep to and parallel to the superior thyroid artery and supplies the cricothyroid muscle and the inferior constrictor. It is noteworthy that the cricothyroid gets a different supply to the other laryngeal muscles. Hilton called the cricothyroid muscle the 'tuning-fork of the larynx'. This muscle is a tensor of the vocal cords. When a sound is about to be uttered the external laryngeal nerve carries instructions to the cricothyroid as to the degree of tension of the cords necessary to produce the required inflection; the other motor impulses must take the longer route to the larynx via the recurrent nerves. When these reach their destination the larynx is already 'tuned' for the sound.

The vagal trunk itself gives off in the neck: (1) Two superior cervical cardiac nerves; (2) the right recurrent nerve.

THE SUPERIOR CERVICAL CARDIAC BRANCHES of the vagus, two in number, run down in the carotid sheath. On the right side, five cervical cardiac nerves (two superior cardiac branches of the vagus, the cardiac branches of the superior, middle, and inferior cervical sympathetic ganglia) cross the first part of the subclavian artery and are then joined by the cardiac branch of the right recurrent nerve on their way to the deep cardiac plexus. On the left side the cardiac nerves are anterior to the subclavian, and two of them, the superior cervical cardiac branch of the sympathetic and the inferior cervical cardiac branch of the vagus, go to the superficial cardiac plexus.

THE RECURRENT NERVE: On the *right* side this nerve arises as the vagus crosses the subclavian artery. It hooks round that vessel, and, passing up behind the common carotid, reaches the groove between the oesophagus and trachea, and, running along the medial surface of the lobe of the thyroid gland, disappears under the lower border of the inferior constrictor, behind the cricothyroid joint, into the larynx, being called the inferior laryngeal nerve. It is accompanied under the constrictor by the inferior laryngeal branch of the inferior thyroid artery, and is motor to all the muscles of the larynx except the cricothyroid. On the *left* side, when it enters the neck the recurrent nerve already lies in the groove between the trachea and oesophagus.

The recurrent nerves supply the *inferior cervical cardiac branches* of the vagus to the deep cardiac plexus, and in addition to supplying the muscles of the larynx, they give branches to the inferior constrictor, trachea, and oesophagus.

Eleventh: Spinal Accessory Nerve: Consists really of a spinal nerve and a cerebral nerve.

The cerebral portion joins the ganglion nodosum of the vagus and is distributed through the vagus. It supplies all the striped muscle which the vagus innervates, i.e., larynx, pharynx, soft palate, and also the inhibitory nerve to the heart.

The spinal part of the spinal accessory nerve descends between the internal jugular and internal carotid, then turns and passes over or under the internal jugular, to cross the transverse process of the atlas. It passes under the posterior belly of the digastric and the occipital artery, and enters the anterior border of the sternomastoid muscle (*Fig.* 144). It emerges from the posterior border of this muscle and in this situation is related to certain glands of the upper deep cervical chain, which drain the pharyngeal tonsil (adenoids). When enlarged, e.g., tuberculous adenitis, these glands actually envelop the nerve, and it is in danger during excision of such glands. The nerve then crosses the posterior triangle, enters the trapezius, and ends in the substance of this muscle at the lowest point of origin of the trapezius (i.e., 12th thoracic vertebral spine).

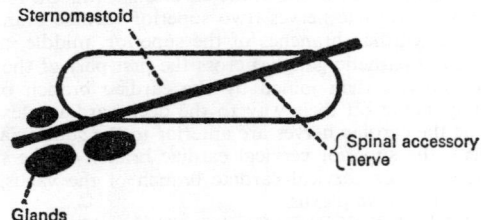

Fig. 144.—Transverse section through right sternomastoid. Relation of glands draining adenoids to spinal accessory nerve.

The spinal part of the spinal accessory nerve supplies, therefore, only the sternomastoid and the trapezius. Whilst in the sternomastoid it communicates with C. 2, and in the trapezius with C. 3 and 4. Where it is crossed by the occipital artery, the artery gives off a sternomastoid branch which accompanies the nerve into the sternomastoid muscle. Sir Harold Stiles stressed the value of this bloodvessel as the surgeon's guide to the nerve in operations in this region.

Twelfth: Hypoglossal Nerve: Emerges from the hypoglossal canal just in front of the foramen magnum, and passes medial both to the internal jugular and the internal carotid. It then curves laterally, working round the ganglion nodosum of the vagus, and comes to lie in front in the groove between the internal carotid and internal jugular. (The vagus lies in the groove between these two vessels behind.) At the lower border of the digastric the nerve crosses both carotids, hooking round the origin of the occipital artery from the external carotid, lies on the hyoglossus deep to the submaxillary gland, and at the anterior border of this muscle it enters the genioglossus and breaks up into its terminal branches. It is a purely motor nerve.

The hypoglossal supplies all the intrinsic and extrinsic muscles of the tongue except the palatoglossus. It therefore supplies all the muscles whose names end in -glossus, except the palatoglossus. It supplies also the geniohyoid and the thyrohyoid. The nerve to the thyrohyoid is a separate branch, so named.

The hypoglossal receives a communication from the first cervical nerve. At the point where it hooks round the occipital artery it gives off a nerve which is called the descendens hypoglossi. This nerve takes part in the formation of the ansa hypoglossi, and it, together with the nerves to the thyrohyoid and geniohyoid, is derived from the fibres which the hypoglossal receives from C.1.

Because of the proximity of facial, accessory, and hypoglossal nerves at the base of the skull, one or other of the two latter is used in the operation of anastomosis to the facial nerve in cases of paralysis of the face.

The Cervical Sympathetic

This nerve-trunk (*Fig.* 145) lies in the prevertebral fascia between the carotid sheath in front and the prevertebral muscles (longus colli and capitis) behind. At its lower part it is continuous with the sympathetic

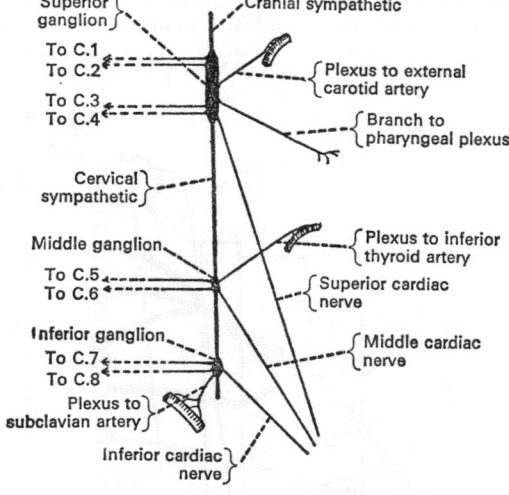

Fig. 145.—The cervical sympathetic.

trunk in the thorax; above, it is continued into the skull as a plexus of nerves round the internal carotid artery, which is sometimes called the cranial sympathetic.

156 A SYNOPSIS OF SURGICAL ANATOMY

Ganglia: There are three ganglia on the cervical sympathetic trunk. The upper and lower are large, the middle small. Each of the three ganglia gives: (1) Grey rami communicantes to the cervical nerves; (2) A cardiac nerve; and (3) A plexus to an artery. White rami communicantes are not given off in the neck.

THE SUPERIOR CERVICAL SYMPATHETIC GANGLION: The largest ganglion in the neck. It lies in front of the transverse processes of the 2nd and 3rd cervical vertebrae on the longus capitis, behind the carotid sheath. It gives: (1) Grey rami to C. 1–4; (2) A plexus to the external carotid; (3) The superior cardiac nerve; (4) The pharyngeal branch to the pharyngeal plexus. In addition, the plexus round the internal carotid leaves its upper end, and it communicates with the vagus, glossopharyngeal, and hypoglossal nerves.

THE MIDDLE CERVICAL GANGLION: The smallest of the three. Lies on the 6th cervical vertebra, in front of or behind the inferior thyroid artery. It is always present. It was formerly described as being frequently absent. This is because the ganglion sometimes occupies a lower position, near the inferior ganglion, of which it was considered a part. It gives: (1) Grey rami to C. 5, 6; (2) A

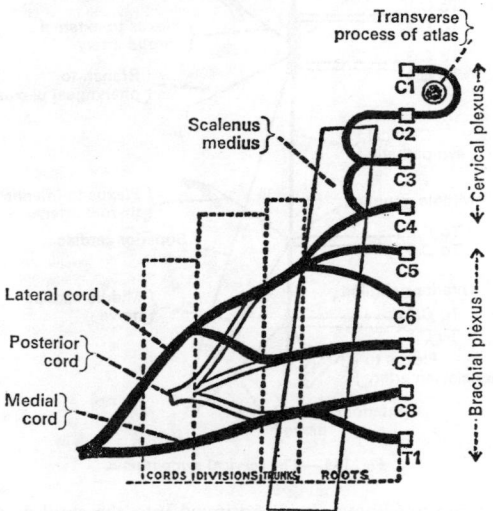

Fig. 146.—To show continuity of cervical and brachial plexuses and their relationship to the middle scalene.

plexus to the inferior thyroid artery; (3) The middle cardiac nerve. It is connected to the inferior ganglion by two or more filaments, one of which crosses the subclavian artery and is called the ansa subclavia (Vieussens).

THE INFERIOR CERVICAL GANGLION: This is large, and lies *behind* the vertebral artery between the neck of the first rib and the transverse process of the 7th cervical vertebra. It gives: (1) Grey rami to C. 7, 8; (2) A plexus to the subclavian artery and its branches; (3) The inferior cardiac nerve.

The Plexuses on the Scalenus Medius

There are four plexuses in the neck. Three are nervous: the cervical, brachial, and pharyngeal. One is venous: the pharyngeal. The first two of these lie on the middle scalene, the other two lie on the middle constrictor.

The cervical plexus is a plexus of *loops*, the brachial plexus is a plexus of *cords* (*Fig.* 146). The cervical plexus supplies skin and muscles of the neck and the diaphragm. The brachial plexus supplies the upper limb.

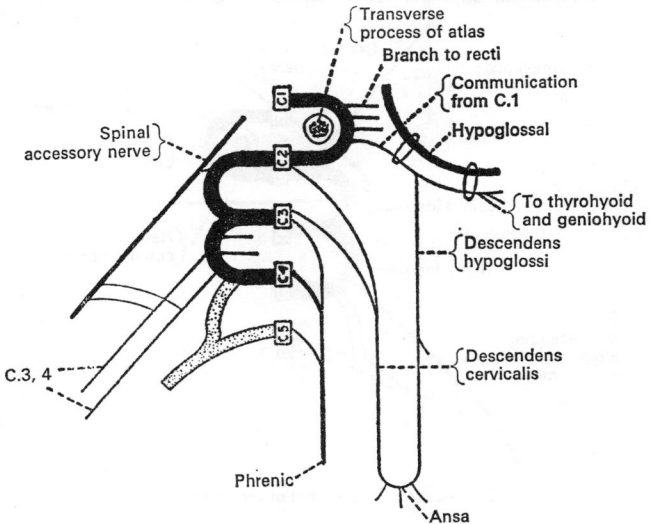

Fig. 147.—Cervical plexus and ansa hypoglossi. Observe that first loop of plexus is directed forwards.

Both plexuses are formed by anterior divisions of spinal nerves. Anterior divisions of spinal nerves have a tendency to form plexuses, e.g., cervical, brachial, lumbar, sacral. The posterior divisions have no such tendency.

158   A SYNOPSIS OF SURGICAL ANATOMY

Cervical Plexus: Lies on the scalenus medius and levator angulae scapulae under cover of the sternomastoid. It is formed by the upper four cervical nerves, each of which divides into two, except the first. The first nerve joins the upper branch of C. 2, the adjoining upper and lower branches fuse, and the lower branch of C. 4 joins C. 5 in the formation of the brachial plexus. In this way three loops are formed, the first of which is directed *forwards* in front of the transverse process of the atlas, the other two are directed backwards (*Fig.* 147).

BRANCHES OF THE CERVICAL PLEXUS: The branches of the plexus consist of two groups, superficial (cutaneous) and deep (muscular). The deep branches are divided into anterior and posterior.

SUPERFICIAL (*Fig.* 148):

Nervus cutaneus colli	C. 2, 3
Small occipital nerve	C. 2
Great auricular nerve	C. 2, 3
Descending supraclavicular nerves	C. 3, 4

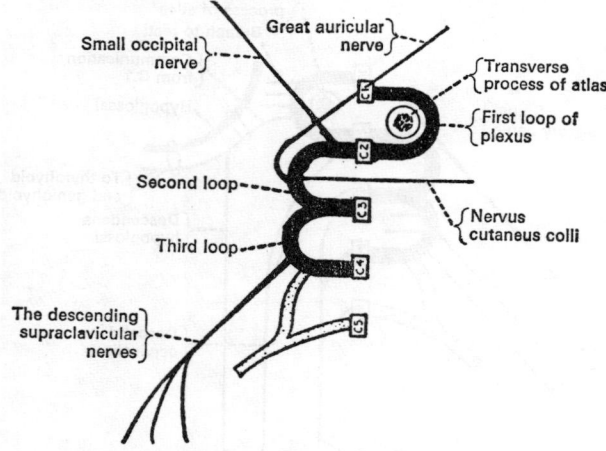

Fig. 148.—Cutaneous branches of cervical plexus.

DEEP:

Anterior:

Phrenic nerve	C. 3, 4, 5
Muscular branches to:	
Thyrohyoid	C. 1
Geniohyoid	C. 1

Rectus capitis lateralis	C. 1
Rectus capitis anterior	C. 1
Longus capitis	C. 1–4
Longus colli	C. 3–8
Scalenus anterior	C. 4–6
Intertransversales	C. 1–8

Posterior:

Sternomastoid	C. 2
Levator scapulae	C. 3, 4
Trapezius	C. 3, 4
Scalenus medius	C. 3–7

COMMUNICATING

1. With sympathetic: Each of the four nerves taking part in the formation of the plexus receives a grey ramus communicans from the superior cervical sympathetic ganglion.

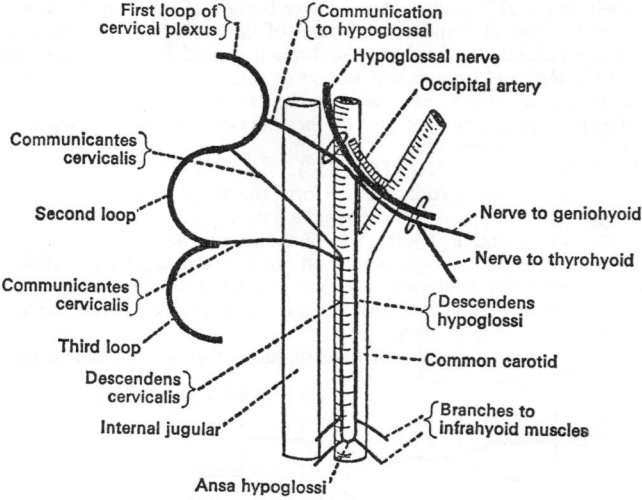

Fig. 149.—The ansa hypoglossi.

2. With hypoglossal from C. 1. This nerve may be called the communicans hypoglossi. It joins the hypoglossal and after a short course with this nerve, leaves it as the nerve to geniohyoid, thyrohyoid, and the descendens hypoglossi nerve. The latter nerve runs down on the front of the carotid sheath, and having supplied the anterior belly of the omohyoid, it joins

160 A SYNOPSIS OF SURGICAL ANATOMY

the descendens cervicalis nerve (formed by the junction of the communicantes cervicalis nerves from C. 2, 3) to form a loop, lying in front of the carotid sheath, known as the ansa hypoglossi (*Fig.* 149). This loop supplies the sternohyoid, sternothyroid, and the posterior belly of the omohyoid. The ansa hypoglossi is derived therefore from C. 1, 2, 3.

Brachial Plexus: This is a plexus of cords. It concerns the doctor more than any other plexus in the body, because of its liability to violence both at birth and subsequently, whether this be traumatic or operative. It is made up of the anterior rami of C. 5, 6, 7, and 8 and T. 1, with communications from C. 4 and T. 2. It consists of roots, trunks, divisions, cords, and branches. The roots and trunks lie in the neck, the divisions behind the clavicle, and the cords and branches in the axilla. Therefore the subclavian artery is related to roots and trunks, and the axillary to cords and branches. The cords end by giving off their terminal branches at the lower border of the pectoralis minor, therefore the first and second parts of the axillary artery are related to cords, and the third part to branches; and for the same reason all the terminal branches of the cords (i.e., all the long nerves to the arm and forearm) *commence at the lower border of the pectoralis minor*. A description of any of these nerves should commence with a statement of this fact.

PLAN OF THE PLEXUS (*Fig.* 150):

A
- C. 5 and 6 roots join to form the *upper trunk*.
- C. 7 alone forms the *middle trunk*.
- C. 8 and T. 1 join to form the *lower trunk*.

B   Each trunk divides into an anterior and a posterior division.

C
- All the posterior divisions join to form the *posterior cord*.
- The upper two anterior divisions join to form the outer or *lateral cord*.
- The lowest anterior division alone forms the inner or *medial cord*.

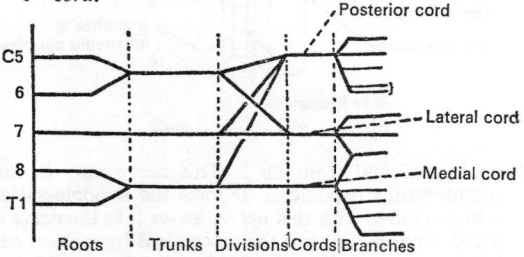

Fig. 150.—Diagram showing method of construction of brachial plexus. The constituent parts—roots, trunks, divisions, cords, and branches—are indicated.

NERVES

The plexus gives off three sets of branches: (1) Branches from the roots; (2) Branches from the trunks; (3) Branches from the cords.

1. BRANCHES FROM THE ROOTS:
   a. The long thoracic nerve (Bell) C. 5, 6, 7
   b. The dorsalis scapulae nerve C. 5
   c. Muscular branches to the three scaleni and longus colli.

2. BRANCHES FROM THE TRUNKS: Only two, both from upper trunk, both begin with 's'.
   a. Suprascapular nerve, C. 5, 6.
   b. Subclavius nerve, C. 5, 6.

   BRANCHES FROM THE CORDS:
   Medial Cord:
   Medial head of median C. 8, T. 1
   Medial anterior thoracic C. 8, T. 1
   Ulnar nerve C. 8, T. 1
   Medial cutaneous of forearm C. 8, T. 1
   Medial cutaneous of arm T. 1
   Lateral Cord:
   Lateral anterior thoracic C. 5, 6, 7
   Lateral head of median C. 5, 6, 7
   Musculocutaneous C. 5, 6, 7
   Posterior Cord:
   Radial C. 5, 6, 7, 8, T. 1
   Axillary C. 5, 6
   Thoracodorsal C. 6, 7, 8
   Subscapular: upper and lower C. 5, 6

RELATIONSHIP:
ABOVE THE CLAVICLE:
   Anterior:
   Skin.
   Superficial fascia and platysma.
   Branches of supraclavicular nerves.
   Deep fascia (roof of posterior triangle).
   External jugular vein and some of its tributaries.
   Omohyoid: posterior belly.
   Transverse cervical artery.
   Nerve to subclavius.
   Third part of subclavian artery in front of the lowest trunk.
   Transverse scapular artery.
   Clavicle.
   Posterior:
   Scalenus medius.
   Long thoracic nerve.

162 A SYNOPSIS OF SURGICAL ANATOMY

Inferior: The lowest trunk lies on the first rib, marking it, sandwiched between the subclavian artery in front and the scalenus medius behind.

IN THE AXILLA:

Anterior:
Skin with superficial fascia and platysma.
Supraclavicular nerves.
Pectoralis major and minor.
Costocoracoid membrane.
Cephalic vein.
Branches of thoraco-acromial artery.
Axillary artery and vein.

Posterior:
Serratus anterior.
Long thoracic nerve.
Fat between serratus and subscapularis.
Subscapularis.

Most of the branches of the plexus are grouped round the third part of the axillary artery (*Fig.* 151). The artery and plexus are covered proximally by the skin, fascia, and pectoralis major; distally by skin and fascia only. The medial head of the median nerve crosses the artery from within out to join

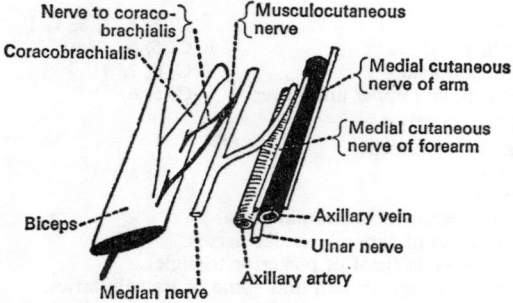

Fig. 151.—Relations of third part of axillary artery to branches of brachial plexus.

the outer head, so that the formed median nerve is lateral to the artery. The musculocutaneous nerve is lateral to the median. In the groove between the artery and the vein, there is in front the medial cutaneous nerve of the forearm, and behind the ulnar nerve. Along the inner border of the vein is the medial cutaneous nerve of the arm.

The radial and axillary nerves both separate the axillary artery from the subscapularis. The radial alone separates it from the latissimus dorsi and teres major.

ERB'S POINT: The spot where six nerves meet (*Fig.* 152): The *fifth and sixth cervical roots* join to form the upper trunk, which is very short, gives off the suprascapular nerve and the nerve to subclavius, and then divides into anterior and posterior divisions. It is here that the upper trunk usually stretches or tears in the upper-arm type (Erb's) of birth paralysis.

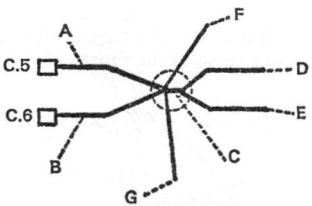

Fig. 152.—The dotted circle is Erb's point. The following nerves meet here: A and B, The fifth and sixth roots of the brachial plexus going to form C, the upper trunk of the brachial plexus; D and E, Anterior and posterior divisions of the upper trunk; F, Suprascapular nerve; G, Nerve to subclavius.

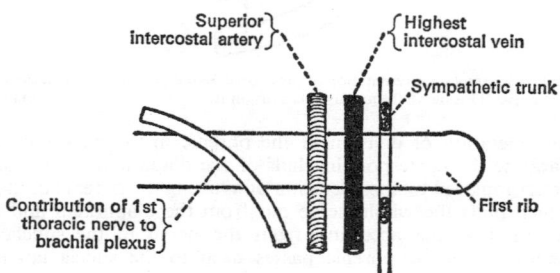

Fig. 153.—Anterior relations of neck of right first rib. The contribution from T.1 to the brachial plexus is tightly stretched across the rib.

CERVICAL RIB: The *eighth cervical and first thoracic* nerves which join to form the lowest trunk do so accurately at the anterior border of the scalenus medius, just above the first rib. It is this nerve therefore (the lowest trunk) that is pressed upon when it is elevated by a cervical rib forcing its way between the nerve and the first rib.

The nerve symptoms usually due to cervical rib may be produced by a normal first rib when the lowest trunk is abnormally stretched across it (*Fig.* 153). This arises when the plexus is *postfixed*, which implies that the communication to the plexus from T. 2 is abnormally large, so that the plexus may be said to be pushed one spinal segment lower down. This means that the lowest trunk is subjected to great pressure where it crosses the first rib.

The plexus is said to be *prefixed* when it is one nerve (cord segment) higher than usual and the C. 4 contribution is abnormally large.

The contribution which is given by T. 2 to the plexus is made up largely of sympathetic (autonomic) nerve-fibres.

COMMUNICATION WITH PHRENIC NERVE: The *nerve to the subclavius* from C. 5 or C. 5 and 6 has considerable importance from the fact that it may carry a large contribution to the phrenic which only joins that nerve in the thorax (*Fig.* 154). For this reason

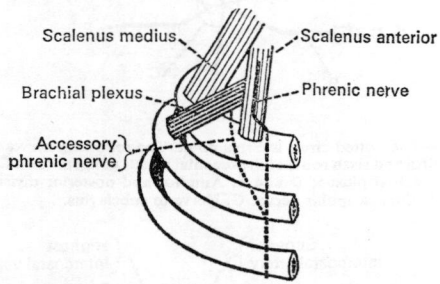

Fig. 154.—Schematic representation of the course frequently taken by an accessory phrenic nerve. This nerve frequently takes origin from the nerve to the subclavius.

the operation of division of the phrenic in the neck may fail to paralyse the corresponding half of the diaphragm. It is therefore better replaced by the operation of avulsing the phrenic in the neck, which pulls the whole nerve out from the diaphragm and makes certain that the accession from the nerve to the subclavius is removed. As the phrenic passes deep to the subclavian (or innominate) vein, whereas the accessory phrenic crosses anterior to the subclavian vein, the nerves between them embrace the vein, which has been damaged in avulsing the nerve, with fatal results.

IV. THE CUTANEOUS NERVES OF THE TRUNK

These are:
FRONT:
1. Descending supraclavicular nerves—C. 3 and 4.
2. Anterior rami of thoracic nerves—T. 2–12.
3. Lumbar—L. 1.

BACK: Posterior rami of:
C. 2, 3, 4, and 5.
T. 1–12.
L. 1–3.
Sacral and coccygeal.

Arrangement of Spinal Nerves: Each spinal nerve arises from the cord by two roots. The anterior is small and motor, the posterior is large and sensory and has a ganglion on it. These join to form a mixed spinal nerve. After a short course, during which it gives off a recurrent twig, the mixed spinal nerve divides into anterior and posterior rami or divisions. The anterior rami are large and have a tendency to form plexuses (cervical, brachial, lumbar, sacral, pudendal). The posterior rami are smaller and do not form plexuses.

THE RECURRENT NERVE (OF LUSCHKA) (*Fig.* 155): This is also called the sinu-vertebral nerve or the meningeal branch. It comes off the spinal nerve near the origin of the white ramus communicans and re-enters the spinal cord through the intervertebral foramen, to give a sensory supply to the posterior longitudinal ligament, periosteum, dura mater, and a sympathetic component to the blood-vessels in the region. Stimulation of this nerve, as with stretching of the posterior longitudinal ligament in protrusion of the intervertebral discs, results in backache.

THE POSTERIOR RAMI: These divide into medial and lateral branches, with the exception of the first nerve of the series and the last three, i.e., Cervical 1, Sacral 4, 5, Coccygeal 1. These nerves supply the skin and the muscles of the back. Above the level of the sixth thoracic spine the cutaneous nerves come from the medial branches of the posterior divisions, and emerge a thumb's breadth from the spines of the vertebrae, in the groove between the spinalis and longissimus columns of the sacrospinalis. The lateral branches do not become cutaneous, and are exhausted in the supply of muscles. Below the level of T. 6 the conditions are reversed. The medial branches of the posterior divisions are exhausted in the supply of muscles, while the lateral branches supply the skin. They emerge almost a hand's breadth from the middle line, in the groove between the longissimus and iliocostalis masses. Certain of the posterior divisions of the spinal nerves give no cutaneous branches. These are C. 1, 6, 7, and 8, and L. 4 and 5.

C. 1 supplies the muscles of the suboccipital triangle and does not become cutaneous.[1] C. 6, 7, and 8 lie on a deeper plane than C. 2, 3, 4, and 5. These latter lie between the semispinalis capitis and cervicis. The former lie deep to semispinalis cervicis and therefore never succeed in reaching the skin. L. 4 and 5 give no cutaneous nerves.

[1] Rarely a branch may be given to the skin at the junction of the back of the neck with the hindmost portion of the scalp.

The lumbar, sacral, and coccygeal regions are supplied by filaments from the posterior divisions of the lumbar, sacral, and coccygeal nerves.

THE ANTERIOR DIVISIONS:

THORACIC: A typical thoracic mixed nerve gives off its posterior division, and the anterior division continues on as an *intercostal nerve*. This gives some muscular branches. It gives in addition two cutaneous branches (*Fig*. 155).

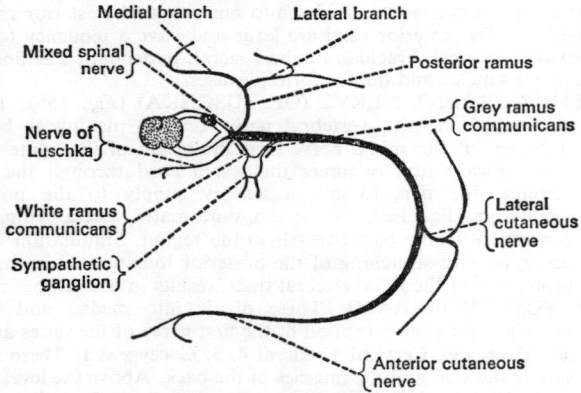

Fig. 155.—Anatomy of a thoracic nerve.

The *lateral cutaneous nerve* emerges in the mid-axillary line, and divides into anterior and posterior branches which supply the side of the chest. The *anterior cutaneous nerve* is the termination of the intercostal, and appears at the inner end of an intercostal space, where it supplies the skin on the sternum and front of the chest.

T. 1 is mostly expended by its contribution to the brachial plexus. The first intercostal nerve is therefore very small, and gives neither lateral nor anterior cutaneous branches. The descending supraclavicular nerves (C. 3 and 4) supply the skin over the first intercostal space. The second intercostal nerve gives off lateral and anterior cutaneous branches. Its lateral cutaneous branch does not divide into two, but crosses the axilla as the intercostobrachial nerve which supplies the skin of the posteromedial aspect of the arm as far as the elbow. The lateral cutaneous branch of the last thoracic nerve crosses the iliac crest and supplies the upper part of the skin of the buttock.

Although the intercostal nerves are *oblique*, the area of skin supplied by any one of them is *horizontal*, and Head has shown that before anaesthesia is evident in the region of their distribution at least three contiguous intercostal nerves must be divided.

The seventh intercostal supplies the epigastrium.

The tenth intercostal supplies the umbilical region.

The twelfth thoracic supplies the region midway between the umbilicus and pubis.

The iliohypogastric (L. 1) supplies the hypogastrium.

The intercostal nerves gain the abdominal wall by passing under the costal margin between the slips of the diaphragm. They run forward between internal oblique and transversus abdominis, supply them, then pierce the posterior rectus sheath, run deep to the rectus for a little distance, enter and supply it, and end as anterior cutaneous nerves. In incisions through the rectus, if these are made more than 3·8 cm. from the midline, all the intercostal nerves in the track of the cut will be divided and the rectus paralysed over that area.

The upper six intercostal nerves reach the inner end of the intercostal spaces, and not the middle line of the body. For that reason a swelling over the centre of the sternum cannot be a cold abscess tracking round from the spine along the intercostal nerve, as such a collection cannot extend more medially than the lateral edge of the sternum.

Segmental Nerve-supply of the Body: This implies the mapping out on the surface of the body of the areas supplied by each posterior nerve-root (*Fig.* 156).

The following account is that given by Sir James Purves-Stewart[1]:

'In the trunk the cutaneous root-areas run mainly horizontally; whereas in the upper limbs they run longitudinally, parallel to the axis of the limb; whilst in the lower limbs, anteriorly, they run from above downwards, and posteriorly, from below upwards. Finally, the genital organs, innervated by the third and fourth sacral roots, are suspended, as it were, amongst strangers, viz., in the neighbourhood of the second and third lumbar areas.

'The teaching of these areas can be simplified as follows: Let us regard the body as a long cylinder, beginning above the head (innervated by the trigeminal nerve), and ending below at the coccyx (*Fig.* 157). If this body had no limbs, everything would be easy, and we might represent the various root-areas as a series of horizontal dermatomes running from above downwards. The upper extremities, growing outwards horizontally from the trunk in the cervicothoracic region, carry with them the corresponding root areas, which run in long strips parallel to the long axis of the limbs, the thumbs being

[1] *The Diagnosis of Nervous Diseases*, 1924, 48, 50. London.

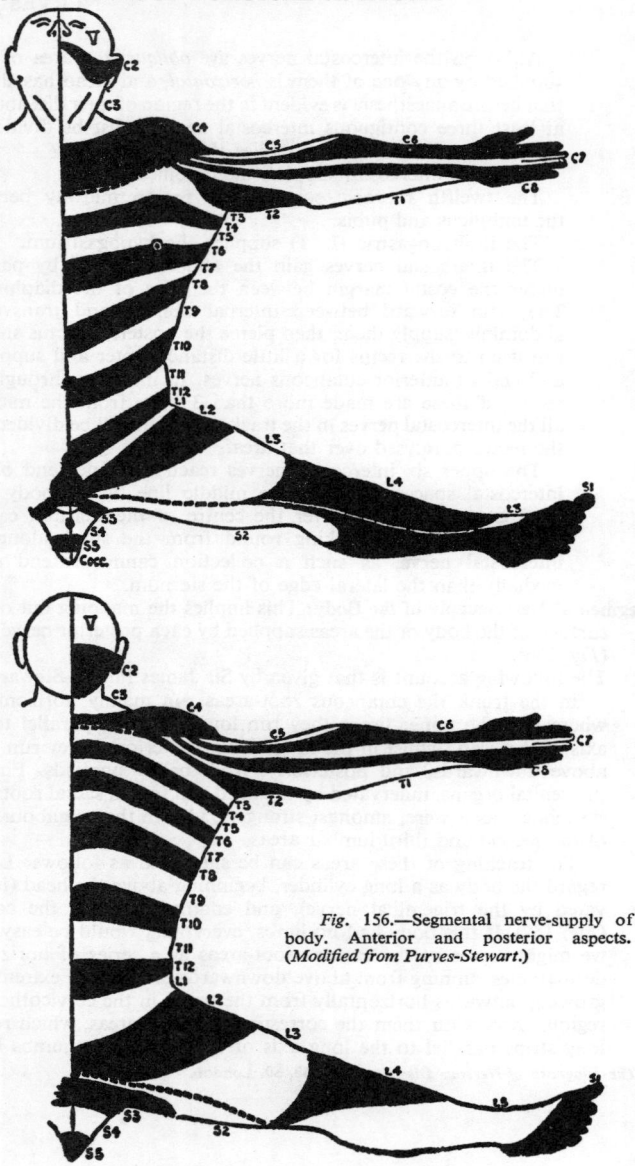

Fig. 156.—Segmental nerve-supply of body. Anterior and posterior aspects. (*Modified from Purves-Stewart.*)

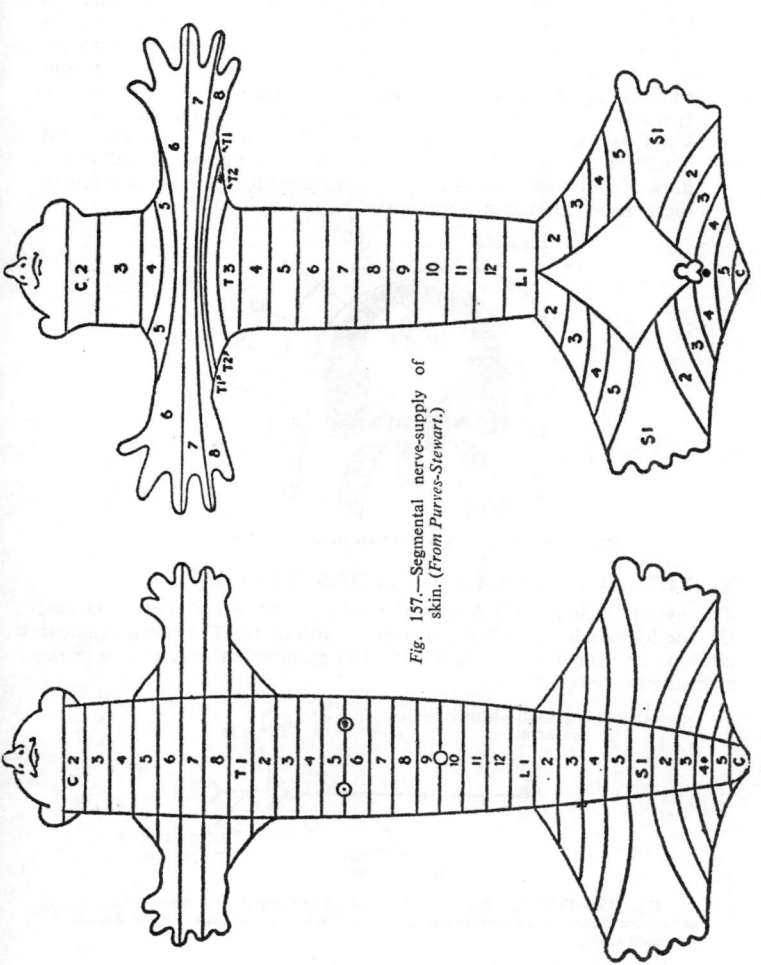

Fig. 157.—Segmental nerve-supply of skin. (*From Purves-Stewart.*)

directed upwards ... The lower limbs may also be represented as horizontal outgrowths, so as to place the great toes uppermost. In this position the cutaneous root areas run from above downwards, the pre-axial roots running along the anterior aspect and the post-axial roots along the posterior aspect, always from above downwards. It is essential in this scheme to retain a small projecting tail with the lower sacrococcygeal root-areas (*Fig.* 158). In the fully developed condition this tail, of course, is embedded in the posterior wall of the anus. Finally, the genital organs, innervated by the third and fourth sacral roots, are inclined forwards.'

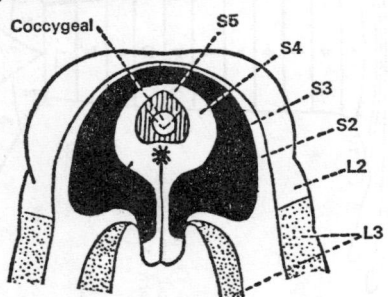

Fig. 158.—Sacrococcygeal root-areas. (*After Purves-Stewart.*)

V. THE AUTONOMIC NERVOUS SYSTEM

This system includes: (1) A central portion: (*a*) Cortical representation; (*b*) The hypothalamus. (2) A peripheral portion: (*a*) The thoracolumbar outflow, or sympathetic system; (*b*) The craniosacral outflow, or parasympathetic system.

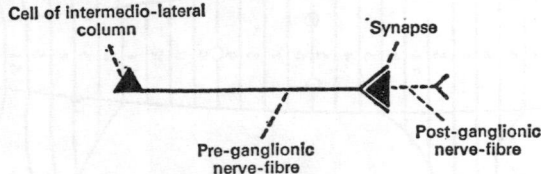

Fig. 159.—Diagram to show that in the parasympathetic system the preganglionic fibre is long and synapses with a single short postganglionic fibre—localized effect.

Functions of the Autonomic Nervous System: The cerebrospinal nerves and the parasympathetic produce localized accurate effects. The sympathetic nerves produce widespread diffuse results. How ingeniously this is effected is shown in *Figs.* 159 and 160, where it will be seen that whereas the parasympathetic preganglionic neurone synapses with but one postganglionic neurone, the preganglionic sympathetic fibre synapses with twenty or more postganglionic neurones. As Sir W. Langdon Brown[1] has it, 'the secret of the arrangement of the sympathetic nervous system is its adaption to produce, as easily and as speedily as possible, generalized effects'.

The sympathetic or thoracolumbar outflow is catabolic in function and activates the body for defence. The parasympathetic is designed more to serve the comforts of the body, being anabolic in function. Sympathetic and parasympathetic are frequently distributed to the same organ, e.g., eye, bladder. When such is the case their functions are antagonistic (Gaskell).

Stimulation of the thoracolumbar outflow results in dilatation of the pupil, increase in the heart-rate, constriction of the visceral blood-vessels, stimulation of the sweat-glands, erection of the hairs, and inhibition of peristalsis.

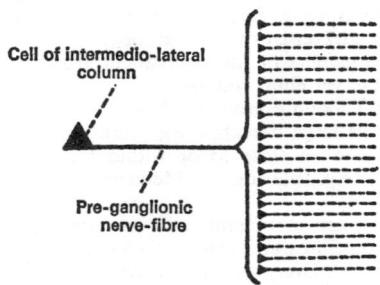

Fig. 160.—Note how on the sympathetic side of the autonomic system the preganglionic fibre synapses with numerous postganglionic fibres—diffuse effect.

The cranial parasympathetic is mainly intended for the supply of the heart and the alimentary canal, and its outgrowths, i.e., lungs, liver, gall-bladder, and pancreas. It is motor and secretory to the alimentary canal and its derivatives, but inhibitory to the heart. Furthermore, it causes constriction of the pupil and the secretion of saliva.

The sacral outflow of the parasympathetic is 'a mechanism for emptying' (Cannon), i.e., it is motor to the bladder and rectum and is the nerve concerned in the erection of the penis. It may here be mentioned that all the vasomotor nerves in the body arise from the

---

[1] *The Sympathetic Nervous System in Disease*, 1920, 6. London.

thoracolumbar outflow T. 1 to L. 2, and all the inhibitory nerves to the gut arise within the same part of the cord. Two clinical facts follow from this:

1. The great fall in blood-pressure which often attends the employment of spinal anaesthesia is due to the fact that the anaesthetic paralyses the vasoconstrictor nerves.

2. That type of paralysis of the bowel (paralytic ileus) which sometimes follows operations is occasionally due to overaction or unopposed action of the thoracolumbar outflow which contains all the inhibitory nerves to the gut.

Plan of the Peripheral Autonomic System: This system is made up of: (1) Preganglionic fibres; (2) Ganglia; (3) Postganglionic fibres.

PREGANGLIONIC FIBRES: These are small *medullated* nerve fibres incorporated with certain of the cranial and spinal nerves. After a course, long in the case of the cranial nerves, and short in the case of the spinal nerves, these fibres leave the cranial or spinal nerves with which they have been incorporated, and run an independent course to the ganglia of the autonomic system. The preganglionic fibres which arise from spinal nerves form the *white rami communicantes*.

GANGLIA: These consist of three groups:

LATERAL: The ganglia of the sympathetic trunk which lie on either side of the vertebral column.

COLLATERAL: These are grouped about the aorta and in relation to some of its large branches, e.g., carotids.

TERMINAL: These lie close to or within the structures which they innervate, e.g., plexuses of Meissner and Auerbach in the gut wall.

These ganglia are *distributing stations* merely. They contain no association fibres and cannot therefore function in any way as 'little brains'. Every autonomic nerve-fibre going from the brain or cord has one cell-station or synapse between its origin and its ultimate destination. This cell-station may be in a lateral, collateral, or terminal ganglion, but there is never less than one synapse and never more than one. The only apparent exception is in the case of the adrenal glands. The preganglionic fibres run directly to the medulla, no synapse intervening. If it be remembered that the medulla of the adrenal is developed from nerve tissue, it will be understood that the medulla itself represents the synapse and postganglionic fibre.

POSTGANGLIONIC FIBRES: These form the second relay of autonomic fibres, i.e., those fibres which take over the nerve impulse distal to the single cell-station which has been seen to occur in the course of all the autonomic nerves. They are non-medullated, and to this group belong all the grey rami communicantes. These fibres pass to the viscera via the blood-vessels and reach the more

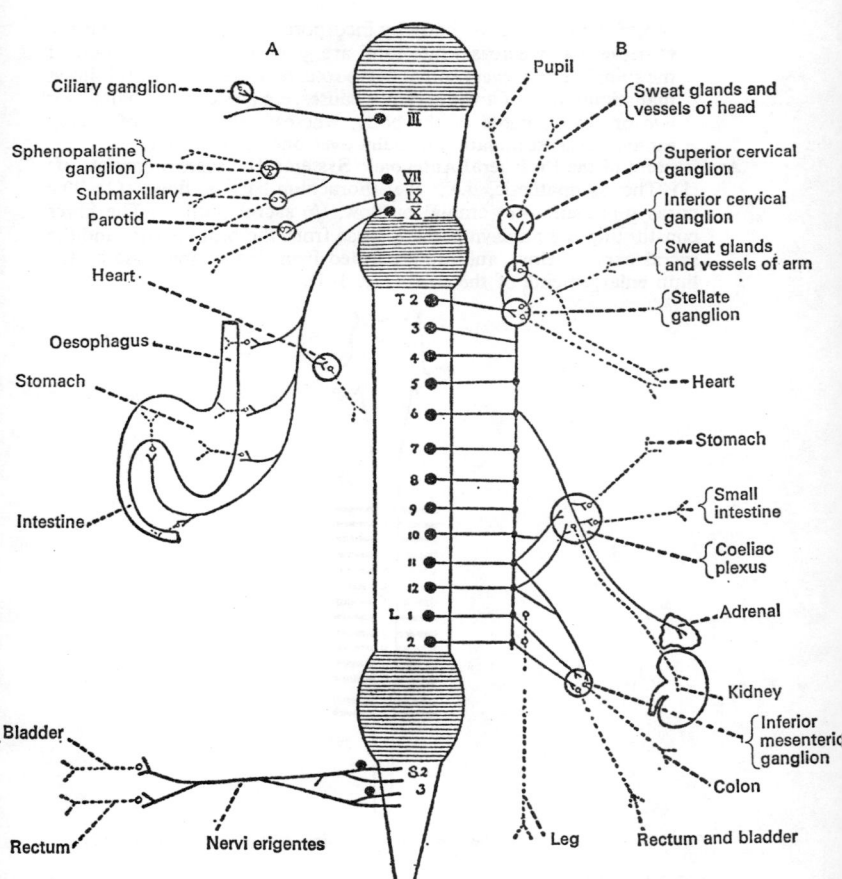

Fig. 161.—Plan of autonomic nervous system. The thoracolumbar outflow is separated from the bulbosacral outflow by the cervical and lumbar limb enlargements of the cord. Preganglionic fibres are shown as uninterrupted lines, postganglionic fibres as broken lines. A, Parasympathetic; B, Sympathetic. (*Re-drawn from 'The Sympathetic Nervous System in Disease', by W. Langdon Brown.*)

174 A SYNOPSIS OF SURGICAL ANATOMY

superficial parts of the body by incorporation in the spinal nerves. Observe that whereas white rami are given off only by certain of the spinal nerves, every spinal nerve receives a grey ramus. It follows that stimulation of a white ramus causes, e.g., erection of hairs over five or six segments of the body, whereas stimulation of a grey ramus causes stimulation of hairs over one segment only.

Architecture of the Peripheral Autonomic System: The system consists of: (1) The sympathetic, i.e., the thoracolumbar outflow; (2) The parasympathetic—(*a*) cranial outflow, (*b*) sacral outflow. The fibres constituting the parasympathetic arise from the brain above, and the sacral nerves below, and are separated from the sympathetic by the limb enlargements of the cord (*Fig.* 161).

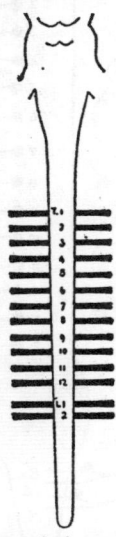

Fig. 162.—The origin of the sympathetic portion of the autonomic system.

THORACOLUMBAR OUTFLOW (Sympathetic): *Fig.* 162 shows the extent and essential simplicity of the spinal origin of this system. It consists of the white rami communicantes excepting only the two from S. 2, 3 which constitute the parasympathetic sacral outflow. They arise from the first thoracic to the second lumbar nerve inclusive. The fibres take origin from cells in the visceral or lateral column of the spinal cord and pass out with the anterior nerve-root and the mixed spinal nerve. Very soon they leave this nerve and pursue an independent course as white rami communicantes to the sympathetic ganglionic trunk. Here many of them end in synapses. The splanchnic branches of the sympathetic trunk are, however, made up of white fibres which run straight through the lateral ganglia to the coeliac plexus, where their cell-stations are situated.

CRANIOSACRAL OUTFLOW (Parasympathetic) (*Fig.* 163):

THE CRANIAL OUTFLOW: Autonomic fibres are found in the following cranial nerves: (1) Oculomotor; (2) Facial; (3) Glossopharyngeal; (4) Vagus.

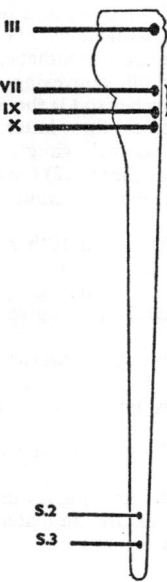

Fig. 163.—The origin of the parasympathetic system.

THE SACRAL OUTFLOW: Two white rami communicantes constitute the sacral outflow. They are also called the nervi erigentes. These arise from S. 2 and 3, or S. 3 and 4. Whereas most of the fibres constituting the thoracolumbar outflow end, i.e., have their cell-stations, in the lateral ganglia, those constituting the cranial and sacral outflows have no relation to the sympathetic ganglionic chain and end in the collateral or terminal ganglia.

GANGLIA:

THE LATERAL GANGLIA or sympathetic chain of ganglia comprise two ganglionated cords, one on each side of the vertebral column, extending from the 2nd cervical vertebra to the coccyx.

There are three cervical, eleven thoracic, four lumbar, and four sacral ganglia, united together by nerve-fibres. White rami are distributed to all the ganglia from the first thoracic to the second lumbar inclusive. Grey rami pass from the lateral ganglia to every one of the spinal nerves. Some ganglia give off several grey rami, e.g., the superior cervical give off four. The grey rami carry vasomotor, pilomotor, and secretory fibres to the sweat-glands. The cervical ganglia give: (1) grey rami to all the cervical nerves; (2) the cranial sympathetic, which follows the internal carotid into the skull, conveying amongst others the dilator pupillae fibres; branches to (3) the pharynx, (4) the thyroid, and (5) the cardiac plexuses: these latter convey the accelerator nerve to the heart. The thoracic ganglia give: (1) grey rami to the thoracic nerves; branches to (2) the aortic and (3) the pulmonary plexuses, and to (4) the splanchnic nerves. These latter are three on each side:

Great splanchnic from 5th–10th ganglia goes to coeliac plexus.
Lesser   „   „   10th–11th   „   „   „   „
Least (imus) „   „   12th ganglion   „   renal   „

The lumbar and sacral ganglia give grey rami to the lumbar and sacral nerves.

COLLATERAL GANGLIA OR SYMPATHETIC PLEXUSES:

In the Thorax:

The cardiac plexus lying below and behind the arch of the aorta.

The pulmonary plexus lying in front of and behind the root of the lung.

The oesophageal plexus lying around the oesophagus.

These three plexuses are intimately associated with the vagi, and to a lesser extent with the lateral ganglia.

In the Abdomen:

The coeliac plexus is situated around the origin of the coeliac artery, there being a large nerve mass on each side of this vessel known as the coeliac ganglion.

This plexus is continuous with a network of sympathetic nerves in relation to the aorta—the aortic plexus.

Numerous branches accompany the blood-vessels arising from the aorta and are known by the same names, e.g., phrenic, adrenal, renal plexuses, etc.

The splanchnic nerves run to the coeliac plexus, which also receives branches from the vagi.

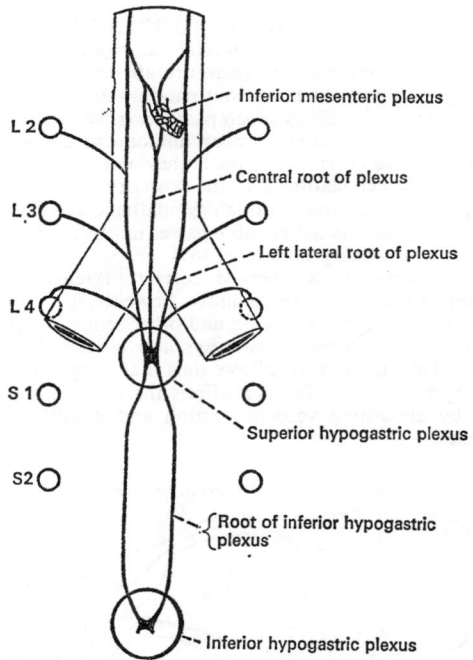

Fig. 164.—Showing the superior and inferior hypogastric plexuses and the method of their formation. The small circles are part of the lateral chain of sympathetic ganglia.

The nerves from these plexuses run to the abdominal viscera via the blood-vessels.

The superior hypogastric or presacral plexus lies in front of the sacral promontory. It is formed by strands from the lower end of the aortic plexus, receiving also branches from the ganglionated trunk on each side. The plexus divides into two nerves which run down on either side of the rectum to form, behind the base of the bladder, the inferior hypogastric plexus. This plexus supplies the bladder, rectum, and internal and external genitalia (*Fig.* 164).

TERMINAL GANGLIA: These lie in the walls of organs such as the bowel and bladder, and little is known about them. These plexuses may contain a mechanism for purely local reflex action.

178 A SYNOPSIS OF SURGICAL ANATOMY

AFFERENT SIDE OF THE AUTONOMIC SYSTEM: Although knowledge on this matter is still far from complete, it is now definitely established that there are afferent autonomic pathways conveying fibres which transmit painful sensations. It is of interest to note that these fibres which pass along the peripheral autonomic routes take a precisely similar anatomical course to the fibres subserving somatic pain, once they enter the central nervous system. The cell-station is in the posterior root ganglion, the long peripheral fibre passes through sympathetic ganglia to its origin in the viscus, and the central fibre passes up the cord precisely as does the somatic sensory fibre (*Fig.* 165).

The foregoing statement is correct in regard to the sensory supply of the viscera. In the limbs, however, it is now believed that all sensations conveying pain and other sensory impressions travel via cerebrospinal nerve pathways and do not thus pass through sympathetic ganglia. It follows thus that ganglionectomy can only influence pain in so far as it affects the vascular supply to a limb, i.e., by abolishing vasoconstriction and pathological vasomotor reflexes.

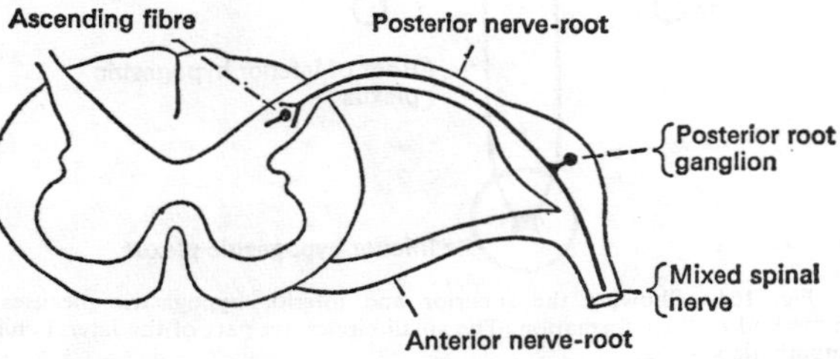

Fig. 165.—To show that the viscero-sensory or afferent autonomic fibre takes a precisely similar course to the afferent somatic fibre.

The receptor end-organ is identical with that of the somatic pain fibre. These autonomic sensory fibres are collectively spoken of as viscero-sensory. The nature of visceral pain is well known. Despite the fact that the stimuli necessary to evoke it are so different from those which evoke somatic pain, it has recently been contended that there is no essential difference in the actual physiology or nature of such pain sensations from those arising from muscles and tendons on the somatic side, but that the apparent differences are due to the fact that the viscera are not so richly supplied with sensory nerves as are more superficial structures, and are also more protected from noxious stimuli and that their response to such stimuli is therefore different. It is of considerable practical importance to note that all afferent visceral fibres (excepting those from bladder, prostate, uterine cervix, and lower colon, which pass to the cord via the nervi erigentes) enter the cord between its first thoracic and second lumbar segments (area of origin of white rami communicantes). The fibres concerned are here collected into comparatively small compass and can be attacked surgically if necessary, to interrupt the appropriate pathway of pain, either in the lateral sympathetic ganglia or in the posterior nerve-roots. Note that the vagus does not convey sensations of visceral pain from below the diaphragm and that it is therefore unnecessary to anaesthetize it in operations on the viscera which it supplies.

This matter will be dealt with further in the section dealing with the surgery of the sympathetic system. In this place the writer would like to put on record his indebtedness to the writings of White and Smithwick,[1] who have so ably simplified a difficult subject.

Chapter XXI

MUSCLES

I. CERTAIN IMPORTANT MUSCLES[2]

The arrangements and actions of certain muscles are not always understood and require clarification.

Pharyngeal Constrictors: The constrictors of the pharynx are arranged like three flower pots fitting into each other (*Fig.* 166, A). They have a continuous origin from—

1. The lower third of the posterior border of the medial pterygoid plate
2. The pterygomandibular raphe
3. The sides of the tongue
4. The mucous membrane of the mouth
5. The mylohyoid line

} Origin of superior constrictor

6. The stylohyoid ligament
7. The hyoid bone

} Origin of middle constrictor

---

[1] *The Autonomic Nervous System*, 1942. London.
[2] The muscles mentioned in Section I are not inter-related and have been included to describe special features or tests.

8. The thyroid cartilage } Origin of inferior constrictor
9. The cricoid cartilage

The middle constrictor arises from the two sides of the angle formed by the stylohyoid ligament and the great horn of the hyoid bone (*Fig.* 166, B).

The superior constrictor arises above this, and the inferior comes from the cartilages below. The muscles are inserted into a median raphe situated posteriorly, the superior constrictor reaching the pharyngeal tubercle at the base of the skull. At the side of the pharynx between the upper border of the highest constrictor and the base of the skull the pharyngeal aponeurosis is exposed (pharyngobasilar fascia). Here lies the auditory tube sandwiched between the levator palati medially and the tensor palati laterally. All three structures pierce the pharyngeal aponeurosis.

It is important to realize that the pharyngeal aponeurosis is the middle coat of the pharynx, lying within or internal to the muscular coat.

NERVE-SUPPLY OF THE CONSTRICTORS: The constrictors are all supplied by the pharyngeal plexus (through the accessory part of the spinal accessory). The inferior constrictor has two additional nerves, the external and recurrent laryngeal branches of the vagus.

The stylopharyngeus muscle enters the wall of the pharynx between the superior and middle constrictors; here it meets the palatopharyngeus muscle and is inserted with it into the posterior border of the thyroid cartilage.

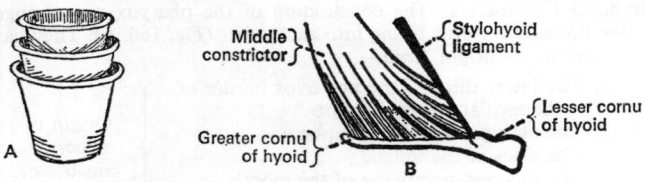

Fig. 166.—A, The pharyngeal constrictors are arranged like three flower pots fitting into each other. B, Origin of middle constrictor.

PLEXUSES SITUATED ON THE OUTER SURFACE OF THE MIDDLE CONSTRICTOR: There are two of these: (1) The pharyngeal plexus of nerves; (2) The pharyngeal plexus of veins.

THE PHARYNGEAL PLEXUS OF NERVES is formed by the pharyngeal branch of the vagus together with branches from the glossopharyngeal and sympathetic. The nerves leaving the plexus pierce

MUSCLES 181

the pharyngeal wall to supply its muscles and mucous membrane, also the soft palate.

THE PHARYNGEAL PLEXUS OF VEINS drains into the internal jugular opposite the angle of the jaw by one or two vessels which pass outwards between the two carotids.

Postural Activity: It has been found that certain muscles which are concerned in keeping the trunk erect have a very special physiological property called 'postural activity'. This implies that their activity is constantly greater than that of other muscles which do not participate in this quality. These muscles are the sacrospinalis, glutei, quadriceps, sartorius, and to some extent the calf muscles. The practical application of this fact is seen in cases of infantile paralysis where it is found that the loss of muscles possessing postural activity cannot be supplied by transplanting muscles without this type of activity. Thus in paralysis of the quadriceps, the transplantation of the biceps into the patella to replace it is often a failure, because the biceps is not endowed with postural activity (Elmslie[1]). It is thought that a special centre governing this function exists in the cord.

Serratus Anterior:

ACTIONS:

1. In the first 90° of abduction at the shoulder-joint, the muscle, together with the trapezius, fixes the scapula, while the deltoid abducts the arm.
2. In the second 90° of abduction, the muscle rotates the scapula, while the deltoid fixes the humerus at a right angle, and the trapezius prevents all scapular movement excepting rotation round a central axis.
3. The muscle is the strongest protractor of the upper extremity, i.e., it pulls the scapula forward and with the scapula the humerus. It is therefore the boxer's muscle, being the motive force in a forward punch.

TEST: Let the patient face a wall with his hand on the side to be tested against the wall, and his arm at his side with elbow flexed. Let him now push his body away from the wall with this hand. If the muscle is paralysed, the vertebral border of the scapula will stand out from the chest wall, i.e., winging of the scapula.

Flexor Digitorum Sublimis: A valuable test for the function of this muscle as distinct from that of the flexor digitorum profundus is described by Graham Apley.[2] The patient's hand is laid on the table palm upwards. The surgeon holds the fingers flat on the table with the exception of the one to be tested and asks the patient to flex this finger. If the sublimis is strong it flexes the second phalanx, leaving the distal joint straight and so freely movable that to the examiner it feels

---

[1] *Modern Operative Surgery*, edited by Carson, 1931, **1**, 115.
[2] Apley, A. Graham, *Br. med. J.*, 1956, **1**, 25.

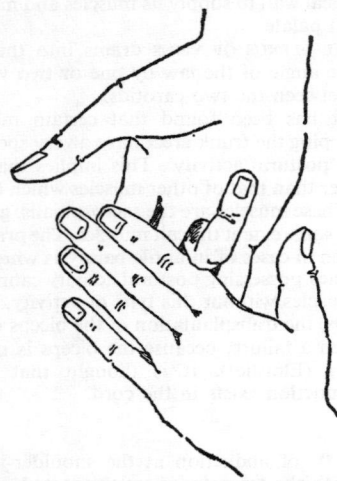

Fig. 167.—Testing the integrity of the flexor digitorum sublimis. (*By courtesy of Apley and the Editor of the 'British Medical Journal'.*)

flail. If, however, the sublimis is weak or paralysed, the profundus flexes the finger at both interphalangeal joints. In consequence the distal phalanx is bent and not flail.

The explanation given is that in a normal hand the profundus acts *en masse* to bend all fingers at all joints. In the above tests the surgeon's hand prevents this mass action and only the sublimis is available to flex the finger and therefore the last joint is straight and flail (*Fig.* 167).

Muscles producing Abduction and Adduction of the Hand: These movements are performed by the extensors and flexors of the wrist acting together. This can be appreciated if during these actions the wrist on that side is encircled by the examiner's hand. The tendons on front and back of the wrist are felt acting in concert.

Intrinsic Muscles of the Hand:

SMALL MUSCLES OF THE THUMB:

ABDUCTOR POLLICIS BREVIS: An important muscle.

Action: It pulls the thumb directly forward away from the palm in a plane at right angles to the palm (*Fig.* 168).

OPPONENS:

Action: It enables the pad of the last phalanx of the thumb to be approximated to that of any other finger.

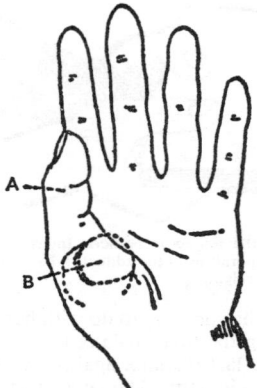

Fig. 168.—Action of abductor pollicis brevis. A, Thumb in line with fingers. B, Thumb pulled directly forwards by the short abductor at right angles to plane of palm.

The abductor pollicis brevis and opponens are together responsible for the action of rotating the thumb opposite the index finger for the pincer action in picking up objects.

ADDUCTOR POLLICIS:

Action: It pulls the thumb across the palm in a plane parallel to the palm (*Fig.* 169).

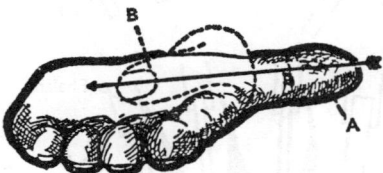

Fig. 169.—Hand seen end on, showing that action of adductor pollicis is to draw the thumb transversely across palm in the direction shown by arrow. A, Thumb abducted; B, Thumb adducted.

Test (Froment's sign, 1914): Give the patient a thin book and tell him to grasp it firmly between the last phalanges of the thumb and forefinger. If the muscle is acting, the thumb will be straight. If the muscle is not acting, the last phalanx of the thumb will be fully flexed (*Fig.* 170). The reason is that though

184 A SYNOPSIS OF SURGICAL ANATOMY

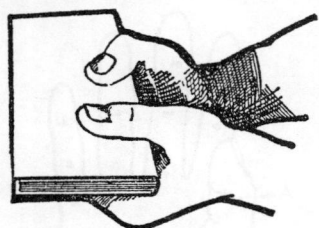

Fig. 170.—Testing the adductor pollicis. Interphalangeal joint of upper thumb is flexed, showing paralysis of the adductor. In the lower thumb it is acting normally and thumb is straight.

the adductor has nothing to do with flexion of the last phalanx, yet by pulling the first phalanx towards the palm, it opposes flexion of the last phalanx against resistance. This is the best test for the adductor. The muscle is supplied by the deep branch of the ulnar nerve.

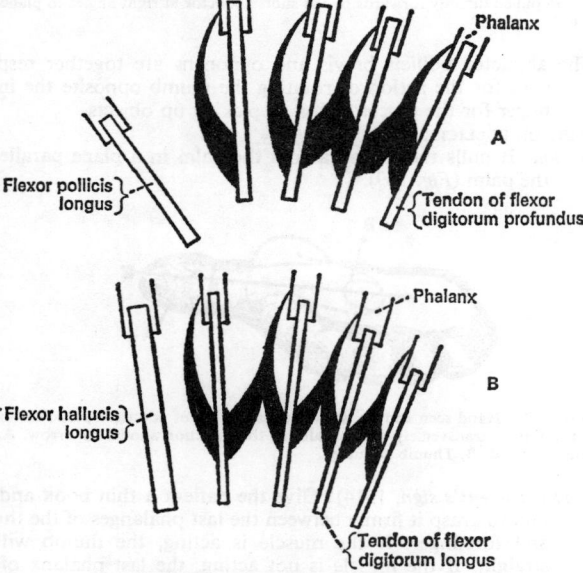

Fig. 171.—The lumbricals. A, In the hand. B, In the foot.

II. THE LUMBRICALS AND INTEROSSEI

Lumbricals: Four in each hand and foot. They *arise* from the tendons of the flexor profundus in the hand and flexor digitorum longus in the foot (*Fig.* 171). The only differences in hand and foot are: (1) The fact that the 2nd lumbrical comes from one tendon in the hand and two in the foot; and (2) The tendons wind round to the back to be attached to the extensor expansion and the base of the first phalanx. In the hand they wind round the thumb side of the fingers (lateral). In the foot they wind round the big-toe side of the toes (medial).

Interossei: The attachments of these muscles are a never-ceasing source of worry to the student. No effort should be made to memorize their origins and insertions, as these can be supplied by remembering certain facts governing their attachments.

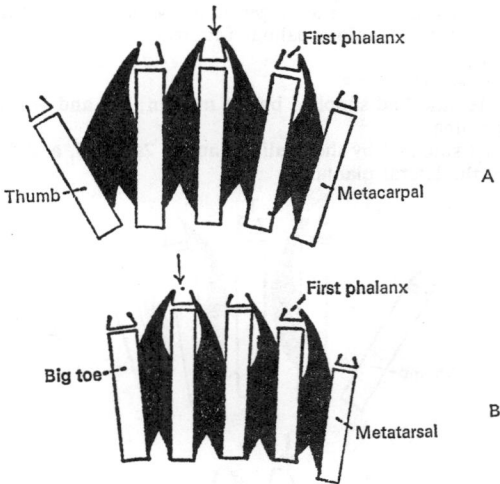

Fig. 172.—The dorsal interossei. A, In the hand. B, In the foot. The arrows indicate the central axis.

1. There are seven interossei in each hand and in each foot.
2. Four are dorsal, of which each arises from two adjacent bones (metacarpals or metatarsals).
    Three are palmar, of which each arises from one bone only (metacarpal or metatarsal).
3. The dorsal interossei are abductors from the central axis.
4. The palmar interossei are adductors towards the axis.

186 A SYNOPSIS OF SURGICAL ANATOMY

5. The axis of abduction and adduction is—
   IN THE HAND—an imaginary line passing through the third digit.
   IN THE FOOT—an imaginary line passing through the second digit.
6. The palmar, plantar, and dorsal interossei are attached to the dorsal extensor expansion and the bases of the first phalanges.
7. In both the hand and foot the interossei are the extensors of the second and third phalanges of the fingers and toes.
8. The interossei only produce axial deviation of the fingers when the first phalanx is extended.

With these facts in mind the attachments of the muscles can be readily supplied.

The muscles are best represented by a simple scheme (*Figs.* 172 and 173). Note that the thumb and great toe have no interossei inserted into them, as they have abductors and adductors of their own. The little finger and toe have abductors but not adductors, therefore palmar interossei go to them.

Nerve-supply:
   LUMBRICALS:
   HAND: 1st and 2nd supplied by the median; 3rd and 4th supplied by the ulnar.
   FOOT: 1st supplied by the medial plantar; 2nd, 3rd, and 4th supplied by the lateral plantar.

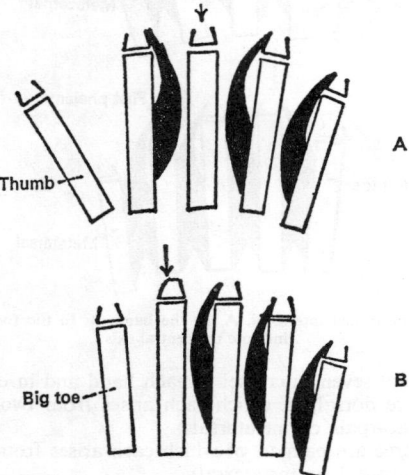

Fig. 173.—The palmar and plantar interossei. A, In the hand. B, In the foot. The arrows indicate the central axis.

MUSCLES 187

INTEROSSEI:
> HAND: All are supplied by the deep branch of the ulnar nerve.
> FOOT: All are supplied by the lateral plantar nerve.
> Occasionally the 1st, or 1st and 2nd dorsal interossei in the hand may be supplied by the median nerve.
> The median is the nerve mainly responsible for *coarse movements* of the hand, as it supplies most of the long muscles on the front of the forearm. It is the 'labourer's' nerve.
> The ulnar is the nerve mainly responsible for the *fine movements* of the hand, as it supplies most of the small muscles of the hand. It is the 'musician's' nerve (hence the old name for the lumbricals was musculi fidicinales).

Actions: These are the same in hand and foot.
> LUMBRICALS: Flex the first phalanges. Their opponents are: the extensor digitorum communis in the hand, the extensor digitorum longus in the foot.
>> Observe that though a lumbrical is hardly as big as the earthworm from which it takes its name, yet it is opposed by a muscle which extends from the humerus. Also flexion is a stronger action than extension.
> The extensores digitorum in the hand and foot have as their prime function extension of the first phalanx (*Fig.* 174). When, however, the knuckles are bent, extension of the second and third phalanges is a combined function of the long extensors and the intrinsic muscles of the hand (or foot).

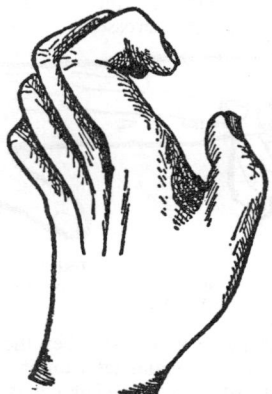

Fig. 174.—Shows that the prime function of the **extensor digitorum communis** is extension of the first phalanx.

188 A SYNOPSIS OF SURGICAL ANATOMY

INTEROSSEI: Besides being abductors and adductors, the interossei are extensors of the middle and terminal phalanges.

Explanation: The interossei are inserted into the extensor tendon expansion at the back of the first phalanx. The firm attachment of the extensor to the back of the first phalanx is the

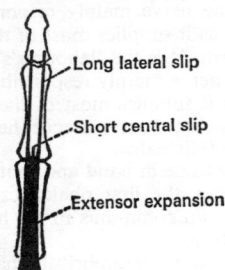

Fig. 175.—Showing that the extensor expansion at the back of the first phalanx breaks up into one short central and two long lateral processes.

insertion of the extensor tendon proper, and the extensor, therefore, extends this phalanx and does nothing more. The extensor tendon divides into three slips, one short central and two long laterals (*Fig.* 175). These slips are really extensions of the interossei tendons, and go to be inserted into the second and third phalanges, which are therefore extended by the interossei.

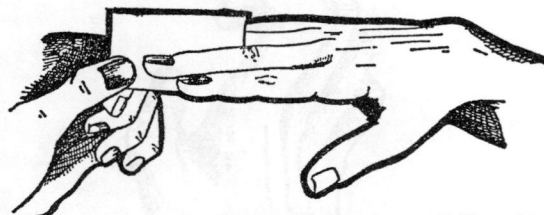

Fig. 176.—Test for interossei. The wrist should be dorsiflexed to cut out the action of the long flexors of the fingers.

If the ulnar nerve which supplies the interossei is paralysed, the two distal phalanges cannot be extended.

The opponents of the interossei acting as extensors are the flexores digitorum sublimis (which flexes the second phalanx) and profundus (which flexes the third phalanx).

TEST: The muscles are best tested by letting the patient grasp a piece of paper between the sides of two adjacent fingers. If the muscles are acting, this paper will be firmly held and some resistance will be offered to its withdrawal (*Fig.* 176). Extension of the second and third phalanges is also a test for the muscles.

RÉSUMÉ:

	Flexed by	*Extended by*
1st phalanx	Lumbrical	Extensor digitorum
2nd ,,	Sublimis	Interossei
3rd ,,	Profundus	Interossei

The matter, however, is not quite so simple as this. It has been stated, in the author's opinion correctly, that with the hand fully flexed at the wrist, the extensor digitorum extends the second and third phalanges. When the wrist is dorsiflexed these phalanges are extended by the interossei.

The small muscles of the thumb are abductor, adductor, flexor brevis, opponens.

The small muscles of the big toe are abductor, adductor, flexor brevis (no opponens).

The small muscles of the fifth finger are abductor (no adductor), flexor brevis, opponens.

The small muscles of the fifth toe are abductor (no adductor), flexor brevis (no opponens).

III. THE DEEP MUSCLES OF THE BACK[1]

These muscles lie between the posterior and middle layers of the lumbodorsal fascia in the lumbar region and between the thoracic part of the lumbodorsal fascia and ribs and transverse processes of the vertebrae in the thoracic region. There are two great muscle groups: (1) Sacrospinalis group; (2) Transversus spinalis group.

Plan of arrangement of the muscles (*Fig.* 177):

	SACROSPINALIS GROUP	TRANSVERSUS SPINALIS GROUP
Width	A muscle mass as broad as the palm of the hand	As broad as the thumb
Lateral Extent	From the spines of the vertebrae to the angles of the ribs	From the spines of the vertebrae to the tips of the transverse processes
Vertical Extent	From the 4th piece of the sacrum to the mastoid process of the occipital bone	From the 4th piece of the sacrum to the occipital bone

(*continued overleaf*)

---

[1] This section is based on the lucid teaching of Professor Wright, of the London Hospital Medical School. The classification appeared, I am informed, in Macalister's *Text-book of Anatomy*, 1889.

190 A SYNOPSIS OF SURGICAL ANATOMY

	SACROSPINALIS GROUP	TRANSVERSUS SPINALIS GROUP
Composition	Three muscle groups placed side by side like 3 fingers—000	Three muscle groups placed one on top of the other like the constituents of a 0 sandwich—0 0
Nerve-supply	Is segmental from the posterior divisions of the spinal nerves	Is segmental from the posterior divisions of the spinal nerves

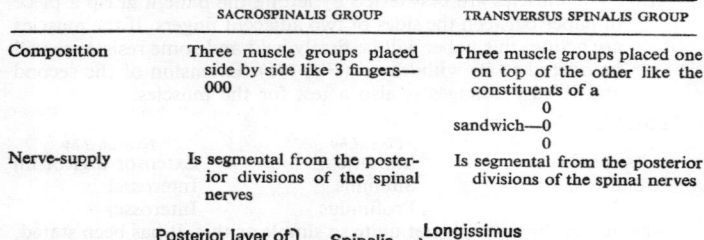

Fig. 177.—Showing on the reader's left the arrangement of the transversus spinalis muscle mass and on the right the arrangement of the sacrospinalis mass.

It will be seen that owing to the nature of their nerve-supply these muscles may be cut across without damaging any but the part cut. The cutting across of most other muscles entails paralysis of the part distal to the division owing to section of nerves, excepting only other segmental muscles such as the rectus abdominis.

Sacrospinalis:

ORIGIN: From the surfaces of a cave formed between the back of the sacrum and the aponeurosis of origin of the sacrospinalis. This aponeurosis has a U-shaped attachment (*Fig.* 178). The inner limb of the U is attached to the spines of the sacral and lumbar vertebrae, outer limb to the iliac crest and posterior sacro-iliac ligaments, connecting limb to the back of the sacrum.

THE APONEUROSIS OF ORIGIN OF THE SACROSPINALIS is a composite aponeurosis, the tendinous structures which go to assist in its formation being:
1. Posterior layer of the lumbodorsal fascia.
2. Tendinous origin latissimus dorsi.
3. Tendinous origin serratus posterior inferior.
4. Tendinous origin gluteus maximus.
5. Sacrotuberous ligament.

MUSCLE GROUPS: The muscle divides into three groups of muscles lying side by side between the angles of the ribs and spines of vertebrae (*Fig.* 179):

MUSCLES 191

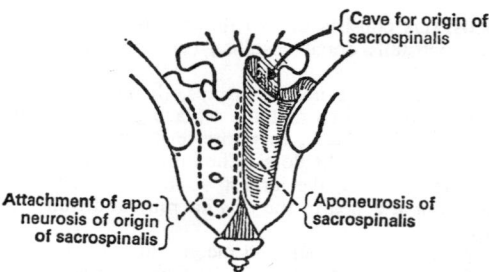

Fig. 178.—Back of the sacrum showing on the left the U-shaped attachment of the aponeurosis of origin of the sacrospinalis; on the right is shown the cave formed by this aponeurosis and the sacrum which gives origin to the muscle.

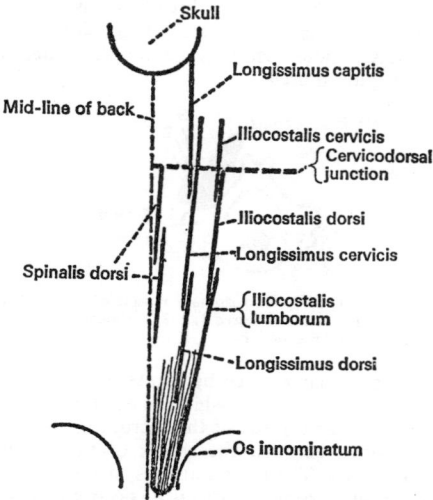

Fig. 179.—Arrangement of muscles comprising sacrospinalis group. Observe that only three slender muscles reach the neck.

1. SPINALIS consists of: (*a*) spinalis lumborum, (*b*) spinalis dorsi, (*c*) spinalis cervicis.
2. LONGISSIMUS consists of: (*a*) longissimus dorsi, (*b*) longissimus cervicis, (*c*) longissimus capitis.

192 A SYNOPSIS OF SURGICAL ANATOMY

3. ILIOCOSTALIS consists of: (a) iliocostalis lumborum (iliocostalis), (b) iliocostalis dorsi (costalis), (c) iliocostalis cervicis (costalis cervicalis).

Each of these three muscle groups, therefore, is subdivided into three relays arranged so that the replacing muscle is always medial to the muscle it replaces; therefore, e.g., the iliocostalis cervicis is medial to the iliocostalis dorsi. The iliocostalis group is attached to ribs. The longissimus, the largest of the three, has a herring-bone pattern, being attached to the ribs laterally and transverse processes medially.

The spinalis is very small and inconstant, and goes from spines to spines. Frequently only the spinalis dorsi is present.

Of this huge powerful muscle only three of the relays succeed in reaching the neck (*Fig.* 180), and only one reaches the skull. The three relays which reach the neck are so slender that they are shaped like three ribbons placed with their surfaces in contact, presenting a medial and a lateral surface. The three 'ribbons' of muscles are, from medial to lateral, longissimus capitis, longissimus cervicis, and iliocostalis cervicis. These ribbons lie on the outer surface of the semispinalis capitis muscle.

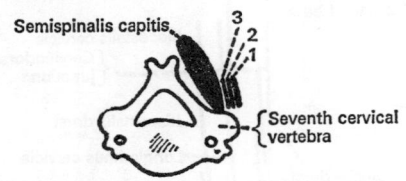

Fig. 180.—The parts of the sacrospinalis muscle mass which reach the neck are shown as three black lines numbered 1, 2, 3. 1, Iliocostalis cervicis. 2, Longissimus cervicis. 3, Longissimus capitis.

Transversus Spinalis: A name given by Professor Wright to designate the group of three muscle systems which lie deep to the sacrospinalis and extend from the fourth piece of the sacrum to the skull, and fill the thumb-like groove between the spines of the vertebrae and their transverse processes. The three muscle systems lie one on top of the other. The muscles from superficial to deep are: (1) Semispinalis—dorsi, cervicis, capitis; (2) Multifidus; (3) Rotatores.

All these muscles arise *laterally* from portions of the vertebral arch (laminae, or transverse processes, or articular processes) and go to the spines of the vertebrae *medially* (rotatores go from transverse processes to laminae). The rotatores occur in the dorsal region only. The multifidus occurs from the fourth piece of the sacrum to the 2nd cervical spine. The semispinalis is found in the thoracic and cervical regions. The semispinalis dorsi arises from the lower thoracic transverse processes and goes to the upper thoracic spines. The semispinalis cervicis arises from the upper thoracic transverse processes and goes to the cervical spines. The semispinalis capitis arises from the upper thoracic transverse processes and lower cervical articular processes and goes to the thumb-shaped area on the occipital bone between the superior and inferior nuchal lines.

THE SEMISPINALIS CAPITIS was called *complexus* because of its complicated structure. It is an important landmark at the back of the neck, and may be recognized by the fact that: (1) It is very large; (2) It is liberally 'splashed' with tendinous fibres; (3) Its fibres are vertical; (4) Its outer border is its origin and is fixed; (5) Its inner border is free; (6) It is pierced by the great occipital nerve; (7) It forms the roof of the suboccipital triangle; (8) The splenius muscle crosses it mediolaterally like a strap binding it down; (9) There is an arterial anastomosis round the muscle.

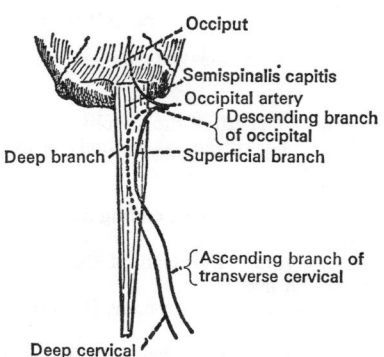

Fig. 181.—The anastomosis round the semispinalis capitis muscle.

THE ANASTOMOSIS ROUND THE SEMISPINALIS CAPITIS (*Fig.* 181):

On its Dorsal Surface: The ascending branch of the transverse cervical inosculates with the superficial division of the descending branch of the occipital artery.

On its Ventral Surface (between the semispinalis capitis and the semispinalis cervicis): The deep cervical (from costocervical branch of subclavian) anastomoses with the deep division of the descending branch of the occipital.

All the relevant facts regarding the sacrospinalis and the transversus spinalis have been enumerated, and this is one of the few

194 A SYNOPSIS OF SURGICAL ANATOMY

situations in the body where the exact detail of muscle attachments is neither useful nor necessary to the practical anatomist.

IV. THE DIAPHRAGMS OF THE BODY

These are: (1) The diaphragm of the floor of the mouth—muscular; (2) The diaphragm of the upper aperture of the thorax—fascial; (3) The diaphragm of the lower aperture of the thorax—musculotendinous; (4) The diaphragm of the pelvis—muscular; (5) The urogenital diaphragm—musculofascial.

Diaphragm of the Floor of the Mouth: This is a muscular diaphragm and is formed by the two mylohyoid muscles (*Fig.* 182).

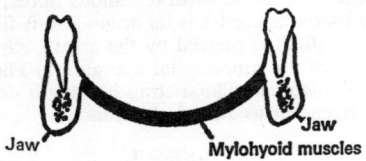

Fig. 182.—The diaphragm of the mouth.

MYLOHYOID:

ORIGIN: From the whole length of the mylohyoid line of the mandible (oblique line on inner surface of the body of the mandible).

INSERTION:
1. Body of hyoid.
2. Chiefly into a median raphe extending from the symphysis menti to the hyoid.

NERVE TO THE MYLOHYOID: A branch of the inferior alveolar (3rd division of the 5th nerve).

ACTION: Elevates the hyoid and the tongue. Its fibres run down and in.

RELATIONS:
On its Under Surface: Anterior belly of the digastric, crossing it obliquely.

It forms the anterior part of the floor of the submaxillary triangle, supporting here the submaxillary salivary gland and some of the submaxillary lymph-glands. The two muscles form the whole floor of the submental triangle, and the lymph-glands of the same name lie on the muscles. The mylohyoid vessels and nerve lie on it. Just under the skin is the platysma with the mandibular branch of the 7th nerve deep to it.

On its Upper Surface:
Muscles: Geniohyoid, genioglossus, hyoglossus.
Salivary Glands: The deep part of the submaxillary gland and the sublingual gland, and their ducts.

MUSCLES 195

Nerves and Vessels: The lingual nerve, the hypoglossal nerve and its vena comitans, the sublingual artery.

Mucous membrane of the floor of the mouth covers the origin of the muscle posteriorly.

The mylohyoid muscles together form a muscular hammock supporting the tongue and the structures on the floor of the mouth.

The anterior borders of the muscles are connected along the median raphe. The posterior borders are free. Lenthal Cheatle showed that the lymphatics draining the tongue which pierce the mylohyoid and tongue muscles are of exceptionally large calibre, so that in cancer of the tongue the cancer cells pass through the lymph-vessels without being held up in them. Secondary growths are therefore unlikely to occur in the muscles of the floor of the mouth, but tend to occur in the lymph-glands, the thorough removal of the latter being therefore of much greater importance than of the former.

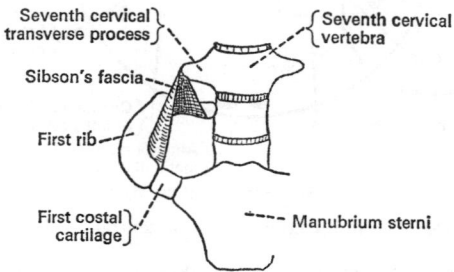

Fig. 183.—The diaphragm of the upper aperture of the thorax—Sibson's fascia.

Diaphragm of the Upper Aperture of the Thorax (*Fig.* 183): This is a fascial diaphragm, also called Sibson's fascia (suprapleural membrane), covering in the lateral part of the upper thoracic aperture. It protects the cervical dome of the pleura, which is attached to its under surface. The fascia, spreading out like a fan from the transverse process of the 7th cervical vertebra, is attached to the inner border of the 1st rib.

Diaphragm of the Lower Aperture of the Thorax: This is formed by the diaphragm muscle. It completely shuts off the thoracic and abdominal cavities from each other (*Fig.* 184).

ORIGIN:

ANTERIOR: By two slips from the xiphoid process.

LATERAL: From the inner surfaces of the lower six cartilages, interdigitating with the transversus abdominis.

POSTERIOR:
1. From medial and lateral lumbocostal arches and median arcuate ligament.
2. By two crura from the bodies of the upper three lumbar vertebrae.

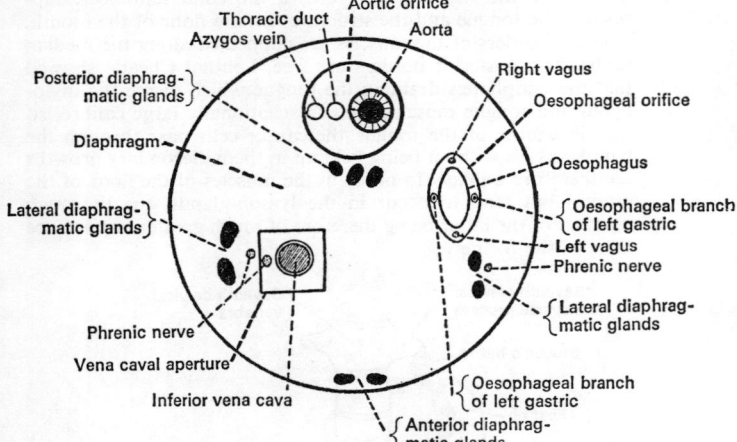

Fig. 184.—Upper surface of the diaphragm.

INSERTION: The fibres converge on a central tendon shaped like a trefoil leaf.

NERVE-SUPPLY: C. 3, 4, and 5, through phrenic (mixed). Lower intercostal nerves (sensory). The diaphragm is developed in the neck, hence its supply from cervical nerves.

ACTION: It is the chief muscle of respiration.

RELATIONS:
UPPER SURFACE: Pleura and lung each side, pericardium and heart between these.

CIRCUMFERENTIALLY: Costal cartilages, ribs and internal intercostal muscle, quadratus and psoas muscles.

LOWER SURFACE: Liver and stomach, spleen and kidney. The adrenals, the kidneys, and the pancreas lie on the crura. Much of the superior surface of the muscle is covered by pleura, and most of the inferior surface by peritoneum. A part of the posterior surface of the kidneys and the bare area of the liver are in direct contact with the muscle, no serous membrane intervening. Disease of the kidney or liver may spread through to the chest at these unprotected areas.

MUSCLES 197

OPENINGS IN THE DIAPHRAGM: The three large openings in the diaphragm are:

NAME OF OPENING	LEVEL	SHAPE	POSITION
Inferior vena caval	8T	Square	Slightly to right of median plane
Oesophageal	10T	Oval	Slightly to left of median plane
Aortic	12T	Round	Central

CAVAL OPENING: Transmits the inferior vena cava and half of the right phrenic nerve (the nerve first pierces the muscle and then supplies it).

OESOPHAGEAL OPENING: This opening is strengthened by the crura interlacing around it. In addition to the oesophagus it transmits the right and left vagi and the oesophageal branches of the left gastric artery with the accompanying veins. These vessels communicate here with the oesophageal branches of the aorta. This is one of the sites where portal and systemic circulations communicate. In obstruction to the veins in the liver (cirrhosis), therefore, these veins at the lower end of the oesophagus become very dilated and varicose, and frequently rupture.

The left vagus passes through the anterior angle of the oval, the right vagus through the posterior angle. The left vagus is anterior because it is going to supply the anterosuperior surface of the stomach, whereas the right vagus is destined for the postero-inferior surface. The alimentary canal is at an early developmental stage a median tube with right and left sides. The right vagus supplies the right side, the left supplies the left side; with the outgrowth of the liver the stomach rotates so that its left side becomes uppermost, carrying its nerve-supply with it.

AORTIC OPENING: Lies between the crura; the aortic orifice is completed by the median arcuate ligament which connects the crura. Three unpaired structures pass through it. From right to left these are the vena azygos major, the thoracic duct, and the aorta.

SMALLER ORIFICES IN THE DIAPHRAGM:

Between xiphoid slip and that from the 7th costal cartilage: Superior epigastric vessels pass.

Between the slips from the 7th and 8th costal cartilages: Musculo-phrenic vessels pass.

Between each pair of the remaining slips: One of the lower five intercostal vessels and nerves pass.

Behind the lateral lumbocostal arch: Last thoracic nerve and subcostal vessels pass.

Behind the medial lumbocostal arch: The sympathetic trunk passes.

Each crus is pierced by: The great, lesser, and least splanchnic nerves.

The left crus is pierced in addition by: The vena hemi-azygos.

Pelvic Diaphragm: This is formed by the levatores ani and coccygei muscles (*Fig.* 185).

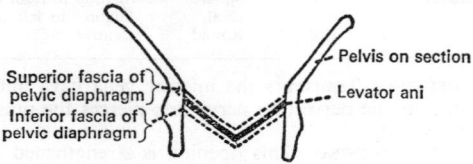

Fig. 185.—Pelvic diaphragm.

LEVATOR ANI: Separates the pelvic cavity from the ischiorectal fossae.
- ORIGIN: Bone in front and behind (the pubic bone and spine of ischium); fascia between these points (the parietal layer of pelvic fascia).
- INSERTION: The central point of perineum, side of anal canal between the external and internal sphincters, anococcygeal body (a fibrous mass between the tip of the coccyx and anus), and the coccyx.
- NERVES: Sacral 2, 3, and 4.
- ACTION: Raises the pelvic floor and assists in defaecation. It forms one of the vaginal sphincters.
- RELATIONS:
    The Pelvic Surface is related to the pelvic viscera.
    The Perineal Surface forms the inner wall of the ischiorectal fossa.
    The Posterior Margin is in contact with the anterior margin of the coccygeus.
    The Anterior Margins are separated by a triangular gap in which lies the prostate in the male, the vagina in the female.

COCCYGEUS: Lies on the sacrospinous ligament, which is merely a delamination of the muscle which has degenerated into a ligament. Both structures have therefore the same attachments.
- ORIGIN: Spine of ischium.
- INSERTION: The last piece of the sacrum, the first piece of the coccyx.
- NERVE: As levator.

The pelvic diaphragm has the unique and supremely important function of supporting the whole weight of the superincumbent viscera when the body is erect. In four-footed animals this weight comes on the anterior abdominal wall. Hernias through the muscle, such as prolapse of the rectum or uterus, are frequent.

Urogenital Diaphragm or Triangular Ligament: This consists of two muscles, the sphincter urethrae membranaceae, in which lies the membranous part of the urethra (1·8 cm. long), and the deep transverse perineus. These muscles are enveloped in two layers of fascia, the fasciae superior and inferior of the urogenital disphragm (upper and lower layers of the triangular ligament), forming the deep perineal pouch (*Fig.* 186).

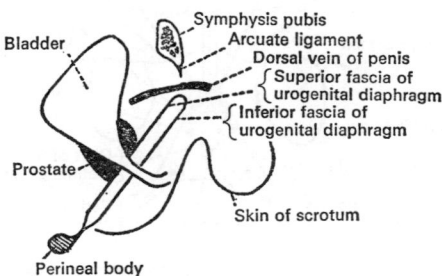

Fig. 186.—Vertical section of urogenital diaphragm.

MUSCLES:

THE SPHINCTER URETHRAE MEMBRANACEAE: Arises from ramus of pubis. Its fibres surround the urethra. When the sphincter vesicae (internal sphincter) is destroyed, as after the operation of prostatectomy, the sphincter urethrae membranaceae is the only sphincter left to the urethra, and is competent to control urination.

THE DEEP TRANSVERSE PERINEUS: Arises from the junction of ischial and pubic rami and is inserted into a median raphe behind the sphincter.

FASCIAE:

SUPERIOR: Is derived from the parietal layer of pelvic fascia.
  Attachments:
    Laterally to the conjoined ischiopubic rami.
    Anteriorly and posteriorly to the fascia inferior of the diaphragm.
    Superiorly to the fascial sheath of prostate.
  Pierced by: The urethra in the male, the vagina and urethra in the female.

INFERIOR: Is not triangular but trapezoid.
  Attachments:
    Laterally to the conjoined ischiopubic rami.
    Posteriorly fuses with the superior fascia and Colles's fascia (i.e., the deep layer of the superficial fascia of the perineum).

Anteriorly fuses with the superior fascia to form the transverse ligament of the pubis. Passing over this ligament the deep dorsal vein of the penis goes to the pudendal plexus (*Fig.* 187).

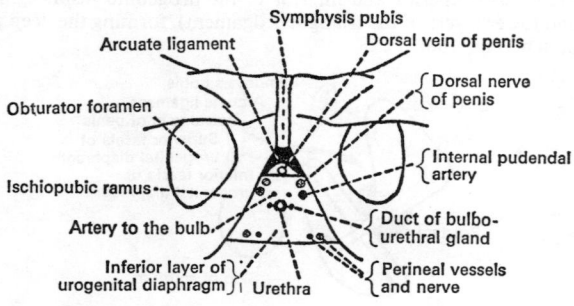

Fig. 187.—The urogenital diaphragm seen from below.

Pierced by:
  At base: Perineal nerve. The internal pudendal artery and the dorsal nerve of the penis insinuate themselves between the two layers of the urogenital diaphragm where they blend behind.
  At margins: Internal pudendal artery, dorsal nerve of penis.
  Centre: The urethra, the ducts of the bulbo-urethral glands, arteries to the bulb.
  In female the vagina pierces it in addition to the above.
The inferior surface of the fascia is related to the muscles of the superficial perineal pouch.
BETWEEN THE TWO LAYERS ARE:
  Membranous urethra.
  Sphincter urethrae membranaceae.
  Bulbo-urethral glands (Cowper's) in male, the vagina in female.
  Internal pudendal arteries.
  Arteries to bulb.
  A plexus of veins.
  The dorsal nerve of the penis or clitoris.
The ducts of the bulbo-urethral glands in the male pierce the inferior fascia and enter the urethra 2·5 cm. distal to the fascia. In the female the greater vestibular glands (Bartholinian) do not lie between the two layers of fascia but beneath the inferior layer, so that the ducts do not have to pierce the fascia.

V. INTRICATE MOVEMENTS AT SHOULDER, KNEE, AND FOOT

Joint movements other than these are simple to understand. The mechanisms of the shoulder, knee, and foot movements are more difficult of comprehension.

Abduction at the Shoulder: The upper limb may be abducted through a range of two right angles (180°) from the side of the body. Four muscles are concerned in this movement, the supraspinatus, deltoid, trapezius, and serratus anterior. In the first 90° of abduction the movement occurs at the shoulder-joint, in the second 90° of abduction the movement occurs at the sternoclavicular joint.[1]

THE FIRST 90°: The deltoid moves the upper limb into this position. To do this the scapula must be fixed to the chest wall so firmly that it cannot move sideways or rotate. Two muscles so fix it—the trapezius and the serratus anterior—to give the deltoid a fixed point on which to contract. The only other muscle which is possibly capable of some power of abduction through the first 90° is the supraspinatus. With a deltoid out of action the arm cannot be abducted except very exceptionally where the supraspinatus is able to perform the function.

Moseley[2] states that electromyographic studies in cases with proved complete ruptures of the supraspinatus tendon have suggested that the supraspinatus alone initiates the first 20–30° of abduction. If, however, in acute cases, local anaesthesia is infiltrated to remove the protective pain reflex, full shoulder movement is obtained, proving that the supraspinatus is not essential to initiate abduction. The power to maintain abduction at 90° is, however, seriously impaired owing to the loss of fixation of the fulcrum of the humerus which supraspinatus function supplies. In support of this statement is the observation that after division of the suprascapular nerve the deltoid is able to abduct the arm.

THE SECOND 90°: The humerus can abduct on the scapula only to 90° (*Fig.* 188). It is then stopped by impinging on the acromion process. Should the humerus be forced to a greater angle from the side of the body, one of two things must obviously happen: (1) The humerus breaks where the acromion touches it; or (2) The head of the humerus is forced through the lower part of the capsule of the shoulder-joint (dislocation).

---

[1] Lockhart has shown by observation of movements at the shoulder-joint in different positions that some scapular movement occurs during the first 90° of abduction, and by radiography that there is some humeroglenoid movement during the second 90° of abduction. This article (*J. Anat.*, Lond., 1930, April, 288) should be consulted by all those interested. For teaching purposes we feel that the classical account of the mechanism of abduction given in the text is sufficiently near the truth.

[2] Moseley, H. F., *Br. J. Surg.*, 1951, 38, 340.

Abduct the humerus to 90°, put a finger over the sternoclavicular joint, and continue abduction; the movement will be felt to occur at the *sternoclavicular joint,* and is therefore a movement of the shoulder-girdle (scapula and clavicle), the humerus being firmly fixed and held in 90° of abduction. The muscle which fixes the humerus at 90° is the deltoid.

The movement of the shoulder-girdle is a rotation of the lower angle of the scapula outwards, carrying the clavicle with it. This is performed by the serratus anterior. To enable the serratus to rotate the lower angle of the scapula outwards and so force the glenoid cavity with the humerus in contact with it through the second 90° of abduction, the scapula must be capable of rotating round its own centre, exactly as though it were fixed to the chest by a nail through its middle. The trapezius is the nail and so fixes it, whilst the serratus causes it to rotate. Five of the eight digitations of the serratus are inserted into the lower angle of the scapula, proving how important a function of the serratus is rotation of the scapula.

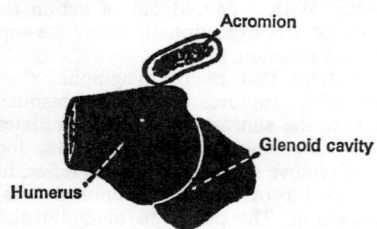

Fig. 188.—Showing that abduction of the humerus beyond a right-angle is prevented by its surgical neck impinging on the acromion process.

Martin[1] has drawn attention to a most important phase of abduction at the shoulder-joint which has escaped previous observers. With the arms at the sides of the body, flex the elbows to a right-angle with the forearms pointing directly forward. Abduct the arm as far as possible. Observe that abduction is only possible to a *right-angle* (90°). Now, with the arms hanging at the sides, the elbows flexed to a right-angle and the forearms in the coronal plane (i.e., pointing directly outwards), again abduct; observe that abduction is now possible through two right-angles (180°) (*Fig.* 189). What is the explanation? Towards the end of the first 90° the great tuberosity of the humerus impinges on the acromion, further abduction only being possible if the arm rotates outwards through 90° to allow the tuberosity to escape from the

[1] *Br. J. Surg.*, 1932, 20, 61.

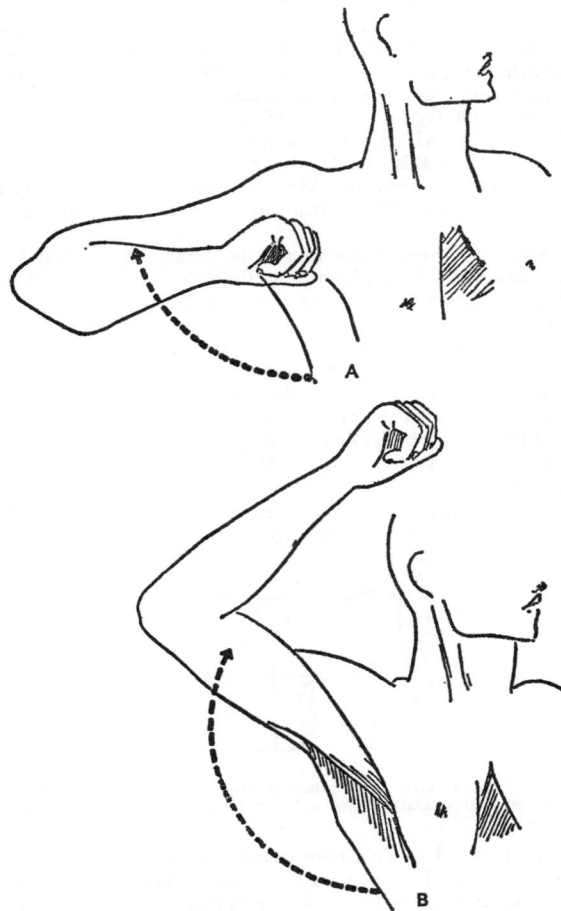

Fig. 189.—A, When the arm is rotated inwards, abduction at the shoulder is limited to 90°. B, With the arm rotated out, abduction can take place to 180°, i.e., until it is perpendicular.

impediment offered by the acromion process. Full abduction of the arm is, therefore, accompanied by lateral rotation of the humerus through 90°. The significant practical application of Martin's observation is that inability to rotate the arm outward will, *ipso facto*, result in inability to carry out the second 90° of abduction. The power of rotation requires, therefore, to be carefully examined in every case of injury in the region of the shoulder.

EFFECTS OF PARALYSIS OF MUSCLES CONCERNED:

1. THE DELTOID: If this muscle be out of action, the person cannot abduct the arm from the side, except in an occasional very rare instance where the supraspinatus becomes capable of the task.

2. THE SERRATUS: Should this muscle be paralysed, the first 90° of abduction can be performed by the deltoid, the scapula being fixed by the trapezius, though the scapula becomes winged, i.e., its vertebral border and lower angle project out from the chest wall. The second 90° cannot be carried out.

3. THE TRAPEZIUS: Should this muscle be out of action, the arm can be abducted by the deltoid through the first 90°, the scapula being fixed by the serratus. The second 90° cannot be performed. If now the scapula be firmly pressed by the examiner's hand against the chest wall so that it can rotate under the hand but not move sideways, the patient is able to perform the second 90° of abduction. The hand takes the place of the 'nail' by permitting rotation but not lateral mobility of the scapula.

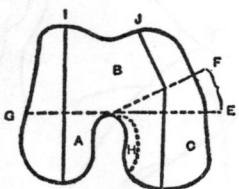

Fig. 190.—Condyles of femur with cartilage in situ. Areas marked out are explained in text, with special reference to 'locking-home' action of knee-joint.

Rotation at the Knee-joint: This joint admits of flexion and extension. At the very end of extension a slight amount of inward rotation of the femur on the tibia takes place. At the beginning of flexion a slight amount of outward rotation of the femur on the tibia occurs. The markings on the lower end of the femur with its cartilage in situ demonstrate this (*Fig.* 190). The axis of the outer condyle (I) is straight, that of the inner condyle (J) is curved, to enable it to rotate.

A is the surface for the outer condyle of the tibia. B is the surface for the patella. C is the surface for the inner condyle of the tibia. When the extension itself is complete the anterior edges of the menisci of the knee-joint rest in the slight grooves G and E. The movement of the outer condyles is completed; the inner condyle of the femur, however, rotates inward through the arc FE, so that the anterior border of the inner meniscus rests in the groove F. The joint is now locked. The muscles can be relaxed, yet the bony lock makes the lower limb quite stable. Thus one may stand at attention for a long time with relaxed quadriceps muscles. The reverse movement occurs when the knee is flexed. If the foot is off the ground, the joint is unlocked by the tibia rotating inward on the femur. The popliteus and semimembranosus, acting from above, perform this action. If the foot is fixed on the ground, the femur rotates outward to unlock the joint, this action being performed by the popliteus acting from below.

The childish game of tapping the back of the knee of an unsuspecting playmate involves this anatomy. The tap is the physiological stimulus to the unlocking muscles to contract, and the person, taken off his guard, falls to the ground.

The area H has nothing to do with the locking mechanism. It comes into contact with a similar area on the inner side of the articular surface of the patella in full flexion at the knee, the patella rotating slightly outwards in this position.

Inversion and Eversion of the Foot: The ankle-joint transmits more weight than any other joint in the body. It is therefore a very stable joint, which property entails limited mobility. The only movements possible at the joint, therefore, are flexion and extension. The movements of abduction, adduction, inversion, and eversion take place below the ankle-joint, at the mediotarsal and subtaloid joints.

INVERSION: Rotating the sole of the foot inwards round the long axis of the foot is performed by the tibialis anterior and posterior. The flexors of the toes assist.

EVERSION: Rotating the sole outwards around the long axis of the foot:
1. WHEN THE FOOT IS PLANTAR-FLEXED: The three peronei—longus, brevis, and tertius—perform the movement.
2. WHEN THE FOOT IS DORSIFLEXED: The movement is performed by the extensor digitorum longus.

This is easily verified. Plantar-flex the foot and evert strongly; the strain is felt on the outer side of the leg over the peronei. Now dorsiflex and evert, no strain is felt over the peronei, but the extensor longus is seen and felt to be in strong action. This was discovered by orthopaedic surgeons, who found that if the extensor digitorum longus was paralysed, the foot could be everted in plantar flexion but not in dorsiflexion.

In *congenital club-foot* (talipes equinovarus), the object of treatment is to get the foot dorsiflexed and everted. It is of the first importance, then, to develop the muscle which does this, the extensor digitorum longus. It is useless putting the foot in the correct position if this muscle is not strong enough to hold it there.

Chapter XXII

FASCIAE

I. THE FASCIA COLLI

THE deep fascia of the neck is of profound surgical importance. It consists essentially of three layers: (1) The general investing layer of fascia; (2) The pretracheal fascia; and (3) The prevertebral fascia. The arrangement is the simplest possible, as the diagram indicates (*Fig.* 191).

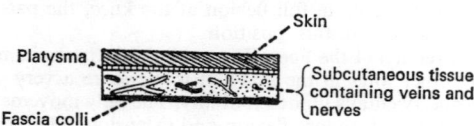

Fig. 191.—Plan of fascia colli.

General Investing Layer: This layer, which corresponds to the deep fascia in any other region, is remarkable for the frequency with which it splits into two. Its superficial relations are of much importance. The platysma muscle is superficial to it. Between the fascia and this muscle lie the superficial veins (anterior and external jugulars) and cutaneous nerves of the neck. The student is usually forgetful of the fact that the muscle must be cut before the veins are seen (*Fig.* 192). Incisions in the neck bleed freely before the deep fascia is cut, as the retraction of the divided platysma holds the cut veins open and they are thus prevented from retraction because of their attachment to the surface of the fascia. Once the deep fascia is divided, the veins are able to retract and most of the oozing stops. In sewing up a neck wound the surgeon is careful to approximate the deep fascia and platysma. Should this precaution be neglected the scar will stretch, as the divided platysma exerts a constant distraction on it.

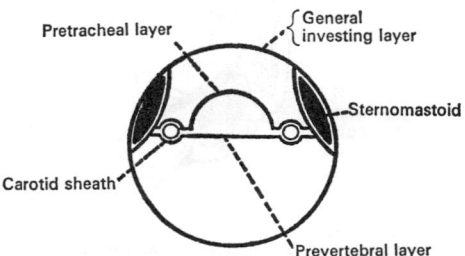

Fig. 192.—Relationship of integuments of neck.

ARRANGEMENT OF THE GENERAL INVESTING LAYER: Posteriorly, where it is thin and weak, it is attached to the ligamentum nuchae. It splits immediately to enclose the trapezius, at the anterior border of which it reunites to form the dense fascial roof to the posterior triangle. Reaching the posterior border of the sternomastoid, the fascia again divides and ensheathes this muscle, and then the two layers rejoin and continue onwards as the roof of the anterior triangle (*Fig.* 192).

The fascia is terminated above and below by attachments to bone:

ATTACHMENTS ABOVE:
1. External occipital protuberance.
2. Superior nuchal line.
3. Base of mastoid process.
4. Zygomatic arch.
5. Lower border of mandible.

ATTACHMENTS BELOW:
1. Spine of scapula and acromion process.
2. Clavicle.
3. Manubrium sterni.

The fascia splits above to enclose two of the salivary glands:
1. SUBMAXILLARY GLAND INVESTMENT: At the lower border of the submaxillary salivary gland the fascial roof of the anterior triangle splits to ensheathe this gland. The layer of fascia superficial to the gland is attached to the lower border of the mandible. The layer which passes deep to the gland is attached to the mylohyoid line on the inner surface of the same bone (*Fig.* 193). Observe the fact that the submaxillary lymph-glands are in actual contact with the salivary gland, being inside its sheath. For this reason the surgeon, in removing this group of lymph-glands for conditions such as carcinoma or tuberculosis,

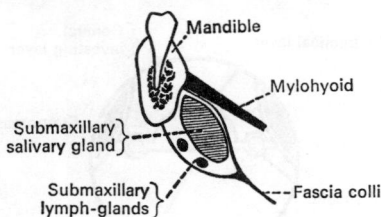

Fig. 193.—To show splitting of general investing layer of fascia colli to enclose the submaxillary salivary and lymph-glands.

must remove the salivary gland as well. D. M. Blair[1] has drawn attention to the fact that lymphoid tissue may occur *within* the actual capsule of the salivary gland. This fact may account for cases of tuberculosis apparently primary in the submaxillary salivary gland, and is an added argument in favour of removal of this gland in cases of cancer of the floor of the mouth and tongue.

2. THE PAROTID INVESTMENT: Behind the angle of the mandible is a gap between this bone and the mastoid process, which gap is occupied by the parotid gland. At the lower pole of this gland the general investing layer splits to ensheathe it. The deeper of the two layers passes up under the gland to be attached to the base of the skull; the more superficial layer passes up anterior to the masseter muscle to be attached to the lower border of the zygomatic arch. It is this layer which is called the parotideo-masseteric fascia. It is of great strength and density, which accounts for the severe pain produced by inflammatory swellings of the parotid, as these cause tension beneath the fascia, e.g., mumps. This layer forms the deep fascia of the posterior part of the cheek. The rest of the face is devoid of deep fascia. That part of the parotid sheath which binds the styloid process to the angle of the mandible is called the stylomandibular ligament. It separates the parotid and submaxillary glands, and is pierced by the cervical part of the external maxillary artery. In excising a submaxillary gland the careful surgeon secures the artery before dividing it, otherwise the vessel may retract through the stylomandibular ligament and cause serious bleeding before it can be controlled (Stiles).

The general investing layer of fascia splits below to form two spaces:

1. Where it forms the lower part of the roof of the posterior triangle the fascia splits into two layers both of which are attached to the clavicle. Between these two layers are found:

---

[1] *Br. med. J.*, 1929, **1**, 443.

a. Portions of the descending supraclavicular nerves (becoming superficial).
   b. A portion of the external jugular vein (becoming deep).
   c. Lymphatics and cutaneous vessels.
 2. Where it forms the lower part of the roof of the anterior triangle the fascia splits to form the suprasternal space (the space of Burns). The layers pass down to be attached, one to the anterior, the other to the posterior border of the manubrium sterni. Between these two layers are found:
   a. The sternal heads of the sternomastoid muscles.
   b. The communication between the anterior jugular veins.
   c. A lymph-gland.
   d. The interclavicular ligament.

To recapitulate: the general investing layer of the fascia colli:
 1. Splits to enclose *two muscles*: trapezius, sternomastoid.
 2. Splits to enclose *two salivary glands:* submaxillary, parotid.
 3. Splits to form *two spaces*: in the roof of the posterior triangle; in the suprasternal space.

CAROTID SHEATH: The general investing layer gives off, on the deep surface of the sternomastoid, two sheets of fascia, the pretracheal and the prevertebral fasciae. Between these two layers near their origins are found the common carotid artery, the internal jugular vein, and the vagus nerve (the carotid system). The fascia immediately surrounding these structures is the carotid sheath. It is obvious, therefore, that both the pretracheal and the prevertebral fasciae assist in the formation of the sheath.

Pretracheal Fascia:

HORIZONTAL EXTENT: It passes across the front of the carotid system, and then meeting the thyroid gland it splits to enclose it.

VERTICAL EXTENT: The fascia passes up in front of the larynx, ending above by being attached to the hyoid bone. It is bound down to the cricoid and thyroid cartilages. Passing down in front of the trachea, it ends below by blending with the fibrous pericardium over the great vessels in the superior mediastinum.

The thyroid gland moves up and down with the larynx in swallowing because the pretracheal fascia fixes it to the laryngeal cartilages. The sheath which this fascia gives to the thyroid gland is weakest, or may even be absent, over the posterior surfaces of the lateral lobes. Enlargements of the gland may therefore extend backwards in this line of least resistance, coming into relation with the oesophagus or pharynx and giving little surface indication of their presence (Stiles). The pretracheal fascia gives off (like the prevertebral layer) one single fascial process—the fascia of the depressors. This is a thin sheet of fascia which passes in front of the sternohyoid, sternothyroid, and omohyoid muscles. It is this layer which binds

210 A SYNOPSIS OF SURGICAL ANATOMY

down the intermediate tendon of the omohyoid to the clavicle. This is a definite fascia landmark in operations on the thyroid gland.

Prevertebral Fascia:

HORIZONTAL EXTENT: Commencing from the deep surface of the sternomastoid, this process passes posterior to the carotid system, the pharynx, larynx, oesophagus, and trachea, but in front of the vertebrae and the prevertebral muscles.

VERTICAL EXTENT: The fascia is attached above to the base of the skull. Below it extends into the superior mediastinum of the thorax, fading away on its posterior wall.

This layer of fascia is the posterior boundary, as the pretracheal layer is the anterior wall, of a space to which Sir Harold Stiles gave the happy name of 'the visceral compartment of the neck'. It will be seen that all the viscera of the neck—pharynx, larynx, trachea, and thyroid—are contained in this compartment.

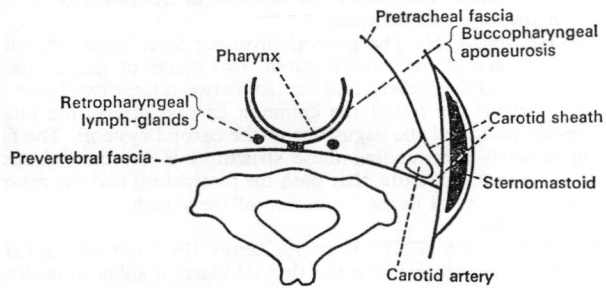

Fig. 194.—Showing how upper part of pharynx is bound to prevertebral fascia in *midline* by buccopharyngeal aponeurosis. Note also formation of carotid sheath.

BUCCOPHARYNGEAL FASCIA: This is a layer of connective tissue found at the sides and back of the pharynx. It has this single important physical relationship, viz., that it binds the middle line of the back of the pharynx firmly to the prevertebral fascia (*Fig.* 194). This fact is of diagnostic significance in the condition known as *retropharyngeal abscess*. Such a collection may occur in one of two anatomical sites (*Fig.* 195):

1. THE ACUTE TYPE: This occurs in front of the prevertebral fascia in relation to one of the retropharyngeal lymph-glands which lie in front of this fascia. Such an abscess remains *on one side of the middle line* because of the attachment of the buccopharyngeal fascia to the prevertebral fascia.

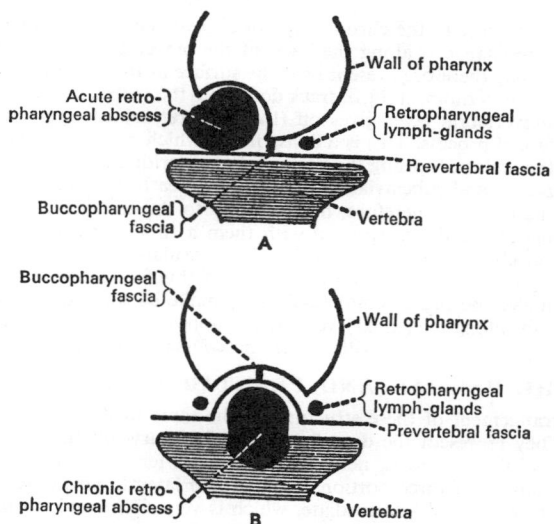

Fig. 195.—Diagrams to show that acute retropharyngeal abscess (A) presents in pharynx to one side of midline, whereas chronic abscess (B) presents centrally.

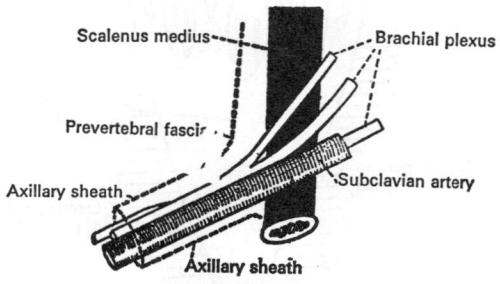

Fig. 196.—Formation of axillary sheath.

2. THE CHRONIC TYPE: This abscess forms in relation to disease (usually tuberculosis) of a cervical vertebra and is therefore behind the prevertebral fascia. *It is central in position* and bulges into the pharynx in the midline, in contrast to the acute abscess, which is lateral in situation. It will be seen that should the

pressure in the chronic type of abscess increase, the line of least resistance is along the back of the prevertebral fascia. The pus may therefore present near the surface at the posterior border of the sternomastoid, or track down into the thorax behind the fascia.

The prevertebral layer gives off (like the pretracheal layer) one single fascial process. This is a dense fascia which passes backwards over the scaleni, forming the floor of the posterior triangle. The brachial plexus and subclavian artery lie underneath this floor. On leaving the triangle, therefore, on their way to the axilla, these structures pierce the floor, carrying with them a tubular sheath of the prevertebral fascia (*Fig.* 196). This is the axillary sheath, which extends right down to the elbow. Because of this fact a collection of fluid under the prevertebral fascia may make its way down this fascial tube along the axillary vessels, and appear first as a swelling on the outer wall of the axilla along the course of the artery.

II. THE PALMAR AND PLANTAR FASCIAE

The arrangement of these structures is the same in the hand and in the foot. They represent the deep fascia of other parts of the body and are superficial to the vessels, nerves, muscles, and tendons. In each case the fascia consists of three portions: medial and lateral, which are relatively thin and weak; and intermediate, which is very dense and strong.

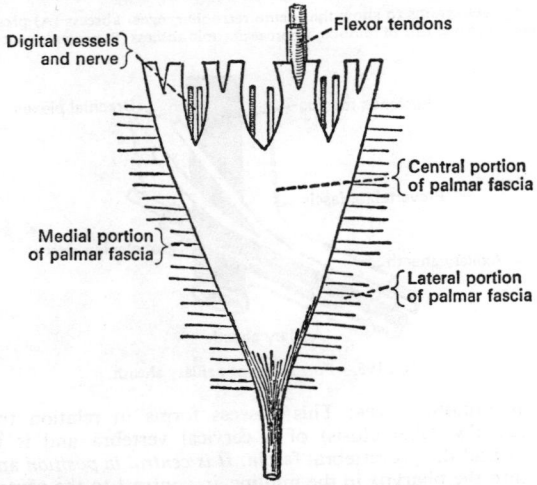

Fig. 197.—General arrangement of palmar fascia. The central triangular process is seen dividing into four digital processes, each of which splits into two.

FASCIAE 213

The Medial Process covers the hypothenar eminence in the hand. In the foot it covers the more superficial muscles of the great toe.

The Lateral Process covers the thenar eminence in the hand and the more superficial muscles of the little toe in the foot. The lateral process of the fascia in the foot is thickened along its posterior part by a dense band of fascia which extends from the outer process of the tuberosity of the calcaneus to the base of the fifth metatarsal bone. It is representative of a muscle which had the same connexions—the extensor of the metatarsal bone of the fifth digit.

The Central or Intermediate Part: Its arrangement corresponds closely in the hand and foot, excepting that in the hand it is related to the inner four digits only, whereas in the foot it is related to all five toes.

ARRANGEMENT IN THE HAND (*Fig.* 197): The fascia is triangular in shape.

THE APEX OF THE TRIANGLE: Attached to the transverse carpal ligament and the palmaris longus tendon.

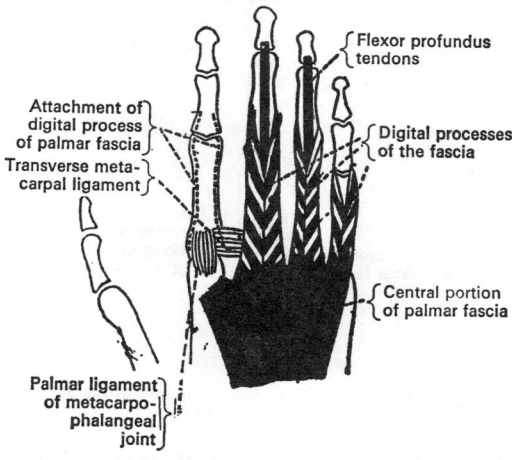

Fig. 198.—To show precise arrangement of digital processes of palmar fascia. Over index finger fascia and flexors are removed and dotted lines show attachments of palmar fascia to sides of first and second phalanges and to transverse ligament. Over middle and ring fingers fascia and flexors are in situ. Over the little finger the flexors are not shown.

THE BASE OF THE TRIANGLE: Divides opposite the heads of the metacarpal bones into four slips, one going to each of the four fingers. The site of division is strengthened by transverse fibres, the general direction of the fibres of the fascia being longitudinal. Passing between these slips are the vessels and nerves going to the fingers, and the lumbrical muscles. Each slip divides into two processes, between which pass the flexor tendons. These processes diverge and dip down to be attached to:

1. The transverse metacarpal ligament (*see* p. 215).
2. The fibrous flexor sheath.
3. The whole length of the inner and outer borders of the first phalanx of the digit (*Figs.* 198, 199).
4. The proximal part of the inner and outer borders of the second phalanx of the digit.

This attachment is of great surgical importance. In advanced cases of pathological contracture of the palmar fascia—Dupuytren (1832)—the first and second phalanges of the fingers are acutely flexed because the palmar fascia is attached to them. The third phalanx is extended as the fascia has no attachment to it. The condition is essentially bilateral.

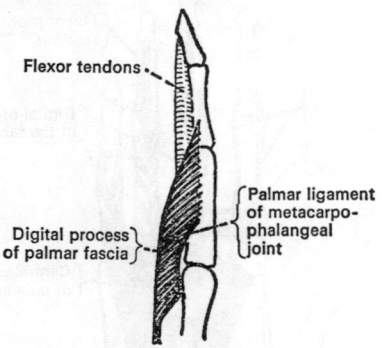

Fig. 199.—Attachment of one of the digital processes of the palmar fascia seen from the side.

In the sole this disease—fibrosis of the plantar fascia—is quite different and often misdiagnosed. It presents as a nodule on the inner border of the foot in the hollow forming the top of the arch. Here the fascia is most likely to be injured in stresses applied to the sole. There is no contracture of the toes because of the feeble or absent attachment of the slips of the plantar fascia to the phalanges. The skin is not contracted as the plantar fascia is not as intimately attached to the skin as obtains in the palm.

By its edges the intermediate portion of the palmar fascia is attached to the thin medial and lateral parts. From these margins of union two septa dip down to be attached to the fascia covering the interossei. By these two partitions the hand is divided into three compartments: (1) A medial, containing the hypothenar muscles; (2) A lateral, containing the thenar muscles; (3) An intermediate, containing the superficial volar arch and its branches, the tendons of the sublimis and profundus digitorum, with the lumbrical muscles and branches of the median nerve. The intermediate portion of the palmar fascia is related therefore by its deep surface to the structures in the intermediate compartment. Its superficial surface is related to fat and to small cutaneous vessels and nerves.

The intermediate process of plantar fascia behaves in a precisely similar fashion to the intermediate process of palmar fascia, excepting that it divides into five processes. Its attachment posteriorly is to the medial process of the tuberosity of the calcaneus. Anteriorly its attachments to the phalanges are weak or absent.

The Transverse Metacarpal Ligament: The transverse metacarpal ligament binds the four fingers together. It is attached to the palmar (volar accessory) ligaments of the metacarpophalangeal joints and prevents separation of the four inner metacarpal bones from each other. The transverse metatarsal ligament has a precisely similar arrangement except that it binds together all five metatarsals. The interossei are dorsal to this ligament; the lumbricals, flexor tendons, and palmar or plantar vessels and nerves are volar to the ligament.

III. THE LUMBODORSAL FASCIA

The lumbodorsal fascia consists of three strong layers of fascia, anterior, middle, and posterior, which fill in the gap between the 12th rib and the iliac crest. The posterior and middle layers are very dense and strong; the

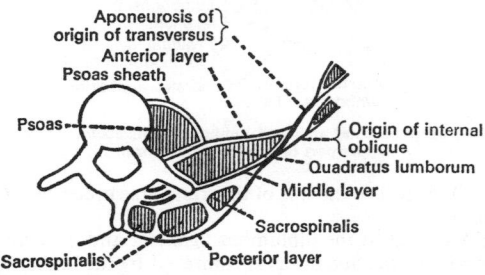

Fig. 200.—Lumbodorsal fascia and psoas sheath.

anterior layer is not so strong. Between the posterior and middle layers are the sacrospinalis and transversus spinalis muscles; between the anterior and middle layers is the quadratus lumborum. The three layers fuse laterally to form a dense tendinous structure which forms the aponeurosis of origin of the transversus abdominis muscle. From the lateral surface of this aponeurosis the internal oblique muscle receives an origin (*Fig.* 200).

Attachments of the Anterior Layer:

ABOVE: Attached medially to the 1st lumbar transverse process, laterally to the 12th rib (in front of the quadratus), forming the lateral lumbocostal arch, from the upper border of which the diaphragm arises, and behind which the 12th thoracic nerve and subcostal vessels pass into the abdominal wall.

MEDIAL: The ridges on the anterior surfaces of the lumbar transverse processes which can often be felt and seen. This ridge is near, though not actually at, the root of the transverse process.

BELOW: The iliolumbar ligament and iliac crest.

The kidney lies on the fascia, and its fascia, the renal fascia, blends with it. The 12th thoracic nerve and subcostal vessels and the iliohypogastric and ilio-inguinal nerves lie between this fascia and the quadratus muscle in exactly the same way that the phrenic nerve in the neck lies between the scalenus anterior muscle and the prevertebral fascia.

Attachments of the Middle Layer:

ABOVE: Attached to the 12th rib laterally and the 1st lumbar transverse process medially (behind the quadratus), forming the lumbocostal *ligament*.

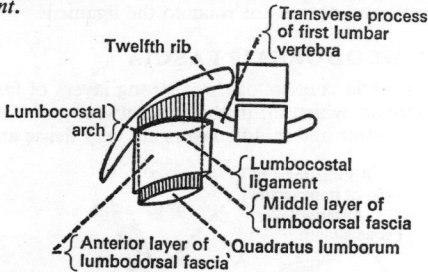

Fig. 201.—Lumbocostal arch and lumbocostal ligament, which embrace upper part of quadratus lumborum.

MEDIAL: Attached to the tips of the transverse processes of the lumbar vertebrae.

BELOW: Attached to the iliolumbar ligament and iliac crest.

The upper part of the quadratus is embraced by the lateral lumbocostal arch in front and the lumbocostal ligament behind (*Fig.* 201).

FASCIAE 217

Attachments of the Posterior Layer:
  MEDIAL: Spines of vertebrae (lumbar, sacral, thoracic).
  BELOW: The iliac crest.
  ABOVE: Extends to the upper part of the thorax as the *thoracic part of the lumbodorsal fascia*.

Attachments of the Thoracic Part of the Lumbodorsal Fascia:
  MEDIAL: Spines of the thoracic vertebrae.
  LATERAL: The angles of the ribs.
  ABOVE: It fuses with the fasciae of the neck. The serratus posterior inferior *arises from* the posterior layer of lumbodorsal fascia below. The thoracic portion of the fascia passes into the neck *deep to* the serratus posterior superior.

Sheath of the Psoas: A membranous 'stocking' round the muscle, which, in disease, may become as strong as the posterior layer of lumbodorsal fascia (*Fig.* 202).

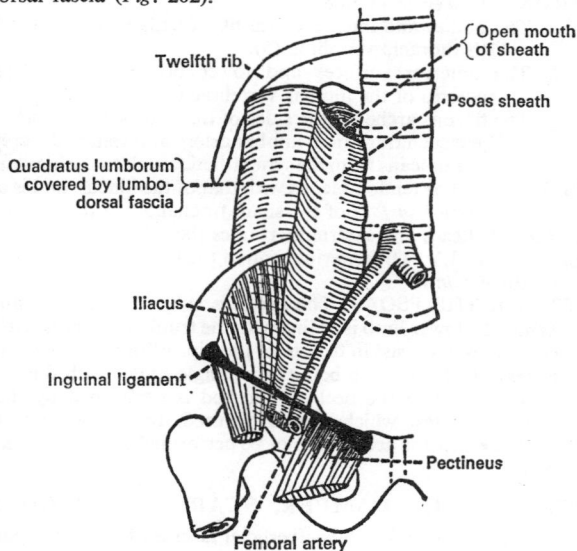

Fig. 202.—The psoas sheath.

ATTACHMENTS:
  MEDIAL: The bodies of the lumbar vertebrae.
  LATERAL: Blends with the anterior layer of the lumbodorsal fascia above and the fascia iliaca below.

BELOW: Extends behind the femoral artery into the thigh, where it blends with the psoas tendon.

ABOVE: It is held open by its upper attachment to the body of the 2nd lumbar vertebra medially and the 1st lumbar transverse process laterally. This upper edge forms the medial lumbocostal arch, and the diaphragm arises from it. It is a funnel-shaped orifice opening into the posterior mediastinum of the thorax. Pus tracking down from thoracic vertebrae (in tuberculous spondylitis) enters this funnel and is directed by the psoas sheath into the thigh, where it presents behind and on each side of the femoral vessels. Such a collection of pus may, however, rupture higher up into the anterior compartment of the lumbodorsal fascia or under the fascia iliaca.

Psoas Major Muscle:
ORIGINS: Fifteen in number:
  a. The bodies and intervertebral fibrocartilages of the lumbar and 12th thoracic vertebrae (5).
  b. The anterior surfaces and lower borders of the transverse processes of the lumbar vertebrae (5).
  c. The fibrous arches at the sides of the bodies of the vertebrae (5). These each transmit a lumbar artery and vein and a grey ramus communicans from the sympathetic trunk to the lumbar nerves.

INSERTION: The tendon blends with that of the iliacus, and is attached to the *anterior surface* of the small trochanter of the femur.

ACTION: It flexes and externally rotates the thigh.

NERVE-SUPPLY: The anterior rami of the lumbar nerves. The lumbar plexus lies *in* it.

TEST FOR THE PSOAS: The psoas is subject to sprains and tears. When the lower limb is in line with the trunk, the rectus femoris and other muscles assist in flexion of the hip. With the patient sitting up in bed, the lower limb being at an angle of 90° with the trunk, the action of lifting the heel off the bed is performed by the psoas. This is the test which should be used. In severe injuries to the muscle either the action cannot be performed or it is associated with pain.

IV. FASCIAE OF CAMPER, SCARPA, AND COLLES

These are names applied to the superficial fasciae of the lower part of the anterior abdominal wall and perineum.

Fasciae of Scarpa and Camper: Midway between the umbilicus and pubis the superficial fascia is condensed on its deep surface to form a membranous layer—the fascia of Scarpa. Sandwiched in between the skin and this fascial condensation is fat which corresponds to and is continuous with the subcutaneous fat of the body generally. This fat receives in this situation the name of Camper's fascia (*Fig.* 203).

FASCIAE

The fasciae of Camper and Scarpa may be compared to a piece of surgeon's lint. The smooth side is Scarpa's fascia, the rough side is Camper's fascia. They can only be separated with a knife, excepting just below the inguinal ligament, where they are separated by the lymph-glands and cutaneous vessels of the groin (*Fig.* 204).

Just below the subcutaneous abdominal ring (external ring) Camper's fascia gives place to the dartos muscle of the scrotum, which, like the platysma, is a muscle of the superficial fascia. There is no subcutaneous fat in the penis or scrotum.

THE DARTOS: Gives a muscle sheath to the penis and to each testicle. The muscle is much more extensive than is usually thought and is responsible for the corrugations of the scrotal skin.

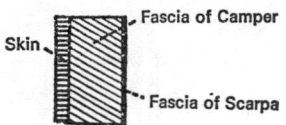

Fig. 203.—To show nature of fasciae over lower abdominal wall.

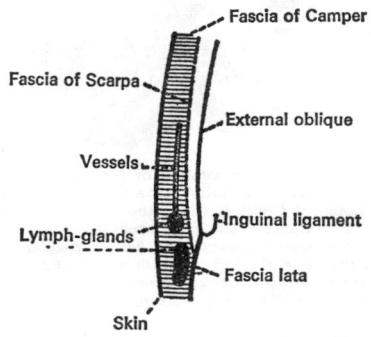

Fig. 204.—Fasciae of Scarpa and Camper. The lymph-glands and vessels interposed between these two layers at the inguinal region are shown.

THE ATTACHMENTS OF SCARPA'S FASCIA:
ABOVE: The fascia fades away midway between the pubis and umbilicus above, and in the lumbar region at the sides.

BELOW:
    Medial: Just below the subcutaneous or external abdominal ring the fascia changes its name to fascia of Colles.

Lateral: The fascia is attached to the deep fascia of the thigh—the fascia lata—just below the inguinal ligament. This attachment is about 5 cm. below the anterior superior iliac spine, and just below the pubic spine.

Because of this attachment to the fascia lata fluid tracking down from above under the superficial fascia cannot extend farther into the thigh than the line of this attachment.

Fascia of Colles: Just below the subcutaneous inguinal ring Scarpa's fascia changes its name to Colles's fascia. This extends over the penis and scrotum, giving a fascial covering to each; it then covers the muscles in the superficial compartment of the perineum (*Fig.* 205).

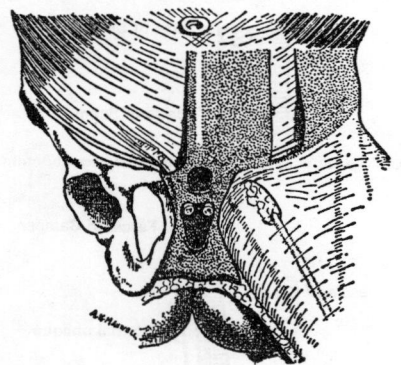

Fig. 205.—A masterly representation of the continuity of the fasciae of Scarpa (above the groin) and of Colles (below the level of the groin). The upper aperture in the fascia of Colles is where the penis passes through the fascia carrying a fascial sheath with it. The lower opening is where the spermatic cords pass through carrying a similar investment. Note particularly that the fascia of Scarpa does not fuse with the rectus sheath and external oblique superiorly, although the drawing suggests it. (*By kind permission of Professor Lockhart and the publishers of Cunningham's 'Textbook of Anatomy'.*)

ATTACHMENTS:

LATERAL: It is attached to the conjoined ramus of the ischium and pubis.

BELOW: It is attached to the posterior border of the urogenital diaphragm.

ABOVE: It is continuous with the fascia of Scarpa.

MEDIAL: It is continuous with its fellow of the opposite side.

The fascia sends a median septum to be attached to the perineal muscles.
This septum is not complete, and fluid may pass through it from one side to the other.

Practical Points:
  RELATION OF SPERMATIC CORD: The spermatic cord passes
    into the scrotum deep to the fasciae of Scarpa and Colles.
  EXTRAVASATION OF FLUID: If fluid is extravasated under the
    fascia of Colles in the perineum from rupture of the urethra in this
    region, such fluid may extend only as follows:
    DOWNWARDS: It can extend only to the lower border of the urogenital
      diaphragm, as here the fascia of Colles fuses with the base of this
      diaphragm.
    LATERALLY: It may extend through the median septum as far as the
      conjoined ischiopubic rami because the fascia of Colles is attached
      here.
    UPWARDS: It may extend over the penis and scrotum because they are
      covered by the fascia of Colles.
      It may extend up alongside the spermatic cord on to the
      abdominal wall because the fascia of Colles is not bound down
      to the pubis in this region.
      Once fluid gains the anterior abdominal wall, it may extend
      down just over the inguinal ligament, until it is held up by the
      attachment of Scarpa's fascia to the fascia lata. The fluid may
      extend upward to any extent, even to the axillae, in the plane
      between the superficial and deep fasciae.

V. THE PELVIC FASCIA

The pelvic fascia is an essentially simple structure. It consists of two layers:
(1) Parietal—membranous and strong; (2) Visceral—connective-tissue-like.
The Parietal Layer: Is merely the layer of wall-paper which lines the walls
  of the room formed by the true pelvis. The obturator internus muscle
  is between the wall and the wall-paper. The part of the fascia covering
  this muscle is confusingly and unnecessarily called the obturator fascia.
  ATTACHMENTS OF THE FASCIA:
    ANTERIOR: The anterior limit of the fascia is along a line extending
      from the pelvic brim to the back of the pubis. This line begins at
      the pelvic brim at the level of the junction of the lower and middle
      third of the external iliac vessels, and is not straight, as it loops
      downwards to allow the obturator nerve and vessels to get to the
      obturator foramen without having to pierce it (*Fig.* 206).
    SUPERIOR: The fascia blends with the psoas sheath at the pelvic brim.
    POSTERIOR: The fascia extends behind the rectum, lining the hollow
      of the sacrum and becoming continuous with its fellow of the
      opposite side. It extends back in front of the piriformis and sacral
      plexus of nerves, and its outer surface is bound down to the
      margins of the small and great sacrosciatic foramina as it crosses
      them. In other words, the wall-paper covers the cracks in the wall
      made by these foramina.

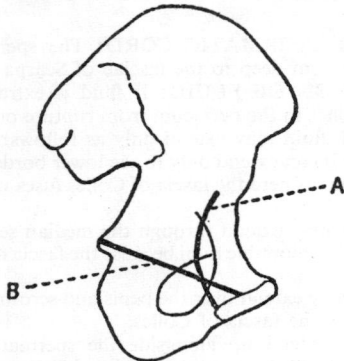

Fig. 206.—Showing how anterior attachment (A) of parietal layer of pelvic fascia and attachment of visceral layer (B) to side wall of pelvis cross like an X.

INFERIOR: The fascia extends down over the obturator internus, and many of its fibres end by being attached to the bony rim of the pelvic outlet (the conjoined ischiopubic ramus). Certain fibres, however, bridge the gap between the ischiopubic rami and form the *superior layer of the urogenital diaphragm* (upper layer of triangular ligament).

The inferior layer of the urogenital diaphragm has nothing to do with the pelvic fascia. At one time during evolution the pelvis had no gap beneath the symphysis. This was filled by a mass of bone. With the advent of mammals there was insufficient room at the pelvic outlet for the passage of the foetal head: the bony mass became replaced by fascia—*the inferior fascia of the urogenital diaphragm*. This is therefore the morphological representative of this one-time bony layer.

Attached to the inner surface of the wall-paper are two structures;
(1) The levator ani; and (2) The visceral layer of pelvic fascia.

The Visceral Layer: The parietal layer is closely applied to the walls of the pelvic cavity. The visceral layer is attached to the parietal merely by its edge. This edge of the visceral layer is attached along a line extending from the back of the pubis to the ischial spine (these are also the limits of the levator ani attachments). In *Fig.* 206 this line of attachment is seen. It is also apparent that this line crosses the anterior limit of attachment of the parietal layer. The two fasciae thus cross like an X behind the pubis.

The visceral layer (*Fig.* 207) extends horizontally into the cavity of the pelvis from this line of attachment and gives fascial sheaths to:

FASCIAE 223

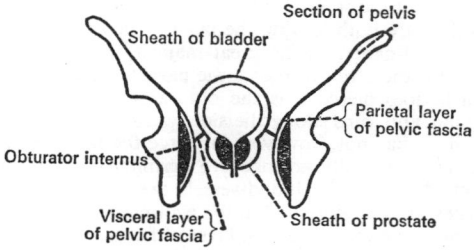

Fig. 207.—Coronal section of pelvis showing parietal and visceral layers of pelvic fascia.

(1) The rectum; (2) The bladder; (3) The prostate.

In the female the arrangement of the visceral layer of pelvic fascia is somewhat different. The fascia ensheathes bladder, urethra, vagina, and rectum. A fairly well-defined layer of the fascia extends down in front of the vagina and a second layer between rectum and vagina.

Of considerable importance is that part of the fascia which radiates fanwise from the cervico-vaginal junction to the side wall of the pelvis, forming the transverse ligament of the cervix, retinaculum uteri, or ligament of Mackenrodt (see PROLAPSE OF THE UTERUS, p. 717).

Nature shows great economy of labour in the manner in which the various structures are disposed of at the sides of the true pelvis (Fig. 208). The arrangement from external to internal is as follows:

1. Bone (wall of pelvis).
2. Parietal muscles (obturator internus and piriformis).
3. The sacral plexus of nerves.
4. The parietal pelvic fascia.
5. The blood-vessels.
6. The peritoneum.

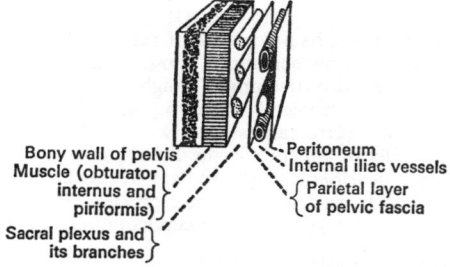

Fig. 208.—Isometric view of arrangement of structures on side wall of pelvis.

Observe that the obturator internus and piriformis are outside the wallpaper, as they are both leaving the pelvis. The sacral nerves are also outside the wall-paper, as the great majority are leaving the pelvis. They have not therefore to pierce the parietal fascia. The only large nerve which does pierce it is the obturator. This pierces the wallpaper behind and runs along the side wall of the pelvis. To get out of the pelvis it has not, however, to pierce the fascia a second time, as the fascia is specially arranged to permit it to cross its anterior attachment. Most of the blood-vessels are destined for the pelvic viscera. They are therefore within the wall-paper. Those going out of the pelvis must pierce the parietal layer of fascia.

Arising from the inner surface of the parietal layer of fascia at the side of the pelvis is the levator ani. The two levatores project inwards, one from each side, forming the pelvic diaphragm. They have each a fascial sheath. The part of the sheath on their upper surfaces is called the superior fascia of the pelvic diaphragm. The part of the sheath on their inferior surfaces is called the inferior fascia of the diaphragm, or the anal fascia. These names merely denote the sheaths of the muscles.

The above description of the pelvic fascia is somewhat different from that usually given, and is justified by its simplicity.

Chapter XXIII

BONES

I. ACCESSORY RIBS

Cervical Rib: Keith[1] has shown that there is always a rudiment of a cervical rib in the fetus. This usually entirely disappears, but in 1 or 2 per cent of cases it may persist throughout life. In only a part of this percentage does it ever give rise to symptoms. (It will be observed that in its constancy in the fetus, its percentage of occurrence in the adult, and the fact that it may only sometimes cause symptoms, it corresponds closely to a Meckel's diverticulum.) Though cervical ribs are frequently bilateral, symptoms are usually found on one side only.

A typical cervical vertebra possesses two tubercles on the transverse process. The anterior tubercle is the homologue of a rib, and may attain excessive development and remain free as a cervical rib, or it may be fused with the true transverse process. Sargent[2] has noted five types of rudimentary ribs at the cervicothoracic junction:

---

[1] Treves and Keith. *Surgical Applied Anatomy*, 184.
[2] *Surgical Applied Anatomy*, 205.

1. An excessively large costal process of the 7th cervical vertebra. It is unjointed, fused with the transverse process behind, and prolonged down as a fibrous band, attached to the 1st rib behind the scalene tubercle. This is the commonest abnormality.
2. A short cervical rib, with costocentral and costotransverse articulations with the vertebra, continued on as a fibrous band as in (1).
3. A jointed rib, carrying the 8th cervical nerve root on its bony portion, also connected with the 1st thoracic rib by a fibrous band.
4. A jointed rib, the anterior end being fused with, or articulating with, the 1st rib. The anterior and middle scaleni may be attached to such a rib.
5. The 1st thoracic rib is incomplete, its anterior end being replaced by a fibrous band.

Types 1 and 5 may not be visible in radiographs. Wood Jones states that prefixation of the plexus is apt to be associated with a 7th cervical rib and postfixation with an abnormal first thoracic rib.

The fibrous band causes more symptoms than the rib itself.

When the rib is longer than 5 cm. the subclavian artery and brachial plexus cross it on their way to the axilla and are elevated by it. This elevation has been mistaken for an exostosis, and for an aneurysm when the artery is pushed forward.

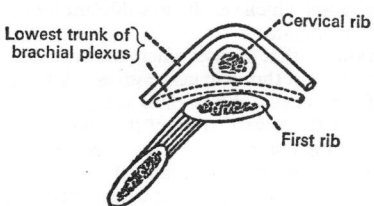

Fig. 209.—To show how a cervical rib may cause traction on the lowest trunk of the brachial plexus by angulating it. Dotted line shows normal position of trunk, which has been elevated by a cervical rib in this case.

The lowest trunk of the brachial plexus (C. 8, T. 1) lies in the subclavian groove on the upper surface of a normal first rib and is responsible for this groove (Wood Jones[1]). When a cervical rib exists it elevates this trunk which is already tautly stretched over the rib, and may in this fashion cause interference with its conduction (*Fig.* 209). This occurs when the nerve is fully stretched by the completion of growth, i.e., 20 to 30 years, or in later years when through worry, etc.,

[1] *Proc. R. Soc. Med.* (Clin. Sect.), 1895, Feb. 14, 1913.

the muscles holding up the shoulder lose their tone. Thus Head spoke of this type of sufferer from cervical rib neuritis as 'widows who take to washing'. There is then numbness on the ulnar side of the forearm and wasting of the small muscles of the hand. In 60 per cent of the cases there is no alteration in common sensibility.

Sargent classifies the symptoms of cervical rib as being referable to damage to:—
1. The somatic afferent nerves—e.g., neuralgia, cutaneous and deep sensory disturbance.
2. The somatic efferent fibres—e.g., muscular weakness, wasting, and electrical changes.
3. The sympathetic fibres—e.g., circulatory changes, such as coldness, cyanosis, oedema; and paraesthesiae such as tingling, numbness, coldness, or swelling.

Ross[1] states that a cervical rib can give rise to nervous or vascular symptoms but not to both. Vascular symptoms are produced by a complete rib, whereas a short one, continued forward by a fibrous band, may cause symptoms referable to nerve compression. The explanation given is that with a complete rib the plexus is prefixed and therefore not compressed whereas the artery has no such latitude. When the aneurysm affects the subclavian artery as the result of compression or angulation by the rib or anterior scalene muscle, it is always beyond the area of compression. It is caused by turbulence set up within the vessel which results in sufficient lateral pressure to cause dilatation or aneurysm.

It has been shown that in cases where the brachial plexus is postfixed, i.e., where the second thoracic nerve gives a large contribution to the formation of the plexus, the normal 1st rib may produce symptoms from pressure on the lowest trunk of the plexus. In such cases the part of the rib causing the pressure may have to be removed with its periosteum (to prevent its re-formation).

The elevation of the whole thorax which occurs in cases of advanced emphysema may cause sufficient raising of the 1st rib to produce pressure on the lowest trunk of the plexus, which results in the symptoms usually associated with cervical rib.

Pressure at the Cervicobrachial Junction: This lucid term is the title of an essay by Telford and Mottershead.[2] It serves well to group under one head a number of different anatomical conditions which produce a welter of clinical pictures which are difficult to disentangle and which are the cause of much confusion. The terms 'cervical rib' or 'scalenous anterior syndrome' are most commonly applied to the condition, but the former is often absent and it is doubtful if the latter condition exists.

---

[1] Ross, J. Patterson, *Ann. Surg.*, 1959, 150, 340.
[2] Telford, E. D., and Mottershead, S., *J. Bone Jt Surg.*, 1948, 30B, May, No. 2, 249.

Walshe[1] illuminates the perplexing situation. He points out how many and varied may be the factors producing the pressure. There are developmental ones such as the segmental origin of the brachial plexus. If the 4th cervical nerve makes a large contribution to its formation—prefixed plexus—a cervical rib may exist (although this is not an essential condition for its presence); if the 2nd thoracic nerve sends an important component—a postfixed plexus—the 1st rib may be imperfectly formed. Cervicothoracic scoliosis may throw the 1st rib and collar-bone into a propinquity which results in pressure on the neurovascular bundle. As Walshe points out the essence of the matter is the existence of an abnormal upper thoracic outlet. Add now the physiological activity normally occurring here: the thorax moves up and down about 23,000 times a day, the clavicle moves with each arm movement, head and neck movements also enter the picture. If the shoulder-girdle sags as happens often enough in weak-muscled, fatigued, or overworked people (usually women) the neurovascular bundle is pulled downwards on the sloping 1st rib and thus traction is effected, and this will always be greatest on the lowest trunk of the plexus. Such traction necessarily pulls this nerve-trunk and the subclavian artery hard up against the anterior scalene, which is then a mechanical compressing factor but only a secondary one. This author considers that under the conditions mentioned the artery becomes bound down by fibrous tissue thus fixing it and allowing of damage which may cause vascular symptoms or even aneurysmal dilatation. This explanation attributes the vascular disturbances to the mechanical factors outlined and not to irritation of sympathetic nerve fibres in the lowest trunk of the plexus. The authorities mentioned in this section share the views of many others that there can be no justification for the preoperative diagnosis of the scalene syndrome. Should this muscle play a part in the pathology it is either a secondary one as indicated above, or due to the existence of a lateral prolongation of its tendon of insertion which may act as a compressing factor (Telford and Mottershead) (*Fig.* 210). It is apparent from the foregoing that any part the anterior scalene may play in cases of cervicobrachial pressure is purely a passive one and the factor of spasm does not arise.

Telford and Mottershead are of the opinion that in persons with normal anatomy neither the brachial plexus nor the subclavian artery can be compressed against the 1st rib by the clavicle. When, however, some factor arises which narrows the clavicle–1st rib interval, such as cervicothoracic scoliosis, then the neurovascular bundle may be subjected to compression and removal of the 1st rib will relieve it. White and others[2] draw attention to the congenital anomalies of the

---

[1] Walshe, F. M. R., *Diseases of the Nervous System*, 4th ed., 1945. 236. Edinburgh.
White, James C., Poppel, M. H., and Adams, Ralph, *Surgery Gynec. Obstet.*, 1945, 31, 643.

1st thoracic rib. They show that in such cases this structure is usually poorly developed ending freely in the muscles or joining the 2nd rib by synostosis or pseudarthrosis. They state that the abnormality cannot be distinguished from a cervical rib on purely clinical grounds.

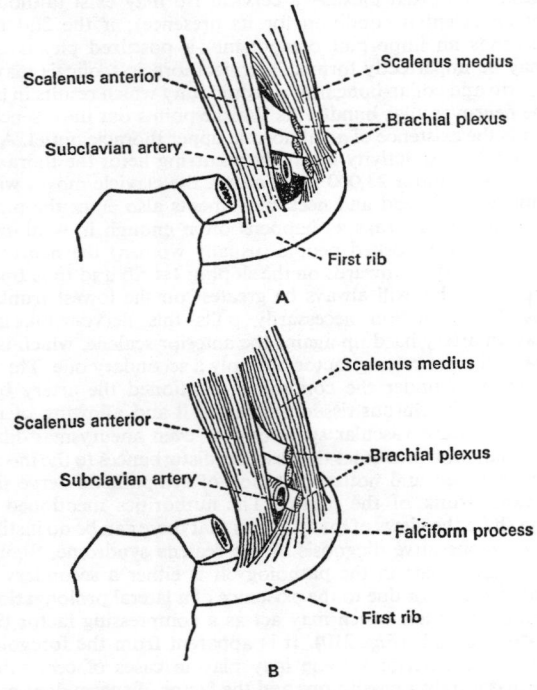

Fig. 210.—In A the normal anatomy is shown. In B is illustrated the manner in which the neurovascular bundle is compressed by a falciform process of the tendon of insertion of scalenus medius. (*Re-drawn from Telford and Mottershead.*)

The very important observation is made that the neuralgia from a 1st thoracic rib is usually much more widespread than that from a cervical rib due to the fact that the former rib is longer and deforms the thoracic outlet more than the latter.

To the picture thus described must be added:

1. Neuralgia due to prolapse of one of the cervical intervertebral discs.

2. Encroachment by bone on cervical nerves where they enter the intervertebral foramina such as is so commonly seen in cervical osteoarthritis. Under certain circumstances the dural sheath of the spinal nerve (just before it enters the intervertebral foramen) may compress the nerve and cause motor or sensory disturbances.

3. Peripheral neuritis, muscle dystrophies, etc.

It is apparent how complex the differential diagnosis may be, how great the need for meticulous study of the case, and how wise the advice of Telford and Mottershead who enjoin that operation should not be undertaken with any preconceived rigid ideas but through exposure sufficiently generous to allow of thorough investigation of the cause of pressure.

Lumbar Rib: An accessory rib may occur at the other end of the thorax. Usually this takes the form of a short rib articulating with the 1st lumbar vertebra (*Fig.* 211). Cases have been recorded where such a rib

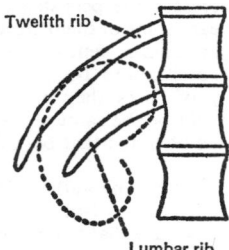

Fig. 211.—Relation of a lumbar rib to the kidney.

(which forms a direct posterior relation of the kidney) has produced constant backache because of its close relation to the kidney. The removal of the rib has caused the disappearance of the symptoms.

II. OTHER ACCESSORY BONES

Thurstan Holland[1] remarks: 'Formerly the importance of the presence of these small ossicles was purely academic and anatomical, and all the knowledge about them was gained from anatomical specimens. The advent of X-rays, however, made it possible to demonstrate their presence during life; and owing to the facts that radiologically they may simulate injuries or be the site of certain diseases, an accurate knowledge of these ossicles, especially in view of such Acts as the Workmen's Compensation Act, became of great practical importance'.

---

[1] 'The Accessory Bones of the Foot', *The Robert Jones Birthday Volume*, 157. The whole of the facts dealing with the accessory bones of the foot are taken from this article.

The same authority, in stressing the importance of these bones in the foot, makes the important statement that though similar ossicles do occur in the hand, they are so seldom shown by X-rays that they cannot compare in radiological interest with those in the foot, some of which are comparatively common and can be easily demonstrated. Apart from the mere radiological interest, the practical importance of such bones in the foot far outstrips that of those sometimes seen in the hand.

The student will find it profitable at this point to read 'Homologies of the Carpus and Tarsus', on p. 240.

CLASSIFICATION: Accessory bones are divisible into two classes:
1. SESAMOID BONES: These are regular constituents of the skeleton.
2. TRUE ACCESSORY BONES: These are small occasional ossicles which occur in definite sites. It is of importance to note 'that whilst these bones are sometimes quite separate entities, they may also be represented by protrusion from an adjacent bone with which they are incorporated' (Thurstan Holland).

ORIGIN: The bones represent the persistence of embryonic vestiges which usually disappear. Some of them are always present in certain animals. They develop from a 'centre' present about the tenth to twelfth year of life, ossification being complete by adolescence. In the vast majority of cases they are *bilateral*. They may be unilateral. They may not be the same shape or size in the two feet or hands. The moral is obvious: that both feet or hands should be radiographed.

IMPORTANCE: To quote the same author: 'All these bones are not necessarily important from the X-ray point of view, and this for two reasons. Some are so rare that from a practical point they have little or no radiological significance, whilst others do not lend themselves to demonstration by X-rays even when they are present. Notwithstanding this, however, it should be laid down as a golden rule of radiology, that if any unusual bone deposit is shown in either a foot or a hand, whether it is a separate shadow or whether it is caused by an unusual projection from an otherwise normal bone, care should be taken in reaching a definite diagnosis, and the possibility of an accessory bone, separate or incorporated, should be considered.'

FREQUENCY: Pfitzner states that 25 per cent of human feet show one or other of these ossicles. Only the commoner accessory bones will be described.

Accessory Bones of the Foot (*Fig.* 212): These are as follows:
1. Os tibiale externum.
2. Os trigonum, or accessory astragalus.
3. Os Vesalianum tarsi.
4. Secondary os calcis.
5. Secondary cuboid.
6. Astragalo-scaphoid bone of Pirie.
7. Intermetatarseum.
8. Os intercuneiforme.

BONES 231

9. Os paracuneiforme of Cameron and Carlier.
10. Os uncinatum.
11. Astragalus secundarius.
12. Os subtibiale.
13. Os sustenaculum proprium.
14. Peroneal process of the os calcis.
15. Sesamum peronaeum.
16. Sesamoids of flexor hallucis brevis.
17. Trochlear process of head of astragalus.
18. Process from middle of upper surface of astragalus.
19. Spurs on the os calcis.
20. Spurs on the phalanges.

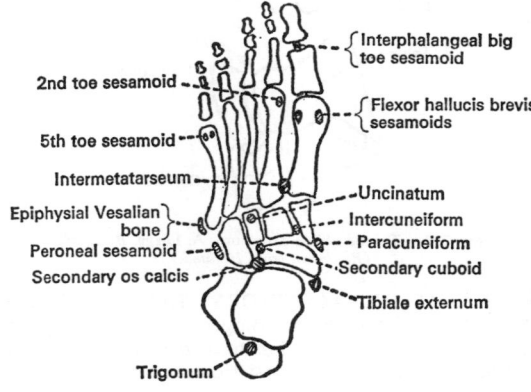

Fig. 212.—Accessory bones of the foot. (*After Thurstan Holland.*)

OS TIBIALE EXTERNUM OR ACCESSORY NAVICULAR (OR SCAPHOID) (*Fig.* 213): Note that, despite the name, the bone occurs on the *internal* border of the foot. It occurs in 10 to 12 per cent of persons, being very definitely related to the tuberosity of the navicular. It occurs, therefore, on the inner aspect of the navicular. It is usually bilateral, but may be unilateral. It is frequently described as a sesamoid in the tendon of the tibialis posterior. There are several unsettled points in connexion with the bone:

RELATIONSHIP TO TENDON OF TIBIALIS POSTERIOR: Some say the bone is enclosed in the tendon, others that though it may be involved in the tendon, it is never enclosed in it.

RELATIONSHIP TO TUBEROSITY OF THE NAVICULAR: There is doubt whether it is incorporated with the navicular, or whether it is a separate entity. In the author's cases it appeared in every instance to be a separation of the tubercle of a hypertrophied navicular.

ASSOCIATED SYMPTOMS: It is often associated with pain and redness over the part. The author agrees with Isadore Zadek[1] that the presence of the bone is associated with a weak and painful foot.

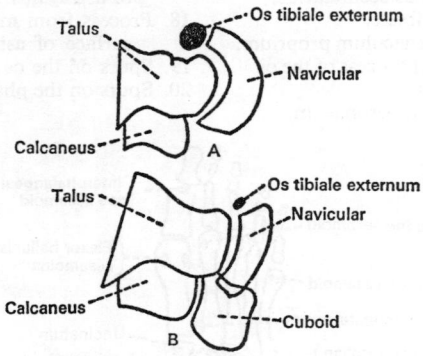

Fig. 213.—The os tibiale externum. A, Large. B, Small. (*Re-drawn from Holland.*)

OS TRIGONUM OR ACCESSORY TALUS (ASTRAGALUS)

(*Fig. 214*): This bone, the homologue of the os intermedium of the primitive tarsus and of the lunate in the carpus, exists usually as the lateral tubercle of the posterior border of the astragalus or

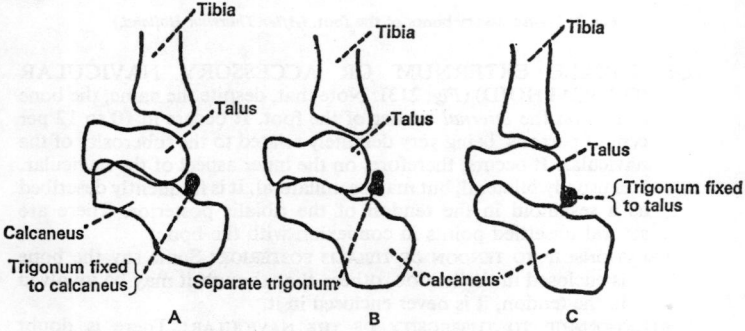

Fig. 214.—The os trigonum. A, Os trigonum fused to calcaneus. B, Separate os trigonum. C, Trigonum fused to talus. (*Re-drawn from Holland.*)

[1] *J. Bone Jt. Surg.*, 1926, 8, 618.

BONES 233

talus. In other words, the keystone of the human tarsus, the talus, is a composite bone made up of a fusion of the os tibiale with the os intermedium. In 7 per cent of cases the lateral tubercle is a separate bone which is known as the os trigonum. It is a constant bone in the wombat (Holland). In a radiograph it is seen as a separate ossicle in the angle between the posterior border of the talus and the upper surface of the calcaneus. Holland points out that very exceptionally the ossicle may be fused with the upper surface of the calcaneus.

OS VESALIANUM TARSI (*Fig.* 215): Much controversy has centred round this ossicle. Thurstan Holland has reduced the matter to

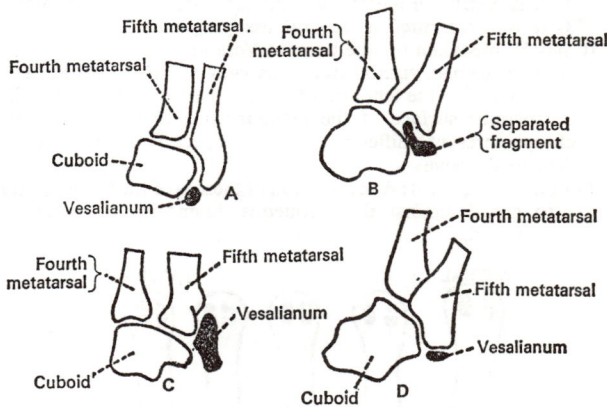

Fig. 215.—The os Vesalianum. A, Bone of Vesalius. B, Fracture of tuberosity of 5th metatarsal. C, Bone of Vesalius consisting of the whole tuberosity of the 5th metatarsal. D, The os Vesalianum as described by Vesalius. (*Re-drawn from Holland.*)

lucidity. According to this author three varieties of separate bone formation may be found at the base of the 5th metatarsal:

1. A true epiphysis, seen only in childhood, disappearing at puberty, when it fuses with the shaft of the bone. It is always bilateral.
2. The epiphysis just described fails to fuse, and exists separately throughout adult life. It consists of a large part or the whole of what normally constitutes the tuberosity of the 5th metatarsal. It is rare and generally bilateral.
3. A very small ossicle persists throughout life adjacent to the tip of the tuberosity, which in itself is quite well formed. The rarest of the three. It may be unilateral or bilateral. Holland considers this to be the bone described by Vesalius.

The base of the 5th metatarsal is often injured, notably in the 'dancing fracture' of Sir Robert Jones. It is obviously of the first importance to be able to distinguish a fracture from an abnormal ossification.

SESAMOIDS OF THE FOOT:

1. PERONEAL SESAMOID:

   Position: This bone lies in the tendon of the peroneus longus where this tendon grooves the outer border of the cuboid. It is always bilateral.

   Variations:
   1. It is very small—a mere dot—'the small peroneal sesamoid'.
   2. It is nearly an inch long—'the large peroneal sesamoid'.
   3. It is represented as several ossifying nuclei.

   It may be mistaken for the bone of Vesalius.

2. SESAMOIDS OF THE FLEXOR HALLUCIS BREVIS: These two bones, one in each half of the tendon of the short flexor of the big toe, lie on the plantar surface of the metatarsophalangeal joint, and are always present, differing in this respect from all the bones described above.

   Variations (Fig. 216): A recognition of these is of the first importance to guard against the erroneous diagnosis of fracture of a sesamoid.

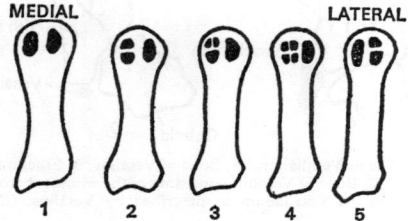

Fig. 216.—To show the variations in the sesamoids of the great toe. (*See* text.)

   a. The inner sesamoid may consist of two, three, or four bony areas. When in two pieces the line of cleavage is transverse: when in three pieces, one of the two pieces is also divided longitudinally. When four pieces exist each half is divided longitudinally.

   b. The outer sesamoid is much more rarely divided, and then only into two pieces.

   When either of the conditions described in (*a*) and (*b*) exists developmentally, *the same state of affairs will be found in the other foot.*

Though division of the sesamoid is common, fracture is rare. It follows that both feet should invariably be X-rayed if a suspicion exists of fracture of a sesamoid.

3. OCCASIONAL SESAMOIDS: In addition to the peroneal and flexor brevis hallucis sesamoids, others are sometimes found:
   a. A sesamoid on the plantar surface of the interphalangeal joint of the big toe.
   b. A sesamoid on the inner side of the second metatarsophalangeal joint.
   c. A sesamoid on the outer side of the 5th metatarsophalangeal joint.
   d. A sesamoid on the inner side of the 5th metatarsophalangeal joint.
   e. A sesamoid opposite the distal interphalangeal joint of the second toe.
   f. A sesamoid opposite the metatarsophalangeal joint of the fourth toe.

TROCHLEAR PROCESS OF THE TALUS (*Fig.* 217): A bony spur may project upwards from any part of the upper surface

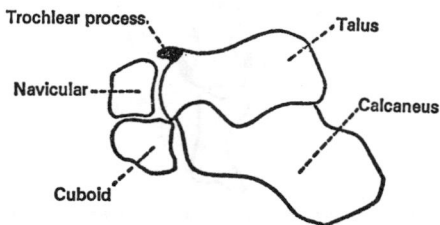

Fig. 217.—Trochlear process of talus. (*Re-drawn from Holland.*)

of the neck of the talus (i.e., in front of the tibia). Though often the result of an osteoarthritis of the midtarsal joint, Holland thinks it is sometimes developmental in origin.

CALCANEAL SPURS (*Fig.* 218): These are always pathological, and occur in rheumatic conditions which give rise to fibrositis. They are specially common as a late result of gonorrhoea. They do not always cause symptoms. A spur may be fractured and will then appear as a separate ossicle. As they are shown in a radiograph only in lateral views of the foot, they appear as thin spikes, but when exposed at operation they are often quite broad.

POSITION:
   a. On the under-surface of the bone, extending from the front of the tuberosity into the plantar fascia.

b. On the under-surface of the bone, further back than (*a*).
c. On the posterior surface of the bone at the insertion of the tendo Achillis.

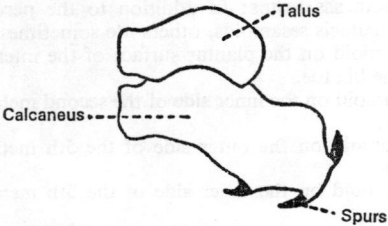

Fig. 218.—Varieties of calcaneal spurs. (*Re-drawn from Holland.*)

PHALANGEAL SPURS (*Fig.* 219): These are found on any of the distal phalanges, especially that of the great toe. They grow from either side of the base of the phalanx, may get large, and usually do not cause symptoms.

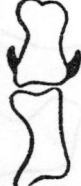

Fig. 219.—Phalangeal spurs. (*Re-drawn from Holland.*)

Accessory Bones of the Hand: These are neither as numerous nor as important as those of the foot. Furthermore, less is known about them. They are classified as follows: (1) True accessory bones; (2) Sesamoid bones.

TRUE ACCESSORY BONES (*Fig.* 220): These are as follows:
1. Os triangulare.
2. Os centrale.
3. Os styloideum.
4. Os Vesalianum.
5. Os para-trapezium.
6. Os radiale externum.
7. Os ulnare externum.
8. Bipartite bones: (*a*) navicular, (*b*) triquetrum, (*c*) pisiform.

As all these anomalies are rare they are not further commented on.

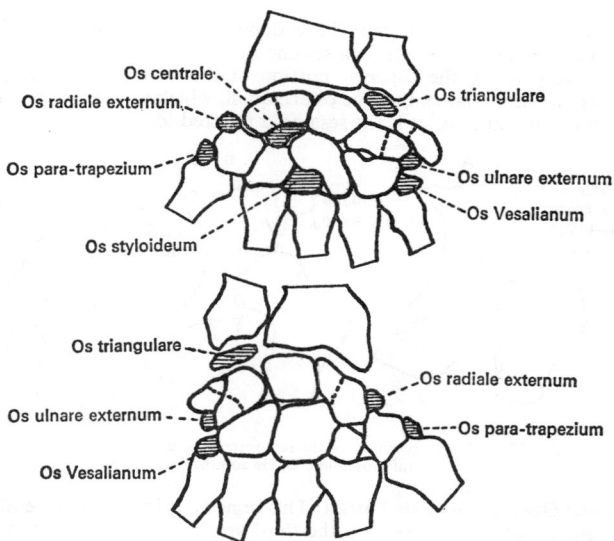

Fig. 220.—Accessory bones of the hand. Upper figure: Dorsal aspect of carpus. Lower figure: Palmar aspect of carpus. The navicular, pisiform, and triquetrum, which are crossed by interrupted lines, may sometimes be bipartite. The carpal bones shown stippled are accessory.

Sesamoid of the Rectus Femoris: This bone is important, as it may be mistaken for a fracture. It is not described in anatomical or surgical works, and is referred to by radiologists as the so acetabuli, a name which is quite erroneous, though unfortunately sanctioned by custom. During the ossification of the acetabulum a centre of ossification appears in the Y-shaped cartilage which separates the three constituent parts of that socket. This centre, called the os acetabuli, assists in the formation of the pubic part of the socket, but fuses with the other bones in the neighbourhood at puberty. In radiographs of the hip-joint a small nodule of bone is frequently seen just below the anterior inferior iliac spine. Radiologists call this the os acetabuli. It is a sesamoid bone in the reflected head of the rectus femoris and in no wise comparable to the true os acetabuli. It is seen in adult hip-joints long after acetabular ossification is complete (*Fig.* 221).

The anterior inferior iliac spine may be avulsed by the powerful iliofemoral ligament. It is obvious, therefore, that compensation cases may centre, as they have done, round the question whether a loose portion of bone is a sesamoid or a fracture.

Very rarely the superior portion of the acetabulum may persist as a separate bone, the true os acetabuli, which is *in* the hip-joint and not external to it, as is the sesamoid referred to.

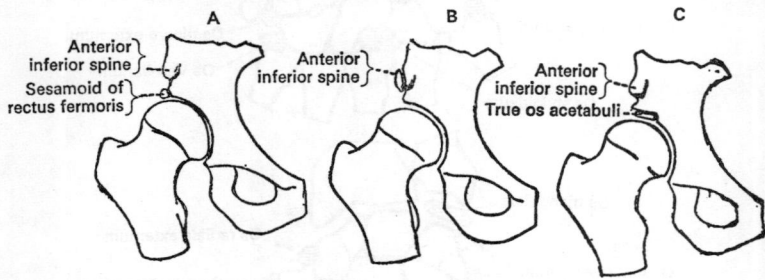

Fig. 221.—A, The sesamoid of the rectus femoris. B, Avulsed anterior inferior spine. C, Os acetabuli.

Unusual Ossification of the Patella: This bone is ossified from several bony granules,[1] which appear in the third year to form, as a rule, a single ossific centre, and ossification is complete about puberty.

VARIATIONS:
1. The bone may be absent.
2. The bone may be rudimentary.

The existence of either condition is usually associated with imperfect development of the quadriceps muscle.[2]

Extremely rarely[3] the upper, outer part of the patella may be almost or completely separate from the remainder of the bone (*Fig.* 222). There may even be several separate ossicles in this situation. (We have observed this type of developmental variation so often as to be convinced that it is not excessively rare.) It is often referred to as bipartite or tripartite patella. It is important to note that the abnormality is *bilateral*, thus excluding the possibility that it may be mistaken for fracture.

'*Emargination*' is the term used when the upper outer angle of the patella is absent and a notch exists there.

Note also that the patella does sometimes ossify from two centres.

Patella Cubiti: This is a rare condition due to failure of fusion of the upper epiphysis of the ulna, which persists as a loose bone in the tendon of

---

[1] Piersol, G. A., *Human Anatomy*, 1918, 400. Philadephia.
[2] Albeé, F. H., *Orthopaedic and Reconstruction Surgery*, 1919, 912. Philadelphia.
[3] C. Thurstan Holland, *J. Anat.*, 1921, 55, 235.

BONES 239

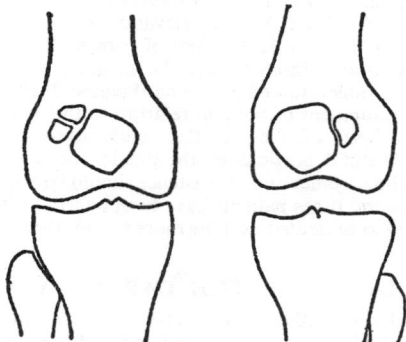

Fig. 222.—Unusual, though important, methods of ossification of the patella. On the reader's left ossification from three centres is shown; on the right there are only two.

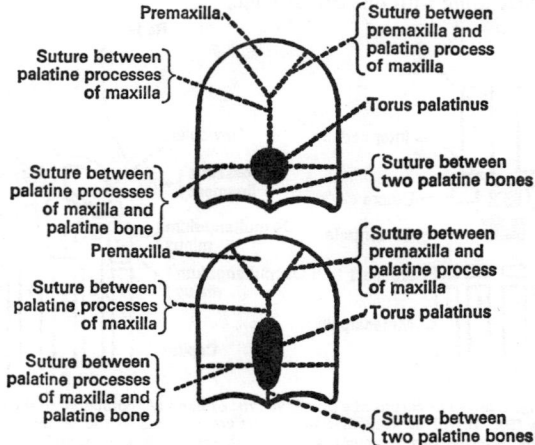

Fig. 223.—The torus palatinus. Two usual shapes are figured. Observe the relationship of the prominence to the maxillary and palatine sutures.

the triceps. Care must be taken not to confuse the condition with that of failure of union of a fractured olecranon.

Torus Palatinus (*Fig.* 223): A bony elevation of the hard palate; not uncommon, occuring in 22 per cent of persons (Nacke[1]).

It is not a tumour, though it may be mistaken for such, but a bony eminence or a ridge situated on the hard palate. It is due merely to an excessive development of bone in relation to the suture between the palatine processes of the maxillae, particularly at their junction with the horizontal portions of the palate bones. This prominence is of clinical importance and its existence should be much better known than it is. Several times patients have been referred with the diagnosis of sarcoma who presented nothing more serious than a well-developed torus.

III. HOMOLOGIES OF THE CARPUS AND TARSUS

The human hand is primitive in type. The wing of a bird or the fin of a whale are more highly specialized. Both hand and foot in the human are based on a common plan of construction.

Hand (*Fig.* 224):

PRIMITIVE CARPUS: This is made up of:

A proximal row of three bones—radiale below radius, ulnare below ulna, and a bone between the two, the os intermedium.

A distal row, the carpalia, is numbered 1 to 5, each bone articulating with one carpal bone.

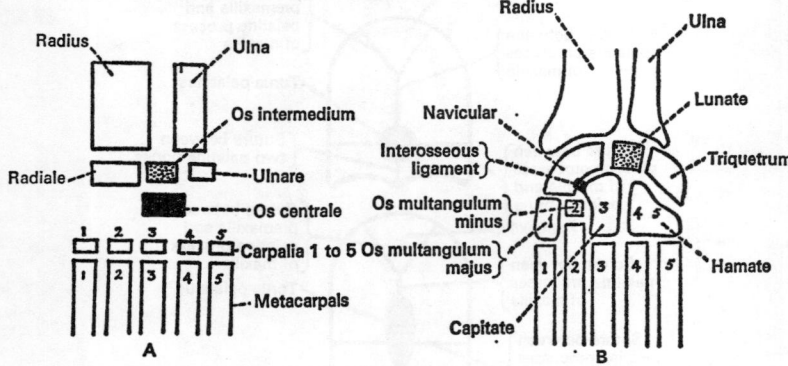

Fig. 224.—The carpus of a primitive type of hand (A) compared to the human carpus (B). It will be seen that the lunate corresponds to the os intermedium and the interosseous ligament shown in black in B corresponds to the os centrale in A.

[1] Nacke, *Neurol. Centralb.*, 1893, June 15.

BONES 241

Between the first and second rows is a single bone—the os centrale.

HUMAN CARPUS: Compare this with the above. It consists of two rows of bones—

First Row—

	Navicular	Lunate	Triquetrum
corresponding to	Radiale	Os intermedium	Ulnare

Second Row—

	Multangulum majus	Multangulum minus	Capitate	Hamate
corresponding to	Carpalia 1	2	3	4 and 5

The hamate articulates with two metacarpals and represents the fusion of carpalia 4 and 5.

OS CENTRALE: The first and second rows of bones in the human carpus are united by anterior and posterior ligaments and by only one interosseous ligament, that joining the navicular and os capitatum. This, with the small part of the navicular to which it is attached, is the representative of the os centrale. In early foetal life the lower medial corner of the navicular is a separate cartilaginous nodule and is the representative of the os centrale. It may remain as a separate bone, but usually fuses with the navicular.

Foot (*Fig.* 225):

PRIMITIVE TARSUS: Built on exactly the same plan as the carpus, i.e., two rows of bones with an intervening bone:

First row—tibiale below tibia, fibulare below fibula, the os intermedium between.

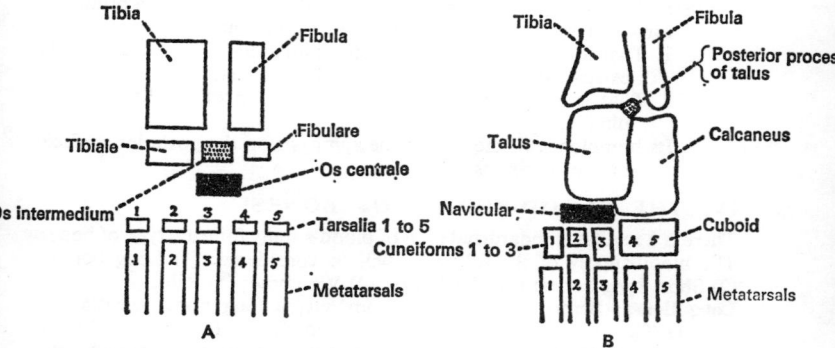

Fig. 225.—A comparison of the primitive tarsus (A) with the human tarsus (B). Observe that the posterior process of the talus (stippled) is homologous with the os intermedium of the primitive tarsus and the lunate in the hand, whereas the navicular (black) in the foot corresponds to the os centrale of the primitive tarsus and the corresponding ligament in the hand.

Second tow—tarsalia 1–5.

Between the two rows is the os centrale.

HUMAN TARSUS: Two rows of bones—a bone between the two:

First Row—

	Talus	Calcaneus
corresponding to	Tibiale	Fibulare

Second Row—

	3 Cuneiforms	Cuboid
corresponding to	Tarsalia 1–3	Fusion of tarsalia 4 and 5

The cuboid articulates with two metatarsals.

The navicular is the representative of the os centrale.

The *os intermedium* is represented by the lateral tubercle of the talus, which may sometimes be separate, and is then called the 'os trigonum'.

Homologies of the Carpus and Tarsus: Both being derived from the same plan:

CARPAL BONES			TARSAL BONES
Navicular	corresponds to		Talus
Lunate	,,	,,	Os trigonum
Triquetrum	,,	,,	Calcaneus
Multangulum majus	,,	,,	1st Cuneiform
Multangulum minus	,,	,,	2nd Cuneiform
Capitate	,,	,,	3rd Cuneiform
Hamate	,,	,,	Cuboid
Interosseous ligament between navicular and capitate, and inferior angle of navicular	,,	,,	Navicular

PISIFORM: There is no representative of the pisiform in the primitive carpus. Two views are held as to its significance:
1. That it is the remains of a post-minimal digit, i.e., a digit which existed on the ulnar side of the little finger.
2. That it is a sesamoid bone in the tendon of the flexor carpi ulnaris.

Its homologue in the foot is the epiphysis on the posterior surface of the calcaneus.

IV. THE BLOOD-SUPPLY OF BONES[1]

There is a regular standardized plan of blood-supply for each type of bone. The blood-supply of the following will be considered: (1) Long bones; (2) Short long bones; (3) Flat bones; (4) Vertebrae; (5) Ribs.

Long Bones: Before ossification is complete, a long bone consists of:
(1) The shaft or diaphysis; (2) The epiphysis; (3) The epiphysial cartilage; (4) The metaphysis, i.e., the part of the shaft immediately on the diaphysial side of the epiphysial cartilage—in other words it is *the end of the diaphysis*.

---

[1] This knowledge we owe to the work of Lexer.

BONES 243

THE METAPHYSIS has important characteristics when considered from a surgical point of view:
  a. It is the area of greatest growth activity in the bone.
  b. It has an extremely profuse blood-supply, as the different sets of blood-vessels supplying the bone anastomose in this region. It has been aptly called 'a lake of blood'.
  c. The muscles, tendons, and joint capsules and ligaments are attached to or near it, so that it is an area which is very likely to suffer damage in strains, whether these come directly through the bone or through the ligaments, etc., attached to the metaphysis.
  d. Because of its great vascularity, and the delicate nature of the lamellae of which it is composed, 'separation of epiphysis' takes place through the part of the metaphysis which abuts immediately on the epiphysial cartilage. As this cartilage is separated from the shaft with the epiphysis, growth in length at the injured end of the bone completely stops unless the fragments be replaced in continuity again. Ollier has shown that a very common type of injury to growing bones is a 'juxta-epiphysial strain', i.e., an injury causing some damage to the metaphysis, stopping short of actual separation of the epiphysis.
  e. A part of the metaphysis is often inside the capsule of a joint, so that disease of the metaphysis is very likely to invade the joint in such circumstances, or vice versa.

THE BLOOD-SUPPLY OF A LONG BONE is derived from the following four sources (*Fig.* 226):
  1. NUTRIENT ARTERY: Before entering the bone, this vessel is very tortuous, the object of the tortuosity being to allow movement without damage to the nutrient vessel and to break the blood-pressure. On entering the bone the vessel divides into two branches, one running towards each end of the bone. These are called the 'nutritiae'. Each soon divides into a leash of parallel vessels which run to the metaphysis.
  2. JUXTA-EPIPHYSIAL VESSELS OF LEXER: These are numerous small vessels derived from the anastomosis round the joint. They pierce the metaphysis along the line of the attachment of the joint capsule.
  3. EPIPHYSIAL VESSELS: In those cases where the capsule is attached to the epiphysis and not to the metaphysis, the juxta-epiphysial vessels are replaced by the epiphysial vessels, which arise in exactly the same way as the juxta-epiphysial vessels do from the anastomosis round the joint. Some of these vessels may pierce the epiphysial cartilage and reach the metaphysis.
  4. PERIOSTEAL VESSELS: The periosteum has a rich blood-supply, from which many little vessels go to pierce the bone.

244 A SYNOPSIS OF SURGICAL ANATOMY

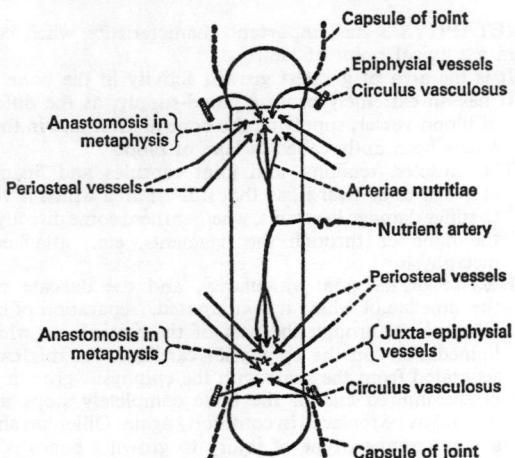

Fig. 226.—Schematic representation of the blood-supply of a long bone. Observe the tortuosity of the nutrient artery and the parallel nutritiae.

All these four sets of vessels come into communication at the metaphysis, which is thus an extremely vascular zone.

Short Long Bones (*Fig.* 227): These bones have a single epiphysis and therefore a single metaphysis.

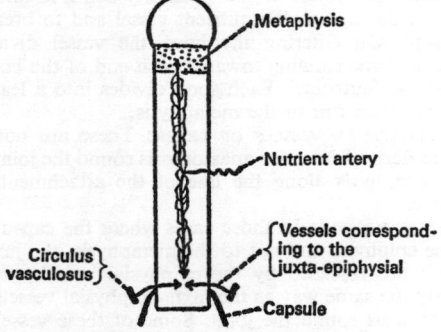

Fig. 227.—Blood-supply of a short long bone. The periosteal vessels are omitted for simplicity. Only blood-supply of end devoid of epiphysis is shown. At epiphysial end blood-supply corresponds to that at end of a long bone.

1. The nutrient vessel on entering the shaft breaks up into a plexus immediately.
2. At the epiphysial end of the bone the blood-supply is arranged exactly as in the long bones.
3. At the other end (no epiphysis), there are no juxta-epiphysial vessels, and only vessels corresponding to the epiphysial vessels exist.
4. The periosteal vessels assist in the supply.

Flat Bones: E.g., scapula (*Fig.* 228), ilium.
1. A nutrient vessel, or vessels, enters and breaks up into branches which ramify all over the bone.
2. The periosteal blood-supply is profuse and important.

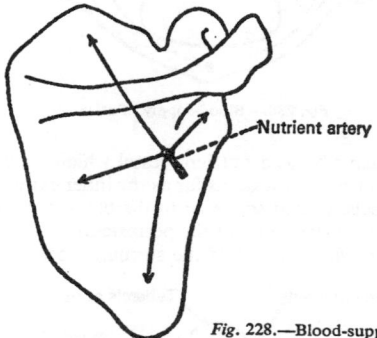

Fig. 228.—Blood-supply of scapula.

Vertebrae (*Fig.* 229):
BODY:
1. Two large vessels enter the body from behind.
2. Smaller vessels enter the body from in front.

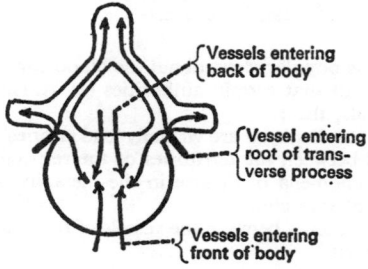

Fig. 229.—Blood-supply of a vertebra.

ARCH:
3. A vessel enters at the root of the transverse process and sends branches to lamina, pedicle, spine, and transverse process.

THE ATLAS, having no body, receives only the third group, i.e., a vessel enters the base of each transverse process (*Fig.* 230).

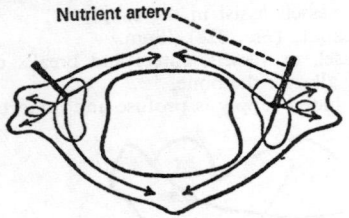

Fig. 230.—Blood-supply of atlas.

Ribs (*Fig.* 231): Each rib has a nutrient vessel which enters it just beyond the tubercle and runs forward as far as the inner extremity of the bone. Periosteal vessels, of course, assist in the blood-supply. The practical point may here be stressed that the periosteum of the ribs strips easily from the bone, whereas that of the sternum does not.

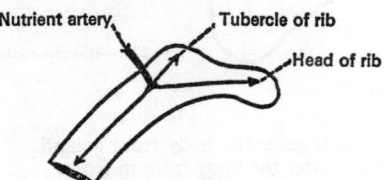

Fig. 231.—Blood-supply of a rib.

While these are the popular views about the blood-supply of bones, it is necessary to point out that certain authorities (H. A. Harris[1]) allege, on experimental grounds, that:
1. The vessels of the diaphysis are virtually 'end arteries' with but a poor anastomosis between the territories of the respective end arteries. Thus the phenomena of disease in the metaphysis are essentially phenomena of infarction.
2. *No anastomosis* occurs between the vessels of the diaphysis and those of the epiphysis.

[1] *J. Anat.*, 1929, Oct., 64, 3.

V. OSSIFICATION

Certain features of the development of bone have clinical and surgical applications.

Skull: Centres of ossification, additional to the usual ones, may appear in the membrane from which the vault of the skull develops, and give rise to small bones situated between the named ones. These are the so-called *Wormian bones*. They are most common where the occipital bone joins the parietals (lambdoidal suture).

METOPIC SUTURE: Ossification may fail to extend across the membrane which at an early stage unites the two halves of the frontal bone. This results in a vertical suture called the 'metopic suture', which occurs in 8 per cent of skulls.

Mandible: A bone developed in membrane. It is the second bone in the body to begin to ossify. A single centre appears in each half at the 6th week. All traces of the symphysial cartilage are gone at birth.

Clavicle[1] (*Fig.* 232): The ossification of the clavicle is more complicated than was at one time thought. Fawcett[2] has shown that during the 7th week two centres of chondrification appear quite close to each other at the junction of the outer third with the inner two-thirds. Centres of ossification soon appear in these foci and the two ossific centres soon unite. From this double centre ossification spreads towards the acromion and towards the sternum, being preceded by a formation of cartilage. At the 18th year a secondary centre appears in cartilage at the sternal end of the bone. This epiphysis unites at the age of 25. It is intracapsular.

The clavicle is the first bone to ossify and its epiphysis is the last to appear.

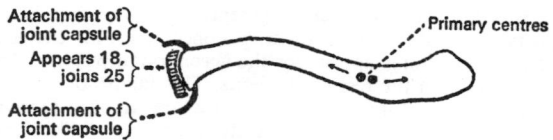

Fig. 232.—Ossification of clavicle (Fawcett). Observe the two primary centres at the junction of the middle and outer thirds of the bone. They soon fuse. The arrows show how ossification extends from the centre.

The elucidation of the development of the clavicle has enabled the many variations to which the bone is subject to be better understood:
1. The clavicle may be absent.
2. The outer one-third may be absent.

---

[1] I would express my thanks for the facts set out here to Professor Fawcett, who supplied them.
[2] Fawcett, E., *J. Anat.*, 1913, **47**, 225.

248 A SYNOPSIS OF SURGICAL ANATOMY

3. The inner two-thirds may be absent—half as often as (2).
4. A fissure of small or great extent may divide the outer one-third from the inner two-thirds.
5. The rhomboid fossa of the collar bone was described by Pendergrass and Hodes.[1] This is an unusual X-ray appearance in the clavicle(s) of adult males which resembles an erosion of part of the bone. It is situated on the inferior surface of one or both clavicles in the area of attachment of the costoclavicular (rhomboid) ligament. It is a broad rough surface about an inch long, commencing about a centimetre from the sternoclavicular joint. The appreciation of this anomaly is important as in an X-ray picture it resembles a destructive bone lesion (*Fig.* 233).

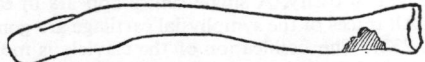

Fig. 233.—The rhomboid fossa of the clavicle.

It will be readily seen how easily these anomalies are explicable in the light of the facts regarding the development of the bone which are set out above.

Sternum and Sacrum:
5 *vertebrae* form the sacrum.
4 *sternebrae* form the body of the sternum.
In each case the union of the constituent bones takes place from below upwards between the ages of 18 and 25.

Scapula: Has a complicated development. The only fact of practical importance in this development is concerned with the acromion. Two or more centres appear for the acromion at puberty. They may fail to unite with the rest of the bone. This failure of union may be interpreted in an X-ray picture as a fracture. In such cases a radiograph of the acromion of the opposite side will in all likelihood show the same failure of union.

Long Bones of the Limbs:
LAW OF OSSIFICATION: Where a bone has an epiphysis at either end, the epiphysis which is the first to appear is the last to join; and the epiphysis which is the last to appear is the first to join. The fibula is the only exception to this rule.

Growth continues longest at the shoulder and wrist in the upper limb, and longest at the knee in the lower limb. That means that the epiphyses of—

---

[1] Pendergrass, E. P., and Hodes, P. J., *Am. J. Roentg.*, 1937, 38, 152.

BONES 249

The upper end of the humerus
The lower end of the radius
The lower end of the ulna
The upper end of the tibia
The lower end of the femur
} unite later than the epiphyses at the other end of these bones.

This fact is of importance in the following respects:
1. The nutrient foramina of the limb bones are directed according to the rhyme "to the elbow I go, from the knee I flee". The nutrient foramina are originally directed in the opposite direction to that which they take in the adult, but, growth being more active at the shoulder, wrist, and knee, the arteries are pushed farther and farther away from these ends of the bones, and ultimately the foramina are deflected towards the other (and slower growing) ones.
2. Sarcoma is commonest at the lower end of the femur and upper end of the tibia. The epiphyses here unite later than those of any other limb bone. It has been suggested that this fact may have something to do with the common occurrence of malignancy at these sites (Kolodny[1]).

OS INNOMINATUM: By the fusion of its three constituent elements at the acetabulum, this becomes one bone at the age of 12 to 16 years (*Fig.* 234). The skeletal maturity of the vertebral column may

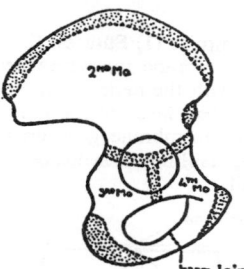

Fig. 234.—Ossification of os innominatum. Dates of appearance of primary centres for the three constituent parts of the bone are shown in the figure. Portions developed from secondary centres, five in number, are stippled. These centres appear at puberty and fuse between the ages of 18 and 25, except triradiate strip of cartilage in acetabulum, which is completely ossified by 16, through the intervention of a secondary centre known as the os acetabuli.

be assessed by the progress of ossification in the secondary centre of the crest of the ilium—the iliac apophysis. Ossification begins at the anterior superior iliac spine and extends backwards. When it reaches the posterior superior spine ossification of the vertebral

[1] *Bone Sarcoma*, 1927, Chicago.

column is complete. Radiographs supply the information which is a guide in the handling of cases of structural scoliosis, as lateral curvature of the spinal column usually ceases to progress when the column is skeletally mature.

The secondary centre for the lower end of the femur occurs in the 9th month just before birth. It indicates that the infant has developed to a viable size and is therefore of important medicolegal significance.

Chapter XXIV

JOINTS, TENDON-SHEATHS, AND BURSAE

I. JOINTS

BONES may be united by fibrous, cartilaginous, or tube-like connexions, and joints are therefore classified as fibrous, cartilaginous, or synovial. Movement between the related bone ends is not implicit in the definition of a joint.

Description:

FIBROUS JOINTS: Comprise (1) Sutures, (2) Syndesmoses.

1. SUTURES: Sutural membrane intervenes between the two bones, and is connected with the periosteum on the outer surface and the outer or periosteal layer of the dura on the inner surface. Ossification in the membrane goes on till the two bones are completely fused, resulting in synostosis (*Fig.* 235). These only occur in the skull.

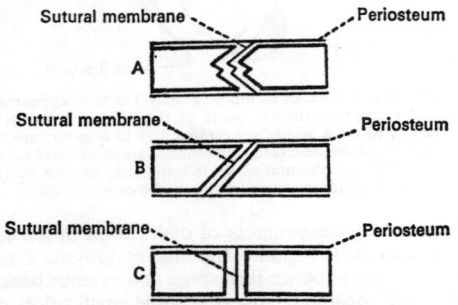

Fig. 235.—Sutural joints. A, Sutura serrata. B, Sutura squamosa. C, Sutura harmonia.

> a. *Serrata:* E.g., two parietals articulating with each other at interparietal suture.
> b. *Squamosa:* Overlapping edges, e.g., parietal and squamous temporal.
> c. *Harmonia:* Two flat surfaces in contact, e.g., between two maxillary bones.
> 2. SYNDESMOSES: The bony surfaces are united (*a*) by interosseous ligaments, e.g., inferior tibiofibular joint, and ligamenta flava of the vertebrae, or (*b*) by an interosseous ligament such as occurs in the forearm and leg. A slight amount of movement is possible. They persist throughout life (*Fig.* 236).

CARTILAGINOUS JOINTS: These are (1) Primary or (2) Secondary.
> 1. PRIMARY (synchondrosis): The related bones are united by a plate of hyaline cartilage. They are immovable and all disappear by synostosis, e.g., the junction of the diaphysis and epiphysis of a growing bone (*Fig.* 237).

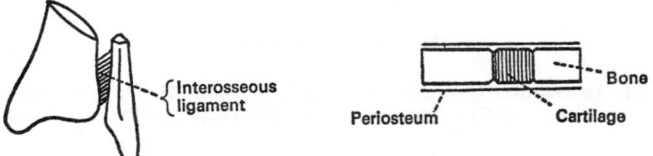

Fig. 236.—The tibiofibular syndesmosis, a variety of amphiarthrosis (diagrammatic).

Fig. 237.—Synchondrosis.

> 2. SECONDARY (amphiarthrosis): These joints occur only in the median plane, e.g., between the vertebral bodies or the pubic symphysis. The bone-ends are covered by articular (hyaline) cartilage and connected by an intervening disc of fibrocartilage connected with the periosteum of the bones (*Fig.* 238).

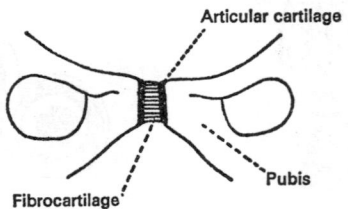

Fig. 238.—Symphysis pubis, a variety of amphiarthrosis.

252 A SYNOPSIS OF SURGICAL ANATOMY

SYNOVIAL JOINTS (DIARTHROSES): The two bone-ends are covered by articular cartilage. They are connected by a fibrous capsule continuous with the periosteum of the bones. It is often strengthened by accessory ligaments. The inner surface of the capsule and all intra-articular structures which are not covered with cartilage are covered by synovial membrane, which secretes an oily fluid—synovial fluid (*Fig.* 239).

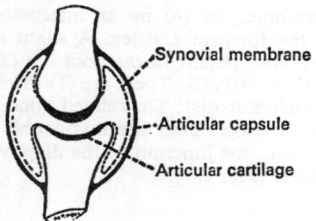

Fig. 239.—Synovial or diarthrodial joint.

1. ARTHRODIAL (*Fig.* 240): Flat surfaces in contact. The bones permit simple gliding movements, e.g., intercarpal joints.

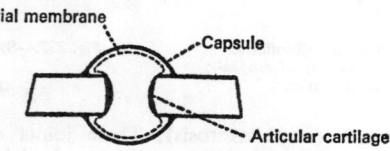

Fig. 240.—Arthrodial joint.

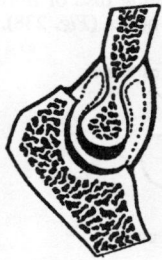

Fig. 241.—Hinge joint.

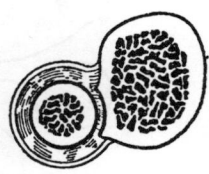

Fig. 242.—Pivot joint
Superior radio-ulnar joint.

JOINTS, TENDON-SHEATHS, AND BURSAE

2. GINGLYMUS OR HINGE (*Fig.* 241): Movement around a transverse axis, e.g., humerus and ulna.
3. TROCHOID OR PIVOT (*Fig.* 242): A pivot-like process turning within a ring: e.g., upper radio-ulnar joint; another example is dens of 2nd cervical vertebra with the atlas.
4. CONDYLOID (*Fig.* 243): A condyle received into an elliptical cavity. It allows flexion, extension, adduction and abduction, and a combination of these, circumduction, but no rotation round a central axis: e.g., wrist-joint.

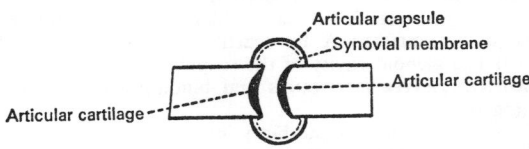

Fig. 243.—Condyloid joint.

5. SELLARIS (ephippial or saddle) (*Fig.* 244): Opposing surfaces both concavo-convex. Permits same movement as condyloid: e.g., the carpometacarpal joint of the thumb. The wide range of movements of the thumb is due to the nature of this joint; compare restricted range of movements of big toe where the tarsometatarsal joint is a simple condyloid one.

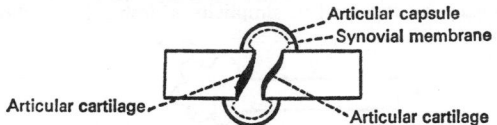

Fig. 244.—Ephippial joint.

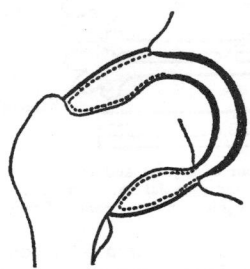

Fig. 245.—Ball-and-socket joint.

254 A SYNOPSIS OF SURGICAL ANATOMY

6. ENARTHROSIS (ball and socket) (*Fig.* 245): The globular head fits into a cup-like cavity. It can move in every direction round a common centre, e.g., hip- and shoulder-joints.

Intra-articular Structures: These are found in certain joints:

CARTILAGINOUS STRUCTURES:
1. ARTICULAR DISCS (*see below*):
    a. Complete: (i) In mandibular joint; (ii) In the sternoclavicular joint; (iii) Between the distal end of the ulna and carpus.
    b. Incomplete: In the acromioclavicular joints.
2. ARTICULAR MENISCI: Semilunar cartilages of the knee-joint.
3. LABRUM GLENOIDALE: A fibrocartilaginous ring which deepens (*a*) The glenoid cavity of the scapula; (*b*) The acetabulum.
4. LIGAMENTS TRAVERSING JOINTS and binding articulating surfaces together.
    a. Ligamentum teres of the hip-joint.
    b. Cruciate ligaments of the knee.
    c. Intra-articular ligaments of the heads of the 2nd to the 9th ribs. Such may be found at the chondrosternal joints also.

MUSCLE TENDONS arising inside the capsule of the joint:
1. The long head of the biceps at the shoulder-joint.
2. The tendon of the popliteus at the knee-joint.

Articular Discs: To appreciate their origin the development of a joint must be reviewed.

DEVELOPMENT OF JOINTS: For simplicity a limb joint is chosen (*Fig.* 246).

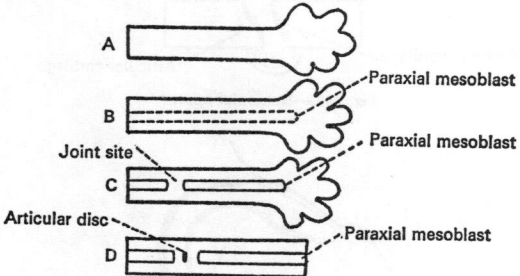

Fig. 246.—Development of a joint and articular disc. A, The limb bud. B, The limb bud showing the paraxial bar of mesoblast. C, Degeneration of paraxial bar at site of future joint. D, Appearance of articular disc.

1. At a very early stage the limb bone consists of a sausage-like projection. The skin of the sausage is ectodermal. Its contents form a homogeneous mass which is mesodermal.

2. A condensation of this mesoblast occurs round the longitudinal axis of the limb—*the paraxial bar of mesoblast*. This is going to form the future skeleton of the limb.
3. The paraxial bar degenerates at the site of the future joints of the limb, the two parts of the bar remaining connected by the fibrous membrane which encloses the bar. This fibrous membrane forms the periosteum of the bones and the capsule of the joint. Hence the two are continuous with each other.
4. If the developing joint is the site of an intra-articular disc, a small portion of the paraxial bar remains intact in the line of the joint.

FUNCTIONS OF INTRA-ARTICULAR DISCS:
1. To act as a buffer and absorb shocks. The complete ones are found at ulnacarpal, sternoclavicular, and temporomandibular joints, where shocks are commonly received.

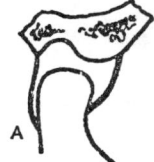 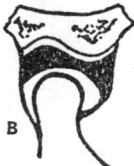

Fig. 247.—Showing how an articular disc renders irregular joint surfaces harmonious. A, Temporomandibular joint without articular disc. B, Temporomandibular joint with articular disc in situ.

2. To make a more harmonious articulation, e.g., temporomandibular joints. The glenoid cavity of the temporal bone is saddle-shaped. The head of the mandible is convex. The disc harmonizes the two surfaces (*Fig. 247*).
3. They strengthen the joint, comprising one of its accessory ligaments.

Hilton enunciated a great law: A joint is supplied by the same nerves which supply the muscles crossing the joint and the skin over the joint. In joint disease, therefore, the irritation of the nerves causes a reflex spasm of the muscles which fixes the joint in the position of greatest comfort, and may cause pain referred to the overlying skin.

II. TENDON-SHEATHS AND BURSAE

Tendon-sheaths occur in and near the foot and hand. Bursae occur around the shoulder and elbow in the upper limb and around the hip and knee in the lower limb. Such exceptions as occur to this rule are for the most part insignificant and will be alluded to below.

TENDON-SHEATHS

Tendon-sheaths are all arranged on the same plan, viz., the tendon is invested by a glistening endothelial-lined membrane which plays inside a second endothelial-lined membrane, the two layers being joined at their extremities. The sheath forms a sac closed at both ends (*Fig.* 248).

Hand: Over the phalanges the flexor tendons have fibrous sheaths and mucous sheaths.

FIBROUS SHEATH: Forms with the bones an osteofascial tunnel which retains the tendon in place. It is attached to the medial and lateral borders of the phalanges, where it is strong, and to the ligaments of the joints of the fingers, where it is weak, to allow freedom of movement. The palmar (or plantar) fascia is attached to the fibrous sheaths over the whole length of the first and the base of the second phalanx.

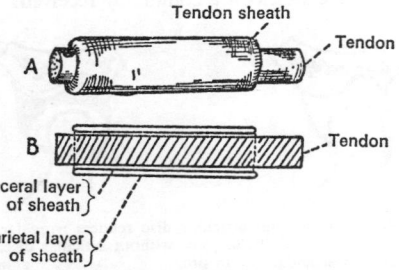

Fig. 248.—The arrangement of a tendon-sheath. A, Closed sheath. B, Sheath on section.

MUCOUS SHEATHS:

ANTERIOR: The sublimis and profundus slips to each of the 2nd, 3rd, 4th, and 5th digits have a common sheath which extends from the neck of the metacarpal bone to the base of the third phalanx, where the profundus ends. Over the middle third of the metacarpals these tendons, with the exception of those to the 5th digit, have no sheaths. Proximal to this the tendons are invested by another sheath which extends upwards as far as 2·5 cm. above the wrist-joint (*Fig.* 249). The sheath investing the tendons to the 5th digit continues proximally without interruption to join the common flexor sheath at the wrist. The common flexor sheath with its extension along the little finger tendons is the *ulnar bursa*.

Not infrequently there may be an interruption in the ulnar bursa, the arrangement of the sheaths being identical with that of the other fingers. A tenosynovitis of the little finger would

JOINTS, TENDON-SHEATHS, AND BURSAE 257

in such cases be held up by such an interruption to the weal of the person concerned. In operating on any case of tenosynovitis, then, a rule-of-thumb method should never be followed, but the arrangement of the sheath be carefully examined in a bloodless field and the operation planned accordingly.

The tendon of the thumb has a sheath which extends from the base of the last phalanx to a point 2·5 cm. above the upper

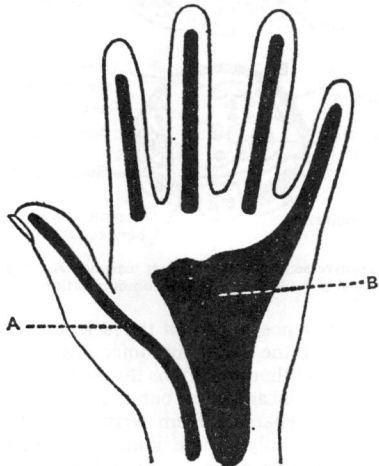

Fig. 249.—Synovial sheaths of flexor tendons of wrist and fingers. **A**, Radial bursa, or synovial sheath of flexor longus pollicis. **B**, Ulnar bursa, or synovial sheath of flexores sublimis and profundus at wrist, and its extension to little finger.

border of the wrist-joint. This is called the *radial bursa*. The flexor carpi radialis has a sheath which extends from a point 2·5 cm. above the wrist to the insertion of the tendon.

The radial and ulnar bursae pass under the flexor retinaculum (transverse carpal ligament). Their relation to each other here is of great importance (*Fig.* 250).

1. They may be quite separate from each other.
2. They communicate with each other in 50 per cent of cases (Poirier): (*a*) Directly; (*b*) Through a separate sheath for the tendons of the index finger. Some writers place this intercommunication of the bursae as high as 80 per cent. This fact is obviously of great moment in cases of infection extending along a sheath. The infection will easily spread to other sheaths in the event of a communication existing.

258 A SYNOPSIS OF SURGICAL ANATOMY

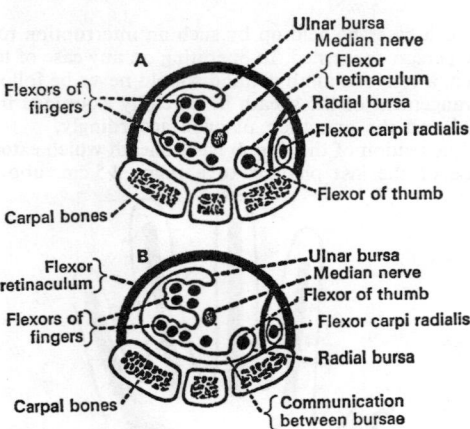

Fig. 250.—Transverse sections through carpus. A, The usual distinct arrangement of radial and ulnar bursae. B, Communication between the bursae.

Thus in tenosynovitis of the little finger the infection may spread up the sheath and infect the synovial sheath of the finger and thumb tendons through such a communication.

The radial and ulnar bursae lie on the front of the carpus and are separated from wrist and intercarpal joints by ligaments only. These joints may on occasion become infected from suppuration in the bursae.

POSTERIOR: Between the extensor retinaculum (dorsal carpal ligament) and the bones there are six compartments, each of which contains a mucous sheath for the tendons traversing the compartment. From lateral to medial these are:

1. One sheath for abductor pollicis longus and extensor pollicis brevis.
2. One sheath for extensores carpi radialis longus and brevis.
3. One sheath for extensor pollicis longus.
4. One sheath for the communis digitorum and extensor indicis proprius.
5. One sheath for the extensor minimi digiti.
6. One sheath for the extensor carpi ulnaris.

All these sheaths begin 2·5 cm. proximal to the dorsal carpal ligament. They extend:

1. To about the middle of the metacarpal bones in the case of the tendons going to the phalanges, excepting tendons of the thumb.

JOINTS, TENDON-SHEATHS, AND BURSAE

2. To the base of the metacarpal bones in the case of the tendons going to the metacarpals, and to a similar extent for the tendons of the thumb.

On the phalanges the extensors are quite devoid of sheaths.

STENOSING TENOVAGINITIS:

IN THE HAND: Tendon-sheaths are found where a tendon is considerably angulated when in action. The object is to secure maximum function and to avoid bow-string effects. The tendons affected by stenosis have strong fibrous sheaths. They are the abductor pollicis longus and extensor pollicis brevis, which lie in a common sheath where they cross the base of the radial styloid; the finger flexors at the metacarpophalangeal joints (trigger finger); and the flexor pollicis longus at a similar level. Although trigger finger may occur in infants, tendon-sheath narrowing is usually a disease of early and mid-adult life. It is due to frequent repetitive movements such as wringing clothes, typing, etc. It may thus be an occupational disease. It afflicts women ten times as often as men. The tendon-sheath becomes thickened and sometimes the tendon also. It is satisfactorily treated by incising the sheath.

IN THE FOOT: The peroneal retinaculum behind and below the lateral malleolus may also become disproportionate to the enclosed peronei. This causes pain on inversion of the foot or walking. It is cured by slitting up the thickened tendon-sheath.

Foot:

MUCOUS SHEATHS:

ANTERIOR: Three separate sheaths are found (*Fig.* 251):

The sheath of the tibialis anterior extends from upper border of transverse ligament of leg to just below the ankle-joint.

The sheaths of the extensor hallucis longus and extensor digitorum longus extend from the level of the malleoli to the base of the metatarsal bones.

MEDIAL: Three sheaths are found (*Fig.* 252):

Sheath of tibialis posterior extends from 5 cm. above the medial malleolus to the site of insertion of the tendon at the tuberosity of the navicular.

The sheaths of the flexor hallucis longus and flexor digitorum longus extend from the medial malleolus to the middle of the sole. Near the heads of the metatarsals these tendons acquire new sheaths which are arranged over the phalanges in a precisely similar manner to what obtains in the fingers.

LATERAL (*Fig.* 253): The peroneus longus and the brevis are enclosed in a sheath which extends 5 cm. above the tip of the malleolus and 5 cm. below it. Above the malleolus, where the tendons lie together, the sheath is single. Where they diverge below, the sheath gives each a separate investment.

260 A SYNOPSIS OF SURGICAL ANATOMY

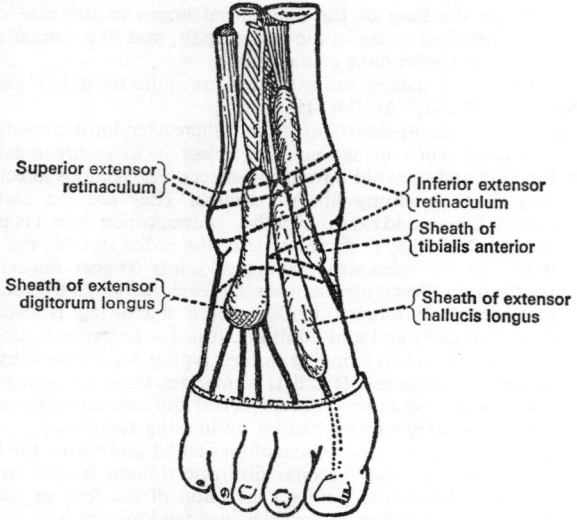

Fig. 251.—Tendon-sheaths on front of ankle.

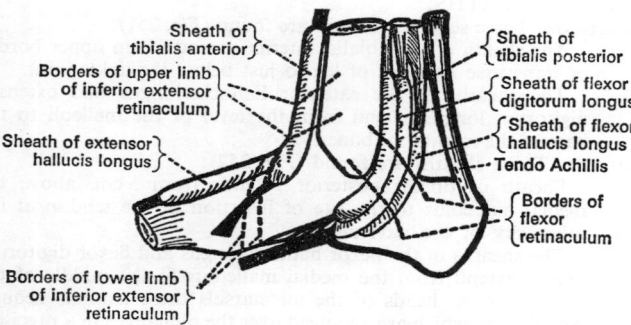

Fig. 252.—Tendon-sheaths on front and inner side of ankle.

POSTERIOR: The tendo Achillis has a definite sheath, which extends upwards for about 7·5 cm. from the insertion of the tendon to the calcaneus. Inflammation of this sheath is one of the causes of pain at the insertion of the tendo Achillis—so-called 'achillodynia'.

JOINTS, TENDON-SHEATHS, AND BURSAE 261

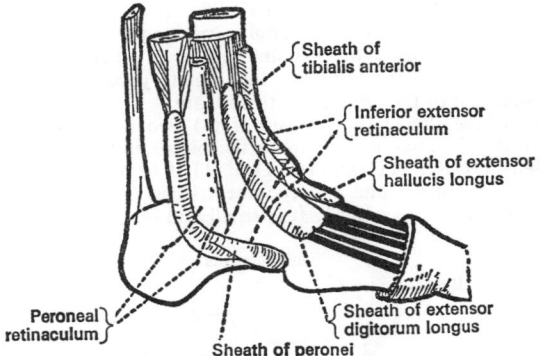

Fig. 253.—Tendon-sheaths on front and outer side of ankle.

BURSAE

Fibrous sacs lined with synovial membrane that secrete synovial fluid.

Bursae around the Shoulders: These are: (1) Subdeltoid and subacromial; (2) Subscapular; (3) Bursa under the infraspinatus; (4) The synovial sheath of the long head of the biceps.

The subscapular bursa and the synovial sheath of the long head of the biceps always communicate with the shoulder-joint.

The bursa under the infraspinatus may communicate with the shoulder-joint.

The subacromial bursa and the subdeltoid bursa may communicate with the shoulder-joint (10 per cent of cases).

SUBDELTOID AND SUBACROMIAL BURSAE: These bursae form one large cavity separating the deltoid from the upper part of the shaft of the humerus below and intervening between the under-surface of the acromion and the tuberosities of the humerus above. It disappears entirely under the acromion in right-angled abduction. This fact is utilized in distinguishing subdeltoid bursitis from other lesions round the joint. Pressure just below the acromion over the deltoid with the arm by the side causes pain if bursitis exists. Pressure over the same point with the arm abducted to a right angle causes no pain, because the bursa has disappeared under the acromion (Dawbarn's sign).

SUBSCAPULAR BURSA: This is between the subscapularis on the one hand and the front of the neck of the scapula and the base of the coracoid on the other.

SUB-INFRASPINATUS BURSA: Not always present. It separates the infraspinatus from the back of the neck of the scapula.

262 A SYNOPSIS OF SURGICAL ANATOMY

SYNOVIAL SHEATH OF THE BICEPS: The tendon of the long head of the biceps carries a tubular prolongation of the synovial membrane of the shoulder-joint with it, as it lies in the intertubercular sulcus of the humerus. Inflammatory fluid in the joint may spread out of the joint along this sheath.

Bursae around the Elbow: These consist of: (1) Two in relation to the triceps insertion; (2) Two in relation to the biceps insertion.

BURSAE IN RELATION TO THE TRICEPS INSERTION (*Fig.* 254): An upper one between the triceps tendon and the upper surface of the olecranon. It is small and of little importance.

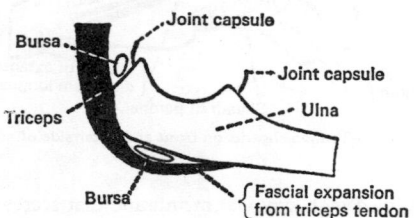

Fig. 254.—Bursae in relation to triceps insertion.

A lower one between the triceps expansion and subcutaneous triangular area on the dorsal surface of the olecranon. It is large and very important. Acute inflammation of this bursa, or of the corresponding bursa at the knee, the prepatellar, may cause a widespread 'sympathetic' inflammation of the surrounding soft parts.

BURSAE IN RELATION TO THE BICEPS INSERTION: These are both small. One separates the biceps tendon from the smooth anterior part of the bicipital tuberosity of the radius, the other separates the tendon from the oblique cord.

Bursae around the Hip: These are: (1) Subgluteal; (2) Subpsoas.

SUBGLUTEAL (*Fig.* 255):

FOUR UNDER THE GLUTEUS MAXIMUS:
 1. Between the gluteus maximus and the smooth part of the ilium lying between the posterior curved line and the outer lip of the iliac crest.
 2. Between the gluteus maximus and the lower part of the outer aspect of the great trochanter of the femur. It is large.
 3. Between the gluteus maximus and the ischial tuberosity. It may enlarge in persons who follow sedentary occupations (weaver's bottom). It is small and often absent.
 4. Between the tendon of the gluteus maximus and vastus lateralis.

ONE UNDER THE GLUTEUS MEDIUS: Between it and the upper part of the lateral aspect of the great trochanter.

ONE UNDER THE GLUTEUS MINIMUS: In relation to its insertion into the front of the great trochanter.

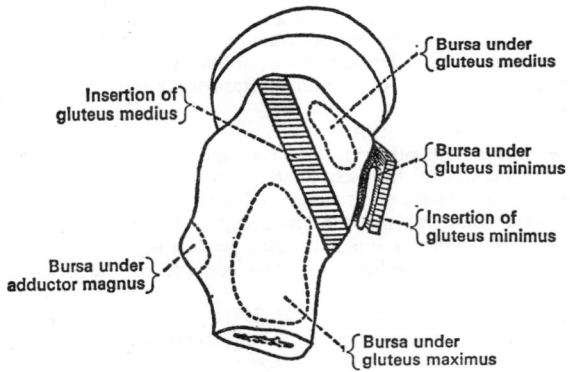

Fig. 255.—Bursae on great trochanter of femur.

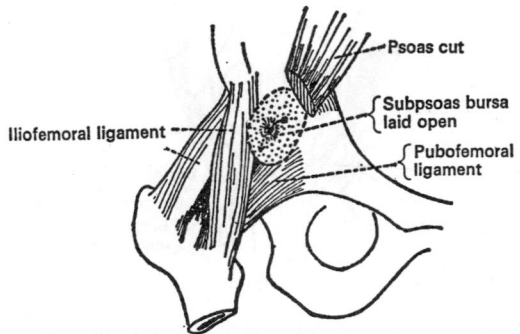

Fig. 256.—Showing a communication between the subpsoas bursa and the hip-joint.

SUBPSOAS (*Fig.* 256): This bursa is found between the iliopectineal eminence and the psoas tendon. It is important. In 10 per cent of cases it communicates with the hip-joint through the thin part of the capsule between the iliofemoral and pubofemoral ligaments.

Bursae around the Knee-joint: There are twelve: two are posterior; three are medial; three are lateral; four are anterior.

TWO POSTERIOR BURSAE: One between each head of origin of the gastrocnemius and the capsule of the joint. They often communicate with the joint. The bursa between the inner head of the gastrocnemius and the capsule sends a prolongation between the gastrocnemius and semimembranosus. This bursa is often enlarged, forming a swelling at the inner side of the popliteal space, which is spoken of as enlargement of the semimembranosus bursa. This bursa may become immense.

THREE MEDIAL BURSAE:
1. Separating the sartorius, gracilis, and semitendinosus from the tibial collateral ligament as they cross it.
2. and 3. Separating the tendon of the semimembranosus from the tibial collateral ligament medially and the head of the tibia laterally. The semimembranosus tendon is sandwiched between the ligament medially and the condyle of the tibia laterally (*Fig.* 257).

THREE LATERAL BURSAE (*Fig.* 257):
1. Between the biceps tendon and the fibular collateral ligament.
2. Between the fibular collateral ligament and the popliteus tendon.

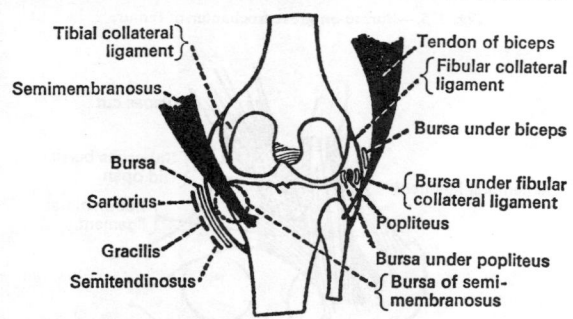

Fig. 257.—Bursae on inner and outer aspects of knee-joint.

3. Between the popliteus tendon and the lateral condyle of the femur. This bursa is really a tube of synovial membrane round the popliteus tendon like that around the long head of the biceps at the shoulder-joint. The bursa therefore communicates with the joint.

FOUR ANTERIOR BURSAE (*Fig.* 258):
1. THE SUPRAPATELLAR BURSA lies between the anterior surface of the lower part of the femur and the deep surface of the quadriceps muscle. It extends exactly three finger-breadths above the upper

border of the patella when the limb is at rest in extension. It always communicates with the knee-joint. For this reason it is always cleared away in excisions of the joint for tuberculosis. It may, however, become shut off from the rest of the joint cavity by disease.

2. PREPATELLAR BURSA: The bursa of housemaid's knee. It lies in front of the lower half of the patella and the upper half of the patellar ligament; exactly in the same area where the patellar nerve plexus is situated, the latter being between the bursa and the skin. This bursa is called *housemaid's knee* because, in scrubbing, the hands rest on the floor, bringing the bursa into contact

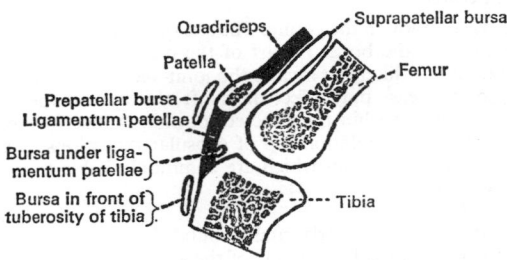

Fig. 258.—Bursae on front of knee-joint.

with the ground. This often causes inflammation—bursitis. Such a bursa may get very large and drop by its weight much below its original situation. Priests do not get prepatellar bursitis, because when they kneel in the upright position the bursa is not brought into contact with the ground.

3. Between the patellar ligament and the tibia.
4. Between the skin and the smooth lower part of the tuberosity of the tibia.

Several other anterior bursae are described. They are inconstant and unimportant.

The prepatellar, suprapatellar, and bursa between the inner head of the gastrocnemius and the semimembranosus are much the most important of the bursae around the knee-joint.

Adventitious Bursae: These do not normally exist, but appear over bony situations which are subject to much friction or pressure.

1. TAILOR'S ANKLE: Over the subcutaneous area above the lateral malleolus a large bursa often appears in tailors who sit in the cross-legged position, thus bringing this area in contact with the table.
2. PORTER'S SHOULDER: Between the upper surface of the clavicle and skin in those who carry loads on the shoulder.

3. **WEAVER'S BOTTOM**: Between the gluteus maximus and the ischial tuberosity.
4. **BUNION**: From pressure of faulty shoes over the medial part of the head of the first metatarsal bone.
5. **CALCANEAL**: Between the posterior part of its under-surface and the skin.
6. **KYPHOTIC**: Over the prominent part of the vertebral spinous processes and the skin in some cases of kyphotic curvature of the spine.

III. EPIPHYSIAL LINES AND CAPSULAR REFLECTIONS

Bone disease is common in the young. The site of election for its occurrence is the metaphysis of the bone. If part of the metaphysis is inside a joint capsule, the disease is likely to invade the joint—a serious matter. On the other hand, joint disease may affect the shaft of a bone if the metaphysis of that bone is partly within the affected joint. It is therefore of the first importance to know the relationship of capsular reflections to epiphysial lines in those joints and bones which are commonly liable to infection.

Humerus (*Fig.* 259):

UPPER END:

EPIPHYSIAL LINE: Runs horizontally round the upper end of the bone at the level of the lowest part of the articular surface of the head.

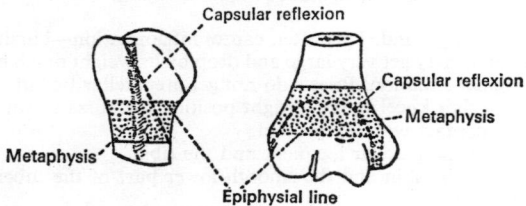

Fig. 259.—Relations of metaphyses and capsular reflections of humerus.

CAPSULE: Is attached above to the anatomical neck. Below it is attached to the shaft an inch below the lowest part of the articular surface of the head.

The metaphysis is therefore partly intracapsular.

LOWER END:

EPIPHYSIAL LINE: A horizontal line at the level of the lateral epicondyle of the bone. The inner epicondyle has a separate epiphysis—a tongue of shaft intervening between the epiphysis of the inner epicondyle and that of the rest of the lower end of the bone.

JOINTS, TENDON-SHEATHS, AND BURSAE

CAPSULE:
  Anterior: Follows the margin of the coronoid and radial fossae.
  Posterior: Follows the distal half of the margin of the olecranon fossa, crossing the floor of the fossa at its middle.
  Medial and Lateral: Attached 0·6 cm. from the articular margins.
  The metaphysis is therefore partly intracapsular.

Radius (*Fig.* 260):
  UPPER END:
    EPIPHYSIS: The head forms the epiphysis.
    CAPSULE: Is attached to the neck of the bone.
    The metaphysis is partly intracapsular.
  LOWER END:
    EPIPHYSIS: Is a horizontal line at the level of the upper part of the ulnar notch.

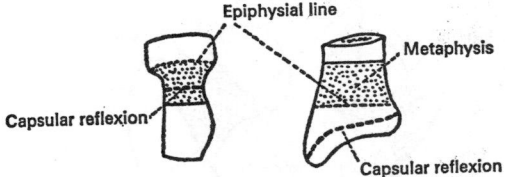

Fig. 260.—Relations of capsular reflections and metaphyses of radius.

  CAPSULE: Is attached very close to the articular margin all the way round.
  The metaphysis is entirely extracapsular.

Ulna (*Fig.* 261):
  UPPER END:
    EPIPHYSIS: Is very variable. It is usually a flake of bone on the upper surface of the olecranon.
    CAPSULE: Is attached near the articular surface in its whole extent.

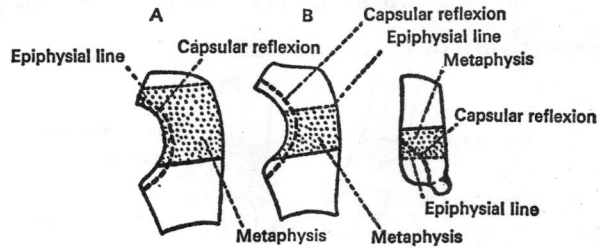

Fig. 261.—To show relations of metaphyses and capsular reflections of ulna. A and B show the small (usual) and large types of upper ulnar epiphyses.

Here the unique condition exists of the epiphysis being entirely extracapsular, so that the whole metaphysis and part of the diaphysis also are related to the capsular line.

LOWER END:

EPIPHYSIS: A horizontal line at the level of the upper extremity of the articular surface for the radius.

CAPSULE: Attached to margins of articular surface except laterally, where it is a little proximal to the radial articular surface. The metaphysis is therefore partly intracapsular.

Femur:

UPPER END (*Fig. 262*):

EPIPHYSIS: The epiphysial line of the head corresponds exactly to its articular margin.

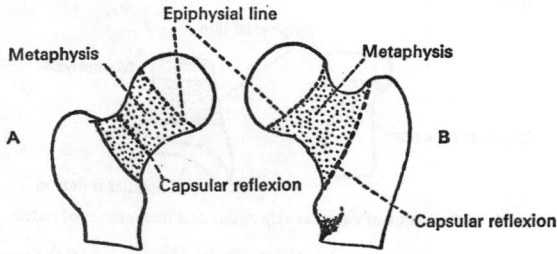

Fig. 262.—Capsular and metaphysial relations of upper end of femur.
A, Anterior. B, Posterior.

CAPSULE:

Anterior: Attached to the spiral line, the whole neck being intracapsular.

Posterior: Attached a finger's breadth medial to the intertrochanteric line, the neck being therefore partly intra- and partly extracapsular.

The metaphysis is entirely intracapsular.

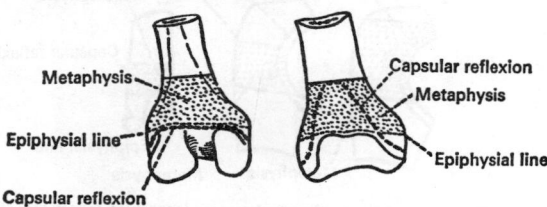

Fig. 263.—Capsular and metaphysial relations of lower end of femur.

LOWER END (*Fig.* 263):
  EPIPHYSIS: An irregular horizontal line round the bone at the level of the upper limit of the articular surface in front and behind. It crosses the middle of the adductor tubercle.
  CAPSULE:
    Posterior: To the articular margin.
    Lateral and Medial: Half a centimetre from the articular margin.
    Anterior: Some distance proximal to the articular margin (usually 5 cm.)
  The metaphysis is intracapsular in front only.

Tibia (*Fig.* 264):
  UPPER END:
    EPIPHYSIS: Is 1·2 cm. from the articular margin. It sends a tongue-shaped process distally to form the upper half of the tuberosity

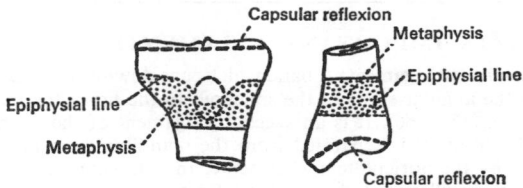

Fig. 264.—Capsular and metaphysial relations of tibia.

  CAPSULE: Is attached to the articular margin.
  The metaphysis is some distance distal to the capsular line.
  LOWER END:
    EPIPHYSIS: Is a horizontal line 0·6 cm. above the broad lower end of the bone.
    CAPSULE: Is attached to the margins of the articular surface.
    As at the upper end, the capsular attachment and metaphysis at the lower end are separated by the whole thickness of the epiphysis. Disease of this bone is therefore very unlikely to affect the joint and vice versa.

Fibula (*Fig.* 265):

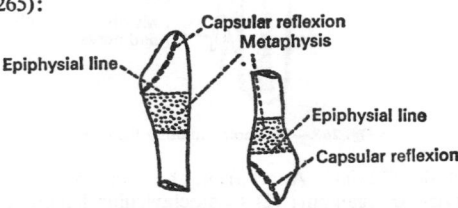

Fig. 265.—Capsular and metaphysial relations of fibula.

EPIPHYSES: At both extremities of the bone the epiphysis is the bulbous end.
CAPSULES: The capsules are attached to the articular margins.
The metaphyses are entirely extracapsular.
The epiphysial line at the lower end is at the level of the ankle-joint. This is important, as disease of the ankle-joint may spread to the shaft of the fibula and vice versa.

Chapter XXV

LIGAMENTS

I. CERTAIN IMPORTANT LIGAMENTS

Sphenomandibular Ligament: A band which runs downwards and outwards from the angular spine of the sphenoid to the lip of the mandibular foramen (*Fig.* 266). It is an accessory ligament of the temporomandibular joint. It is separated from the mandible from above downwards by the auriculotemporal nerve, the pterygoidus externus, the internal maxillary vessels, and the inferior alveolar vessels and nerve.

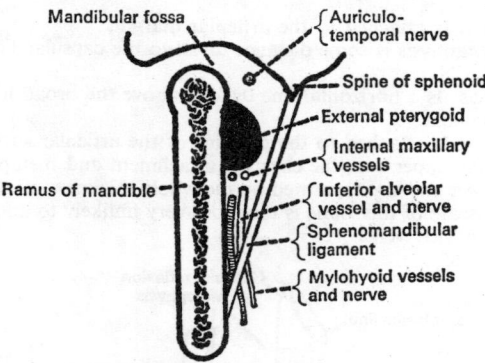

Fig. 266.—Sphenomandibular ligament.

Ligaments of the Clavicle: Apart from the joint capsules there are: (1) Interclavicular ligament; (2) Costoclavicular ligament; (3) Coracoclavicular ligaments.

LIGAMENTS

INTERCLAVICULAR LIGAMENT: A T-shaped ligament attached to the upper aspect of the inner end of each clavicle and to the upper margin of the manubrium sterni (*Fig.* 267).

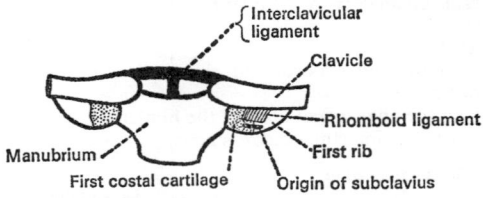

Fig. 267.—Interclavicular and rhomboid ligaments and origin of subclavius muscle.

COSTOCLAVICULAR OR RHOMBOID LIGAMENT: This structure lies behind and medial to the subclavius muscle, being attached to the same structures (*Fig.* 267). Below it is attached to the first rib and costal cartilage, above it is attached to the costal tuberosity of the clavicle; the costocoracoid ligament is attached to its outer border. Posterior to it is the innominate vein.

CORACOCLAVICULAR LIGAMENTS: These are the *conoid* and *trapezoid* ligaments. They suspend much of the weight of the upper limb from the clavicle (*Fig.* 268). The conoid has the shape of an inverted cone. The costocoracoid ligament is attached to it. The

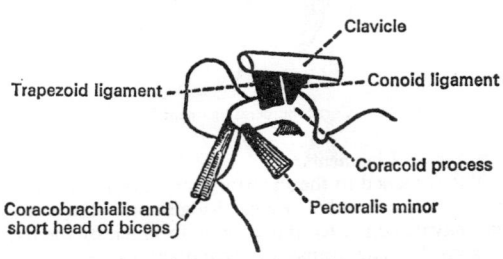

Fig. 268.—Coracoclavicular ligaments.

trapezoid is quadrilateral in shape and lies anterior and external to the conoid, suggested by the first two vowels of the word 'trapezoid'.

Coraco-acromial Ligament: This structure overhangs the shoulder-joint and lies under cover of the anterior fibres of the deltoid. Beneath it is the tendon of the supraspinatus, the subacromial bursa intervening. It is triangular in shape, the base being attached to the posterolateral

272 A SYNOPSIS OF SURGICAL ANATOMY

border of the horizontal part of the coracoid process; the apex is attached to the apex of the acromion. Morphologically it represents a continuation of the biceps tendon.

Coracohumeral Ligament: A ligament accessory to the shoulder-joint (*Fig.* 269).

ATTACHMENTS:
> ABOVE: To the outer border of the vertical part of the coracoid process.
> BELOW: To the anatomical neck of the humerus just behind the upper end of the intertubercular sulcus.

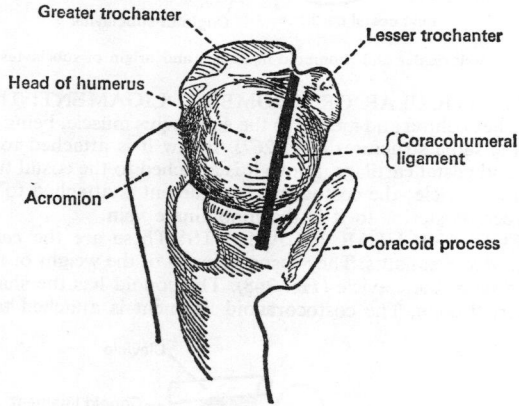

Fig. 269.—Coracohumeral ligament from above.

Transverse Scapular Ligaments:
> SUPERIOR: Attached to the superior margin of the scapula and to the base of the coracoid process. Bridges over the scapular notch, which may be converted into a bony foramen by the ossification of the ligament. The transverse scapular vessels pass over it, the suprascapular nerve passes beneath it (nerve-notch). The omohyoid arises from it.
> INFERIOR: Passes from the lateral border of the spine to the back of the head of the scapula. The vessels and nerves pass deep to it.

Collateral Ligaments of the Elbow-joint (*Fig.* 270):
> RADIAL COLLATERAL LIGAMENT:
> ATTACHMENTS:
>> *Above:* To the distal part of the lateral epicondyle of the humerus.
>> *Below:* To the annular ligament of the head of the radius.

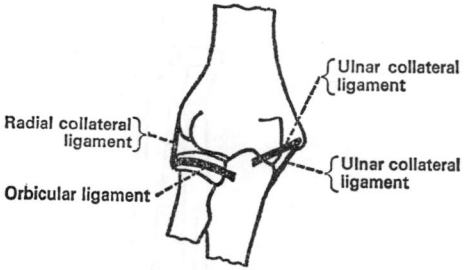

Fig. 270.—Collateral ligaments of elbow-joint.

ULNAR COLLATERAL LIGAMENT:
ATTACHMENTS:
> *Above:* To the distal part of the medial epicondyle of the humerus.
> *Below:* To the medial margins of the olecranon and coronoid processes and to a band which stretches across between these bony processes.

It gives origin to some fibres of the flexor sublimis digitorum. These ligaments play an important part in preventing lateral movement at the elbow-joint. If one of them is broken, there is lateral movement at the joint towards the opposite side.

The Oblique Cord (*Fig.* 271): A band passing down and out from the outer border of the coronoid process of the ulna to the radius just distal to its tuberosity. It is said to represent a degenerate part of the flexor pollicis longus origin.

Interosseous Membrane of the Forearm:
ATTACHMENTS:
> MEDIAL: Lateral border of ulna.
> LATERAL: Medial border of radius.

The fibres of the membrane pass downwards and inwards. Those of the interosseous membrane of the lower limb pass down and out.

FUNCTIONS:
1. Increases the area for the origin of the muscles of the forearm.
2. Breaks the force of shocks transmitted up the radius. These pass from the radius to the ulna along the membrane in a recurrent direction and thence to the humerus (*Fig.* 271).

Between its upper border and the oblique cord is a gap through which the dorsal interosseous vessels pass backwards.

ANTERIOR SURFACE: Gives origin to the flexor pollicis longus and the flexor profundus. Between these two muscles lie the volar interosseous vessels and nerve. The vessels perforate the membrane

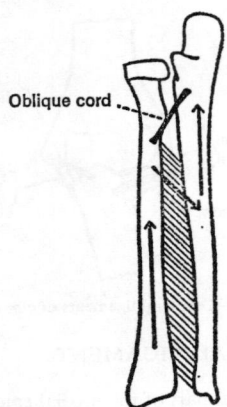

Fig. 271.—To show recurrent course to ulna, via interosseous membrane, taken by shocks transmitted from hand to radius.

near its lower end and then lie on its posterior surface. The lower quarter of the membrane is covered by the pronator quadratus.

POSTERIOR SURFACE: Gives origin to the abductor pollicis longus, extensor pollicis brevis and longus, and extensor indicis proprius. The supinator rests on the proximal part of the membrane. Lying on its distal part are the volar interosseous vessels and dorsal interosseous nerve.

Collateral Ligaments of the Wrist-joint (*Fig. 272*):

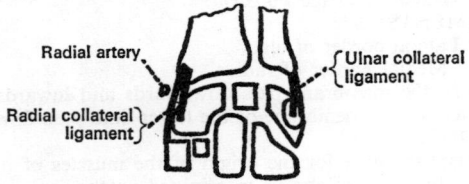

Fig. 272.—Collateral ligaments of wrist-joint.

RADIAL COLLATERAL LIGAMENT: From radial styloid to tuberosity of the navicular and to os multangulum majus. The radial artery crosses it.

ULNAR COLLATERAL LIGAMENT: From styloid process of ulnar to pisiform and triquetrum.

LIGAMENTS 275

Collateral Ligaments of Metacarpophalangeal and Interphalangeal Joints:
Arranged on the same principle as the collateral ligaments at the elbow and wrist. Attached to the side of the head of the proximal bone and to the side of the base of the distal bone. Prevent lateral mobility (*Fig.* 273).

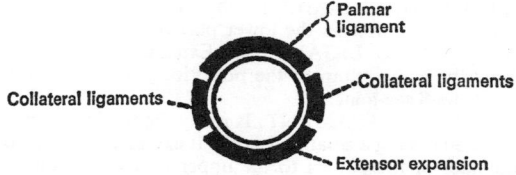

Fig. 273.—Transverse section showing ligaments of a metacarpophalangeal joint.

Palmar Ligaments of Metacarpophalangeal and Interphalangeal Joints:
They are very dense. Attached firmly to the distal bone, and loosely to the proximal bone. If they are torn, they remain attached to the distal bone.

The metatarsophalangeal and interphalangeal joints of the foot have the same arrangement of their ligaments.

Ligaments of the Hip-joint (*Fig.* 274):

ILIOFEMORAL: The strongest ligament in the body. It has the shape of an inverted Y.

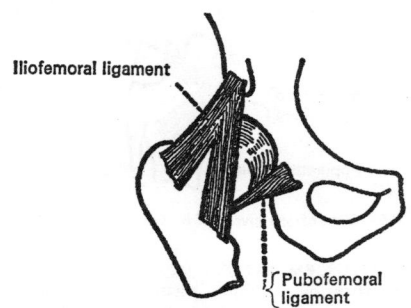

Fig. 274.—Iliofemoral and pubofemoral ligaments of hip-joint.

ATTACHMENTS:

Proximal: Anterior inferior spine of ilium.

Distal: The two limbs are attached to the intertrochanteric line. The ligament is so strong that when subjected to strain it may remain intact, and, instead of the ligament tearing, the anterior inferior

276 A SYNOPSIS OF SURGICAL ANATOMY

spine of the ilium may be wrenched off. Similarly it remains intact as a rule in dislocations of the head of the femur and to some extent governs the position of the head. Such dislocations are called 'regular'; when the ligament is torn the dislocation is referred to as being 'irregular'.

PUBOFEMORAL LIGAMENT: The fibres pass from the superior ramus of the pubis to the lower part of the capsule.

ISCHIOFEMORAL LIGAMENT: Extends from the ischium just below the acetabulum to the posterior part of the capsule.

Ligaments of the Knee-joint:

THE PATELLAR LIGAMENT: Is really the tendon of the quadriceps, the patella being a sesamoid bone. It extends from the lower border and sides of the patella to the upper part of the tuberosity of the tibia, i.e., it is attached to the epiphysis of the tibia. The upper part of the tuberosity may be partly detached by the pull of the tendon.

THE LIGAMENTS OF THE SEMIMEMBRANOSUS: The tendon of the semimembranosus gives off three ligamentous expansions (*Fig.* 275).

1. THE OBLIQUE POPLITEAL LIGAMENT: Strengthens the capsule behind. It passes upwards and outwards from the tendon of the semimembranosus to blend with the capsule. The popliteal vessels lie on it and it is perforated by the azygos geniculate artery.

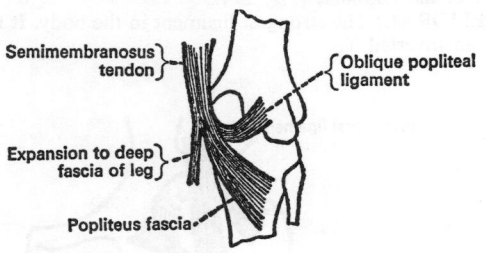

Fig. 275—Expansions given off by tendon of semimembranosus.

2. THE POPLITEUS FASCIA: An expansion from the tendon of the semimembranosus which passes down and out to cover the popliteus. It is attached to the popliteal line of the tibia. The popliteal vessels lie on it and end at its lower border.

3. AN EXPANSION TO THE DEEP FASCIA ON INNER SIDE OF LEG.

THE COLLATERAL LIGAMENTS (*Fig.* 276): These are very strong structures which prevent lateral movements at the joint. If they are torn or even stretched, the integrity of the joint is lost. The fibular collateral ligament is round and cord-like and stands

LIGAMENTS 277

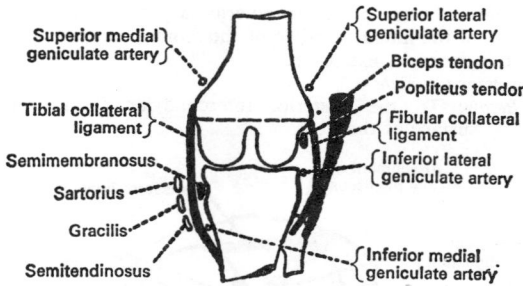

Fig. 276.—Collateral ligaments of knee-joint.

well away from the bone. The tibial collateral ligament is broad and strap-like and is closely applied to the bone. An inferior geniculate artery (from the popliteal) passes under each ligament, running in a forward direction.

ATTACHMENTS:

1. *Fibular Collateral Ligament:*
   Superior: To the lateral epicondyle of the femur just above the groove for the popliteus.
   Inferior: To the head of the fibula anterior to the apex. It divides the biceps tendon into two; the popliteus passes out beneath it.

2. *Tibial Collateral Ligament:*
   Superior: To the medial epicondyle just below the adductor tubercle.
   Inferior: To 3·8 cm. of the medial surface of the tibia commencing 5 cm. from the upper end of the bone.
   It is attached to the medial meniscus. Three tendons cross it: those of the sartorius, gracilis, and semitendinosus. A bursa separates them from the ligament.
   H. A. T. Fairbank[1] points out that, as the result of trauma, the upper attachment of the tibial collateral ligament is injured seven times as often as the lower attachments.

THE CRUCIATE LIGAMENTS: Very powerful cord-like structures. They prevent movement of the two bones on each other in an anteroposterior direction.

ATTACHMENTS (*Fig.* 277):
   Anterior Cruciate:
      Below: To the anterior intercondylar fossa of the tibia.

[1] *Br. med. J.,* 1930, **1**, 582.

Above: To the posterior superior aspect of the medial surface of the lateral condyle of the femur.

It is tense in extension.

Posterior Cruciate:

Below: To the posterior intercondylar fossa and popliteal surface of the tibia.

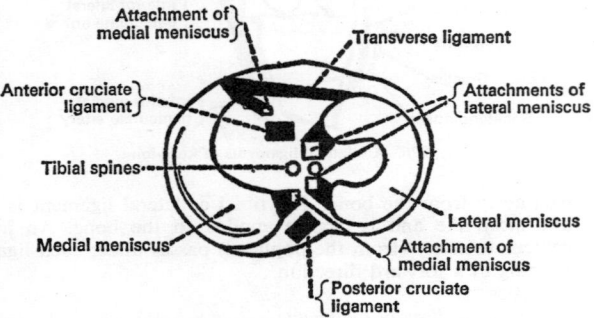

Fig. 277.—Attachments to upper surface of tibia.

Above: To the anterior and inferior aspect of the lateral surface of the medial condyle of the femur. It is joined by a slip from the posterior part of the lateral meniscus (ligament of Wrisberg).

It is tense in flexion.

The anterior cruciate passes backwards and outwards. The posterior cruciate passes inwards and forwards; therefore in opening the knee-joint from the inner side the posterior cruciate is seen first.

The anterior cruciate prevents the tibia from being moved forwards on the femur in extension. The posterior cruciate prevents the tibia from being moved backwards on the femur in flexion.

THE MENISCI (SEMILUNAR CARTILAGES): The one-time belief that the menisci were covered by synovial membrane is known to be erroneous.

METHOD OF FIXATION OF THE MENISCI: ATTACHMENTS (*Fig. 277*):

The medial meniscus is comma-shaped, the broad end being behind; it forms a small segment of a large circle. *The lateral meniscus* is more circular; it forms a segment of a smaller circle.

Extremities: The anterior and posterior ends are attached respectively to the anterior and posterior intercondylar fossae of the tibia.

Peripherally: They are attached to the capsule of the joint. The capsule thus attaches them to the tibia below (short coronary ligaments) and to the femur above (long coronary ligaments).

Anteriorly: Their anterior margins are bound together by the transverse ligament of the knee-joint.

Billington first pointed out that the transverse ligament may be looked upon as the continuation of the peripheral fibres of each meniscus. The more internal fibres of the menisci continue on to be attached to the tibia. It will be obvious that if any force acts on the periphery of the meniscus while the central part is fixed, it will tend to tear longitudinally along a line between the inner and outer sets of fibres. This is a common accident and produces what is known as a 'bucket-handle' tear of the cartilage, the medial one being usually affected (*Fig.* 278).

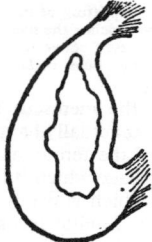

Fig. 278.—'Bucket-handle' type of injury to meniscus.

THE RELATION OF THE TIBIAL COLLATERAL LIGAMENT TO THE MEDIAL MENISCUS: This relationship is an extremely important one and is directly responsible for the fact that injuries to the menisci affect the medial one vastly more commonly than the lateral. The lateral is free to move within a small compass, but this slight degree of mobility is sufficient to ensure its safety. The medial one is fixed at one point by the tibial collateral ligament and because of this anchorage it is so prone to injury (*Fig.* 279). The tibial collateral ligament consists of long and short fibres. The long ones have been described above in giving the attachment of the ligament. The short ones are on the deep surface of the ligament at its posterior part, and they are attached to the margin of the medial meniscus behind its middle and to the condyle of the tibia, thus binding the meniscus to the tibia. Passing forward between these deep fibres and the overlying long or superficial fibres of the tibial collateral ligament is the tendon of the semimembranosus. The medial meniscus being fixed in this way at one point, it follows that if its anterior part is subjected to any strain of a nature

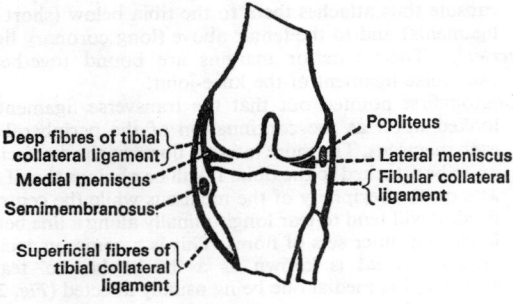

Fig. 279.—Diagram showing splitting of tibial collateral ligament into deep and superficial fibres. The former anchor the medial meniscus, and the tendon of the semimembranosus insinuates itself between the two sets of fibres. The lateral meniscus has no attachment to the fibular collateral ligament.

tending to elongate the meniscus it may tear away from this fixed part. This is what actually happens in many cases (*Fig.* 280). Excessive rotation of the femur on the tibia tears the movable front part of the cartilage which is fixed between the bones away from the back part which is firmly anchored.

RE-FORMATION OF MENISCI: Smilie[1] has shown that when a meniscus is removed a new one is invariably formed from the parietal synovial membrane. Partial removal is similarly followed by regeneration providing the portion removed included the peripheral zone.

Injury of such re-formed menisci is rare because they are more firmly attached and project less far into the joint cavity than the original cartilages.

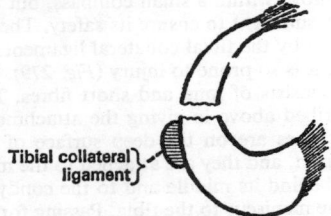

Fig. 280.—Transverse tear of meniscus just in front of its attachment to tibial collateral ligament.

[1] *Br. J. Surg.*, 1944, 31, 398.

Ligaments around the Ankle-joint:
MEDIAL:
DELTOID LIGAMENT: Triangular, with the apex above. It is very powerful (*Fig.* 281).

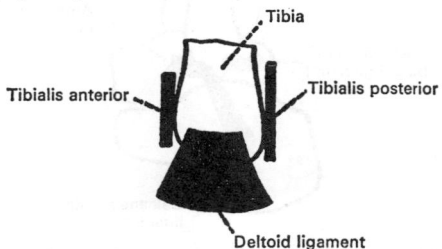

Fig. 281.—Deltoid ligament and tendons of tibial muscles.

Attachments:
  Apex: To the medial malleolus.
  Base: Attached from before back to the tuberosity of the navicular, the inferior calcaneonavicular or spring ligament, neck of the talus, the sustentaculum tali, and body of talus. Its medial surface is crossed by the tendons of the tibialis posterior and the flexor longus digitorum (*Fig.* 282).

LATERAL:
On the outer aspect of the joint are three ligamentous bands which are accessory to the capsule of the joint. They are very frequently injured in sprains, etc., and are of great importance. They are the anterior talofibular, the posterior talofibular, and the calcaneofibular ligaments (*Figs.* 283, 284).

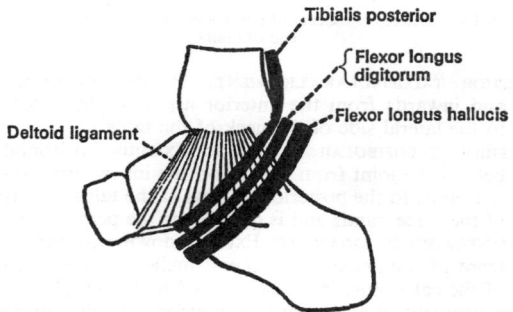

Fig. 282.—Relation of posterior tendons to deltoid ligament of ankle-joint.

282 A SYNOPSIS OF SURGICAL ANATOMY

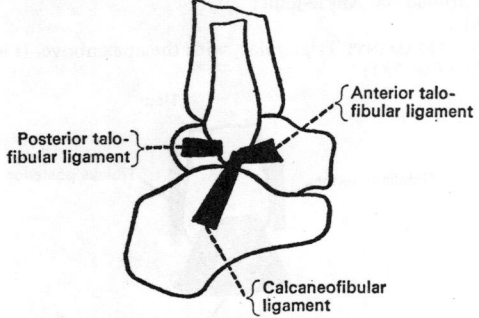

Fig. 283.—Lateral accessory ligaments of ankle-joint. The talofibular ligaments are horizontal, the calcaneofibular is vertical.

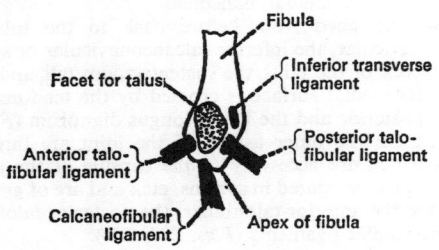

Fig. 284.—Accessory ligaments of ankle-joint which are attached to lower end of fibula.

ANTERIOR TALOFIBULAR LIGAMENT: Passes horizontally forwards and inwards from the anterior aspect of the lateral malleolus to the lateral side of the neck of the talus.

POSTERIOR TALOFIBULAR LIGAMENT: Extends horizontally inwards behind the joint from the pit on the inner surface of the lateral malleolus to the posterior process of the talus. It is the strongest of the three bands and is crossed by the peronei tendons.

CALCANEOFIBULAR LIGAMENT: Extends down and back from just in front of the apex of the lateral malleolus to the lateral surface of the calcaneus. It is also crossed by the peronei.

These ligaments may be torn by injuries, and the correct treatment depends on the exact diagnosis as to which band is injured.

LIGAMENTS 283

Interosseous Membrane of the Leg: The fibres run down and out. It occupies the whole of the gap between the two bones, blending with the capsule of the tibiofibular joint proximally and with the interosseous tibiofibular ligament distally. It is perforated at its proximal part by the anterior tibial vessels, and near its distal end by the perforating branch of the peroneal artery.

ANTERIOR SURFACE: The tibialis anterior, extensor longus digitorum and extensor longus hallucis, and peroneus tertius arise from it. The anterior tibial vessels and deep peroneal nerve lie on it (*Fig.* 285).

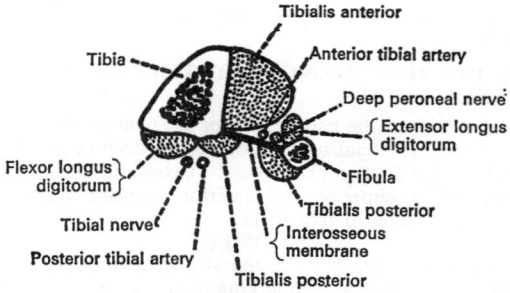

Fig. 285.—Relations of interosseous ligament of leg.

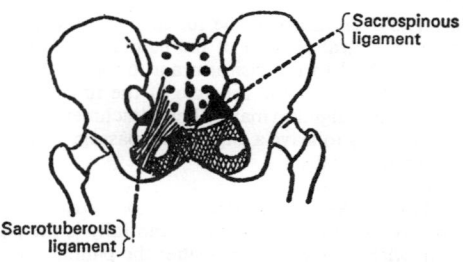

Fig. 286.—Sacrotuberous and sacrospinous ligaments.

POSTERIOR SURFACE: The tibialis posterior and flexor longus hallucis arise from it.

Sacrotuberous Ligament: Bridges the gap between the sacrum and the hip bone. It assists in the formation of the sacrosciatic foramina (*Fig.* 286).
ATTACHMENTS:
ABOVE: Posterior iliac spines, last three pieces of the sacrum, and the side of the coccyx.

BELOW: The medial margin of the ischial tuberosity. A prolongation of the ligament to the ramus of the ischium is called the falciform process.

From its posterior surface the gluteus maximus arises. Its anterior surface forms the posterior wall of the ischiorectal fossa.

Sacrospinous Ligament: Is triangular in shape (*Fig.* 286). The apex is attached to the ischial spine. The base is attached to the side of the coccyx and sacrum. The coccygeus covers its anterior surface. It may be looked upon as a delamination of this muscle (Wright). Its posterior surface is crossed by the internal pudendal vessels and pudendal nerve. The fifth sacral and coccygeal branches of the coccygeal plexus pierce it.

II. THE BINDING BANDS AT THE WRIST AND ANKLE

The tendons acting on the hand and foot are held in place by ligaments which are all merely specialized portions of the deep fascia. There are six such specialized bands: two at the wrist—flexor and extensor retinacula; four at the ankle—superior and inferior extensor retinacula, flexor retinaculum, and peroneal retinacula.

The Wrist

Flexor Retinaculum (*Fig.* 287): Is the size of a 'postage stamp' (to be remembered in the surface marking of the ligament). Like a postage stamp it has two surfaces and four borders.

BORDERS:
SUPERIOR: The deep fascia of the forearm is attached to it.
INFERIOR: The central portion of the palmar fascia is attached here.
MEDIAL: Is attached to the pisiform and hook of the hamate.
LATERAL: Is attached to the tubercle of the navicular and the ridge on the os multangulum majus. This attachment is by two processes so arranged as to leave a gap for the passage of the tendon of the flexor carpi radialis.

SURFACES:
PALMAR: This surface is crossed by those structures entering the palm superficial to the ligament; centrally is the palmaris longus tendon with a nerve on each side: the palmar cutaneous branch of the median on the radial side, the palmar cutaneous branch of the ulnar on the ulnar side. The ulnar vessels and nerve cross the ligament under cover of the pisiform bone. They are held in place by a fascial process named the volar carpal ligament, which is attached to the pisiform medially and the flexor retinaculum laterally. In addition, this surface gives partial insertion to the flexor carpi ulnaris and palmaris longus, and partial origin to all the small muscles of the thenar and hypothenar eminences except the abductor minimi digiti quinti—i.e., the abductor

LIGAMENTS 285

pollicis brevis, the flexor pollicis brevis, opponens pollicis, opponens minimi digiti, flexor brevis minimi digiti, and the palmaris brevis.

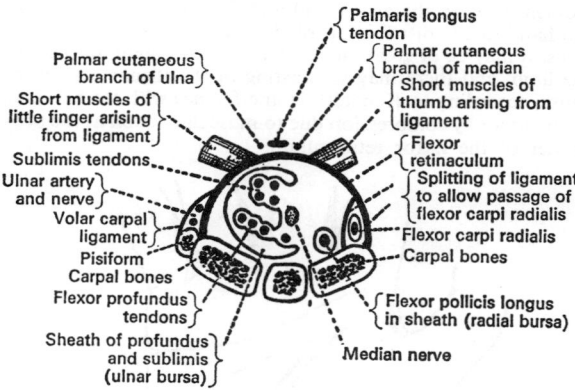

Fig. 287.—The flexor retinaculum.

These muscular attachments entirely hide the volar surface of the ligament, which is much farther from the skin surface than the surgeon is apt to think.

DORSAL: This surface forms with the carpal bones a tunnel. This tunnel is traversed by the flexors of the fingers, sublimis and profundus, the long flexor of the thumb, and the median nerve. The flexors of the fingers are invaginated into a synovial bag (named the ulnar bursa) from its outer side, which bag is therefore open laterally. In this gap lies the median nerve. The arrangement of the tendons under the ligament is as follows:

The sublimis tendons are all separate, being arranged in two pairs: the upper pair consists of one to each of the middle and ring fingers; the lower pair consists of one to each of the index and little fingers.

The profundus tendons: only the slip to the index finger is separate; the other three are still fused and lie medial to the index slip.

The flexor pollicis longus tendon is on the radial side in a separate mucous sheath called the radial bursa. In 50 per cent of cases there is a communication between the radial and ulnar bursae in this situation.

286 A SYNOPSIS OF SURGICAL ANATOMY

The flexor carpi radialis does not go over the ligament and does not go under it, but actually goes through it. It has a separate synovial sheath of its own.

THE CARPAL TUNNEL SYNDROME: Cases occur, usually in women between the ages of 40 and 70, who complain of pain in the hand in the distribution of the median nerve on one or both sides. It may be of great intensity, is worse at night, may extend up the limb, and there may be wasting of the thenar eminence. The cause, according to Kendall[1], is interference with the blood-supply of the nerve by compression due to muscular action at the proximal border of the flexor retinaculum.

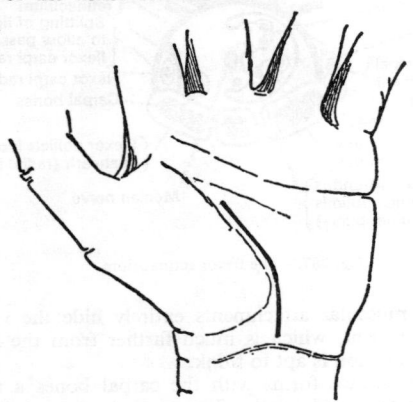

Fig. 288.—Incision for exposing the flexor retinaculum.

It may be cured by division of this retinaculum (*Fig.* 288). Before resorting to surgery, medical measures should be tried as myxoedema, etc., may be responsible for swelling under the ligament.

Some authorities bring this condition into line with stenosing tenovaginitis at the radial styloid and trigger finger, etc.

Extensor Retinaculum (*Fig.* 289): Is oblique in direction at the back of the wrist. It has four borders and two surfaces like the transverse ligament.

BORDERS:
SUPERIOR AND INFERIOR: Are continuous with the deep fascia.
MEDIAL: Is attached to the triquetrum and pisiform.
LATERAL: Is attached to the lower 2·5 cm. of the volar (anterior) border of the radius.

[1] Kendall, D., *Br. med. J.*, 1960, Dec. 3 1633.

It is not attached to the lower end of the ulna by its medial border. If it were, it would interfere with the movements of the radius round the ulna (pronation and supination).

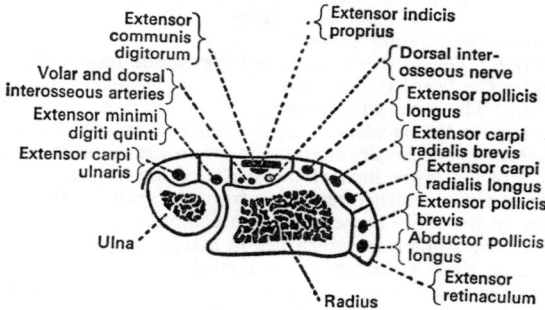

Fig. 289.—Extensor retinaculum and structures passing beneath it.

SURFACES:

DORSAL: Is crossed by veins draining the dorsal carpal arch (i.e., the commencement of cephalic and basilic veins) and by four cutaneous nerves, viz., the dorsal branch of the ulnar nerve, the superficial branch of the radial, and the terminations of the posterior branches of the medial and lateral cutaneous nerves of the forearm.

DEEP OR ANTERIOR: This surface is related to the extensor tendons. Fascial processes pass from it to the radius and ulna, which divide the space between the ligament and the bones into six compartments for the tendons. These six compartments house from lateral to medial:

1. { Abductor pollicis longus.
     Extensor pollicis brevis.
2. { Extensor carpi radialis longus.
     Extensor carpi radialis brevis.
3. Extensor pollicis longus.
4. { Extensor communis digitorum.
     Extensor indicis proprius.
5. Extensor minimi digiti.
6. Extensor carpi ulnaris.

VESSELS AND NERVES: The terminations of the volar and dorsal interosseous arteries and the dorsal interosseous nerve go through the compartment for the extensor communis digitorum, lying between it and the bone.

It is worth observing that beyond the ligament, on the dorsum of the hand, the extensor indicis tendon lies on the ulnar side of the communis slip to the index. So, too, the extensor minimi digiti is on the ulnar side of the communis slip to the fifth digit.

The Ankle

At the ankle the binding bands are:

ANTERIOR: The superior and inferior extensor retinacula.
MEDIAL: The flexor retinaculum.
LATERAL: The peroneal retinacula.

Superior Extensor Retinaculum: This is a thickening of the deep fascia, with which its borders are continuous. Its attachments are the anterior borders of the lower inch of the shafts of the tibia and the fibula. Under it pass the structures going from the front of the leg to the dorsum of the foot. These lie in one common compartment except for the tibialis anterior, which lies in a separate compartment. The relation of these structures from medial to lateral is: The tibialis anterior, extensor hallucis longus, the anterior tibial artery with a vein each side, the deep peroneal nerve, the extensor communis digitorum, and the peroneus tertius.

The superficial surface is crossed by the commencement of the long saphenous vein, the saphenous nerve, and the superficial peroneal nerve.

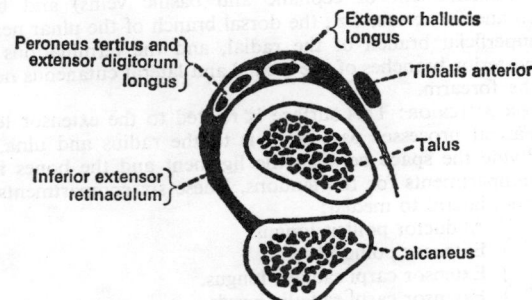

Fig. 290.—Arrangement of inferior extensor retinaculum. Note its relation to tendon of tibialis anterior. (*Re-drawn from Frazer.*)

Inferior Extensor Retinaculum: This is a Y-shaped structure stretching across the foot in the region of the ankle-joint. It is a thickening of the deep fascia.

The *stem* of the Y is attached to the upper surface of the anterior part of the calcaneus (the extensor digitorum brevis also arises from here and therefore takes origin from the ligament as well).

The *upper limb* of the Y is attached to the medial malleolus.

The *lower limb* of the Y blends with the deep fascia on the medial border of the foot (plantar aponeurosis).

The structures passing under this ligament are identical with those passing under the superior extensor retinaculum. They are now, however, grouped into two compartments—a medial for the extensor hallucis longus, and a lateral for the extensor communis and peroneus tertius. These compartments are formed in a different way from the arrangement at the back of the wrist. There septa extend from the ligament to the bone; here the ligament merely splits to form the compartments. The vessels and nerves pass deep to the ligament. The tibialis anterior passes superficial or deep to the inner part of the ligament, not lying in a specialized compartment.

Frazer very aptly likens the ligament to a sling preventing the tendons from prolapsing to the inner side of the foot (*Fig.* 290).

Flexor Retinaculum: Has four borders and two surfaces.

BORDERS:

UPPER: Is continuous with two layers of fascia: the deep fascia of the leg, and the strong fascia which extends between the superficial and deep muscles of the calf.

LOWER: Is continuous with the medial part of the plantar aponeurosis. The abductor hallucis takes origin from it.

LATERAL: Is attached to the tuberosity of the calcaneus.

MEDIAL: Is attached to the medial malleolus.

SURFACES:

SUPERFICIAL OR MEDIAL: Is related to the medial calcaneal vessels and nerves, which first pierce it and then cross it.

DEEP OR LATERAL: Is related to the tendons, vessels, and nerves passing from the back of the leg to the sole of the foot. They lie in a common compartment in the following order from before back: Tibialis posterior, flexor digitorum longus, posterior tibial artery with a vein each side, posterior tibial nerve, and flexor hallucis longus. Each tendon has a separate synovial sheath.

Under the lower part of the ligament the artery and nerve both divide into medial and lateral plantar branches.

Peroneal Retinacula: These are thickenings of the deep fascia (*Fig.* 291).

The *superior* runs from calcaneus to lateral malleolus and binds the two peronei, longus and brevis, to the back of the lateral malleolus in a common compartment.

The brevis is next to the bone.

The *inferior* is attached to the outer surface of the calcaneus. It is divided into two compartments by a septum which is attached to the peroneal tubercle.

The brevis is highest.

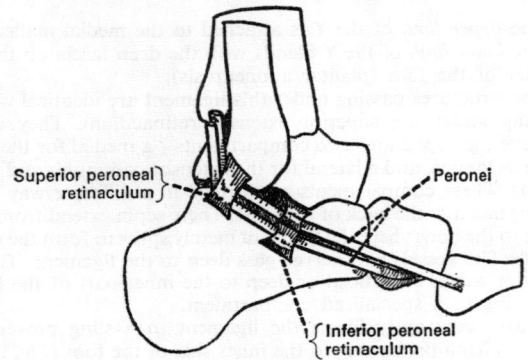

Fig. 291.—The peroneal retinacula.

III. LIGAMENTS AND ARCHES OF THE FOOT

The foot bones are held together by articular capsules (binding adjacent bones), interosseous ligaments, and accessory ligaments.

The *articular capsules* are for the most part weak and do not take a great part in supporting the arch of the foot.

The *interosseous ligaments* bind together the non-articular surfaces of the adjacent bones. They, like the former group, take but a small part in supporting the arches.

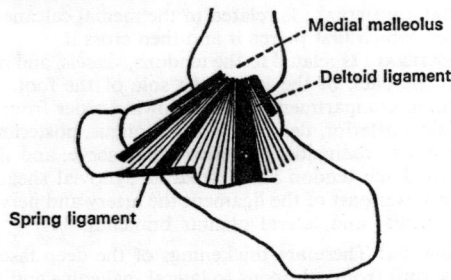

Fig. 292.—Deltoid ligament of ankle-joint and spring ligament.

Accessory Ligaments: These are amongst the most important structures which maintain the arches. They are: (1) The inferior or plantar calcaneonavicular or spring ligament; (2) The long plantar ligament; (3) The short plantar ligament, or plantar calcaneocuboid; (4) The transverse ligament of the heads of the metatarsal bones.

LIGAMENTS

THE PLANTAR CALCANEONAVICULAR OR SPRING LIGAMENT (*Fig.* 292) is a broad, thick, powerful structure. If any ligament can be called *the* most important in the foot, this best deserves the title.

Attachments and relations of the spring ligament:

POSTERIORLY: It is attached to the anterior border of the sustentaculum tali.

ANTERIORLY: It is attached to the plantar surface of the navicular.

INNER BORDER: The deltoid ligament of the ankle-joint is attached to its inner border.

UPPER SURFACE: The head of the talus rests on it and the bone has a flat facet on it made by contact with the ligament.

LOWER SURFACE: Is crossed by the tendon of the tibialis posterior, which supports the ligament.

The ligament is accessory to the joints between the talus, calcaneus, and navicular, and the capsules of the joints round the head of the talus are blended with the ligament. There is therefore a mass of ligamentous tissue around the inner side of the talocalcaneonavicular joint. In the condition of congenital talipes equinovarus this ligamentous tissue may be 2·5 cm. thick, and has been called the talonavicular capsule (Parker[1]). It is one of the most important obstacles to the reduction of the deformity (*Fig.* 293). Elmslie devised an operation for the removal of this

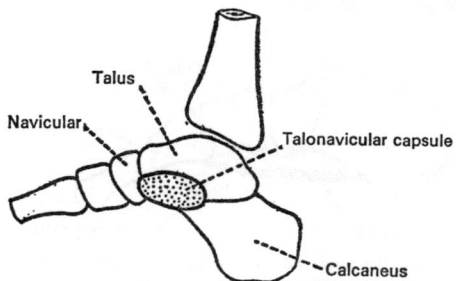

Fig. 293.—Talonavicular capsule (diagrammatic). The deltoid ligament is omitted for clearness.

ligamentous capsule in such circumstances. This ligament supports the keystone of the arch of the foot, the talus. For the arch to drop, as it does in flat-foot, the head of the talus descends, pushing this ligament before it and stretching it. Pain in this condition is

---

[1] Quoted by Jones and Lovett, *Orthopedic Surgery* 581. London.

felt over the ligament, i.e., immediately posterior to the tubercle of the navicular.

LONG PLANTAR LIGAMENT (*Fig.* 294): Is a powerful quadrilateral band which assists in maintaining the longitudinal arch of the foot. Its attachments and relations are:

POSTERIORLY: It is attached to the under-surface of the calcaneus in front of the tuberosity.

ANTERIORLY: It is attached to the ridge on the under-surface of the cuboid and to the bases of the second, third, and fourth metatarsal bones.

UNDER-SURFACE: Is covered by and gives origin to the quadratus plantae, the short flexor of the fifth toe, and the adductor of the great toe.

UPPER SURFACE: Crosses the calcaneocuboid joint and supports it. The short plantar ligament is between it and the joint. The peroneus longus is between it and the cuboid. With the cuboid the ligament forms a tunnel for the tendon.

SHORT PLANTAR LIGAMENT (*Fig.* 294): Binds the under-surfaces of calcaneus and cuboid, lying between these bones and the long plantar ligament.

TRANSVERSE METATARSAL LIGAMENT: Binds the five metatarsals together anteriorly on the plantar aspect, supporting a transverse arch formed by the bones. It prevents 'spreading' of the heads of the metatarsals.

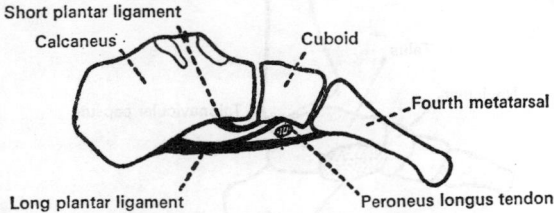

Fig. 294.—Showing the long and short plantar ligaments. and the peroneus longus tendon in the tunnel formed by groove on cuboid and long plantar ligament.

Arches of the Foot: The entire body-weight is supported by the foot. In bearing burdens or jumping from a height the extra strain is taken by the foot. To meet these requirements an elastic structure is supplied which is made up of a great number of little bones held together by ligaments, tendons, and muscles. There are longitudinal and transverse arches.

LONGITUDINAL ARCH: This consists of *inner* and *outer* portions resting on a common pillar posteriorly—the tuberosity of the calcaneus. The inner part of the longitudinal arch is formed by the talus, the navicular, the three cuneiform bones, and the inner three metatarsals and corresponding phalanges. The outer part of the longitudinal arch is formed by the calcaneus, the cuboid, and outer two metatarsals and corresponding phalanges.

The talus is the keystone of the arch. It receives the body-weight and transmits it to the arches below.

The outer part of the longitudinal arch is very low and almost rests on the ground. The inner part is high and only touches the ground behind (tuberosity of calcaneus) and in front (head of first metatarsal bone, i.e., ball of great toe).

The parts of the foot which normally bear the body-weight and transmit it to the ground are therefore the tuberosity of calcaneus, the head of the first metatarsal, and the head of the fifth metatarsal.

The inner border of the foot is normally straight or concave inwards when weight is being borne. When the arch collapses, as it does in flat-foot, this concavity becomes a convexity because the head of the talus projects down into it.

TRANSVERSE ARCHES: The metatarsal and tarsal bones are arranged with a convex curve on the dorsum and a concave one on their plantar aspects. There is therefore normally a series of transverse arches extending from the arch formed by the heads of the metatarsals back to the arch formed by the navicular and the cuboid. In flat-foot the arch drops and becomes flattened out. From the patient's point of view the dropping of the arch formed by the heads of the metatarsals is the most important fact, as the digital vessels and nerves are normally protected by the arch formed by the heads and when it is obliterated the nerves are pressed upon, which results in much pain. This is called *Morton's disease*, or *metatarsalgia*. Sir Robert Jones has shown that the nerve mainly pressed on is the communicating twig between the digital nerve in the third space (medial plantar) and that in the fourth space (lateral plantar). The pressure is caused by the head of the fourth metatarsal bone, and pain is therefore most marked beneath it. If the weight is taken off the heads of the bones by a football bar on the sole of the boot behind the heads, the pain disappears.

SUPPORTS OF THE ARCHES OF THE FOOT: These are: (1) Tendons; (2) Muscles and fascia; (3) Ligaments; (4) Bones.

1. TENDONS: Two powerful tendons form most important 'slings' for the support of the arch; they are the tendons of the peroneus longus and tibialis posterior.

   a. Peroneus Longus: Passes down the outer side of the leg and across the outer side of the foot, turns at right angles on itself, and runs across the sole from lateral to medial, lying in a tunnel formed by the cuboid and the long plantar ligament

294   A SYNOPSIS OF SURGICAL ANATOMY

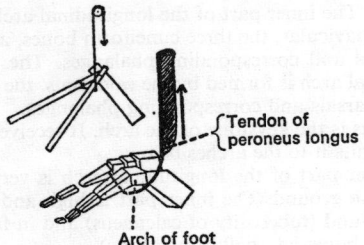

Fig. 295.—To show that the action of the peroneus longus tendon is like that of a pulley holding up the arch of the foot.

(*Fig. 295*). It is inserted into the outer side of the first cuneiform and base of the first metatarsal.

It 'slings' up the longitudinal arch of the foot exactly at its middle.

  b. *Tibialis Posterior:* This muscle has a very similar function to that of the peroneus longus, and balances it on the inner side. The tendon has its main insertion about the middle of the

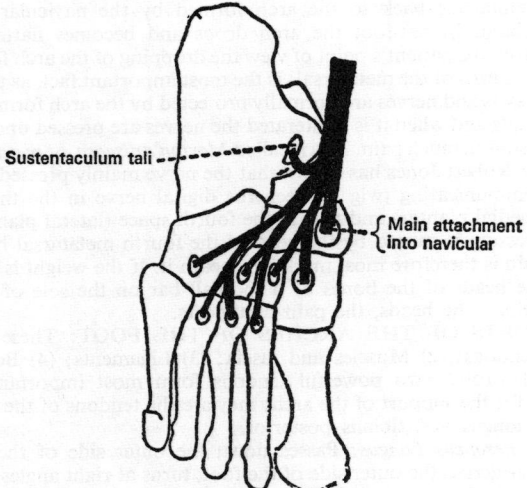

Fig. 296.—Showing attachments of tendon of tibialis posterior.

longitudinal arch to the under-surface of the navicular (*Fig. 296*). It lends additional support to the arch by giving a tendinous slip of insertion to every bone of the tarsus (except the talus), and also to the bases of the second, third, and fourth metatarsal bones.

2. MUSCLES AND FASCIA:

a. Long Muscles: Long flexors of the toes retain to some extent the concavity of the arch.

b. Short Muscles: The intrinsic muscles of the sole of the foot pass mostly in the direction of the longitudinal arch and tend to hold the extremities of the arch together. Muscles, and particularly short muscles, are much better able to withstand strain than inert ligaments—witness the breaking up of the rectus abdominis into short muscles by the tendinous inscriptions, which enable that muscle better to withstand intra-abdominal pressure.[1] So powerful are these short muscles as maintainers of the arch of the foot that they may increase the arch to such a degree as to constitute a deformity, as in the condition of *pes cavus*.

The transverse arch is maintained by the transverse head of the adductor hallucis and to a less extent by its oblique head.

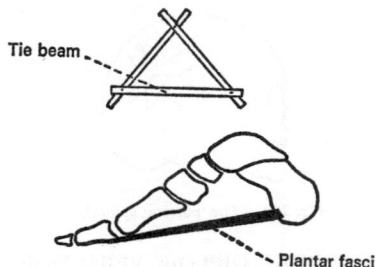

Fig. 297.—Showing that the plantar fascia acts as the 'tie beam' of an arch.

c. Fascia: The intermediate process of the plantar aponeurosis is attached to the extremities of the arch, i.e., the posterior part of the calcaneus behind and the heads of all the metatarsals and the proximal phalanges in front. It acts exactly as the 'tie beam' of a gable, holding the extremities of the arch together (*Fig. 297*).

---

[1] The subluxation of the hip- or knee-joint which so often accompanies the deformities resulting from untreated infantile paralysis is an excellent example of the inability of ligaments to withstand strain.

3. LIGAMENTS: These have been described. It is evidence of the great economy of effort shown in the construction of the body that the ligaments of the dorsum of the foot are relatively weak. On the sole are collected great powerful bands, as here is need for strength to hold the component bones of the arch together.
4. BONES: These are so shaped as to lend some strength to the arch.

Chapter XXVI

VEINS

Diploic Veins: Four trunks on each side drain the diploic plexus, which lies between the inner and outer tables of the skull.
   FRONTAL DIPLOIC VEIN: Drains into the supra-orbital vein by a twig which emerges through a foramen which may be seen in the wall of the supra-orbital notch or foramen.
   ANTERIOR TEMPORAL DIPLOIC VEIN: Drains into the spheno-parietal sinus.

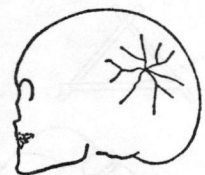

Fig. 298.—The 'parietal spider'.

   POSTERIOR TEMPORAL DIPLOIC VEIN: Drains into the lateral sinus.
   OCCIPITAL DIPLOIC VEIN: Drains into the lateral sinus.
   The bony channels for the diploic veins may be seen in radiographs of the skull and may easily be mistaken for fractures of the bone. In the parietal region they may often be seen distinctly, giving an appearance which has been called the 'parietal spider' (*Fig.* 298).
Emissary Veins: Connect the veins inside the skull with those of the head, neck, or face.
1. VEIN OF THE FORAMEN CAECUM: Connects the commencement of the superior sagittal or longitudinal sinus with the veins of the frontal sinus and root of the nose.

2. **OPHTHALMIC VEINS:** May be looked upon as large emissary veins connecting the supra-orbital and frontal veins of the forehead with the cavernous sinus of the skull.
3. **PARIETAL EMISSARY VEIN:** Connects the veins of the scalp with the superior sagittal sinus.
4. **MASTOID VEIN:** Connects the posterior auricular vein with the transverse sinus. It is a very constant and very important emissary vein.
5. **VEINS OF THE HYPOGLOSSAL CANAL:** Small veins connect the transverse sinus with the deep veins of the neck through the hypoglossal canal.
6. **VEINS OF THE CONDYLOID CANAL:** Small veins connect the transverse sinus with the deep veins of the neck through the condyloid canal.
7. **VEINS OF THE FORAMEN LACERUM:** Connect the cavernous sinus with the pterygoid plexus.
8. **VEINS OF THE FORAMEN OVALE:** Connect the cavernous sinus with the pterygoid plexus.
9. **VEINS OF THE FORAMEN VESALII:** Connect the cavernous sinus with the pterygoid and pharyngeal plexuses.
10. **MIDDLE MENINGEAL VEINS OR SINUSES:** Run with the artery of that name. They may end in the sinuses of the skull or in the pterygoid plexus, being then emissary veins.

Emissary veins are of profound surgical importance, as infection may spread along them into the skull, or out of it. Relatively trifling infected scalp wounds may thus cause death. Though we are convinced that such an occurrence is an unusual surgical event, it is none the less conducive to care in the handling of scalp wounds to recollect that 'if it were not for emissary veins, wounds of the scalp would lose half their significance'.

Blood Sinuses of Cranium: These venous channels lie between the two layers of the dura or between a re-duplication of the inner layer. They receive the venous blood from the brain and drain ultimately into the two internal jugular veins. There are some important matters of applied anatomy in relation to these venous channels:

1. Sinus bleeding is usually consequent on fracture of the skull. This occurrence is infrequent as the channels do not lie in bony grooves with the exception of the lower part of the lateral sinus (sigmoid sinus).
2. Pressure in the sinus is low but is readily raised by coughing, struggling, etc. As the walls of the sinuses are too rigid to collapse, copious bleeding follows wounds of these channels. Traumatic transection of large sinuses may well be fatal.
3. The superior sagittal (longitudinal) sinus is of such outstanding surgical significance that it is dealt with more fully.

ANATOMY: It begins at the crista galli in the midline in the anterior fossa of the skull by the union of small meningeal veins. Here it communicates with the veins of the nose or frontal sinus by emissary veins traversing the foramen caecum. It passes back over the convexity of the brain lying along the attached border of the falx major, and at the level of the inion (external occipital protuberance) or torcular Herophili it turns to one or other side (usually the right) to form the lateral sinus.

TRIBUTARIES: It receives veins from the medial surface of the hemispheres and from the upper halves of their convex lateral surfaces. These veins enter the sinus in the opposite direction to that of the blood-flow in the sinus. The veins from the lower part of the outer surface of the hemispheres drain into the Sylvian system. There is an adequate anastomosis between these two areas of venous drainage.

SUBDURAL HAEMATOMA: The veins entering the sinus must pass through the subdural space. Here they are least protected and may be torn as the result of trauma often of a relatively minor nature. This results in the formation of a subdural haematoma.

Injury to the Superior Sagittal Sinus: Barker[1] draws attenion to the work of Gordon Holmes and Sargent during the first world war. These workers described a characteristic syndrome following injury to the sinus. It has the following features:

1. The head injury may be of a relatively minor nature. Thus there may be no fracture and no loss of consciousness.
2. The outstanding pathological feature is that the related cortical veins are swollen and cannot be emptied by pressure.
3. The clinical syndrome is one of spastic paresis affecting one or more limbs and associated with sensory loss of cortical type in the same area. Unlike the spasticity usually seen in head injury the onset of which is delayed by shock, in the cases here described the spasticity is of immediate onset.
4. The explanation given for the syndrome is that the injury is in the region of the superior longitudinal sinus and that some degree of thrombosis affects it owing to deficient venous drainage. This gives rise to oedema of the part of the cortex related resulting in pathological changes in the cortical nerve tissue.

Anterior Facial Vein: Begins at the side of the root of the nose by the union of the supra-orbital and frontal veins. It passes down, lying more superficial than the external maxillary artery and posterior to it and pursues a less tortuous course. It crosses the masseter and ramus of the jaw, crosses the inferolateral surface of the submaxillary gland, and is joined by the posterior facial in the neck to form the common facial.

---

[1] Barker, G. B., *Br. med. J.*, 1949, June 25, 1113.

Having pierced the deep fascia, the common facial crosses the interna and external carotid arteries and ends in the internal jugular. Rarely it crosses the sternomastoid and ends in the external jugular. In the angle of union of this vein with the internal jugular is situated the main lymph-gland of the tonsil—the tonsillar or jugulodigastric gland.

CONNEXIONS OF THE ANTERIOR FACIAL VEIN:
1. It communicates with the cavernous sinus of the skull through the ophthalmic veins.
2. It communicates with the cavernous sinus of the skull through the deep facial vein which connects the pterygoid plexus with the anterior facial vein by dipping down between the buccinator and masseter. The pterygoid plexus in turn communicates with the cavernous sinus by several emissary veins (*Fig.* 299).

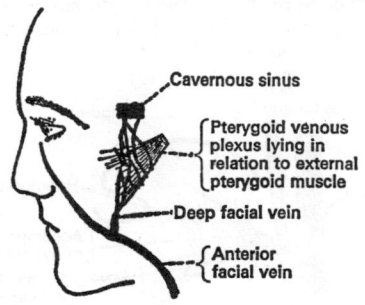

Fig. 299.—Showing the communication between the anterior facial vein and the cavernous sinus inside the skull.

ANATOMICAL POINTS OF SURGICAL MOMENT:
1. The vein has no valves.
2. It lies amongst muscles which by contraction may displace clot in the vein.
3. It drains the 'dangerous area' of the face, i.e., upper lip, septum of nose, and adjacent area (*Fig.* 300).
4. There is no deep fascia here to act as a barrier to the spread of inflammation, and the infective process has ready access to the muscles.

The 'dangerous area' of the face is so named because boils or infections of the face which so commonly occur here deserve the greatest respect from the surgeon. Infection in this region may spread along these venous connexions to the cavernous sinus in the skull and this may have serious consequences.

300 A SYNOPSIS OF SURGICAL ANATOMY

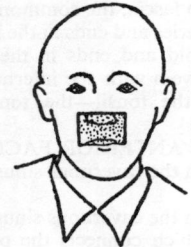

Fig. 300.—Shaded part is 'dangerous area' of face.

Veins of the Tongue: The tongue is drained on each side by four veins all of which pass back in relation to the hyoglossus muscle (*Fig.* 301):
   1. The ranine vein, or the chief vein of the tongue, crosses the anterior surface of the hyoglossus obliquely.

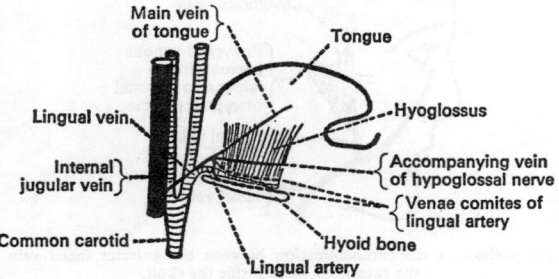

Fig. 301.—Veins draining the tongue.

   2. The vena comes nervi hypoglossi runs with this nerve on the outer surface of the hyoglossus.
   3. The venae comites of the lingual artery—two small veins accompany this artery on the deep surface of the hyoglossus.
   LINGUAL VEIN: Is formed by the fusion of these four radicles at the posterior border of the hyoglossus. The lingual vein then crosses the loop of the lingual artery and both carotids and ends in the internal jugular; sometimes it ends in the common facial.
Jugular Venous System: The following are the jugular veins: (1) Internal; (2) External; (3) Anterior; (4) Oblique; (5) Posterior external.
   INTERNAL JUGULAR VEIN (*Fig.* 302):
   EXTENT: It commences 1·2 cm. below the base of the skull by the union of the transverse sinus with the inferior petrosal sinus.

It ends behind the sternal end of the clavicle by joining the subclavian to form the innominate. It lies lateral to the internal carotid artery above and to the common carotid below. Its relations are therefore similar to those of these vessels. The deep cervical glands are in close relation to the vein. At their lower ends

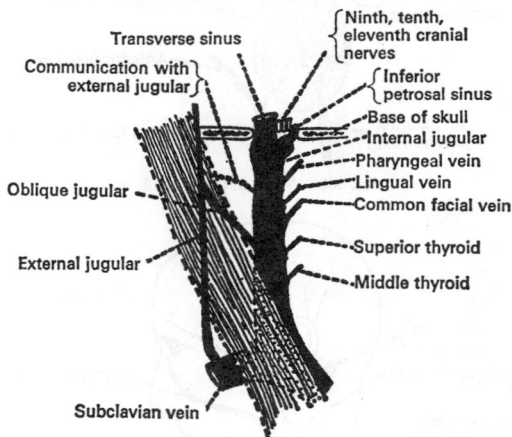

Fig. 302.—Right internal jugular vein.

both internal jugulars trend to the right, so that the right comes to lie farther from the right common carotid while the left vein tends to overlap the left common carotid artery.

TRIBUTARIES: The pharyngeal veins, common facial, and lingual join it in the region of the angle of the jaw. Below these it receives the superior and middle thyroid veins.

EXTERNAL JUGULAR VEIN: The posterior facial vein assists in the formation of two vessels—external jugular and common facial (*Fig.* 303). At its lower end, while in the parotid, the posterior facial divides into anterior and posterior branches. The posterior branch joins the posterior auricular vein to form the external jugular. The anterior branch of the posterior facial joins the anterior facial to form the common facial.

The external jugular vein runs from the angle of the jaw to a point 1·2 cm. above the middle of the clavicle, where it joins the subclavian vein after piercing the fascia forming the roof of the posterior triangle (*Fig.* 304).

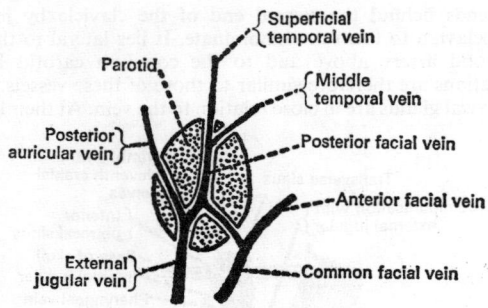

Fig. 303.—Veins in the parotid.

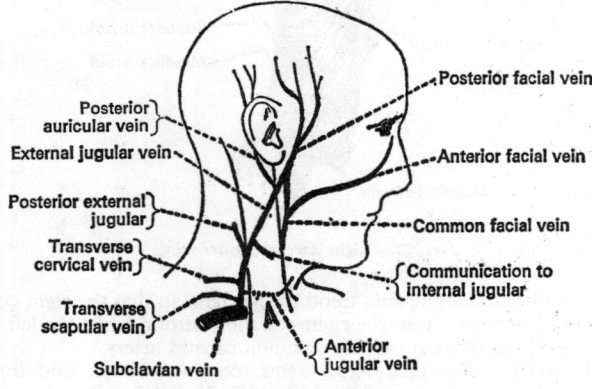

Fig. 304.—External jugular vein.

TRIBUTARIES: Posterior external jugular, anterior jugular, transverse scapular, transverse cervical. The common facial may end in it.

ANTERIOR JUGULAR VEIN: A superficial vein commencing in the submental region, running down on one side of the middle line to just above the sternum, where it communicates with its fellow in the suprasternal space and then turns outward at a right angle to end in the posterior triangle by joining the external jugular. In the transverse part of its course it is sandwiched between the sternomastoid superficially and the depressor muscles of the hyoid bone deeply (*Fig. 305*). It receives small unnamed vessels from the skin and subcutaneous tissues.

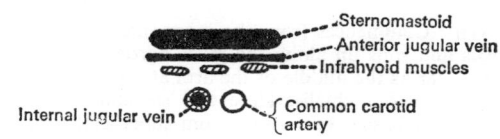

Fig. 305.—Showing position occupied by anterior jugular vein (on right side) in its transverse course.

POSTERIOR EXTERNAL JUGULAR VEIN: An unimportant vessel which commences in the subcutaneous fat of the suboccipital region and crosses the posterior triangle to end in the external jugular about its middle.

OBLIQUE JUGULAR VEIN: The external jugular and internal jugular communicate usually by a small vessel which crosses the sternomastoid. Occasionally a large vein replaces this communication. It crosses the middle third of the sternomastoid obliquely from above downwards and inwards and connects the external jugular with the internal or with the common facial. It will be divided in incisions along the anterior border of the sternomastoid.

Veins of the Upper Limb: These are superficial and deep.

SUPERFICIAL VEINS: Two vessels—cephalic and basilic—are important. They commence in the wrist region by draining the dorsal venous arch at the back of the hand.

CEPHALIC VEIN: Runs up on the outer side of the forearm and arm. In the arm its position is very constant, first along the outer border of the biceps, then in the groove between the deltoid and pectoralis major where it pierces the deep fascia. In the deltopectoral triangle it dips deeply, pierces the costocoracoid membrane, and ends in the axillary vein.

It drains the superficial tissues on the outer side of the shoulder, arm, forearm, and hand. It is the most important venous channel for the return of blood from the upper limb in those cases where the axillary vein has been tied or removed, e.g., some cases of cancer of the breast, and as such the surgeon is careful to preserve it. When the exigencies of the case so require, both the axillary and the cephalic veins may be sacrificed with no ill effects.

The lymphatics from the thumb and forefinger run with it in its whole course.

It may communicate with the external jugular in the posterior triangle by a vessel which crosses the clavicle, and which is in danger of laceration in fractures of the clavicle. This occasional vessel is the remains of a very constant and important connexion in the fetus.

BASILIC VEIN: Commences from the inner side of the dorsal venous plexus and runs up along the inner border of the forearm and arm, as far as the middle of the arm at the level of the insertion of the coracobrachialis. Here two structures pierce the deep fascia: The basilic vein going from superficial to deep and the medial cutaneous nerve of the forearm going from deep to superficial. Having pierced the deep fascia the basilic becomes a vena comes of the brachial artery which already has two accompanying veins. These three vessels join at the lower border of the pectoralis minor to form the axillary vein. The vein is thus shorter than the artery.

COMMUNICATIONS BETWEEN CEPHALIC AND BASILIC VEINS: These take one of two forms (*Fig.* 306): (1) A single vein—the median

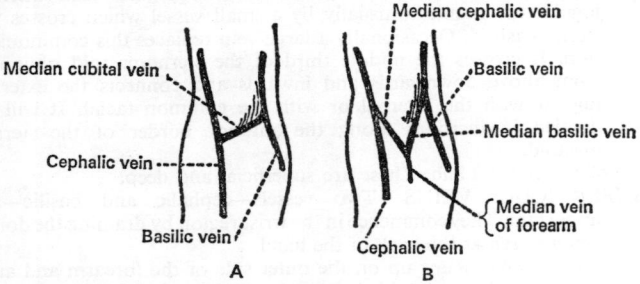

Fig. 306.—Veins at bend of elbow. A, Arranged H Fashion. B, Arranged M fashion.

cubital—crossing the bend of the elbow to connect the two vessels—forming with them the letter H; (2) A more complicated communication forming the letter M. A vessel, called the median vein of the forearm, may exist in the upper half of the forearm lying between the basilic and the cephalic. This bifurcates into two vessels, one going to the basilic called the median basilic, the other to the cephalic called the median cephalic. Where the median vein divides a channel, the profunda (or deep median) vein, joins it, which comes from the deeper structures of the forearm.

The median cephalic and median basilic veins are used for obtaining blood and for giving intravenous injections. The median basilic has important relations.

Deep to it is that accession to the deep fascia given off by the biceps tendon called the lacertus fibrosus. The lacertus separates the vein from the brachial artery and median nerve. The vein *crosses* or *is crossed* by the anterior branch of the medial cutaneous nerve of the forearm, and the nerve may be damaged by the needle or by irritating fluids which enter the subcutaneous tissue instead of the vein, e.g., arsenic. This may produce so much irritation of the nerve as to cause a reflex spasm of the biceps and brachialis, resulting in acute flexion of the forearm which may persist for a long time.

DEEP VEINS: The deep veins of the forearm are venae comites of the arteries.

AXILLARY VEIN: The part of this vein lying in front of the first part of the axillary artery has two important anatomical features: (1) It has a valve here; (2) It is closely related to the subclavius muscle, which touches it—when the arm is above the head the muscle may actually groove the vein.

The importance of these two facts: Cases are sometimes seen where the arm is very swollen and painful owing to thrombosis or clotting of the blood in the axillary vein. This is the condition of thrombosis of the axillary vein—effort thrombosis (*Fig.* 307). In such cases it may be found that the patient has been working

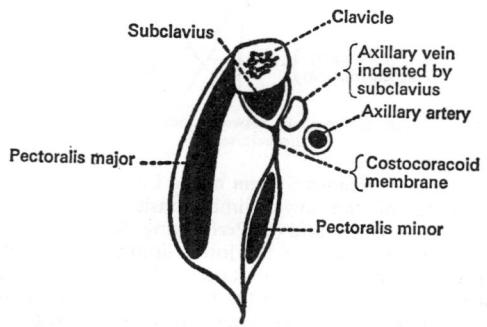

Fig. 307.—Way in which subclavius muscle indents axillary vein in full abduction of arm. This is one of the factors in primary thrombosis of this vein.

with the affected arm raised above his head, as in hanging pictures (strap-hanger's oedema). It is thought that damage is done to the valve in the vein which is injuriously pressed upon by the subclavius muscle. This causes the clotting, which is called primary thrombosis of the axillary vein to distinguish it from the clotting due to disease processes.

This condition is more common in males than in females. It occurs in the third and fourth decades and favours the right side.

Thoraco-epigastric Vein: A vessel which connects the vein of the upper anterior abdominal wall, the superficial epigastric, with the lateral thoracic vein of the axilla (*Fig.* 308). It also communicates with the superficial circumflex iliac and superficial inferior epigastric veins of the lower abdominal wall. It is an important channel for the return of blood to the heart via the superior vena cava in those cases where the inferior vena cava is obliterated (*Fig.* 320). If, however, the superior vena cava is occluded, the blood from the upper limb and head and neck is returned to the heart by the inferior vena cava and traverses this channel (thoraco-epigastric) amongst others. Its valves direct the blood upward above, and downward below (Stiles). These valves may become incompetent when the vessel is enlarged, as in obstruction to the portal vein, or inferior vena cava. The thoraco-epigastric vein communicates with the portal vein through a vein in the round ligament.

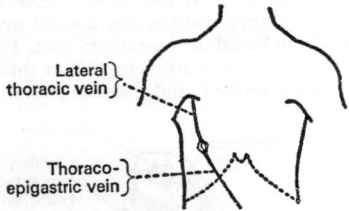

Fig. 308.—Showing anastomosis between thoraco-epigastric and lateral thoracic veins.

Venous System of the Leg[1]

The veins of the lower limb consist of three groups: (1) Superficial, (2) Deep, and (3) Perforating. (*Fig.* 309.)

1. THE SUPERFICIAL VEINS of the lower limb are the long and short saphenous and their tributaries. They have certain special characteristics. They lie in the fat between the skin and the deep fascia, being closer to the latter. The middle coat of these vessels is much thicker than that of other veins, consisting mostly of smooth muscle with some fibrous and elastic tissue.

The Long Saphenous Vein is the longest vein in the body. It commences from the inner part of the dorsal venous arch of the foot, passes in front of medial malleolus straight up to the postero-medial aspect of the knee-joint, and then up to the fossa ovalis or saphenous opening (3·8 cm. below and lateral to pubic tubercle) where it enters the femoral. In palpating this vein in

---

[1] Dodd, H., and Cockett, F. B., *The Pathology and Surgery of the Veins of the Lower Limb*, 1956. Edinburgh and London: Livingstone.

VEINS 307

relation to the knee it is to be found just posterior to the transverse axis of the joint. The saphenous nerve accompanies the vein in the leg. The vein has many tributaries and to be noted particularly are:

a. The posterior arch vein is a large constant vessel which arises from a series of small venous arches connecting the medial ankle perforating veins. These venous arcades receive the delicate venules which drain the skin of the ankle and heel.

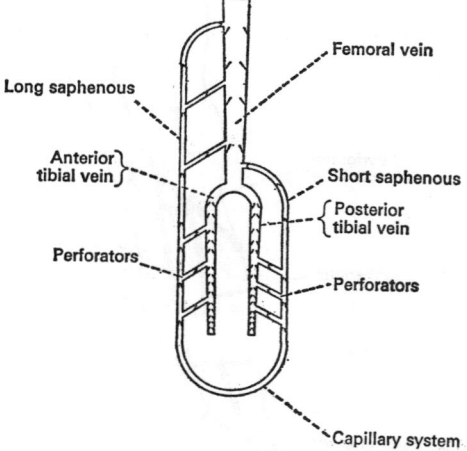

Fig. 309.—Plan of the venous system of the leg. (*By courtesy of Mr. Allen, Department of Anatomy, Medical School, Johannesburg, who drew the figure.*)

It is these small vessels which become dilated in venous incompetence and give rise to the haemangiomatous appearance which obliterates the hollow behind the malleolus and is called the ankle flare. This vessel runs up on the medial aspect of the leg to join the long saphenous below the knee (*Fig.* 310). An anterior vein runs up the front of the leg from the ankle region to join the long saphenous below the knee.

b. The small saphenous vein sends a tributary to it from its upper part. Not infrequently the small saphenous vein itself may end in the long saphenous.

c. The posteromedial and anterolateral veins are large vessels in the thigh which join the saphenous in the upper part of its course (*Fig.* 311). The former is formed by several tributaries from the popliteal area, one of which comes

308 A SYNOPSIS OF SURGICAL ANATOMY

from the short saphenous just before its termination; in fact the short saphenous itself may end in the postero-medial vein. This is an important collateral channel in cases of deep femoral thrombosis. The anterolateral vein runs diagonally from the outer aspect of the knee to join the long saphenous near the fossa ovalis. It lies much nearer the skin than the saphenous vein and may be visible when enlarged. The accessory saphenous vein is an occasional large trunk

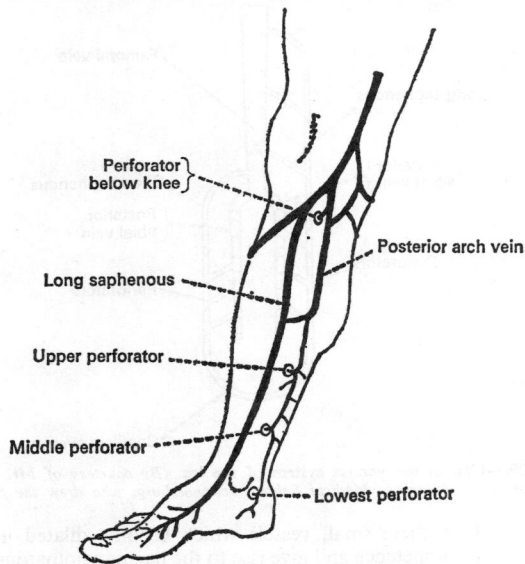

Fig. 310.—The posterior arch vein. (*By courtesy of Dodd and Cockett.*)

which drains skin and fat of upper and inner thigh and enters the long saphenous in its upper part. When present and varicose it may be so large as to require individual surgical attention such as ligature or avulsion.

d. The superficial veins (external pudendal, inferior epigastric, and circumflex iliac) enter the saphenous in a variable manner at the fossa ovalis. In the Trendelenburg or high ligature operation for varicose veins, these apparently insignificant vessels must be ligatured and divided, otherwise varicosity will soon return (*Fig.* 312).

VEINS 309

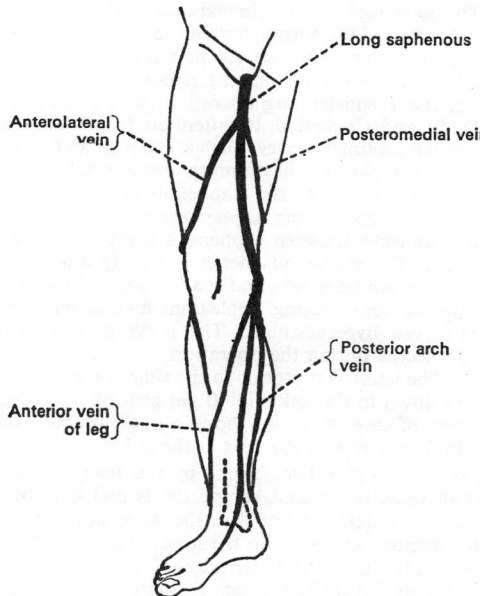

Fig. 311.—The long saphenous vein and its tributaries. (*By courtesy of Dodd and Cockett.*)

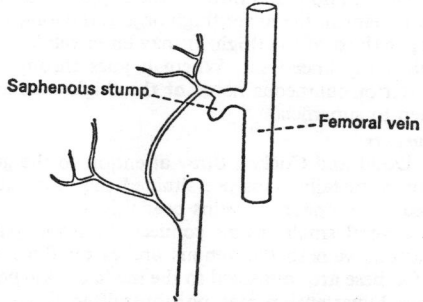

Fig. 312.—Showing how a carelessly performed Trendelenburg operation will not prevent return of varicosity.

 e. The long saphenous vein may enter the femoral 2·5 cm. or more distal to its usual termination. The tributaries it usually receives may go direct to the femoral. This may be a trap for the unwary so that the femoral vein is ligated in error in the Trendelenburg operation (Bevan et al.[1]).

 f. Dodd and Cockett draw attention to an anomalous origin of the profunda artery. Such a vessel arises from the femoral in the region of the foramen ovale, and runs down either above or below the saphenofemoral junction in close relationship to the saphenous termination.

 g. Relationship between saphenous nerve and long saphenous vein: The saphenous nerve is closely associated with the long saphenous vein and may be injured during operations on the vein causing unpleasant anaestheia, hypoaesthesia, or even hyperaesthesia. The nerve must be exposed and protected during the operation.

 The nerve is posterior to the vein at the knee and remains so down to the ankle in 40 per cent of cases, but in 60 per cent of cases it crosses the vein at a variable level in the leg to lie anterior to the vein at the ankle.

The Short Saphenous Vein begins by the fusion of a number of small veins below and behind the lateral malleolus, where it comes into relationship with the large sural nerve which lies just lateral to the vein in the lower third of the leg. The vein then runs along the outer edge of the Achilles tendon, then passes to the midline where it continues until the middle of the popliteal space, where it dips sharply to enter the popliteal vein in most cases.

There are several less usual terminations to the vessel. It may run non-stop through the popliteal space and end in the deep veins in the lower thigh or join the long saphenous in the upper third of the thigh. It may enter the long saphenous just below the knee-joint. Where it goes through the fascia, the posterior cutaneous nerve of the thigh emerges passing from deep to superficial.

Comments:

 a. Dodd and Cockett draw attention to the general rule that the more distally veins are situated the more liberally are they valved. The saphenous veins bear this out.

 b. Several small vessels connect the lower part of the small saphenous vein to the venous arches on the inner side of the leg. As these are connected to the medial ankle perforating veins, venous hypertension may be transmitted to or from the small

---

[1] Bevan, P. G., Green, S. H., and Stammers. F. A. R., *Br. med. J.*, 1956, 1, 610.

saphenous vein depending on which of the systems is incompetent. The upper part of the short saphenous vein communicates with the long saphenous via the posteromedial vein of the thigh. This is also a possible route for the transmission of venous hypertension from one saphenous to the other.

   c. Dodd[1] draws attention to the association of varicosity of the short saphenous vein with varicosity of other tributaries of the popliteal vein, especially the large vessels which drain the two heads of the gastrocnemius muscle. After removal of the varicosities of the short saphenous vein, varicosities of popliteal tributaries may persist. These he calls pseudo-short saphenous veins as they mimic varicosities of the short saphenous itself. He advises generous exposure in dealing with the upper end of the short saphenous vein because of the facts just mentioned, and also because of the vagaries associated with the terminations of this vessel.

   d. Vulval varicose veins in pregnancy: Dodd and Payling Wright[2] comment on the frequency of this condition (23·3 per cent). Most of these cases have incompetent long saphenous veins. The condition is distressing. The sources of such varicosities are:
   i. The long saphenous vein when its tributaries, superficial and deep external pudendal veins, are incompetent.
   ii. Some veins from the labia majora pass with the round ligament through the inguinal canal. They may become varicose and cause a hernia-like swelling in the groin and may also cause a considerable swelling of the labium majus.
   iii. Tributaries of the internal pudendal vein, when enlarged, cause swelling of the perineum and posterior part of the labia. These conditions occur in the latter part of pregnancy and may be sufficiently severe to require operation.

   e. In 90 per cent of cases the short saphenous vein perforates the investing fascia of the leg a variable distance below the popliteal fossa and runs a subfascial course to the popliteal fossa. If in such cases the vein is merely ligated in its subcutaneous position recurrent varicosities will occur because the incompetent upper segment will be left intact. Exploration of the popliteal space will avoid this error.[3]

   f. Relationship between the sural nerve and the short saphenous vein: The sural nerve is usually lateral to the short saphenous vein but in about 20 per cent of cases it is medial to the vein. The nerve often crosses from one side of the vein to the other.

---
[1] Dodd, H., *Br. J. Surg.*, 1959, 46, 520.
[2] Dodd, H., and Payling Wright, H., *Br. med. J.*, 1959, 1, 831.
[3] Moosman, D. A., and Hartwell, S. W., *Surgery Gynec. Obstet.*, 1964, 118, 761.

312 A SYNOPSIS OF SURGICAL ANATOMY

2. THE DEEP VEINS lie amongst and are supported by powerful muscles. These veins are the tibial, peroneal, popliteal, and femoral and their tributaries.

The veins draining the muscles are valved with the notable exception of those in the soleus, the most powerful of the calf muscles. Its veins are of the nature of venous sinuses. They are unvalved and empty segmentally into the posterior tibial and peroneal veins. Some of the perforating veins enter the posterior tibial exactly opposite the entrance of the soleal veins into this vessel (*Fig.* 313).

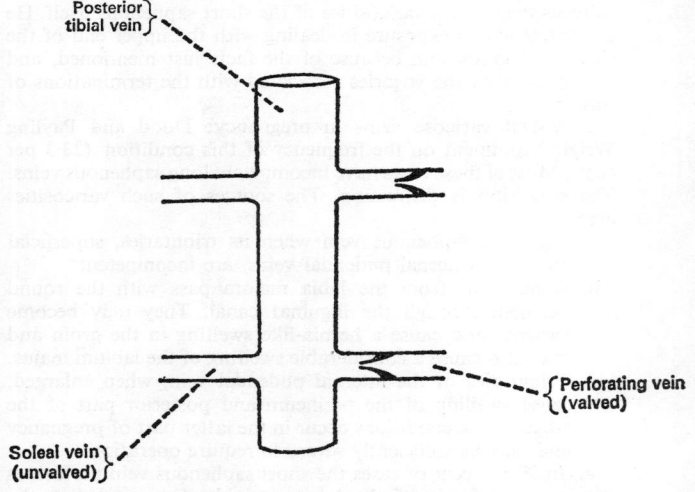

Fig. 313.—The diagram shows soleal and perforating veins entering the posterior tibial vein exactly opposite each other.

Comment:

a. When the calf muscles are at rest, the soleal venous sinuses may be likened to quiet backwaters where blood moves but sluggishly. These are ideal situations for the formation of clots when suitable conditions exist. Most pulmonary emboli begin in this way.

b. Phlebitis, due to inflammation or other cause, commencing in soleal sinuses may extend not only into the posterior tibial vein, but also into the perforating veins and destroy the valves guarding their entrance into the main vessels. The stage is set for the development of venous hypertension and all its dire consequences.

   c. There are no valves in the inferior vena cava and the common iliac veins. In about 80 per cent of people there is a valve in the external iliac vein which protects the saphenofemoral junction against high pressure. The remaining 20 per cent of people with congenital absence of this valve in the external iliac vein, are prone to hypertension in the upper saphenous system and resultant varicose veins commencing at the saphenofemoral junction and proceeding down the vein.[1] This accounts for some cases of varicose veins particularly in young people with a family history of varicose veins.

3. PERFORATING VEINS: These are communicating vessels between the superficial and deep veins.

   Blood is returned to the heart by the *vis-a-tergo* of the circulation and the negative pressure in the thorax. In the lower limbs an additional factor is the calf pump. The muscles of the calf are surrounded by the dense unyielding deep fascia. Every contraction of these powerful muscles, therefore, pumps blood into the deep veins. The blood from the tissues superficial to the deep fascia enters the deep veins through the perforating veins which penetrate this fascia. These are valved near their origin and at their entrance to the deep veins, the latter also being liberally supplied with valves so arranged as to allow for inward flow and for the prevention of reflux.

   When the limb is in action the venous pressure in the deep veins is high and fluctuant; that in the superficial veins falls very low as they are emptied into the calf pump. Should the efficiency of the valve system break down then blood will flow in the reverse direction and venous hypertension occurs. The more distal the breakdown, the greater is the back pressure and the greater the hypertension. This is the genesis of varicose veins and ulceration. Perforating veins are classified as:

a. Indirect: These consist of small superficial vessels which penetrate the deep fascia to connect with a vessel in a muscle, which in turn is connected to one of the deep veins. It is significant that in the ankle region there is little muscle and therefore few indirect perforators, and therefore the return of blood from the superficial tissues is dependent on the direct perforators. Cockett[2] considers this to be one of the most significant factors in the pathology of ankle ulceration.

b. Direct: (i) Long and short saphenous veins. (ii) Smaller perforating veins (*Fig.* 314).

---

[1] Reagan, B., and Folse, R., *Surgery Gynec. Obstet.*, 1971, 132, 15.
[2] Cockett, F. B., *British Surgical Practice, Surgical Progress*, 1958, 13.

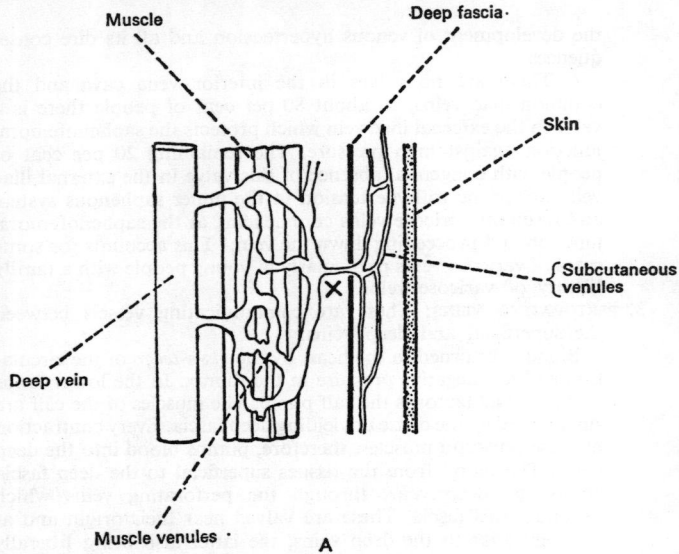
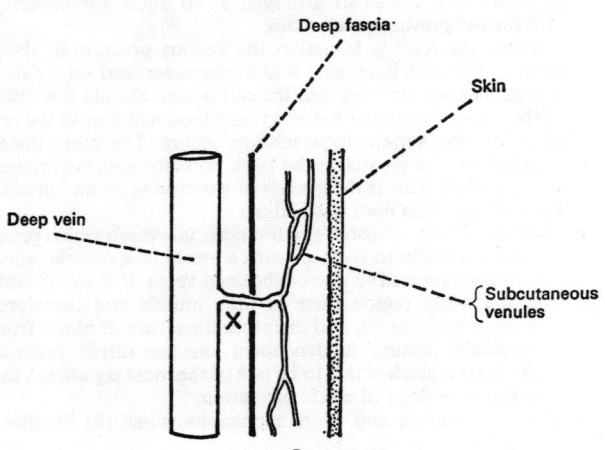

Fig. 314.—A, Diagram of an indirect perforating vein (X). B, Diagram of a direct perforating vein (X).

The long and short saphenous veins are communicating veins between the superficial and deep venous systems of the leg. They are so valved as to prevent flow from deep to superficial systems. When guarding valves become defective venous hypertension becomes evident as varicose veins.

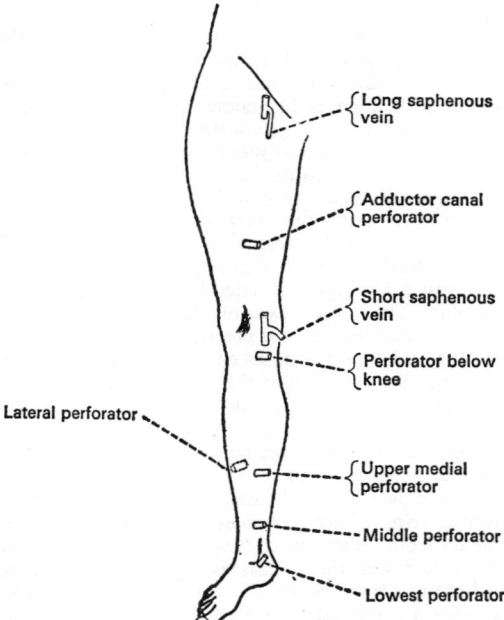

Fig. 315.—The chief perforating veins of the lower limb.

The smaller perforating vessels (i.e., direct) are fairly constantly situated and are of great surgical significance. They do not for the most part connect the saphenous vessels directly to the deep veins. They commence from tributaries of the saphenous vessels and perforate the deep fascia to join the deep veins, being valved at each end, and being accompanied as a rule by a small artery. Dodd and Cockett[1] define them as follows:

[1] Dodd, H., and Cockett, F. B., *The Pathology and Surgery of the Veins of the Lower Limb* 1956. Edinburgh and London: Livingstone.

1. In the thigh: A long constant communicating vein between long saphenous or a tributary in the lower half of the thigh and the femoral vein in Hunter's canal.
2. In the leg:
    a. A communicating vein just distal to the knee connecting the long saphenous or posterior arch vein to the posterior tibial vein.
    b. The ankle perforating veins—(i) internal, (ii) external—are in the lower half of the leg (*Fig.* 315).

There are three internal ankle perforating veins. They connect with a series of venous arcades which characterize the lower part of the large constant posterior arch vein which enters the long saphenous just below the knee. The upper one of the three is found at the junction of middle and lower third of the leg at the posterior medial border of the tibia. It constantly communicates with the long saphenous vein by a small tributary. The middle perforator is about 10 cm. above the tip of the medial malleolus and just behind the tibial margin. The lowest perforator is situated behind and below the medial malleolus. The upper two of these perforators enter the posterior tibial vein at the precise level that one of the (unvalved) soleal venous sinuses enters. Clot arising in the soleal veins can thus extend into the posterior tibial vein and into these perforating veins thus destroying the mechanism which obviates reflux.

A constant lateral direct perforating vein is found on the outer side of the leg at the junction of lower and middle thirds. It connects the small saphenous or one of its tributaries to the peroneal vein. Where it pierces the deep fascia it receives a tributary from the soleus, so that it stands in the same relationship to deep vein thrombosis as the other ankle perforators.

Additional features of the ankle perforating veins are: that they are intimately related to the posterior borders of the tibia and fibula and that they are so valved that in health only an inward flow is possible.

Comment:

a. Dodd and Cockett state: 'It can thus be appreciated that in the erect position the essential venous drainage of what is known clinically as the "ulcer bearing area" is taken directly into the deep veins and not into the saphenous system.'

b. The principle underlying the treatment of varicose veins and venous ulceration is correction of venous hypertension.

The Tourniquet Test[1]: All that is necessary is a piece of rubber tubing. A

---

[1] In the preparation of the ensuing section the author has made use of the valuable article by Charles A. Steiner and Louis H. Palmer, *Ann. Surg.*, 1948, 127, 362.

VEINS 317

diagnosis of varicose veins having been made, the patient lies with the lower limbs exposed:

The limb is elevated above the level of the heart which empties the varicose veins. The tubing is applied round the upper thigh sufficiently firmly to occlude the saphenous but not the femoral vein.

The patient stands:

a. If the varicosities remain empty for 30 seconds the communicating veins are competent; if, however, they fill in this time the communicating veins are incompetent.

b. If the veins remain collapsed as in (a) but fill at once on removal of the tubing, then the saphenofemoral valves are incompetent.

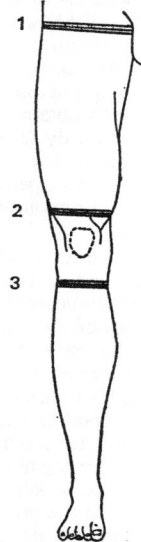

Fig. 316.—The tourniquet test for varicose veins.

c. If the varicosities fill in 30 seconds with the tourniquet in place, but distend even more when it is removed, then both the saphenofemoral and the valves of the perforating veins are incompetent. If the saphenofemoral valve is out of commission the operation of high ligation (Trendelenburg) is indicated. If the valves of the perforating veins are incompetent as determined above it is necessary to determine the level of the inefficiency.

318 A SYNOPSIS OF SURGICAL ANATOMY

   d. The tubing is applied just above the knee instead of higher up. If the leg varicosities remain collapsed, then the incompetent communications lie above the tourniquet and section of the incompetent perforator above the knee will be required. Should the veins, however, fill as rapidly with the tourniquet above the knee as when it is off, then either (i) the small saphenous vein is being filled from the popliteal, or (ii) the valves of the perforating veins below the knee are not functioning.
   e. It then becomes necessary to apply the tubing just below the knee. If now on standing the veins remain empty, then as the small saphenous is compressed by the tourniquet it is obvious that the fault is at the saphenopopliteal junction and the treatment is division of the small saphenous at its entrance to the polpiteal. Should the varicosities fill quickly with the below-knee tourniquet in place it is proof that the perforating veins in the leg are at fault and necessary action may be taken.

Thus by the use of a tourniquet at the top of the thigh, above the knee, and below the knee, it is possible to obtain the information necessary to treat the varicose condition intelligently (*Fig.* 316).

It is apparent from the foregoing that varicose veins are frequently caused by incompetence of the valves of perforating veins. In such cases removal of varicose veins will be disappointing unless the defective perforators are located and divided.

Thrombosis of the Veins of the Lower Limbs: Immobility of the legs during and after an operation and increased coagulability of the blood postoperatively, results in thrombosis in the leg veins, usually commencing in the venous sinuses of the soleus muscle of the calf. Such thrombosis may result in pulmonary embolism and is usually treated by anticoagulants but sometimes may require proximal venous ligation to prevent embolism. This will cause oedema unless the ligation is performed at a site with a good collateral circulation.

   Ligation of the femoral vein has the disadvantage that it may not prevent emboli from the opposite leg nor from the iliac veins but if it is used for this purpose it should be kept in mind that ligation of the superficial femoral vein distal to the profunda vein will leave a good collateral circulation through the profunda vein with very little interference with the venous return from the leg (*Fig.* 317) whereas ligation of the common femoral vein (proximal to the profunda) will will seriously impair venous return.

   It is much less hazardous to tie the common iliac vein because there is a good collateral circulation round this site.

   It is usually desirable to ligate the inferior vena cava below the renal veins to prevent emboli from both sides, and because there is a good collateral (*Fig.* 318) the disability is small unless the thrombosis has occluded the collateral veins.

VEINS 319

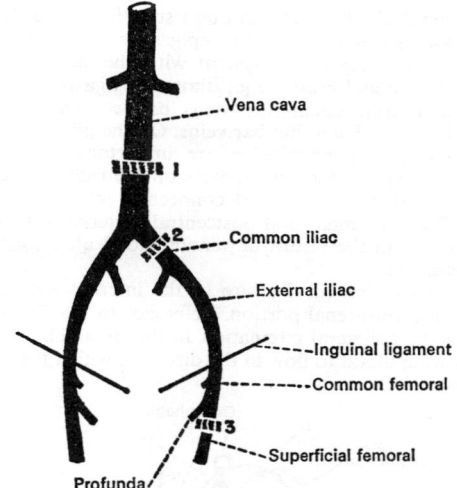

Fig. 317.—Sites of election for ligation of large veins are indicated by numbers.

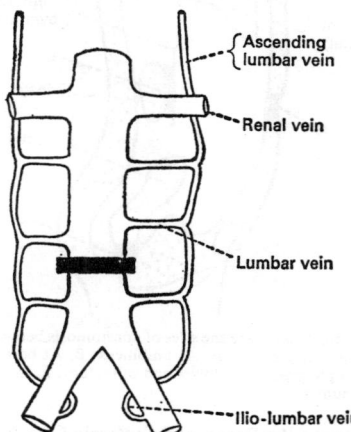

Fig. 318.—The diagram shows part of the venous collateral circulation when the inferior vena cava is tied.

The collateral circulation is through superficial and deep venous channels. The superficial inferior epigastric and circumflex iliac veins connect the saphenous system with the superficial veins of the upper abdominal wall, e.g., thoraco-epigastric. The inferior epigastric and deep circumflex veins connect with the superior epigastric, intercostal, and lumbar veins. On the posterior abdominal wall the ascending lumbar veins are important return pathways becoming, as they do, the vena azygos on the right and the inferior vena hemiazygos on the left and connecting inferior with superior vena cava. The prelaminar and postcentral vertebral venous plexuses also play a part in the return of venous blood after ligature of the inferior vena cava.

The site of election for ligature of the inferior vena cava is the lower part of its infrarenal portion. Reference to *Fig.* 318 shows how generous is the collateral circulation in this area. The veins are not valved, allowing blood to flow in the direction which the local conditions impose.

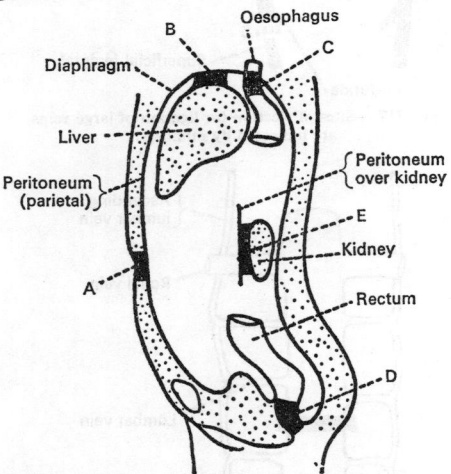

Fig. 319.—The black areas are the sites of anastomosis between the portal and systemic circulations. They occur: A, At umbilicus; B, At bare area of liver; C, At lower end of oesophagus; D, At lower end of rectum; E, In the tissue between kidney and peritoneum.

Communications between the Portal and Systemic Circulations (*Fig.* 319):

These communications are of importance in cases where the portal vein is obstructed, e.g., cirrhosis of the liver, as the portal blood can

find its way to the heart by the venae cavae via these communications. Such communications are found:
1. AT THE LOWER END OF THE OESOPHAGUS: The veins of the stomach (draining to the portal) communicate with the oesophageal veins (draining to the azygos and vena cava). In portal obstruction these veins often become varicose and burst into the oesophagus, causing vomiting of blood and often fatal haemorrhage.
2. AROUND THE UMBILICUS: Veins pass along the falciform ligament to the umbilicus, connecting the veins of the liver (portal) with the veins round the umbilicus (epigastric veins, which are systemic). Enlargement of these may produce a bunch of veins radiating from the umbilicus, which is called the caput Medusae (*Figs.* 320, 321).
3. AT THE LOWER END OF THE RECTUM: Three arteries supply the rectum, and the accompanying veins drain partly to the systemic and partly to the portal circulations. The superior haemorrhoidal vein becomes the inferior mesenteric which is portal. The inferior and middle haemorrhoidal veins empty into the hypogastric which is systemic. In portal obstruction, therefore, the veins in the rectum become dilated, the blood finding its way into the systemic channels. These dilated vessels form *haemorrhoids* or piles, which may therefore be symptomatic of portal obstruction.
4. AT THE BACK OF THE COLON: In front of the kidney small vessels unite the vessels of the peritoneum and colon (portal) with the vessels of the kidney (systemic).
5. BARE AREA OF THE LIVER: Small vessels unite the diaphragmatic veins (systemic) with the liver veins (portal).

Communications between the Portal and Lymphatic Circulations: Postmortem studies have demonstrated lymphatics draining directly into veins and not via the regional lymph-glands. Such observations strike at the basic principle underlying the surgery of malignancy, i.e., that cancer cells travel via lymphatics to the regional gland groups. It is, however, generally accepted that this is only likely to happen if there is obstruction to the onward flow of lymph which increases the intralymphatic pressure. In the case of the systemic circulation it is known, e.g., that some of the lymphatics draining the thymus pass directly into veins.

Valves: Valves are very common in veins, especially in the veins where the blood is carried against gravity. They are absent in the venae cavae, portal, uterine, ovarian, and hepatic veins. The pelvic veins are devoid of valves and have a tendency to form plexuses.

Vertebral System of Veins: It has long been known that a percentage of cases of chronic empyema cause brain abscess by the lodgement of septic emboli. So, too, there occur occasionally instances of carcinoma of the prostate where the vertebral column is riddled with secondaries.

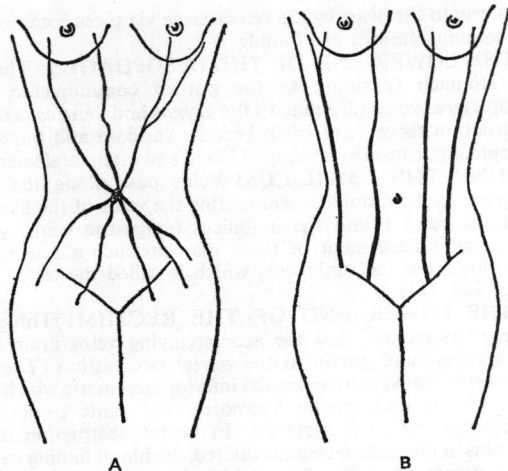

Fig. 320.—The subcutaneous collateral circulation in A, Portal obstruction (caput Medusae). B, Inferior vena caval obstruction.

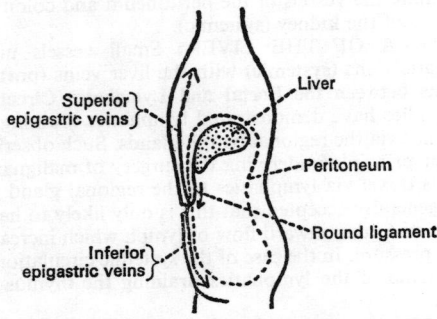

Fig. 321.—In portal obstruction some blood from liver is discharged along veins of round liagment to umbilicus and thence by epigastric veins, as shown by the arrows.

These and some other metastases in which the vehicular pathway of spread has been obscure are explicable by an appreciation of the anatomy of the vertebral venous system—in itself a persistence of the primitive venous plexus of the embryo. There are several plexuses of thin-walled valveless veins in relation to the vertebral bodies. The external vertebral venous plexus consists of anterior vessels in front of the vertebral bodies, and posterior ones on the back of the arches of the vertebrae and in the adjacent muscles. The internal vertebral plexus consists of a postcentral portion and a prelaminar one, each of these sections being drained by two vertical vessels. All these plexuses are in free intercommunication with each other and receive the basivertebral veins draining the bodies of the vertebrae (*Fig.* 322). They are drained by the intervertebral veins which pass through the intervertebral foramina with the spinal nerves. The latter veins also drain the spinal

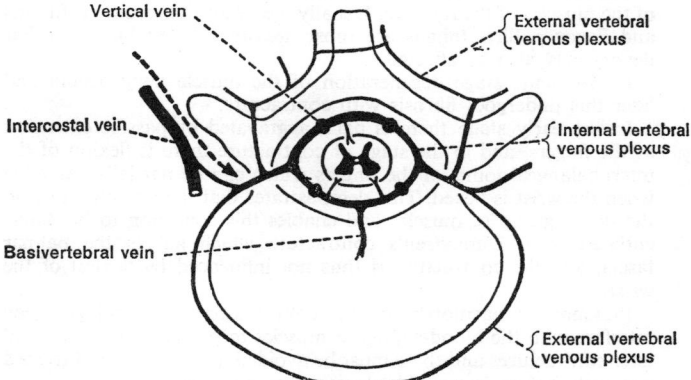

Fig. 322.—The vertebral system of veins.

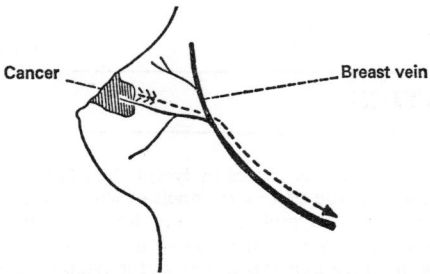

Fig. 323.—Carcinoma of breast. The arrow shows the route taken by an embolus of malignant cells to reach the intercostal vein and thus the vertebral plexus.

cord. These segmental intervertebral veins pour their blood into vertebral, intercostal, lumbar, and lateral sacral veins. They also communicate with veins of the portal system. Thus for example the brain and prostate gland are brought into association by this system. It is apparent that coughing, straining at stool, etc., may dislodge tumour cells or infected emboli from systemic or portal areas into the vertebral venous system. They may gain lodgement in vertebrae, spinal cord, skull, or brain (*Fig*. 323).

Volkmann's Ischaemic Contracture: Following injury of the arm, particularly of the elbow, injury to the brachial artery with associated spasm of the main artery and the collateral circulation results in ischaemia of the muscles of the forearm. Usually the flexor digitorum profundus and flexor pollicis longus are most heavily affected but the other flexors may also be affected.

In the acute stage degeneration of the muscle belly occurs and later this undergoes fibrosis with contracture.

In the early stage there is pain, aggravated by passive extension of the fingers, and in the stage of contracture there is flexion of the interphalangeal joints of the fingers which can be partially extended when the wrist is flexed. This demonstrates that the contracture is in the flexor group of muscles and enables this condition to be differentiated from Dupuytren's contracture which affects the palmar fascia, and the contracture is thus not influenced by flexion of the wrist.

Pressure by haemorrhage and tight plasters or bandages may interfere with the blood-supply of muscles to produce ischaemia and later contractures and these must be avoided, recognized, and treated promptly before irreversible damage has been done.

Chapter XXVII

LYMPHATICS

LYMPH is removed from the tissues by lymphatic channels which drain to regional lymph-nodes, the efferent channels of which in turn drain to more proximal nodes until the lymph eventually drains into the major veins in the root of the neck. However, virtually all nodes have collateral channels which by-pass the node and this accounts for lymphatic metastases at a distance without previous involvement of the primary nodes.[1]

[1] Mahaffy, R. G., *Jl R. Coll. Surg. Edinb.*, 1965, 10, 125.

LYMPH TISSUE OF THE HEAD AND NECK

This consists of: (1) Adenoid tissue; (2) Lymph-glands.

Adenoid Tissue: At the entrance to the pharynx there is grouped a considerable amount of lymphoid tissue which guards the portal into the alimentary canal. This is analogous to the large amount of lymphoid tissue grouped in the lower ileum and appendix which guards the entrance into the large gut. This lymphoid tissue situated at the entrance to the pharynx is grouped in a circular fashion round this part of the gut, and is known as—

WALDEYER'S LYMPHATIC RING (*Fig.* 324), which is constituted as follows:

SUPERIOR: The pharyngeal tonsils or adenoids—a central collection of lymphoid tissue in the roof of the pharynx.

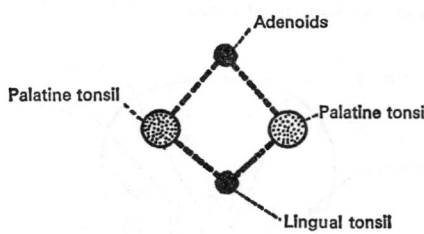

Fig. 324.—Waldeyer's lymphatic ring.

INFERIOR: The lingual tonsil—adenoid tissue situated at the base of the tongue.

LATERALLY: The faucial tonsils, or simply 'tonsils', situated at the isthmus faucium, one on each side. On the side wall of the pharynx is situated scattered lymphoid tissue which completes the ring. This tissue plays a most important part in preventing the entrance of organisms into the body. This is evidenced by the frequency with which hypertrophy and inflammation of the tonsils and adenoids occur. Enlargement of the tonsils does not necessarily mean that these organs are diseased, but merely that they have increased in size in their efforts to cope with infection entering them.

LYMPHATIC DRAINAGE OF WALDEYER'S RING: This adenoid tissue drains into:

1. *The Main Lymph-gland of the Tonsil:* Situated in the angle between the internal jugular and common facial veins just below the angle of the jaw. Other glands in this region assist in the drainage.

326 A SYNOPSIS OF SURGICAL ANATOMY

2. *The Adenoid Glands*, which lie below the tip of the mastoid process under cover of the sternomastoid, receive the lymph from the adenoids (pharyngeal tonsils). These glands become enlarged if the adenoids are diseased. Should they be affected with tuberculosis, it is sometimes necessary to excise the glands, which lie in close relation to the spinal accessory nerve. The nerve may be injured in the process.

Both the main gland of the tonsil and the glands draining the adenoids are members of the upper deep cervical chain of lymph-glands.

Lymph-glands: These consist of: (1) A circular chain of glands; (2) A vertical chain of glands.

1. CIRCULAR CHAIN OF GLANDS (*Fig.* 325): Consists of the following gland groups: (*a*) Occipital; (*b*) Posterior auricular; (*c*) Pre-auricular; (*d*) Parotid; (*e*) Facial; (*f*) Submaxillary; (*g*) Submental; (*h*) Superficial cervical; (*i*) Anterior cervical.

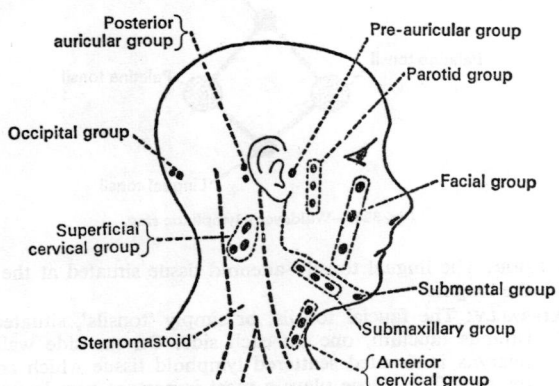

Fig. 325.—The glands of the circular chain.

OCCIPITAL GLANDS: One or two glands situated midway between the mastoid process and the external occipital protuberance. They drain the back of the scalp. The glands lie in close relation to the great occipital nerve, and if enlarged may press on the nerve causing neuralgia in the distribution of the nerve.

POSTERIOR AURICULAR GLANDS: Situated on the mastoid process behind the pinna. They drain the temporal region of the scalp, back of the pinna, and external auditory meatus.

PRE-AURICULAR GLAND: Situated immediately in front of the tragus; the situation is so definite that a swelling not exactly in front of the tragus cannot arise from this gland. The gland lies superficial to the fascia covering the parotid, i.e., the parotideo-masseteric fascia. It drains the outer surface of the pinna and side of the scalp.

PAROTID GLANDS: These glands are situated both in the substance of the parotid salivary gland and deep to it, i.e., between it and the side wall of the pharynx.

The deeper glands drain: (a) The nasopharynx; and (b) The back of the nose. The more superficial receive lymph from: (a) The eyelids; (b) Front of the scalp; (c) External auditory meatus; and (d) Tympanic cavity.

FACIAL GLANDS: Consist of superficial and deep groups.

Superficial Group: Consists of:
   a. *Infra-orbital:* Just below the orbit.
   b. *Buccinator:* On the muscle of this name lateral to the angle of the mouth.
   c. *Supramandibular:* On the mandible in front of the masseter—around the external maxillary artery.

These glands receive lymph from conjunctiva and eyelids, nose, and cheek.

Deep Group: These lie around the internal maxillary vessels in relation to the external pterygoid muscle. They drain: (a) The temporal fossa; (b) Infratemporal fossa; (c) Back of the nose; (d) Pharynx.

SUBMAXILLARY GLANDS: An important group lying in the submaxillary triangle in close relation to the submaxillary salivary gland. The lymph-glands are under the deep fascia in actual contact with the salivary gland. In cancer, therefore, the removal of these lymph-glands necessitates the removal of the salivary gland as well because of this intimate relationship. One of these glands—the gland of Stohr—lies in the S bend which the external maxillary artery makes in crossing the mandible. Choyce[1] has shown that failure to remove this gland in cancer of the tongue may result in recurrence of the disease in this lymph-gland. Small lymph-glands may be actually embedded in the substance of the submaxillary salivary and parotid salivary glands. The submaxillary glands drain: (a) The side of the nose; (b) Inner angle of the eye; (c) The cheek; (d) Angle of the mouth; (e) Whole of the upper lip; (f) Outer part of the lower lip; (g) The gums; (h) Some lymph from the side of the tongue.

SUBMENTAL GLANDS: These lie in the submental triangle. They drain the central part of the lower lip and the floor of the mouth. They receive some lymph from the apex of the tongue.

---

[1] *Modern Operative Surgery*, 1924, 323. London.

SUPERFICIAL CERVICAL GLANDS: These lie on the outer surface of the sternomastoid around the external jugular vein. They drain the parotid region and lower part of the ear.

ANTERIOR CERVICAL GLANDS: These lie near the middle line of the neck in front of the larynx and trachea. They consist of superficial and deep sets of glands.

Superficial Set: Lie in relation to the anterior jugular vein and drain the skin of the neck. They are unimportant.

Deep Set: Consist of:
 a. *The Infrahyoid Glands:* These lie on the thyrohyoid membrane and drain the front of the larynx.
 b. *The Prelaryngeal Glands:* These lie on the cricothyroid ligament and drain the larynx. Trotter has shown that their afferents pass through a small foramen in the middle of the cricothyroid ligament. These glands are often the first to become enlarged in cancer of the larynx. The glands assist in the drainage of the thyroid.
 c. *The Pretracheal Glands:* These lie in relation to the inferior thyroid veins in front of the trachea and drain the thyroid and trachea.

EFFERENTS OF THE CIRCULAR CHAIN: The deep cervical chain receives ultimately all the lymph from the glands enumerated above. It receives the efferents directly from all these gland groups except the facial and submental. The efferents from these two groups pass first to the submaxillary glands.

2. VERTICAL CHAIN OF DEEP CERVICAL GLANDS (*Fig.* 326): This consists of a large number of big glands lying in relation to the

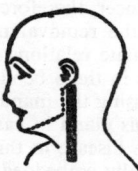

Fig. 326.—The situation of the deep cervical chain of glands is indicated by the black area; this is the vertical chain.

carotid sheath. A few members of this group occupy an outlying position behind the pharynx and are called the retropharyngeal glands. They drain the back of the nose and pharynx and the auditory tube.

The vertical chain of deep cervical glands lies alongside the pharynx, trachea, and oesophagus, and extends from the base of the skull to the root of the neck. They are arbitrarily divided into superior deep cervical and inferior deep cervical groups by the point of bifurcation of the common carotid (or, alternatively, by the omohyoid). The glands of both groups are in very intimate relationship with the internal jugular vein. In removing the glands it is necessary to strip them from the vein and sometimes even to remove part of it. Some of the glands of the inferior group project beyond the posterior border of the sternomastoid into the posterior triangle of the neck. There are a few small glands of this group which lie in the groove between the trachea and oesophagus alongside the recurrent nerve. They are called paratracheal glands and assist in the drainage of the thyroid. Three glands of the deep cervical group are named (*Fig.* 327):

MAIN GLAND OF THE TONSIL (JUGULODIGASTRIC): Below the angle of the jaw in the angle between the internal jugular and common facial veins.

MAIN GLAND OF THE TONGUE: Situated a little lower in the neck at the bifurcation of the common carotid, i.e., just below the great cornu of the hyoid bone.

SUPRA-OMOHYOID GLAND: A gland situated on the common carotid just above the point where the anterior belly of the omohyoid crosses this vessel. It plays a very important part in the lymph drainage of the tongue, receiving some vessels from the apex which take a circuitous route to reach the gland.

The deep cervical glands receive the lymph from the entire head and neck, either directly or indirectly from the glands of the circular chain.

The lymph from the deep cervical chain (i.e., all the lymph from that half of the head and neck) is collected into one trunk—the

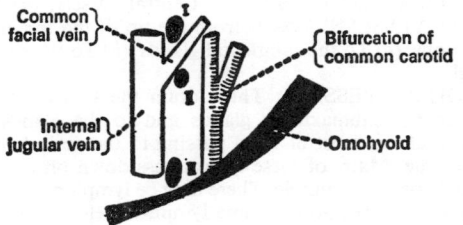

Fig. 327.—Showing three important lymph-glands of the deep cervical chain. I, Tonsillar or jugulodigastric gland; II, Main lymph-gland of tongue; III, Supra-omohyoid gland.

jugular lymph trunk—which leaves the inferior deep cervical glands. On the right side this trunk enters the junction of the subclavian vein and internal jugular vein. On the left side the trunk enters the thoracic duct.

Lymph Drainage of the Lips:
1. The lymphatics of the lips form a fine submucous plexus drained by collecting trunks.
2. There is communication of lymphatics across the midline in the middle area of both lips. Thus (*a*) cancers in or near the midline in both upper and lower lips spread to the glands on both sides. (*b*) Radical surgery in such cases implies removal of the first gland echelon on both sides. (*c*) Glands which are not palpable may be infected with cancer. (*d*) Glands which are palpable may be enlarged merely because of bacterial infection.
3. The lower lip drains to the submental and submaxillary glands, thence to the deep cervical glands.
4. The upper lip and commissures drain to the same gland groups, sometimes to the pre-auricular gland, and directly to higher glands of the deep cervical chain than those reached by the drainage vessels of the lower lip. Thus the upper lip has a more extensive lymph radiation than the lower, this being one factor in the greater gravity of the prognosis in cancer of the upper as compared with the lower lip.
5. An important member of the receiving glands is that lying on the lower border of the mandible on the S bend of the external maxillary (facial) artery.
6. Rouvière[1] has shown that some lymph from the outer third of the lower lip enters the mandible through the mental foramen. Thus cancer of the lip has a direct lymphatic route into the mandible.

Lymph Drainage of the Tongue (*Fig.* 328): The tongue is drained by lymph-vessels which may be divided into four groups: (1) Apical vessels; (2) Marginal vessels; (3) Central vessels; (4) Basal vessels.
1. APICAL VESSELS: Vessels from the tip of the tongue pass in two directions: (*a*) To the submental glands; (*b*) To the supra-omohyoid gland.
2. MARGINAL VESSELS: These drain the side of the tongue and pass to the submaxillary glands and to the glands of the deep cervical chain, most of them passing to the main lymph-glands of the tongue. Many of these trunks pass down on the outer surface of the hyoglossus muscle. There may be lymph nodules lying on the hyoglossus in relation to these lymph-vessels. They are sometimes called lingual glands. They are palpated by one finger in the floor of the mouth, the fingers of the other hand being beneath the jaw bone.
3. CENTRAL VESSELS: These are vessels which drain the area of the tongue on either side of the median raphe (*Fig.* 329). They pass vertically downwards in the midline of the tongue between the

[1] Rouvière, H., *Anatomie des Lymphatiques de l'Homme*, trans. M. J. Tobias, 1938, 24. Ann Arbor: Edward Bros.

LYMPHATICS 331

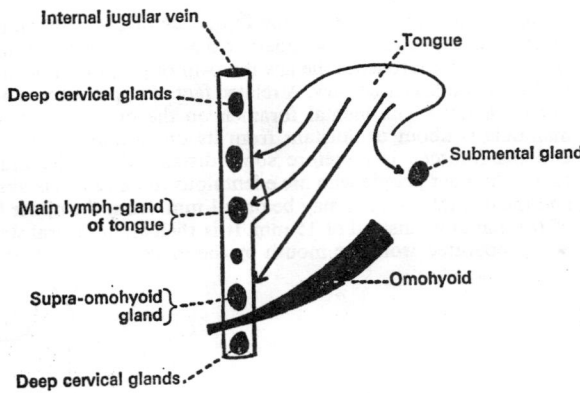

Fig. 328.—Direction of lymph drainage of tongue.

genioglossi muscles and then pass, some to the left and some to the right, to the deep cervical glands.

4. BASAL VESSELS: These trunks drain the posterior part of the tongue. Many of them pass freely from one side of the tongue to the other. They enter the deep cervical glands.

From this description it will be seen that in cancer of the tongue, cancer cells may pass freely to lymphatic glands on both sides of the neck. It is therefore necessary that all the glands receiving lymph from the tongue on both sides of the neck be dealt with in the treatment of cancer of the tongue.

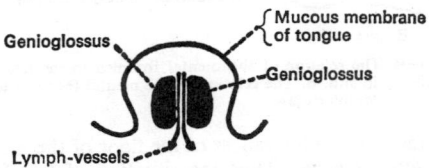

Fig. 329.—Median group of lymphatic vessels of tongue.

Ward and Hendrick[1] state that Polya and associates in 1902 showed that in 50 per cent of normal individuals the lymphatics of the tongue and floor of the mouth pass through the periosteum of the mandible on their way to the lymph-nodes in the submaxillary

[1] Ward, G. E., and Hendrick, J. W., *The Diagnosis and Treatment of Tumours of the Head and Neck*, 1950, 729. Baltimore: Williams & Wilkins.

triangle, thus accounting for the frequency of early attachment of metastases to the jaw. It is apparent that when cancer of the floor of the mouth approaches the jaw removal of part or all of the body of the mandible is necessary. A related fact of importance is pointed out by Byars.[1] The mental foramen on the outer surface of the mandible is about equidistant from its upper and lower borders, and the foramen is therefore some distance from the intra-oral cavity. In older people who are edentulous the alveolus is absorbed and the mental foramen may be only 1 mm. from the upper border of the mandible instead of 15 mm. It is then an intra-oral structure being separated from the mouth by the mucoperiosteum only and

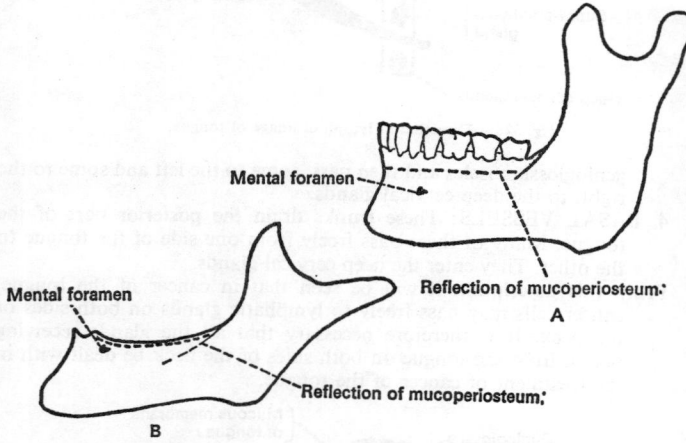

Fig. 330.—A, The relation of the mental foramen to the mucoperiosteum when the teeth are in situ. B, The relation of the mental foramen to the mucoperiosteum in the edentulous jaw.

offers a ready route for cancer of the floor of the mouth to invade the mandibular canal. Thus the situation of this foramen is an important factor in enabling the surgeon to plan the extent of bone removal in cancer of the floor of the mouth encroaching on the jaw. Once the mandibular canal is invaded, nothing short of disarticulation of that side of the jaw is likely to be effective (*Fig.* 330).

The vulnerability of the mandible to cancer: In summary, cancer may involve this bone (*a*) through the lymphatics of the outer third of the lower lip which enter the mental foramen; (*b*) through the

[1] Byars, L. T., *Surgery Gynec. Obstet.*, 1954, 98, 564.

LYMPHATICS

same foramen in cancer of the floor of the mouth, when absorption of the bone in edentulous subjects brings the mucous membrane of the floor of the mouth into contact with the foramen; (c) through the close relationship of the lymphatics of the tongue and floor of the mouth to the periosteum of the bone.

LYMPH-GLANDS OF THE ABDOMEN

These are arranged in two large groups: (1) The parietal lying behind the peritoneum in relation to the large blood-vessels; (2) The visceral, which lie alongside the visceral arteries.

Parietal Glands of the Abdomen: These are arranged in the following groups: (1) External iliac; (2) Common iliac; (3) Hypogastric or internal iliac; (4) Sacral; (5) Lumbar or aortic.

EXTERNAL ILIAC GLANDS (*Fig.* 331): These lie in relation to the external iliac vessels just behind the inguinal ligament. They are divisible into three groups:

LATERAL: External to the vessels.

INTERMEDIATE: Anterior to the vessels. The genitofemoral nerve divides into its two terminal branches behind this gland.

MEDIAL: Internal to the vessels, this gland has prolapsed over the precipice formed by the pelvic brim, lying just below the brim.

The glands receive lymph from: (1) The inguinal glands; (2) The deep lymph-vessels from the anterior abdominal wall below the level of the umbilicus; (3) Glans penis or clitoris; (4) Bladder; (5) Upper part of the vagina; (6) Cervix uteri; (7) Mucous membrane of the urethra and prostate. Their efferents pass to the common iliac glands.

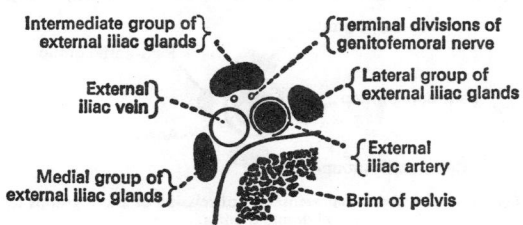

Fig. 331.—The external iliac glands.

COMMON ILIAC GLANDS (*Fig.* 332): Like the preceding group, these glands are arranged in three sets which lie respectively lateral to the artery, behind the artery (cf. external iliac glands), and medial to the artery. They receive the lymph from the external and internal iliac glands. They also receive lymph from the (1) Vagina; (2)

Uterus; (3) Prostate; and (4) Rectum. Their lymph passes to the para-aortic glands.

There is free communication between the two sides of the body in the upper sacral region and at the level of the 1st sacral segment there is a constant communicating vessel.[1]

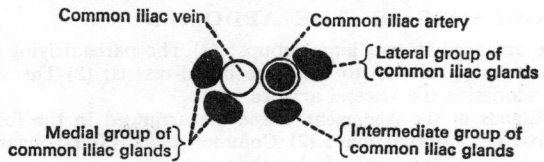

Fig. 332.—The left common iliac glands.

HYPOGASTRIC OR INTERNAL ILIAC GLANDS: These lie in relation to the vessels of the same name. Some of the glands lie alongside the branches of the artery. They receive much of the lymph from the pelvic organs, namely, a large part of the lymph from the: (1) Rectum; (2) Bladder; (3) Urethra; (4) Prostate; (5) Uterus; (6) Buttock. Their efferents pass to the common iliac glands.

SACRAL GLANDS: These lie in the hollow of the sacrum in relation to the sacral blood-vessels. They receive lymph from the: (1) Rectum; (2) Posterior wall of the pelvis. They drain to the aortic glands.

LUMBAR OR AORTIC GLANDS: These consist of many large important glands divided into four groups: (1) Pre-aortic; (2) and (3) Para-aortic right and left; (4) Retro-aortic (*Fig.* 333).

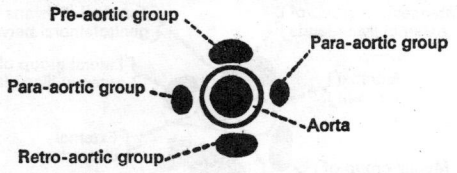

Fig. 333.—Schematic representation of relation of gland groups to abdominal aorta.

1. PRE-AORTIC: These glands lying in front of the great arterial trunk are arranged in three groups: coeliac, and superior and inferior mesenteric. Each group lies on the aorta in relation to the *main stem* of the artery of the same name. They receive lymph from the territories supplied by the blood-vessels after which they are named, i.e., from the gut, liver, spleen, and pancreas. They are

[1] Mahaffy, R. G., *Jl R. Coll. Surg., Edinb.*, 1965, 10, 125.

drained by a single lymph-vessel—the intestinal trunk which enters the cisterna chyli.

2 and 3. PARA-AORTIC: These glands lie at the sides of the aorta. They receive: The efferents of the common iliac glands, i.e., all the lymph from the lower limb, and most of the lymph from the pelvis, the lymphatics from the lateral abdominal wall, kidney, suprarenal, testis, ovary, uterine tube, and body of the uterus.

The efferents of the para-aortic glands unite to form a single trunk on each side, the right and left lumbar lymph-trunks, which unite to form the cisterna chyli. A small portion of the lymph from these glands passes to the retro-aortic and the pre-aortic glands, and some passes up through the crura of the diaphragm to join the thoracic duct in the thorax.

4. RETRO-AORTIC: These are relatively unimportant, receiving some lymph from the other groups of aortic glands and emptying their lymph into the cisterna chyli.

Visceral Lymph-glands of the Abdomen: These lie in relation to the *branches* of the coeliac artery, and the superior and inferior mesenteric arteries. Those in relation to the coeliac artery are arranged in three groups, and have already been described.

SUPERIOR MESENTERIC GLANDS: Numerous glands lying in the mesentery, ileocaecal angle, and transverse mesocolon.

INFERIOR MESENTERIC GLANDS: Lie in relation to the branches of this artery. The lymph-glands of the small and large intestine are arranged in three groups:

1. PROXIMAL: Lie on the arterial trunks going to the gut.
2. INTERMEDIATE: Lie on the large branches of the arterial trunks.
3. DISTAL: Lie amongst the arterial arcades near the wall of the gut or the gut itself.

Peyer's Patches: They are dense collections of lymphoid tissue found in the small intestine. They are well formed in fetal life, increasing in numbers until childhood. After puberty they rapidly become fewer, decreasing in number with advancing years, just as do the lymph follicles of the large intestine.

Before the control of typhoid fever Peyer's patches were common sites of intestinal haemorrhage, ulceration, and perforation.

LYMPH-GLANDS OF THE THORAX

These are arranged into two main groups: (1) Parietal; (2) Visceral.

Parietal Group: Consists of: (1) Anterior, or internal mammary glands; (2) Posterior, or posterior mediastinal glands; (3) Lateral, or intercostal glands; (4) Inferior, or diaphragmatic glands.

INTERNAL MAMMARY GLANDS: These lie alongside the internal mammary vessels, two glands being found in each of the first two intercostal spaces. As a rule glands are not found lower than the third space. They receive lymph from the skin over the breast, from the deep structures forming the abdominal wall above the level of the umbilicus, and from the upper surface of the liver on the right. Their lymph passes by a single trunk on each side into the junction of the subclavian and jugular veins.

POSTERIOR MEDIASTINAL GLANDS: These lie behind the pericardium in relation to the oesophagus and aorta. They drain the: (1) Oesophagus; (2) Diaphragm; and (3) Upper surface of the liver. They drain into the thoracic duct.

LATERAL OR INTERCOSTAL GLANDS: These lie in front of the necks of the ribs or in the posterior ends of the intercostal spaces. They drain the deep structures forming the side and back of the chest. The lymph from the lower four or five spaces drains into the cisterna chyli. That from the upper spaces drains into the thoracic duct on the left and into the right lymph-duct on the right.

DIAPHRAGMATIC GLANDS: These are arranged in four groups—anterior, posterior, and right and left lateral. They all rest on the upper surface of the diaphragm (*see Fig.* 184, p. 196).

ANTERIOR: Lie behind the sternal origin of the diaphragm and the seventh costal cartilage. They receive lymph from the: (1) Upper surface of the liver; and (2) Diaphragm. They drain into the internal mammary glands.

LATERAL: These lie on each side close to the position where the phrenic nerve pierces the diaphragm. They drain the diaphragm and on the right the liver. Their lymph passes to the posterior mediastinal glands.

POSTERIOR: They drain the diaphragm, and their efferents go to the posterior mediastinal glands.

Visceral Glands: Consist of: (1) Superior mediastinal glands; (2) Peri-tracheobronchial glands.

SUPERIOR MEDIASTINAL GLANDS: These glands lie in front of the trachea behind the aortic arch. They drain (1) the trachea and oesophagus, and (2) the heart. A single efferent from these glands unites with the efferent from the peri-tracheobronchial glands to form the bronchomediastinal trunk.

PERI-TRACHEOBRONCHIAL GLANDS (*Fig.* 334): This group comprises many glands, amongst which are some of the largest in the body. It is made up of:

Pre-tracheobronchial glands which lie in front of and lateral to the trachea and bronchi.

Inter-tracheobronchial glands which lie between the two main bronchi.

Interbronchial glands which lie between the divisions of each bronchus at the hilum of and actually in the substance of the lung.

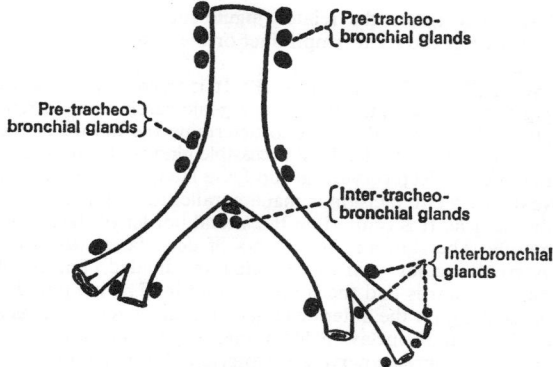

Fig. 334.—The peri-tracheobronchial glands.

These glands drain the lungs and bronchi. A single efferent joins the efferent of the superior mediastinal group to form the bronchomediastinal trunk. This trunk usually opens both on the right and on the left into the junction of the subclavian and internal jugular veins. It may join the right lymph-duct on the right or the thoracic duct on the left.

Lymph Drainage of the Lungs[1]: Lymph converging on the hila of the lungs is not drained in a strictly lobar manner. From the right lung lymph passes directly or indirectly to gland groups related to the bifurcation of the trachea, i.e., inter-tracheobronchial and pre-tracheobronchial glands.

On the left there are three regions of lymph drainage. The superior part of the upper lobe drains to the left pre-tracheobronchial glands. Lymph from the lower part of the upper lobe and upper area of the lower lobe drains to the same gland group, but also to the inter-tracheobronchial glands, passing through them to the right group of pre-tracheobronchial glands. The remaining part of the lower lobe drains also to glands at the tracheal bifurcation and thence to the right pre-tracheobronchial glands.

Some lymph from the glands in relation to the sides of the trachea passes to the inferior deep cervical glands and so to the jugular lymph trunk.

The tracheobronchial glands give rise on each side to a lymph trunk which receives the efferent vessel draining the superior mediastinal gland group—the bronchomediastinal trunk.

---

[1] This account of the lymphatic drainage of the lung is based on the review by Connar, R. G., *Surgery Gynec. Obstet.*, 1955, **101**, 733.

Usually it enters the related jugulo-subclavian junction. It may however enter the right lymph-duct or the thoracic duct according to the side.

PRE-SCALENE GLAND BIOPSY: It is current practice in certain pulmonary diseases, e.g., bronchogenic carcinoma, to remove one of the deep cervical glands to determine the nature of the disease or its operability. The most accessible glands are those members of the inferior deep cervical group lying lateral to the internal jugular vein. A 7·5 cm. incision is made parallel to and about 2 cm. above the clavicle. It is centred on the lateral border of the sternomastoid muscle. The skin and two layers of deep fascia are divided. The external jugular vein is retracted or divided. The omohyoid is pulled upwards and the sternomastoid in. The lymphoid and fatty tissue lying on the anterior scalene muscle is removed, as also that in the jugulo-subclavian junctional angle. The transverse cervical artery and phrenic nerve are protected. All tissue divided is ligated as the area is one rich in lymphatic vessels. Glands can only be felt here clinically in advanced cases, so that the procedure is usually carried out in the absence of lymphadenopathy. The removed tissue contains lymph-glands which are histologically examined.

In 30 per cent of cases the diagnosis is forthcoming for conditions such as cancer of the lung or Boeck's sarcoid. The finding of carcinoma in a lymph-gland in a case of tumour of the lung precludes operation. Usually the ipsilateral scalene fat-pad is removed. It is apparent from the lymphatic drainage of the lower two-thirds of the left lung field that biopsy may need to be bilateral.

Lymphatic Drainage of the Heart[1]:

1. Two plexuses of lymph-vessels are formed in the coronary sulcus around the origin of the right and left coronary arteries.
2. Two lymphatic collecting trunks, anterior and posterior, emerge from these.
3. The anterior trunk runs up on the anterior aspect of the aorta to end in glands of the superior mediastinum. These glands lie between the aortic arch and the left innominate vein.
4. The posterior trunk runs up on the posterior aspect of the pulmonary artery to a gland lying posterior to the aorta and superior vena cava in the angle between them.

LYMPHATIC DRAINAGE OF THE UPPER EXTREMITY

The lymphatic channels of the forearm all converge on the medial side of the upper arm to drain into the lymph-nodes of the upper arm.

These consist of: (1) Supratrochlear; (2) Deltopectoral; (3) Axillary group.

---

[1] This is a brief summary of a paper entitled 'The Lymphatic Drainage of the Heart', by L. R. Shore, *J. Anat.*, 1929, April, 291.

Supratrochlear Gland: This gland lies above the medial epicondyle of the humerus superficial to the deep fascia alongside of the basilic vein. It drains the inner three fingers and inner half of the palm and forearm. Its efferents go to the axillary glands.

Deltopectoral Glands: These lie between the deltoid and pectoralis major just below the clavicle, in relation to the upper part of the cephalic vein. They assist in draining the thumb and index finger and outer side of the hand and forearm. Their efferents go to the apical (infraclavicular) glands of the axilla.

Axillary Glands: These comprise a most important group which drains on each side the breast and the upper limb and the skin of the body from the umbilicus to the clavicle. There are five groups of glands in the axilla (*see Fig.* 27, p. 33):

ANTERIOR GROUP: Glands situated under cover of pectoralis major along the lateral thoracic vessels. They receive most of the lymph from the breast.

POSTERIOR GROUP: Glands situated along the subscapular vessels in relation to the axillary border of the scapula.

LATERAL GROUP: Glands situated along the axillary vein on the inner aspect of the upper part of the humerus.

CENTRAL GROUP: Glands situated in the fat filling the axilla. Much of the lymph from the preceding groups goes to these glands.

APICAL OR INFRACLAVICULAR: Glands situated in the angle between the costocoracoid membrane in front, axillary vein behind, and first intercostal space below. They are of great importance because they receive one vessel directly from the upper part of the mamma and ultimately most of the lymph from the breast (*see also* pp. 33–38).

A single trunk leaves the apical gland group on each side. This is the subclavian trunk. It enters the junction of the jugular and subclavian veins, or may join the thoracic duct on the left.

Red streaks due to inflamed cutaneous lymph-vessels (lymphangitis) are often seen on the front of the forearm. They are readily seen if inflamed, because the cutaneous lymph-vessels lie superficial to the subcutaneous veins, i.e., between them and the skin. These red lines are not seen on the *back* of the forearm, because the lymphatic vessels make their way round to the front or flexor aspect of the limb.

LYMPHATIC DRAINAGE OF THE LOWER EXTREMITY

The leg has a superficial and a deep set of lymphatic channels:

The superficial lymphatics from the medial side of the foot and leg ascend with the long saphenous vein as 10–15 channels to the superficial inguinal nodes. From the lateral side of the foot and leg they ascend and cross in the region of the knee to join the medial group.

The deep lymphatics are few in number, often only a solitary channel, and ascend with the deep blood-vessels to the popliteal nodes and from there along the vessels to the deep inguinal nodes.

There are no communications between the superficial and deep systems.

There are only two constant sets of glands in the lower limb: (1) The popliteal glands; (2) The inguinal glands. Occasionally a gland may be found on the front of the upper part of the interosseous membrane, just where the anterior tibial vessels come through the membrane. It is the anterior tibial gland.

Popliteal Glands: These lie under the deep fascia in the popliteal space. They receive lymph from the skin of the outer side of the leg and foot, and from the deep structures of the foot and leg by means of the lymph-vessels accompanying the anterior and posterior tibial vessels. They receive the lymph from the knee-joint. All the efferents from these glands pass with the popliteal and then with the femoral vein to the deep inguinal lymph-glands.

Inguinal Glands: The authors would like to stress the point that in the infant some of the inguinal glands lie directly over and sometimes even at a higher level than the inguinal ligament; whereas in the adult the glands, though sometimes anterior to the ligament, are usually below the line of the ligament. In the adult, therefore, a swelling above the ligament cannot arise from this gland group, whereas in the child this may be the case.[1]

These glands consist of two groups (*Fig.* 335): (1) Superficial—lying on the fascia lata; (2) Deep—lying beneath the fascia lata.

1. SUPERFICIAL INGUINAL GLANDS: Consist of two sets:

   a. PROXIMAL OR HORIZONTAL SET lying below and parallel to the inguinal ligament.

   This set receives lymph from the skin of the anterior abdominal wall below the level of the umbilicus, from the skin of the

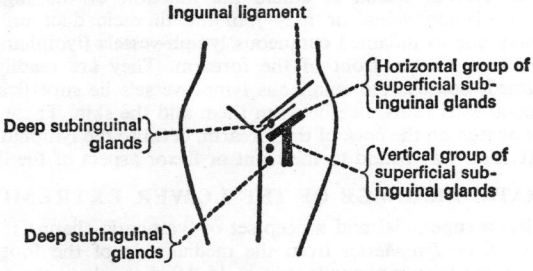

Fig. 335.—Arrangement of lymph-glands at root of thigh.

---

[1] Lejars has encountered glands above the inguinal ligament. (*The Lymphatics*, Poirier, Cuneo, and Delamere, 1903, 117. London.)

penis, scrotum, perineum, and buttock, and from the mucous membrane of the anterior part of the urethra and the anal canal. The lowest parts of the vagina and vulva drain into these glands.

   b. DISTAL OR VERTICAL SET lying alongside the upper end of the long saphenous vein.

      The distal set receives the lymph-vessels accompanying the long saphenous vein. These vessels drain the skin of the entire lower limb excluding that of the outer side of the dorsum of the foot and the back and outer side of the calf. They assist in the drainage of penis, scrotum, and buttock.

These are the only glands in the body which may normally be palpable.

2. DEEP INGUINAL GLANDS: Two or three glands under the fascia lata on the inner aspect of the femoral vein. One lies in the femoral canal. They receive the lymph-vessels running with the femoral vein, also lymph from glans penis or clitoris, and also the lymph from the superficial inguinal glands. The lymph from these glands passes to the external iliac glands.

THE GREAT LYMPH-DUCTS

These comprise: (1) The thoracic duct—single; (2) The right and left subclavian trunks; (3) The right and left bronchomediastinal trunks; (4) The right and left jugular trunks; (5) The right lymph-duct.

These vessels, like all but the very smallest lymphatics, are supplied with bicuspid valves to prevent backflow.

Thoracic Duct: This vessel commences from the upper end of the cisterna chyli. The duct conveys the entire lymph from the body excepting that from the: (1) Right side of the head and neck; (2) Right upper limb; (3) Thoracic wall on the right; (4) Right lung; (5) Right side of the heart; (6) Part of convex surface of the liver; (7) Lower part of the left lung.

      The vessel in the adult is the same length as the spinal cord, viz., 45 cm.

   CISTERNA CHYLI (*Fig.* 336): This lymph sac lies in front of the bodies of the first and second lumbar vertebrae between the aorta and the right crus of the diaphragm. It is present in 50 per cent of cases. It receives three great lymph-trunks, the right and left lumbar and the intestinal. Each of the lumbar trunks is a short vessel which leaves the para-aortic glands to enter the cisterna. The lumbar trunks convey the lymph from the lower limbs, the pelvis including its viscera, kidneys and adrenals, and deep lymphatics of the abdominal walls. The left lumbar trunk reaches the cisterna by passing behind the aorta.

342 A SYNOPSIS OF SURGICAL ANATOMY

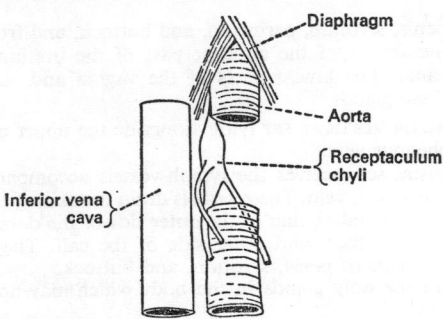

Fig. 336.—The cisterna (receptaculum) chyli.

INTESTINAL TRUNK: Passes from the pre-aortic glands to the cisterna. It conveys lymph from the: (1) Stomach; (2) Pancreas; (3) Spleen; (4) Most of liver; (5) Intestines.

COURSE OF THE THORACIC DUCT:

ABDOMINAL COURSE: Leaving the cisterna, the duct passes through the aortic orifice of the diaphragm, having the vena azygos on its right.

THORACIC COURSE: It runs up in the posterior mediastinum, having the azygos vein on its right and the aorta on its left side. Behind it are the vertebrae, the right intercostal arteries, and the hemiazygos and accessory hemiazygos veins. In front are the oesophagus, diaphragm, and pericardium. The duct, on reaching the 7th thoracic vertebra, begins to cross to the left. It does so very obliquely, reaching the left side at the level of the 5th thoracic vertebra, having crossed behind the oesophagus. It now runs up along the left border of the oesophagus medial to the pleura and behind the left subclavian artery into the neck.

CERVICAL COURSE: In the neck the duct forms an arch which reaches as high as the 7th cervical vertebra. The duct arches behind the 'carotid system' and in front of the 'vertebral system' (Wright), i.e., it passes behind the common carotid, internal jugular, and vagus, and in front of the vertebral artery, vein, and the sympathetic trunk. As the duct arches to the left it also crosses the scalenus anterior and phrenic nerve and the transverse cervical and transverse scapular arteries (*Fig.* 337).

TERMINATION: It usually ends as a single vessel by entering the junction of the left internal jugular and subclavian veins. The opening is guarded by valves to prevent regurgitation of blood into the duct. The duct sometimes divides into two, one vessel

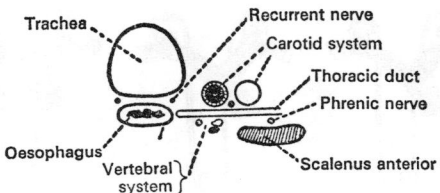

Fig. 337.—Relationship of termination of thoracic duct.

entering the veins on the right side of the head and neck. This is important in wounds of the duct. It used to be thought that if the duct were severed the injury would be fatal. This is not so, for after leaking lymph for a while the patient usually recovers. This indicates that there exist numerous communications with the venous system whereby the lymph in the thoracic duct may enter the circulation.

TRIBUTARIES:

In the Abdomen: The duct receives on either side a trunk from the lateral intercostal lymph-glands of the lower six spaces.

In the Thorax: It receives:
1. A trunk from either side draining the upper lumbar glands which pierces the crus of the diaphragm to join the duct.
2. Efferents from the posterior mediastinal glands.
3. Efferents from the lateral intercostal glands of the upper six left spaces.

In the Neck: It receives:
1. The left jugular lymph-trunk from the left side of the head and neck.
2. The left subclavian lymph-trunk from the left upper limb.
    It may receive:
3. The left bronchomediastinal trunk from the left side of the thorax.

ANOMALIES OF THE THORACIC DUCT: This important channel, discovered by Eustachius (1563), is within the domain of the modern surgeon. It requires protection and the appreciation of the possibility of, and practical implications of, the existence of anomalies.

DEVELOPMENT: At the end of the 2nd month the thoracic duct is a bilateral structure, that on the right lying between the azygos vein and the aorta, and that on the left between the aorta and the hemiazygos. These two channels are connected by many communications passing mainly behind but also in front of the great vessel. Each thoracic duct enters the respective innominate vein (*Fig.* 338).

344 A SYNOPSIS OF SURGICAL ANATOMY

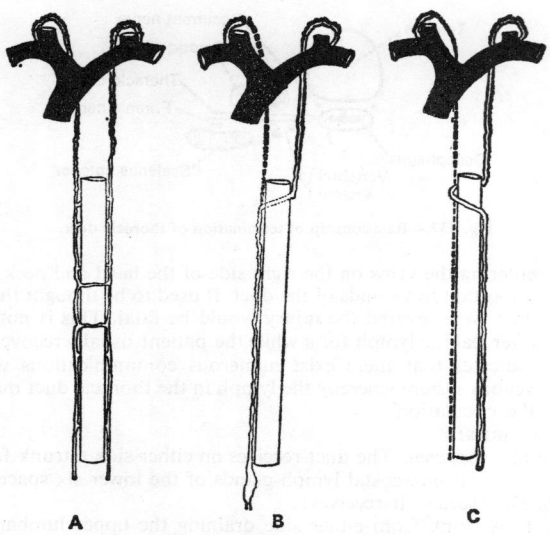

Fig. 338.—The diagram shows the thoracic duct. A, In the 30-mm. embryo. B, The adult pattern. C, An abnormal duct. (*Re-drawn by Dr. E. A. Thomas from Fig.* 3, *H. Butler and K. Balankura,* 'Anat. Rec.' 113, 414.)

The definitive channel as usually described is made up below of part of the right primitive vessel and a retro-aortic communication to what was originally the left duct. It is apparent that many variations may occur. Davis[1] in his classic study described numerous departures from the normal, e.g., (i) the primitive condition persists; (ii) the duct may be double in part and open into the venous system: (*a*) on the left or (*b*) on the right; (iii) the duct may divide into two in its upper part, one branch going left, the other right; (iv) the primitive condition may persist on one or other side.

The duct may terminate singly (77 per cent), doubly (9 per cent), triply (9 per cent), and quadruply (in 5 per cent).

Quite frequently the duct ends in other veins than in the left angulus venosus, e.g., on the left side in the subclavian, internal jugular, or vertebral; on the right in the angulus venosus, the internal jugular, or the subclavian.

[1] Davis, *Am. Jour. Anat.*, 1915, 17, 211.

LYMPHATICS

Right Lymph-duct: This is a short vessel 1·25–2·5 cm. long which runs down on the scalenus anterior to join the junction of the right internal jugular and subclavian veins. It is formed by the union of the right jugular, subclavian, and bronchomediastinal trunks (*Fig.* 339). These vessels may all open separately into the junction between the right subclavian and internal jugular veins.

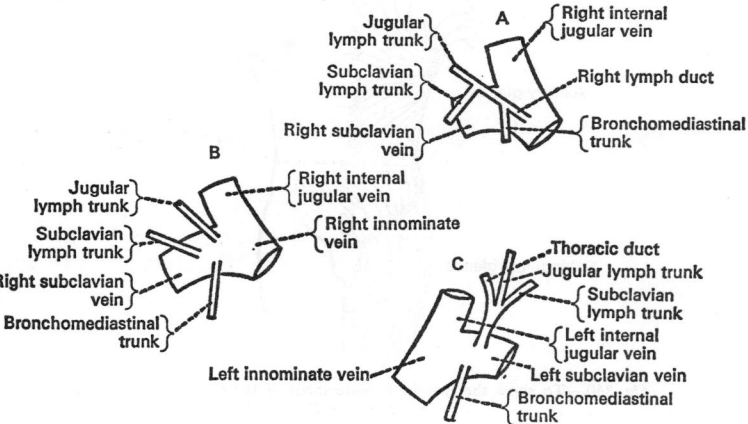

Fig. 339.—Terminations of the great lymph-trunks. A and B, on the right side. C, on the left side.

THE LYMPH PLEXUS ON THE DEEP FASCIA

This is made up of a ramification of lymph-vessels found on the superficial surface of the deep fascia throughout the body. The lymphatic plexus lying on the fascia covering the pectoralis major is thus merely a part of this system. It is important to realize that the lymph from the skin and its appendages drains in the first instance to the plexus of the deep fascia. In cancer of an appendage of the skin, e.g., the breast, radical operation implies, *inter alia*, the removal of that part of the plexus of the deep fascia which is in the neighbourhood of the breast, i.e., the whole of the fascia covering the pectoralis major (*see* p. 36).

THE LYMPHATIC WATERSHEDS OF THE SKIN

Sampson Handley[1] has shown that the lymphatic drainage of the skin and its appendages falls naturally into six great territories. A vertical line through the sagittal plane of the body divides the lymphatic drainage of

[1] *Modern Operative Surgery*, 1924, 424. London.

346 A SYNOPSIS OF SURGICAL ANATOMY

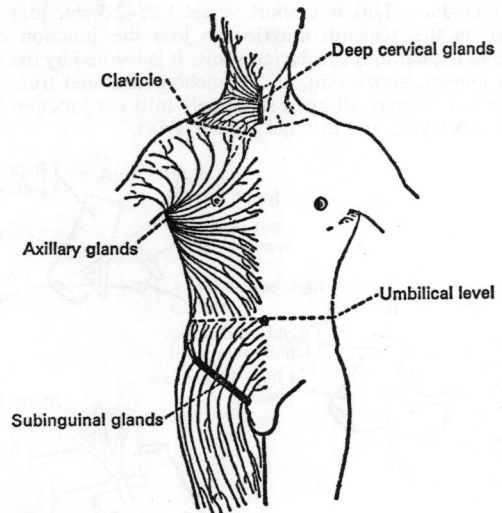

Fig. 340.—To show the lymphatic watersheds of the skin. (*Re-drawn from Sampson Handley.*)

the skin into three areas on each side. There is some communication across the middle line, but it is not free (*Fig.* 340).

The three areas on each side of the body are demarcated from each other by two horizontal lines, one at the level of the clavicle, the other at the level of the umbilicus. These lines are the lymphatic watersheds, and the skin lymph flows in a direction away from them. Each line also represents the meeting-place of two adjacent territories, so that cancer situated on one of these lines may spread by two routes along the lymphatics running away from the watershed. Similarly a cancer situated anywhere in the middle line of the surface of the body may spread in at least two directions because of the lymphatic communication across the midline. Cancer situated at the umbilicus may spread in four directions, viz., towards both axillae and both groins, as lymphatics draining to these glands come into communication at the umbilicus. The importance of these facts is realized when it is remembered that the treatment of cancer is removal of the growth itself *and also removal of the lymphatics and glands which drain the area in which the cancer is situated.*

Chapter XXVIII

IMPORTANT RELATIONS

HILUM OF THE LUNG: From before backwards:
    Vein
    Artery
    Bronchus.

HILUM OF THE KIDNEY: From before backwards:
    Vein
    Artery
    Ureter.

HILUM OF THE LIVER: From before backwards:
    Hepatic duct
    Hepatic artery
    Portal vein.

INTERCOSTAL VESSELS AND NERVES: From above down:
    Vein
    Artery
    Nerve.

OBTURATOR VESSELS AND NERVES: From above down:
    Nerve
    Artery
    Vein.

FEMORAL SHEATH: From medial to lateral:
    Femoral canal
    Femoral vein
    Femoral artery.

AORTIC ORIFICE OF THE DIAPHRAGM: From right to left:
    Azygos vein
    Thoracic duct
    Aorta.

OESOPHAGEAL ORIFICE OF THE DIAPHRAGM: From before back:
    Left vagus
    Oesophagus
    Right vagus.

348 A SYNOPSIS OF SURGICAL ANATOMY

PUDENDAL (ALCOCK'S) CANAL: From above down:
  Dorsal nerve of penis
  Internal pudendal artery
  Perineal division of internal pudendal nerve.

ANTECUBITAL FOSSA: From medial to lateral (N.A.T.):
  Median nerve
  Brachial artery
  Biceps tendon.

FRONT OF WRIST: From medial to lateral:
  Flexor carpi ulnaris
  Ulnar nerve
  Ulnar artery
  Flexor sublimis
  Palmaris longus with median nerve beneath it
  Flexor carpi radialis
  Radial artery.

BACK OF WRIST: From lateral to medial:
  Abductor pollicis longus
  Extensor pollicis brevis
  Extensores carpi radialis longus and brevis
  Extensor pollicis longus
  Extensores communis digitorum and indicis proprius
  Extensor minimi digiti
  Extensor carpi ulnaris.

UNDER SUPERIOR EXTENSOR RETINACULUM: From medial to lateral:
  Tibialis anterior
  Extensor longus hallucis
  Anterior tibial artery
  Deep peroneal nerve
  Extensor digitorum communis
  Peroneus tertius.

UNDER FLEXOR RETINACULUM: From medial to lateral:
  Tibialis posterior
  Flexor digitorum longus
  Posterior tibial artery
  Posterior tibial nerve
  Flexor longus hallucis.

UPPER SURFACE OF THE TIBIA: From before back:
  Transverse ligament
  Medial meniscus (anterior end)
  Anterior cruciate ligament

IMPORTANT RELATIONS

Lateral meniscus (anterior end)
Spines of the tibia
Lateral meniscus (posterior end)
Medial meniscus (posterior end)
Posterior cruciate ligament.

SUPERIOR ORBITAL FISSURE: Above the two heads of the lateral rectus:
Fourth nerve
Frontal and lacrimal branches of ophthalmic division of fifth nerve
Between the two heads of the lateral rectus: in the following order from above down:
Upper division third nerve
Nasociliary nerve
Lower division third nerve
Sixth nerve.

JUGULAR FORAMEN: From before back:
Inferior petrosal sinus
Glossopharyngeal nerve
Vagus and accessory nerves
Transverse (lateral) sinus.

IN THE MIDDLE OF THE FEMORAL TRIANGLE: From before back:
Femoral artery
Femoral vein
Profunda vein
Profunda artery.

IN THE SPERMATIC CORD: From before back (*Fig.* 341):
Pampiniform plexus of veins
Fibrous remnant of processus vaginalis or hernial sac
Ductus deferens.

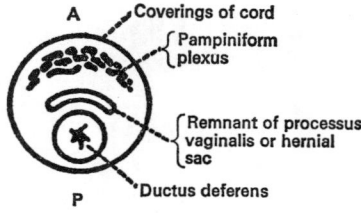

Fig. 341.—Spermatic cord in section. A, Anterior. P, Posterior.

Part II

ANATOMY OF THE ABNORMAL

Chapter XXIX

THE ANATOMY OF CONGENITAL ERRORS

Developmental defects are of considerable social, economic, and surgical importance. A large number of prenatal deaths are due to congenital defects, 2 per cent are recognized at the time of birth and many pass undetected at that time.

I. ERRORS IN THE DEVELOPMENT OF THE HYPOPHYSIS (PITUITARY BODY)

This is developed from two separate parts: (1) A downgrowth from the floor of the third ventricle forms the infundibulum and the nervous part; (2) An upgrowth (Rathke's pouch) from the roof of the primitive pharynx forms the anterior part. The site where this upgrowth took place is represented in the adult on the posterior border of the nasal septum, and may be marked by a recess—a remnant of the pouch of Rathke (*Fig.* 342). In the region of the tuberculum sellae in the anterior fossa of the

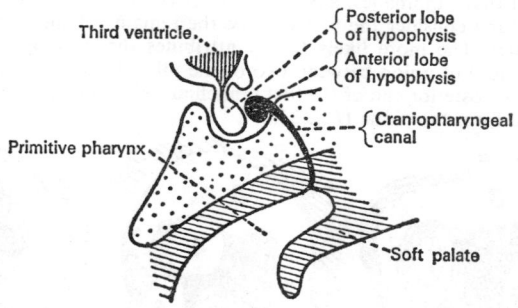

Fig. 342.—Schematic representation of development of hypophysis. The surrounding parts have been shown at a more advanced developmental stage to make the picture clearer.

skull there is sometimes a foramen—craniopharyngeal canal—which marks the upper part of the canal which is made by the upgrowth which goes to form the anterior lobe of the hypophysis. At the site of the pouch of Rathke or along the craniopharyngeal canal, cysts may grow from portions of the upgrowth which have become sequestrated. These are lined with squamous epithelium and are histologically adamantinomata. When they occur in the skull:

354 A SYNOPSIS OF SURGICAL ANATOMY

1. They are likely to damage the hypophysis and cause interference with its function, resulting sometimes in a very fat backward individual without secondary sexual characters—dystrophia adiposogenitalis (Fröhlich's syndrome).
2. They become infiltrated with lime and may be detected with the X-rays in 80 per cent of cases in which such a cyst exists (Cushing).
3. They may press on the optic chiasma and cause bitemporal hemianopia.

II. PRE-AURICULAR FISTULAE[1]

On rare occasions fistulous openings occur on the anterior portion of the prominent rim of the ear, i.e., on the root of the helix. Their incidence is just under 1 per cent and they are bilateral in 23 per cent of cases.

Sir James Paget drew attention in England to these fistulae in 1878.

Sir Arthur Keith stated that a close relationship exists between such fistulae and accessory auricular appendages, and the same observer noted their association with other developmental anomalies, e.g., cleft palate and spina bifida. The fistulae show a strong tendency to occur in different members of the same family.

AETIOLOGY: Observers are agreed as to the developmental nature of these anomalies, albeit they disagree as to their precise genesis. Many consider the fistula to be the remains of the first branchial cleft. The more likely theory attributes the opening to a partial failure of union between two of the tubercles which appear round the posterior end of the first branchial cleft, and which are destined to form the pinna (*Fig.* 343).

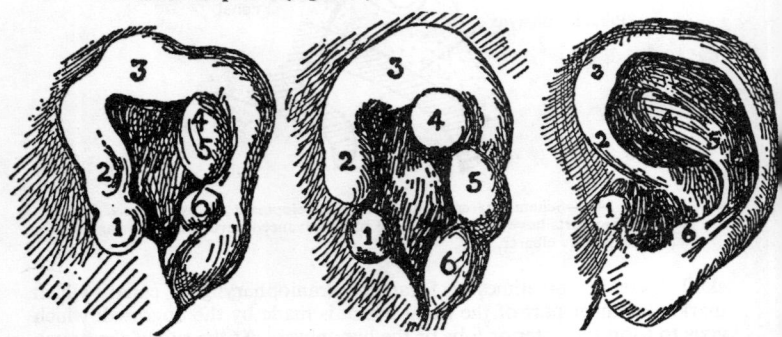

Fig. 343.—Development of auricle. The six tubercles are shown. The usual type of pre-auricular fistula is due to a faulty fusion of tubercles 1 and 2. (*Re-drawn from Prentiss and Arey.*)

[1] For the facts in this section I am indebted to the article on 'Pre-auricular Fistulae', by F. A. R. Stammers, *Br. J. Surg.*, 1926, 14, 359.

THE ANATOMY OF CONGENITAL ERRORS 355

The tubercles are six in number and each takes some part in the formation of the pinna:

Tubercle 1 forms the tragus
" 2 " " crus helicis
" 3 " " helix
" 4 " " antihelix
" 5 " " antitragus
" 6 " " lobule

Now though it is conceivable that any adjacent pair of these tubercles may fail to fuse completely, statistics show that a partial failure of fusion occurs most commonly between tubercles 1 and 2, i.e., such fistulae are found opening between the tragus and crus helicis or on this crus (*Fig.* 344). A bristle can usually be passed for

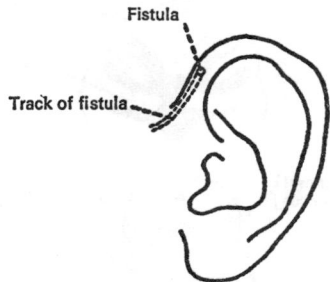

Fig. 344.—Schematic representation of a pre-auricular fistula. The fistulous opening is shown, and also the sinus leading from it. In the figure the orifice of the fistula is shown 1 cm. too high up.

about 0·8 cm. into the fistula. When quiescent it is scarcely noticeable and does not discharge, though a bead of fluid may be expressible. The fistulous track passes downwards and forwards, and when its orifice is blocked the retained secretion may cause a small lump in front of the ear, which may burst, forming an ulcer which will not heal unless the fistulous track be completely excised.

III. HARE-LIP AND CLEFT PALATE

Development of the Face: The face is formed from five processes which surround an opening—the stomodeum—at the anterior end of the embryo (*Fig.* 345). These are: (1) Frontonasal—a single process; (2) Maxillary—one on each side; (3) Mandibular—one on each side.

FRONTONASAL PROCESS: The appearance of the olfactory pits divides the frontonasal process into three: a median—the medial nasal process; and two lateral—the lateral nasal processes. The medial nasal process develops a bulge each side known as the globular process.

MEDIAL NASAL AND GLOBULAR PROCESSES: Form: (1) The septum of the nose; (2) The philtrum of the upper lip; (3) The premaxilla.

LATERAL NASAL PROCESS: Forms the side of the nose. It takes no part in the formation of the upper lip.

MAXILLARY PROCESS: Forms: (1) The cheek and whole upper lip except the philtrum; (2) Most of the upper jaw; (3) The palate.

MANDIBULAR PROCESS: Forms the lower jaw.

These processes fuse round the stomodeum, the site of the future mouth, to form the face.

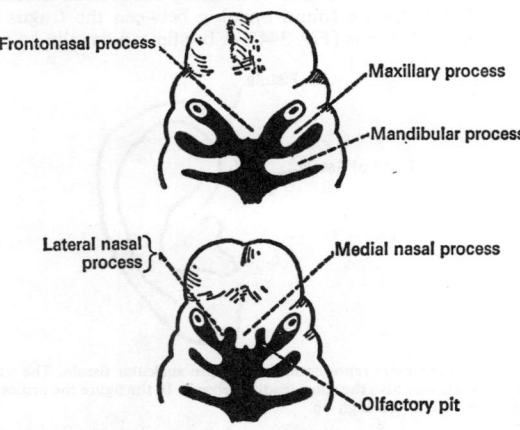

Fig. 345.—Development of face.

Anomalies of Development of the Face: Errors in the fusion of these processes may result in:

Imperfect fusion[1]
- 1. Hare-lip
  - a. Upper (i) central or (ii) lateral
  - b. Lower—central
- 2. Macro- and microstoma
- 3. Cleft palate

Inclusions along the fusion lines
- 1. Sequestration dermoids
- 2. Fibrochondromata

The positions of the original clefts on the fully formed face are seen in *Fig.* 346.

---
[1] There are other types of imperfect fusion than those mentioned. They are purposely excluded because of their great rarity.

THE ANATOMY OF CONGENITAL ERRORS

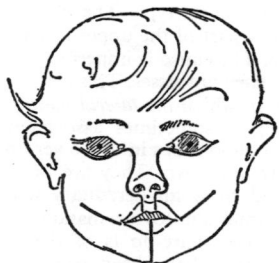

Fig. 346.—The facial fusion lines.

IMPERFECT FUSION:

HARE-LIP:

a. Upper Lip (Fig. 347):

Central: Very rare. Is exactly central. It is due to failure of fusion of the two bulbous extremities of the medial nasal process (the globular processes).

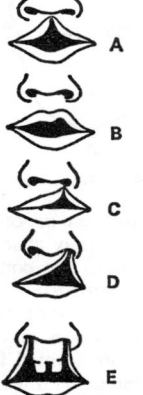

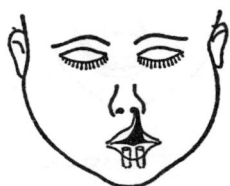

Fig. 348.—Inferior labial sinuses.

Fig. 347.—Types of hare-lip. A, Central hare-lip. B, Hare-lip shown by an indentation of the red margin only. C, Partial hare-lip. D, Complete hare-lip. E, Double hare-lip.

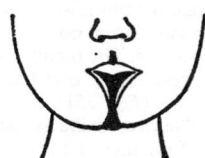

Fig. 349.—Lower hare-lip.

Lateral: The common type. The cleft is between the philtrum (the central part of the upper lip) and the lateral part of the upper lip. The cause is imperfect fusion of the medial nasal and maxillary processes. This cleft is therefore due to failure of fusion in which *the lateral nasal process is not concerned.*

Upper hare-lip is sometimes associated with the presence of two small blind tubes in the lower lip (*Fig.* 348). Their cause is entirely unknown. They are lined with squamous epithelium, and show an hereditary tendency. They are called inferior labial sinuses or mandibular recesses (Sutton).

b. *Lower Lip:* Lower hare-lip is of the greatest rarity. Approximately 100 cases have been recorded. It is exactly central. It is due to failure of fusion of the two mandibular processes (*Fig.* 349).

MACROSTOMA (*Fig.* 350, A): The mouth is formed by the fusion of medial nasal, maxillary, and mandibular processes. Imperfect fusion of maxillary and mandibular processes causes a mouth which is much too large—*macrostoma*. Imperfect fusion is usually on one side only, so that the mouth is *asymmetrical* in addition.

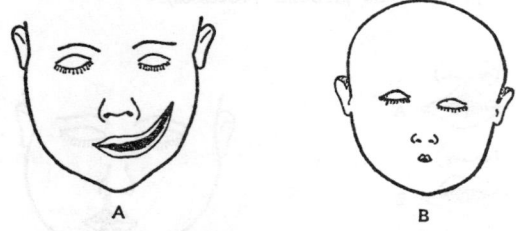

Fig. 350.—A, Macrostoma. B, Microstoma.

MICROSTOMA (*Fig.* 350, B): Excessive fusion of these processes causes a mouth which is too small or may be entirely absent. In this variety all the processes forming the mouth are concerned, so that the abnormally small mouth is *symmetrical*.

CLEFT PALATE: This condition is due to a failure of fusion between the single medial nasal and the two maxillary processes, or between the two latter only. The palate is therefore formed from three processes. The medial nasal forms the premaxilla. Each maxillary process forms one half of the remainder of the hard and soft palates (*Fig.* 351).

The premaxilla is the front part of the upper jaw and carries the four incisor teeth, though sometimes it may only carry two.

Cleft palate may be: (1) Complete; or (2) Incomplete.

THE ANATOMY OF CONGENITAL ERRORS 359

Complete: There is a gap between the two halves of the palate in its entire length, so that nose and mouth are one cavity. In front this gap may pass on one side of the premaxilla or on both

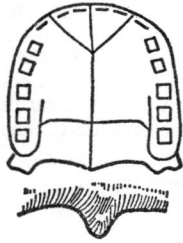

Fig. 351.—The normal palate.

sides. In the latter case the premaxilla is not attached to the palate at all, but hangs down from the septum of the nose some distance in front of (anterior to) where it ought to be (*Fig.* 352).

Incomplete: The two halves of the palate fuse together from before back. The last parts to fuse are the two halves of the uvula. Incomplete fusion therefore may involve: (1) Uvula only—bifid uvula; (2) The whole length of the soft palate; (3) The whole length of the soft palate and the posterior part of the hard palate.

In incomplete fusion, then, the anterior part of the palate is always formed.

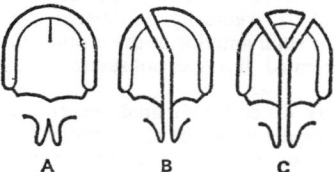

Fig. 352.—Types of cleft palate. A, Cleft of soft palate. B, Complete cleft of palate diverging to one side of premaxilla. C, Complete cleft of palate separating premaxilla from palate.

INCLUSIONS ALONG THE FUSION LINES. TUMOURS:

Epithelium may be isolated in one of the clefts and form a cyst after birth. This is a *sequestration dermoid*. Portions of the deeper tissues, cartilage, or connective tissue may be isolated in one of the cleft lines. This gives rise to a solid tumour—*fibrochondroma*. The determining characteristic of both tumours is that they appear in the line of one of the original clefts (*Fig.* 353). Much the commonest of these tumours is a cyst at the outer angle of the orbit; such a cyst may lie in a depression in the bony wall of the skull, and is sometimes attached to the dura.

DERMOID CYSTS OF THE NOSE: Nydeel and Masson[1] give an account of dermoid cysts of the nose. They quote Grünwald's[2] theory of their development. In the connective tissue covering the cartilage of the nose at birth, the frontal and nasal bones develop. Enclosed between these cartilaginous and bony layers is the prenasal space which extends to the tip of the nose and contains

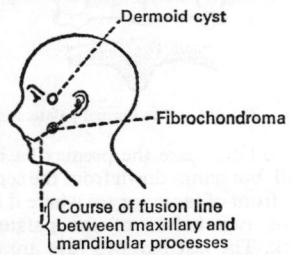

Fig. 353.—Showing common sites of tumours which may arise in connexion with facial fusion lines.

a tubular extension of the dura. Between frontal and nasal bones is a small fontanelle where skin and dura are in contact until separated by formation of bone in the membrane of the fontanelle, the dural communication passing through an aperture, the foramen caecum, which is eventually obliterated except for its internal aperture in the skull anterior to the crista galli. This dural process becomes obliterated. If it does not several developmental anomalies are possible:

a. The tube may distend with fluid—encephalocele.

b. Portions of ectoderm may be entrapped in the prenasal space and form sinuses or dermoid cysts. Thus hair may project from a sinus at the tip of the nose, or a swelling may occur on the dorsum or side of that organ—a dermoid cyst. It will be firmly attached at its base as it extends under the nasal and perhaps also the frontal bones. It will be lined as other dermoids are by squamous epithelium with skin glands in its wall. It may appear at birth or only in later life or it may not be externally apparent. A local removal will be inadequate and extirpation difficult.

[1] Nydeel, C. C., jun., and Masson, J. K., *Ann. Surg.*, 1959, 150, 1007.
[2] Grünwald, L., 'Beiträge zur Kenntnis kongenitaler Geschwülste und Missbildungen an Ohr und Nase', *Z. Ohrenheilk.*, 1910, 60, 270.

IV. BRANCHIAL CYSTS AND FISTULAE

The neck and pharynx are formed from five bars called visceral or branchial arches (*Fig.* 354). Between the bars are depressions both internally and externally. Those internally are called visceral pouches, those externally are the visceral clefts. Between the two is the cleft membrane, which is lined externally with squamous epithelium and internally with columnar epithelium. Each arch has a plate of cartilage, a muscle mass, a nerve, and an artery.

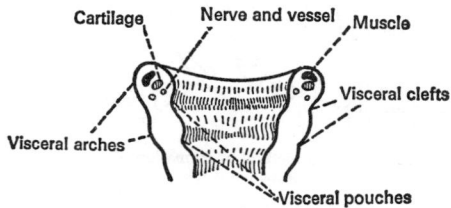

Fig. 354.—Showing arrangement and structure of visceral arches.

The first arch is the mandibular (which takes so large a part in the formation of the face). Its nerve is the mandibular branch of the fifth. The external maxillary is its artery.

The second arch is the hyoid arch. Its nerve is the facial. Its artery is the external carotid.

The third arch is the thyrohyoid arch. Its nerve is the glossopharyngeal. Its artery is the internal carotid.

The fourth and fifth arches are unnamed.

CERVICAL SINUS (OF HIS): The growth of the second arch is much quicker than that of the arches below, so that it soon overhangs them, forming a deep groove—*the cervical sinus* (*Fig.* 355).

Ultimately the overgrown second arch meets the fifth and the two fuse. Now the cervical sinus is a buried space lined by squamous epithelium. It disappears entirely. Should a part of the space persist, it will form a branchial cyst. Should the second arch fail to fuse with the fifth, an opening will be found on the neck at birth—a branchial fistula. Such an orifice will be found along the line of the anterior border of the sternomastoid muscle, its commonest site being just above the sternoclavicular joint. The branchial cyst or fistula will always be separated from the pharynx by a septum which represents the remains of the cleft membrane. In cases of branchial cyst or fistula there may be a diverticulum from the pharynx representing the visceral pouch. This diverticulum often opens just behind the tonsil, and is always separated from the branchial cyst or fistula by a membrane (cleft membrane). His has stated that in those

362 A SYNOPSIS OF SURGICAL ANATOMY

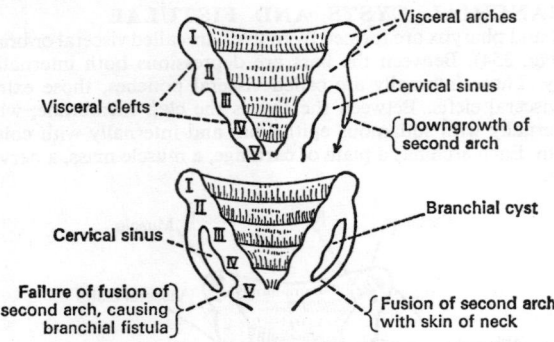

Fig. 355.—Figure illustrating method of formation of a branchial cyst and branchial fistula.

cases where a branchial fistula was reported to lead into the pharynx the surgeon had probably himself destroyed, with his probe, the partition representing the cleft membrane.

In 1956 Frazer showed that the cervical sinus is obliterated from its depth and not by fusion of its edges. A stage is thus reached when the cervical sinus is represented by two depressions, the upper of which communicates with the second cleft and the lower with the third and fourth. This finding adds to the complexities concerning the embryological possibilities connected with the origin of branchial fistulae. There is no final agreement on this matter.

Course of a Branchial Fistula (*Fig.* 356): As the fistula is the remains of the cervical sinus it is below the second arch, and as it usually arises in connexion with the second cleft, it is above the third arch. Now the

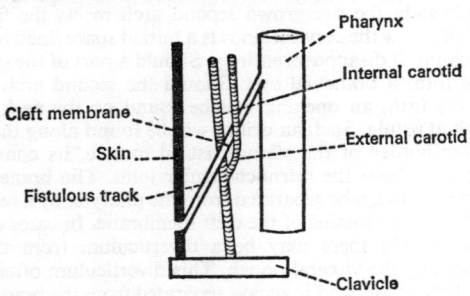

Fig. 356.—Course of a branchial fistula.

nerve of the second arch is the facial, its artery the external carotid. The nerve of the third arch is the ninth, its artery the internal carotid. From its opening on the skin the fistula passes subcutaneously to the level of the upper border of the thyroid cartilage where it pierces the deep fascia. The fistula then passes beneath the posterior belly of the digastric muscle and the stylohyoid, crosses the hypoglossal nerve and internal jugular vein, to traverse the fork of the carotid bifurcation, the external carotid being superficial and the internal carotid deep. It then crosses the glossopharyngeal nerve and the stylopharyngeus muscle to pierce the superior constrictor and to open on the posterior pillar of the fauces behind the tonsil. Wilson[1] stresses certain other features:

1. The site of the opening on the skin surface is not an indication of its cleft origin, as the second, third, and fourth clefts open into the cervical sinus.
2. The so-called 'complete' fistula has a muscular coat continuous externally with the platysma and internally with the palatopharyngeus. If this muscle coat is well developed the fistulous opening is pulled on and puckers on swallowing.
3. Only a part of the vestigial track may remain. Thus a sinus presenting externally may connect with only a short track. Blind internal sinuses resulting from persistence of the pharyngeal pouch rarely cause symptoms and are probably commoner than reported.
4. Fistulae are bilateral in at least 30 per cent of cases. Cysts are usually unilateral.
5. There is a definite familial tendency, and other congenital abnormalities may coexist, such as pre-auricular sinuses, or subcutaneous cartilaginous nodules on one side corresponding in situation to a fistulous opening on the other.

Branchial Cysts: These occur along the line of the anterior border of the sternomastoid, usually in the region of the angle of the jaw. Their relations are similar to those of the fistula. The cyst is lined with squamous epithelium (like the cervical sinus). The fistula is lined with squamous epithelium up to the partition (cleft membrane); medial (internal) to the partition it is lined with ciliated columnar epithelium (which lines the inner surface of the cleft membrane and the visceral pouch).

Anomalies of the First Branchial Cleft: Rankow and Hanford[2] draw attention to such defects. They point out that the ectodermal portion of the first branchial cleft becomes a modified skin and takes part in the formation of the adult external auditory meatus. The corresponding entodermal portion of the first pharyngeal pouch becomes the tympanic cavity of the middle ear and the Eustachian

[1] Wilson, C. P., *Ann. R. Coll. Surg.*, 1955, 17, 1.
[2] Rankow, R. M., and Hanford J. M., *Surgery Gynec. Obstet.*, 1953, 96, 102.

tube. Anomalies of the first branchial cleft are very rare, but their course is so entirely different from fistulae arising from the second cleft that an understanding of the anatomy is implicit to their correct surgical handling. The line of obliteration of the first branchial cleft runs parallel with the mandible and extends from the external auditory meatus to just below the mid-point of the jaw bone. If the skin edges

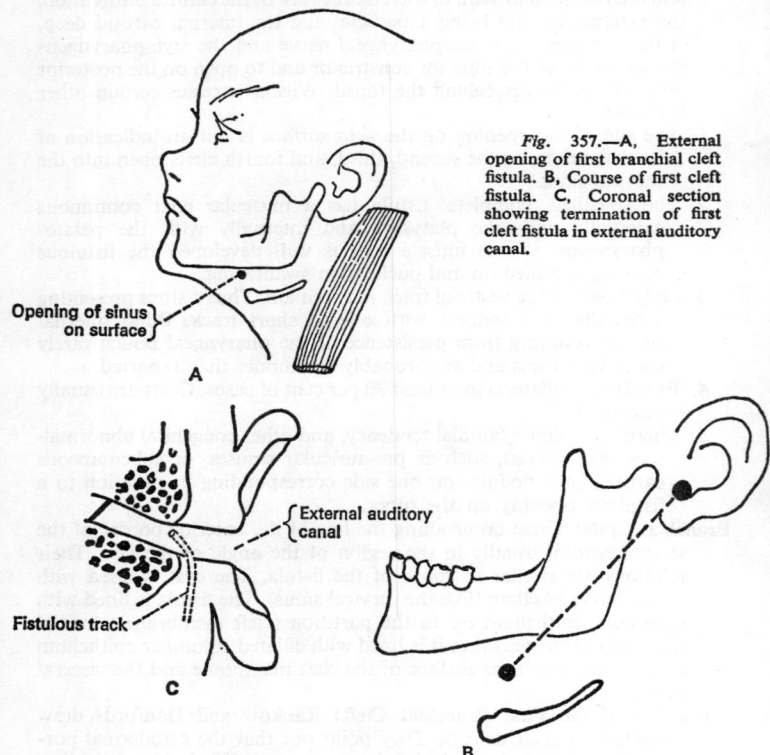

Fig. 357.—A, External opening of first branchial cleft fistula. B, Course of first cleft fistula. C, Coronal section showing termination of first cleft fistula in external auditory canal.

of the first ectodermal groove fuse in the middle of its course, a skin-lined tunnel is formed which is lined throughout by squamous epithelium. The external opening of this channel is situated between the lower border of the mandible and the hyoid bone.

The fistulous track passes inward and upward superficial to the

THE ANATOMY OF CONGENITAL ERRORS 365

posterior belly of the digastric muscle, through the parotid gland and extends to the junction of the bony and cartilaginous portions of the external auditory canal (*Figs.* 357 and 358). Its relationship to the facial nerve varies, being either superficial or deep to the branches of the facial nerve. It would be expected that the track would be superficial to the facial nerve (which is the nerve of the second arch) but the branches of that nerve are taken by their muscles as they migrate to the superficial region of the face over the surface of the first arch, hence the variable relationship of the first cleft to the branches of the facial nerve.

Any portion of the track may persist to form a branchial cyst (of the first cleft) anywhere along its course. Such squamous lined cysts may thus be found in the parotid gland or in the submandibular region.

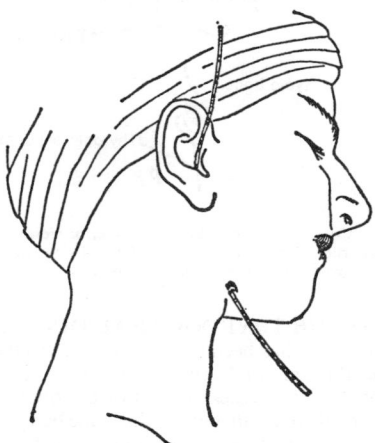

Fig. 358.—Complete auro-cervical fistula.

V. DEVELOPMENTAL ERRORS OF THE THYROID GLAND

Thyroglossal Duct: At the junction of the anterior two-thirds with the posterior one-third of the tongue, there is in the middle line a small depression, the foramen caecum. From the site marked by the foramen there grows down, at an early stage of fetal life, a solid column of cells. This becomes canalized, forming the thyroglossal duct. From this duct is formed the thyroid gland.

COURSE OF THE DUCT: It passes down exactly in the middle line between the genioglossi muscles, as far as the upper border of the thyroid cartilage (*Fig.* 359): it then diverges slightly to one or other side of the middle line, and its course is represented after birth by the pyramidal lobe and the band of muscle or fibrous tissue connecting that lobe to the hyoid.

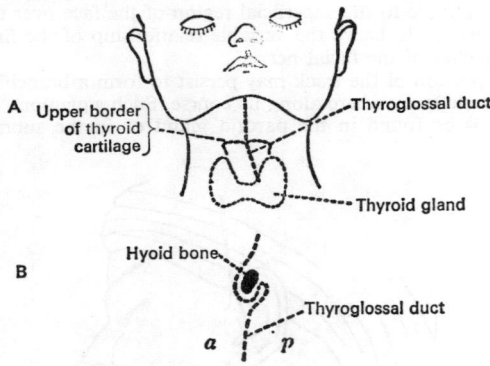

Fig. 359.—A, Course of thyroglossal duct, anterior view; note divergence to left below upper border of thyroid cartilage. B, Lateral view, showing relationship between duct and hyoid bone. *a*, Anterior; *p*, Posterior.

RELATION OF THE THYROGLOSSAL DUCT TO THE HYOID BONE: The point has been long contended whether the duct passes in front of, through, or behind the body of the hyoid. Frazer has shown that the duct passes in front of the body of the hyoid, then takes a recurved course up behind this bone before continuing down. Actually it is the direction of development of the hyoid bone which displaces the tract forwards. In removing the remains of this duct it is essential to remove the part behind the hyoid to ensure total removal. Stiles practised and advised a resection of the middle portion of the body of the hyoid to make certain of this.

ANOMALIES OF THE DUCT: These are : (1) Thyroglossal cysts; (2) Accessory thyroids; (3) Ectopia thyroideae.

THYROGLOSSAL CYSTS: These may occur anywhere on the line of the duct (*Fig.* 360). They are often connected to the foramen caecum by remains of the duct. The removal of the cyst entails the removal of this connexion, or recurrence takes place.

Above the thyroid cartilage cysts, like the duct, are exactly central.

THE ANATOMY OF CONGENITAL ERRORS 367

Below the thyroid cartilage cysts, like the duct, are slightly to one side, usually to the left (Hamilton Bailey[1]).

THYROGLOSSAL FISTULAE: As the thyroglossal duct *never* opens on the skin of the neck at any stage of its development, a congenital thyroglossal fistula is impossible. Such fistulae are therefore of secondary origin due to the bursting or opening of a thyroglossal cyst.

Carcinoma of the Thyroglossal Duct: This condition is rare. In 1964 only 22 cases had been recorded in a review of the literature. All but 1 case were adenocarcinoma of thyroid origin due to inclusion of thyroid tissue in the wall of the duct.

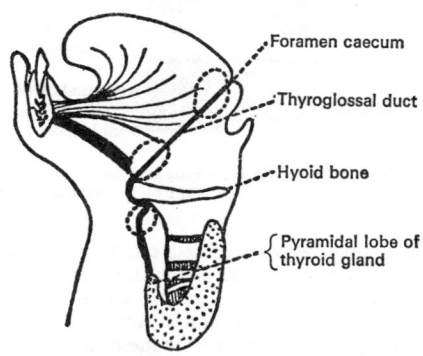

Fig. 360.—Thyroglossal duct, and sites occupied by thyroglossal cysts.

ANOMALIES OF THE GLAND: Accessory or aberrant thyroid tissue may, like thyroglossal cysts, occur in a median situation in the line of development of the gland, in association with a normal thyroid gland. Thus thyroid tissue may occur at the foramen caecum, in the tongue, at the level of the hyoid bone, etc.

Ectopic thyroid tissue lies somewhere in the line of development of the gland other than the normal situation. It is often the only thyroid tissue present. A lingual thyroid lies in the base of the tongue in the region of the foramen caecum. It is rare and in three-fourths of the cases it is the only thyroid tissue present—an ectopic thyroid. Such an ectopic thyroid may occupy a sub-hyoid position and simulate a cyst. Its removal may cause myxoedema. The exhibition of ^{131}I followed by a thyroid scanning will determine whether a normal thyroid exists.

A rare but important anomaly is the absence of one of the lateral lobes of the thyroid.

[1] *Demonstrations of Physical Signs in Clinical Surgery*, 1967, 177. Wright: Bristol.

VI. SPINA BIFIDA

Development of the Spinal Cord and Column

1. In the first days of intra-uterine existence a dorsal groove appears on the surface of the embryo—the neural groove (*Fig.* 361).

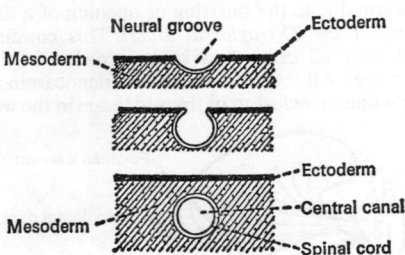

Fig. 361.—Development of spinal cord, showing how neural groove deepens to form cord, which becomes separated from skin by an ingrowth of mesoderm.

2. The neural groove becomes closed off, forming the neural canal. From the walls of this canal the entire central nervous system is developed. Its lumen persists as the central canal (spinal).
3. The neural canal becomes separated from the ectodermal covering of the body by an ingrowth of the mesoderm.
4. Anterior to the neural canal is a solid rod of cells, the notochord (*Fig.* 362).

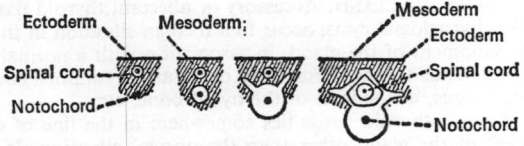

Fig. 362.—Diagrams showing development of vertebral body round notochord and growth of neural arch of vertebra round spinal cord.

5. Round the notochord the vertebral bodies develop.
6. From each of the bodies there extend two projections which grow round the neural canal to form the vertebral arch.
7. The two halves of the arch fuse first in the thoracic region. From there fusion extends up and down.
8. Failure of fusion, i.e., incompleteness of the vertebral arch, constitutes spina bifida.

Types of Spina Bifida:

1. RACHISCHISIS AND MYELOCELE: The neural canal remains open on the surface at stage 1 of development—the spinal cord is therefore exposed at birth on the surface of the body—*rachischisis*. This may be complete throughout the length of the cord or it may be partial. The partial variety is called *myelocele* (*Fig.* 363).

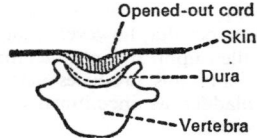

Fig. 363.—Myelocele or partial rachischisis.

2. MENINGOCELE, ETC.: The vertebral arches fail to fuse, so that there is a gap in the bony arch posteriorly, through which the membranes or cord and membranes project. This results in *meningocele* and *syringomyelocele* which are covered by skin. The *meningomyelocele* is only partly covered by skin, the fundus of the sac being covered by a vascular nerve tissue which is connected to the peripheral skin by a serous-like layer probably derived from the pia. This is the commonest type—several varieties exist (*Fig.* 364).

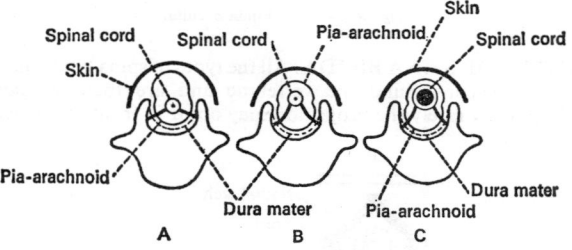

Fig. 364.—Types of spina bifida: A, Meningocele. B, Meningomyelocele. C, Syringomyelocele.

a. MENINGOCELE: The pia and arachnoid protrude as a swelling. The dura stops at the margin of the bony defect.
b. MENINGOMYELOCELE: The cord protrudes as well as the membranes, being pushed out by a collection of fluid anterior to it.
c. SYRINGOMYELOCELE: As (*b*), but the central canal of the cord is dilated to form a cavity filled with fluid.

3. **SPINA BIFIDA OCCULTA**: A small gap exists in one of the vertebral arches, usually in the lumbar or sacral regions. The gap is filled with fibrous tissue. The cord may be adherent to this fibrous tissue. There is, as a rule, no projection on the surface to indicate this defect, though a hairy spot or a tumour may exist. At one stage of growth the spinal cord fills the vertebral canal. Soon the cord lags behind, so that at birth it ends at the 3rd lumbar vertebra (*Fig.* 365). So far development has been normal. In cases of spina bifida occulta, however, usually about the ages 8 to 14, the cord is pulled upon by an attachment to the fibrous plug mentioned above, and this produces nervous symptoms, usually referred to the bladder as incontinence or retention of urine. Club-foot may occur.

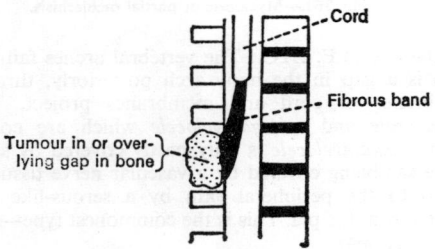

Fig. 365.—Spina bifida occulta.

4. **ANTERIOR SPINA BIFIDA**: All the types of spina bifida mentioned above occur behind the vertebrae and are therefore *posterior*. Extremely rarely the projection may occur in front of the vertebrae

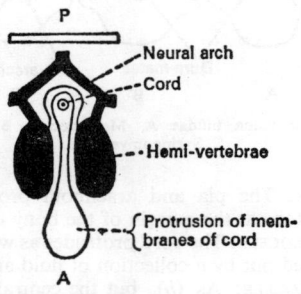

Fig. 366.—Anterior spina bifida. A, Anterior. P, Posterior.

THE ANATOMY OF CONGENITAL ERRORS

and is thought to be due to a defect in the development of the bodies, as a vertebral body consists at a very early stage of two halves which soon join (*Fig.* 366). The failure to join may result in a protrusion of membranes or cord and membranes. It occasionally occurs in the cervical region, where on opening the mouth the posterior wall of the pharynx may be seen to be pushed forward by the tumour. It may occur in the hollow of the sacrum behind the rectum.

VII. ENCEPHALOCELE

Protrusions of brain membranes or brain tissue sometimes occur. The cause is precisely similar to that of spina bifida, i.e., the formation of bone is defective in the skull just as the formation of the vertebral arches is defective in the spine. All are covered by skin.

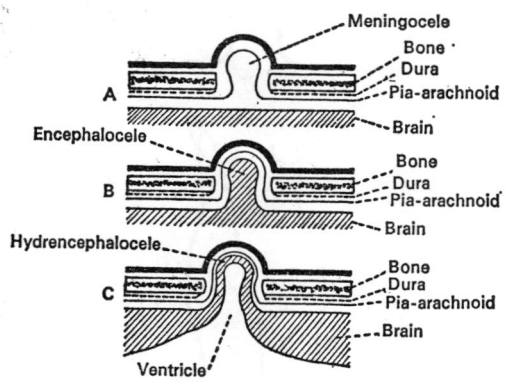

Fig. 367.—Congenital protrusions of cranial contents. A, Meningocele. B, Encephalocele. C, Hydrencephalocele.

Types of Encephalocele (*Fig.* 367):
1. MENINGOCELE: Protrusion of pia-arachnoid occurs through the gap in the bone. The dura stops at the bony margin.
2. ENCEPHALOCELE: The meningeal protrusion contains brain tissue.
3. HYDRENCEPHALOCELE: The brain tissue in the protrusion contains a portion of a ventricle of the brain.

VIII. CONGENITAL ERRORS OF THE BREAST

Development of the Breast: In the very early stages of development there appears on each side of the body an ectodermal ridge known as the 'Milchleisten' (Schultze). These lines extend from axilla to groin

(*Fig.* 368). In the human the whole of this ridge atrophies excepting only a small portion in each pectoral region from which the mammae arise. It is important to realize that these ridges consist of tissue which is potentially mammary, and that failure of the normal disappearance of all of these ridges, excepting such as forms the anlage of the normal breasts, will result in the individual being born with accessory breast tissue. It is also important to note that in the vast majority of cases such mammary tissue lies somewhere in the course of the 'Milchleisten', i.e., along a line extending from the hollow of the arm-pit to the inner part of Scarpa's triangle. The occasional occurrence of accessory breast tissue in situations such as the shoulder or buttock is not explicable on any known embryological data, and must be put down to some unusual developmental process whereby a portion of the milk ridge has become transferred to an ectopic site. Normally, then, that tiny portion of the milk ridge which is going to form the breast

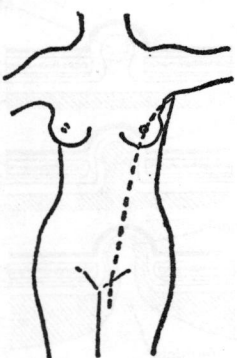

Fig. 368.—The milk line.

enlarges, projecting slightly on the skin and extending deeply in the shape of buds which form long slender tubes from which the ducts and secreting tissue of the breasts are formed. The nipple is either flat or depressed at birth; only later does it project above the surrounding skin.

Congenital Mammary Abnormalities:

1. AMASTIA:

   COMPLETE: An exceedingly rare condition of which only six cases have been recorded. The 'Milchleisten' entirely disappear and the individual is born with no mammary tissue or nipples.

   UNILATERAL: Only one nipple and breast exists. Its genesis is different from that of the bilateral condition, being ascribed to excessive pressure in utero of the arm against the chest region. This hypothesis is supported by the fact that the pectoral muscles of that side are often absent also.

2. POLYMASTIA: In this condition there is more than one breast on one or both sides. It is due to persistence of portions of the milk ridges which usually disappear. Such accessory breasts occur somewhere on this ridge, usually three or four inches below and medial to the normal nipple. In the majority of cases all that is seen is a rudimentary nipple, but it is of importance to realize that there is *always* breast tissue beneath such a nipple. On the other hand, the accessory organ may be well developed, and many instances are recorded of its being used for suckling. Such accessory organs may be single or multiple, symmetrical or asymmetrical. They may occur at the root of the thigh and even in the labium majus where cancer has been reported. Mugebauer reported the case of a patient with ten breasts.

Accessory breasts may exist without ducts. This is particularly the case in the axilla. As accessory mammary tissue is subject to the same physiological changes as normal breasts, swelling of such breasts, which cannot discharge their contents, may lead to great discomfort, and also to great difficulty in diagnosis. These breasts are often mistaken for tumours. We have seen one apparently normal breast which caused much trouble during lactation owing to an entire absence of milk ducts.

Instances are recorded where seepage of breast secretions from the skin overlying accessory breast tissue in the axilla relieves the tension when such tissue is physiologically active. This is understandable when it is recalled that the breasts are developed from modified sebaceous glands possibly of apocrine origin. Accessory mammary tissue in the axilla is very near the skin and feels like a lipoma. As fatty tumours in the axilla are excessively rare, such a mass is more likely to be mammary in origin. In 100,000 admissions to the New York post-graduate hospital no case of axillary lipoma was found (de Cholnoky). Lymph-glands lie deeper and are unlikely to lead to confusion in diagnosis.

3. POLYTHELIA: This condition results from imperfect development of *one* mammary rudiment, and it is not due to multiple rudiments like polymastia. The supernumerary nipples are situated irregularly over the breast and not on the milk ridge.

4. GYNAECOMASTIA: The occurrence of female breasts in the male. The condition is not very uncommon, and though occurring usually at first at adolescence it may develop at any time. Cases have been recorded where such breasts have functioned and have even at times been used for suckling infants.

Supernumerary breasts complete with nipple and areola have the same liability to cancer as normally placed mammae. On the other hand, accessory breast tissue devoid of nipple (aberrant breast tissue) has greater than normal susceptibility to this disease. Despite radical treatment, the prognosis in such cases is very bad.

IX. CONGENITAL ABNORMALITIES OF THE OESOPHAGUS

Development of the Oesophagus (*Fig.* 369): At a very early period the stomach is separated by a mere constriction from the primitive pharynx. This constriction is the future oesophagus. The oesophagus becomes lengthened owing to the development of the lungs, which elongate the constriction greatly. Previous to this elongation, however, the trachea and oesophagus form a single structure. This becomes divided into two by the ingrowth of two lateral septa, which fuse, giving rise to trachea in front and oesophagus behind. The last parts to fuse are the lowest or most distal parts of the two septa. The oesophagus becomes converted into a solid rod of cells, losing its tubular nature. This eventually becomes canalized to form a tube.

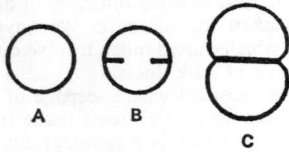

Fig. 369.—Development of oesophagus and trachea. A, at a very early developmental stage the oesophagus and trachea form one structure. B, The ingrowth of two lateral septa. C, The completed development—oesophagus and trachea form two tubes.

Abnormalities (*Fig.* 370):
1. TRACHEO-OESOPHAGEAL FISTULA AND OESOPHAGEAL ATRESIA: Congenital abnormalities may arise if there is interference with the normal development of the trachea and oesophagus. This may take the form of complete atresia of the oesophagus (*Fig.* 370A).

Sometimes there is a fistulous communication between the upper segment of the oesophagus and the trachea (*Fig.* 370B) but in over 80 per cent of cases there is a fistula between the distal segment of the oesophagus and the trachea (*Fig.* 370C). Less commonly both segments communicate with the trachea (*Fig.* 370D) or a lateral communication (H fistula) exists (*Fig.* 370E).

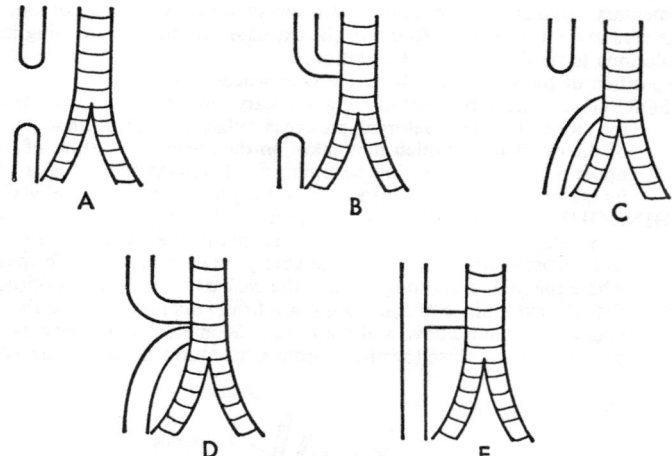

Fig. 370.—Congenital abnormalities of the oesophagus.

X. THE ROTATION OF THE GUT[1]

In the earliest days of development the alimentary canal is represented by a tube suspended in the midline of the abdominal cavity by a ventral and a dorsal mesentery. It consists of three portions, each of which has its own artery, and each of which is destined for a specific function (*see* table *below*).

Departures from the normal situation of the component parts of the foregut and hindgut are exceedingly rare. Errors in the location of the

NAME	EXTENT	ARTERY	FUNCTION
Foregut	Stomach and duodenum as far as the entry of the bile duct	Coeliac axis	Digestive
Midgut	From the ampulla of Vater to the junction of the middle with the left third of the transverse colon—i.e., lower part of duodenum, ileum and jejunum, caecum and appendix, ascending colon, and two-thirds of transverse colon	Superior mesenteric	Absorptive
Hindgut	The left colon—i.e., left third of transverse colon, descending, iliac, and pelvic colons, and rectum	Inferior mesenteric	Excretory

[1] This difficult subject has been rendered easy to understand by the work of Norman Dott. The account given here is therefore essentially a summary compiled from his illuminating article, 'Anomalies of Intestinal Rotation' *Br. J. Surg.*, 1923, 11, 251.

alimentary canal are therefore almost entirely confined to the midgut loop. The reason for this is to be found in the extreme complexity attending its evolutions to attain its normal situation.

Disposition of the Gut before Rotation commences (*Fig.* 371):

FOREGUT: The upper part of the alimentary tube soon bulges to form the stomach. The developing pancreas bulges the dorsal mesentery of the duodenum, which thus takes on the normal curvature of its upper part, at the same time becoming fixed in place by the fusion of its mesentery with the peritoneum of the posterior abdominal wall.

HINDGUT: The upper end of this part of the tube is fixed to the abdominal wall near the origin of the superior mesenteric artery by a condensed part of the dorsal mesentery. Thus a 'flexure' is formed where the mid- and hindgut join—the *colic angle*. It will be noticed that the extremities of the midgut are firmly anchored by the fixed upper duodenum above and the fixed colic angle below. These two points are quite close together, forming the 'duodenocolic isthmus'.

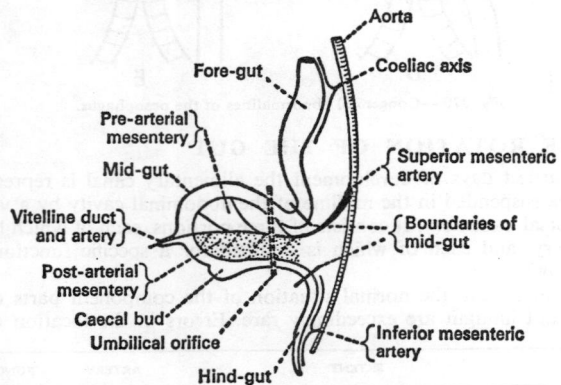

Fig. 371.—Alimentary canal before commencement of rotation. The midgut loop has herniated into the umbilical cord. The dorsal mesentery, suspending the gut from midline of posterior abdominal wall, is not shown. (*After Dott.*)

MIDGUT: There exists at this time a portion of the coelomic (future peritoneal) cavity in the umbilical cord, known as the 'extra-embryonic coelom'. The midgut forms a loop convex forward. It grows so rapidly that the intra-embryonic coelom is too small to hold it, so that part of the loop is extruded into the extra-embryonic coelom in the umbilical cord, forming a *temporary physiological hernia*. Persistence of this extrusion at birth is called an omphalocele. It is covered only by amnion. It occurs approximately once in

5000 births. The cause is unknown. It is often associated with other congenital anomalies. At the apex of the extruded gut is the former site of the vitello-intestinal duct (as it is already obliterated), and here the superior mesenteric artery terminates. The artery of the midgut loop (superior mesenteric) runs from the aorta through the duodenocolic isthmus to the apex of the extruded gut, sending off branches forward to the anterior segment of the midgut loop, and backwards to its posterior segment. The midgut loop and its mesentery still lie in the sagittal plane. The part of the gut in front of the artery is the pre-arterial segment, and its mesentery the pre-arterial mesentery. The gut behind the artery is the post-arterial segment, and its mesentery the post-arterial mesentery. During the fifth week the bud for the caecum and appendix appears *on the post-arterial segment of the loop*. This is the state of affairs at the beginning of the fifth week, and rotation is about to begin.

Chronology of Rotation of the Midgut Loop: *First Stage:* This takes place while the loop lies in the umbilical cord between the fifth and tenth

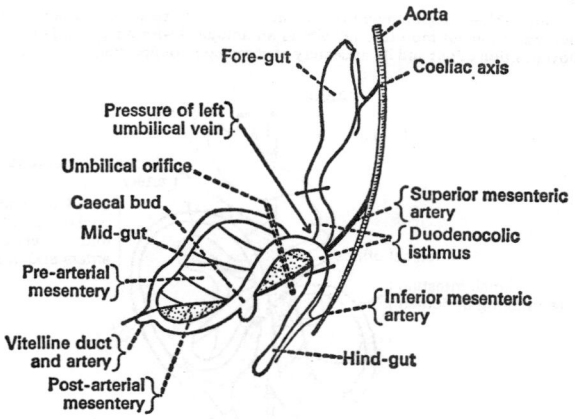

Fig. 372.—The first stage of rotation is occurring. Arrow indicates pressure being exerted by left umbilical vein upon the pre-arterial segment of the loop, forcing it down and to the right. (*After Dott.*)

weeks (Frazer and Robbins[1]). *Second Stage:* This occurs at the tenth to the eleventh week. *Third Stage:* The eleventh week until shortly after birth.

---

[1] 'On the Factors Concerned in causing Rotation of the Intestine in Man', *J. Anat.*, 1915, **50**, 75. Quoted by Dott.

378 A SYNOPSIS OF SURGICAL ANATOMY

FIRST STAGE OF ROTATION: This is largely brought about by the development of the liver. The great growth of its right lobe carries this organ downward and to the right, taking the left umbilical vein (future ligamentum teres) with it (*Fig. 372*). This exercises pressure on the base of the pre-arterial segment of the midgut loop so that this segment is pushed down and to the right. As the pre- and post-arterial segments lie side by side within the narrow confines of the

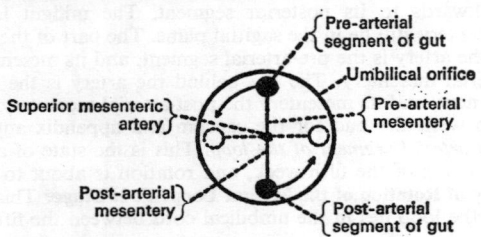

Fig. 373.—Diagrammatic representation of first stage of rotation, showing rotation of midgut loop through 90° in an anti-clockwise direction. Dotted lines show position of gut and its mesentery at completion of first stage of rotation.

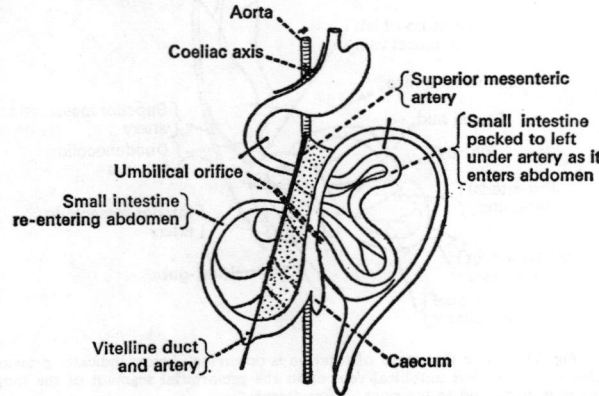

Fig. 374.—Second stage of rotation (ventral aspect). Pre-arterial segment (small intestine) of midgut loop has increased in length disproportionately to post-arterial segment. Caecum and ascending colon have become relatively thick. The physiological umbilical hernia is reducing. Small gut is re-entering abdomen on right side of superior mesenteric vessels and passing to left side of abdomen behind the mesenteric vessels. The vessels are held forward to the umbilicus by the caecum, which still lies outside the umbilicus. (*After Dott.*)

THE ANATOMY OF CONGENITAL ERRORS 379

umbilical segment, the movement of the pre-arterial portion down and to the right forces the post-arterial segment upwards and to the left. The first stage of rotation is complete. The growth of the liver has thus succeeded in rotating the ends of the midgut loop through 90° in an anticlockwise direction (*Fig.* 373).

SECOND STAGE OF ROTATION: About the beginning of the tenth week the midgut loop returns to the abdominal cavity from the umbilical cord. The gut being too bulky to be returned *en masse*, it retreats in a definite order. The pre-arterial portion returns first, commencing with its *proximal portion* (*Fig.* 374). While the pre-arterial segment is returning, the superior mesenteric artery is firmly fixed to the umbilicus by its termination, and is therefore

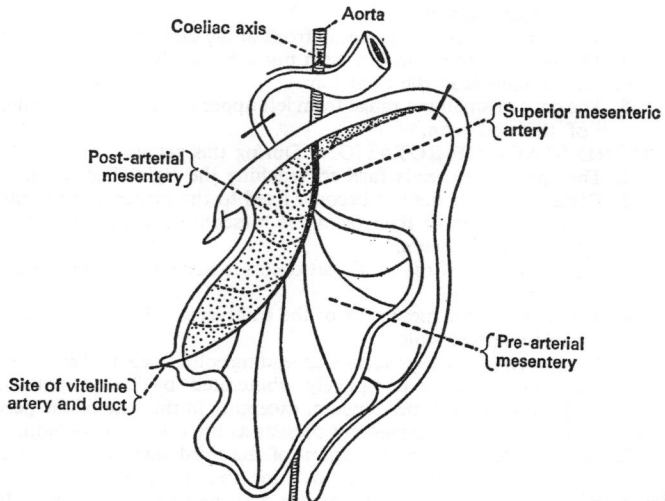

Fig. 375.—Completion of second stage of rotation. Caecum is in contact with posterior abdominal wall in right loin. Midgut loop has rotated on axis of superior mesenteric vessels through 270° from its original sagittal plane. The essentials of the permanent disposition of the viscera have been attained. (*After Dott.*)

stretched like a cord from commencement to termination. The returning small gut enters the abdomen to the *right* of the artery, but the space here being too limited the coils first reduced are pushed to the left behind the taut artery by those following on. By their passage to the left they displace the dorsal mesentery of the hindgut (which occupies the midline) before them, so that the descending colon comes to occupy the left flank and the colic angle is pushed up to form the future splenic flexure. The last coil of the ileum carries the superior mesenteric artery with it as it is reduced. The caecum still lies in the umbilical cord on a plane anterior to the small intestine and its artery. The caecum and right half of the colon now reduce, passing upward and to the right, the colon crossing the pedicle of the small gut at the point of origin of the superior mesenteric artery from the aorta, and the caecum comes to lie under the liver. The subsequent growth elongation of the colon pushes the caecum into the right loin. Now the second stage of rotation is complete (*Fig.* 375). Note that:

1. The duodenum crosses behind the upper part of the superior mesenteric artery.
2. The transverse colon crosses in front of the same part of this vessel.
3. The descending colon has been pushed into the left flank.
4. The caecum is in the right loin.
5. The coils of small gut range from left upper to right lower segments of the abdomen.

THIRD STAGE OF ROTATION: During this stage:

1. The caecum descends further, reaching the right iliac fossa.
2. Certain parts of the gut become fixed to the posterior abdominal wall by fusion of their primitive mesenteries with the posterior parietal peritoneum.
3. The mesentery of the small gut becomes adherent to the posterior abdominal wall.
4. The post-arterial mesentery of the transverse colon persists as the transverse mesocolon.
5. The mesentery of the caecum, ascending colon, hepatic flexure, and hindgut becomes completely obliterated by fusion with the posterior parietal peritoneum, excepting in the case of the pelvic colon, where the mesentery persists as the future mesocolon.

It will be noted that the 'function' of the third stage is the efficient *fixation* of the gut to the posterior abdominal wall.

Errors in Rotation of the Gut: The interest that the rotation of the gut has for the surgeon arises from the fact that errors in this process lead to grave surgical conditions.

The first stage of rotation is never interfered with, except in the condition known as 'extroversion of the cloaca', an entity so rare that it is undeserving of further notice.

The second stage of rotation consists essentially of the reduction of the physiological hernia *in orderly sequence*. Abnormalities of the second stage are due to a departure from this sequence.

Causes of Disorderly Sequence: The bulk of the caecum is an important factor in ensuring its remaining outside the abdomen till the remaining gut is reduced. Undue size of the umbilical ring would not prevent the unduly early return of the caecum. Dott considers this the most probable abnormal factor when the sequence of return is unruly.

During the third or fixation stage of rotation, errors may lead to imperfect fixation.

CLASSIFICATION OF ROTATION ERRORS:

1. DERANGEMENTS OF THE FIRST STAGE OF ROTATION: Extroversion of the cloaca.
2. DERANGEMENTS OF THE SECOND STAGE OF ROTATION:
   a. Non-rotation of the midgut loop.
   b. Reversed rotation of the midgut loop.
   c. Malrotation of the midgut loop.
3. DERANGEMENTS OF THE THIRD STAGE OF ROTATION:
   a. Subhepatic caecum.
   b. Right lumbar caecum.
   c. Pelvic caecum.
   d. Mobile proximal colon.
   e. Volvulus and torsion.

DERANGEMENTS OF SECOND STAGE OF ROTATION:

NON-ROTATION OF THE MIDGUT LOOP: In this condition:
1. The small gut lies chiefly to the right of the midline.
2. The duodenum descends from its normally fixed upper part down along the right side of the superior mesenteric artery.
3. The terminal ileum may:
   a. Cross the midline to reach a left iliac caecum, entering the caecum from its right instead of from its left.
   b. Terminate in the midline in a pelvic caecum.
4. The colon is confined to the left side of the abdomen.
5. Though the gut may become fixed in these abnormal positions, on the other hand no fixative adhesions may occur, so that the whole midgut loop may be suspended in the abdominal cavity by an extremely narrow pedicle which is really the duodenocolic isthmus.

Explanation: The umbilical ring is lax. The colon and caecum are the first constituents of the physiological hernia to reduce. The small gut following displaces the colon to the left and also the superior mesenteric artery.

REVERSED ROTATION OF THE MIDGUT LOOP (*Fig.* 376):
1. The transverse colon crosses behind the superior mesenteric artery.
2. The duodenum crosses in front of the superior mesenteric artery.

Otherwise the intestines are in normal location.

Explanation: The caecum and ascending colon reduce first, passing *behind* the superior mesenteric vessels. The small gut therefore reduces in front of the vessels.

MALROTATION OF THE MIDGUT LOOP: This term is used by Dott to imply irregular defects of rotation.

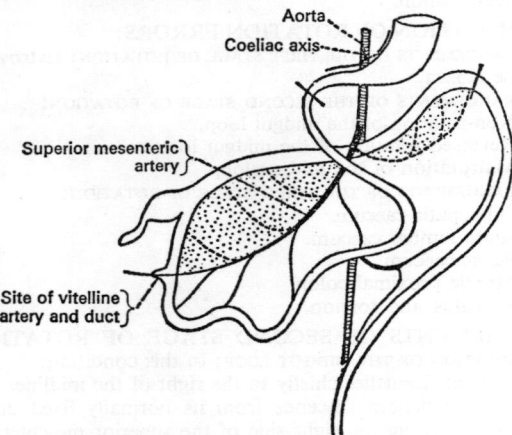

Fig. 376.—Reversed rotation of midgut loop. The midgut has rotated in a clockwise direction through 90° from the original sagittal plane. Thus the colon comes to lie behind the mesenteric vessels and the duodenum in front of them. (*After Dott.*)

DERANGEMENTS OF THIRD STAGE OF ROTATION:

CAECUM: Too early fixation causes imperfect descent of the organ, which may be: (1) Subhepatic; (2) Right lumbar. Deficient fixation causes the caecum to be: (3) Pelvic.

PROXIMAL COLON: Deficient fixation of the post-arterial mesentery causes: (4) Mobile proximal colon.

Pathological Consequences of Anomalies of Rotation:

The following facts are noteworthy:
1. No functional disturbance may result from abnormal fixation.
2. Excessive fixation may cause interference with mobility, kinks, and compression of the bowel.
3. Deficient fixation may cause ptosis, torsion, volvulus.
4. Intestinal obstruction due to volvulus is predisposed to by the existence of abnormal rotation.
5. Such obstruction is particularly likely to occur within the first few days of life. This condition is known as volvulus

THE ANATOMY OF CONGENITAL ERRORS 383

neonatorum. The extent of the twisted gut is great: from the duodenum above to the transverse colon below.

6. Volvulus of the ileocaecal segment is the typical lesion in later life resulting from imperfect rotation or deficient fixation of the gut.

Exomphalos: If the physiological hernia of the midgut loop persists until after birth the condition of exomphalos exists. It may be:

1. COMPLETE: The whole midgut loop occupies the hernial sac.
2. PARTIAL: The caecum and lower ileum lie in the sac.

DISTINCTION FROM TRUE UMBILICAL HERNIA:

1. The sac in exomphalos is a thin, translucent, jelly-like membrane, being really the thinned-out root of the umbilical cord.
2. The vessels of the cord run over the upper surface of the stretched sac, meeting at its apex to form the cord.
3. The sac in true hernia is covered by normal skin.

XI. DUODENAL ILEUS[1]

This term was applied by Wilkie (1921) to cases of constant or intermittent delay in the passage of the duodenal contents, resulting in dilatation of the duodenum, without any obvious cause. He ascribed it to a drag of the

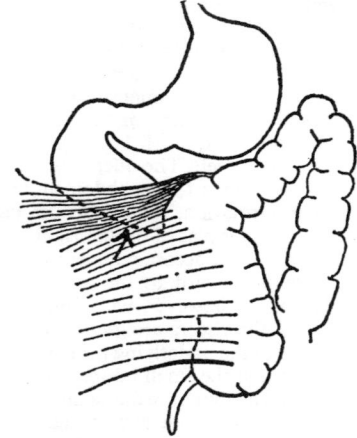

Fig. 377.—Normally placed but mobile right colon has been drawn to the left to show congenital bands (indicated by arrow) passing from the hepatic flexure and mesenteric pedicle across the third part of the duodenum. (*By courtesy of Louw, the Editor and Publishers of the 'Journal of the Royal College of Surgeons of Edinburgh'.*)

---

[1] In the preparation of this sub-section the writer is indebted to J. H. Louw, 'Intestinal Malrotation and Duodenal Ileus', *Jl R. Coll. Surg. Edin.*, 1960, 5, 101.

superior mesenteric vessels compressing the third part of the duodenum at the site where they crossed it—arteriomesenteric pressure.

Ladd (1933) demonstrated that the acute duodenal obstruction of the newborn was caused by abnormal fibrous bands constricting the second part of the duodenum when they were pulled on by an undescended caecum, or one which, though descended, was unattached, permitting a free range of movement (*Fig.* 377).

Ladd and Gross (1941) extended the concept to embrace the type of ileus affecting older children, and Louw et al. (1957) adduce evidence suggesting that the acute ileus of neonates, and the more chronic types affecting older people, are explicable on similar embryological grounds, i.e., duodenal compression by abnormal bands consequent on anomalies of rotation of the midgut loop. Either there is lack of rotation or fixation of the caecum, or there is excessive fixation, so that, even though rotation and fixation are complete and the bowel disposition is normal, yet abnormal fibrous bands constrict the duodenum, usually at its terminal part in the situation of the angulation produced by the ligament of Treitz (*Fig.* 378).

The more chronic types of ileus are episodic and usually affect females. There may be acute attacks of threatened obstruction. X-ray study may show a dilated duodenum in acute attacks, or a normal one in symptom-free periods. Conditions become worse as the patient grows older. Friedman (1946) has shown that the duodenum sags lower with the passage of years, though the duodenojejunal flexure remains fixed in position. Thus the angulation of this bowel junction is intensified.

Treatment consists in division of the constricting bands. This is achieved by delivering the right colon and small bowel out of the abdomen and making traction on them to the left. The offending bands thus exposed are divided and the bowel is returned to the abdomen, being disposed in the primitive condition of non-rotation, the duodenum passing straight into jejunum, the small bowel being placed on the right and the colon on the left. Volvulus is a not-infrequent accompaniment and is corrected.

The procedure is straightforward in the acute duodenal obstruction of the newborn. In the adult, however, with duodenal dilatation, where disposition and fixation of the viscera are grossly abnormal, the operation is a major procedure, though the underlying principles are the same. Again the right half of the colon and the small bowel are delivered on to the left side of the abdominal wall, and the entire duodenum is exposed, constricting bands severed, and the terminal duodenum brought to the right under the mesenteric pedicle straightening out the flexure. A moment's thought will make it clear that, in this operation, the right half of the colon, the second and third part of the duodenum, and the entire mesentery of the small gut must be mobilized so that the bowel may be lifted from the abdomen and the constricting bands released.

Chronic duodenal ileus is associated with duodenal ulcer in 25 per cent of cases and is treated in its own right as the surgeon may elect.

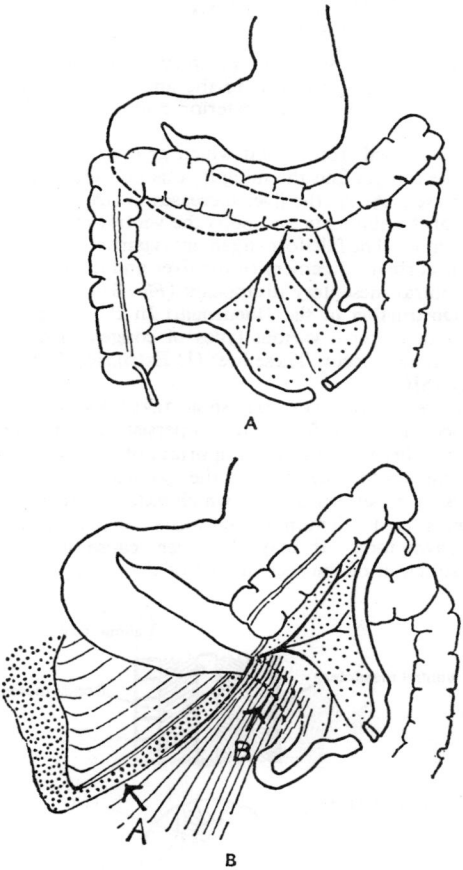

Fig. 378.—A Normally placed and anchored intestines associated with duodenal ileus; B, Mobilization of right colon and division of small bowel anchorage (arrow A). The mobilized colon and small bowel have been retracted to the left and up to show the firm bands compressing the terminal duodenum (arrow B). (*By courtesy of Louw, the Editor and Publishers of the 'Journal of the Royal College of Surgeons of Edinburgh'.*)

XII. CONGENITAL ABNORMALITIES IN THE REGION OF THE JUNCTION OF THE FORE- AND MIDGUT

The gut, at a very early stage in its history, is centrally suspended in the abdominal cavity, being attached to the anterior abdominal wall by the ventral mesentery, and to the posterior abdominal wall by the dorsal mesentery.

The liver is formed from a bud which grows out from the gut at the junction of the foregut and the midgut; this bud grows into and distends the ventral mesentery. As the liver increases in size it extends up into the right region of the abdomen and pulls the ventral mesentery over with it, also the duodenum. The falciform ligament is part of this ventral mesentery, so too are the coronary ligament of the liver and the lesser omentum. The rest of the ventral mesentery disappears (*Fig.* 379).

Congenital Obstruction of the Duodenum: In the region of junction of the mid- and foregut various types of congenital obstruction of the duodenum may occur. These are: (1) Extrinsic; (2) Intrinsic.

1. EXTRINSIC:

   PERSISTENCE OF THE VENTRAL MESENTERY: Parts of this peritoneal process may and frequently do persist, forming peritoneal bands or membranes. The most important of these occasional remnants of the ventral mesentery is the *cystogastrocolic band* (*Fig.* 380). This is a peritoneal fold which extends from the gall-bladder across the duodenum to the transverse colon. It usually produces no symptoms. It may, however, cause complete or partial obstruction of the second part of the duodenum:

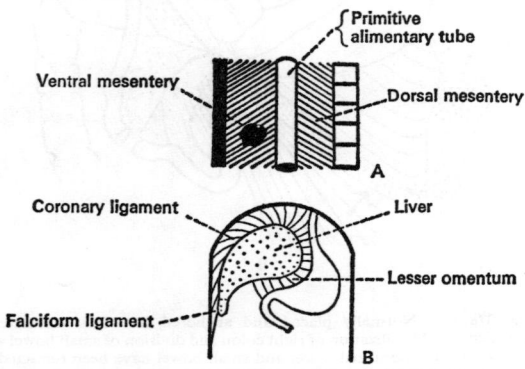

Fig. 379.—A, The primitive alimentary canal suspended by ventral and dorsal mesenteries. B, Remains of ventral mesentery (mesogastrium).

THE ANATOMY OF CONGENITAL ERRORS 387

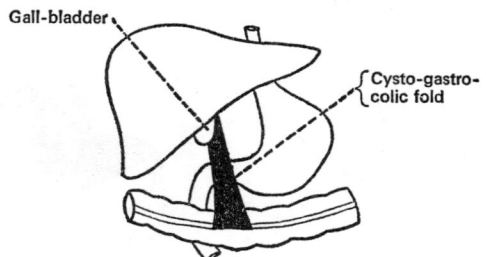

Fig. 380.—The cystogastrocolic fold.

  a. *Complete Obstruction:* The child vomits persistently from birth.
    The stomach stands out in relief. On opening the abdomen a
    tense band is seen to extend from the gall-bladder to the colon,
    crossing and constricting the second part of the duodenum,
    producing the obstruction.
      The condition presents these important differences from
    congenital stenosis of the pylorus:
      i. There is bile in the vomit—in pyloric stenosis there is not.
      ii. The condition is present from birth—in pyloric stenosis
        it commences the second week after birth.
      iii. No tumour is felt as in pyloric stenosis.
  b. *Partial Obstruction:* This is commoner. It may produce
    symptoms:
      i. *At birth:* Producing a lesser degree of the symptoms
        mentioned above.
      ii. *In later life:* Producing pain and vomiting.
2. INTRINSIC: At the site where the bile-duct grows out to form the
liver, narrowing or complete stenosis of the duodenum may occur
(*Fig.* 381). In this connexion the reader is reminded of Bland-Sutton's
generalization that developmental errors tend to occur at the site
of an embryological event.
  Obstruction may also occur elsewhere in the neighbourhood
of the junction of the mid- and foregut, e.g., at the junction of the
stomach and the duodenum, or at the duodenojejunal flexure. It
has been shown[1] that in the second month of development the
passage from the stomach to the duodenum is completely blocked
by proliferation of the epithelium. Vacuoles appear in this
epithelium and then septa stretch across the lumen which
ultimately disappear, thus re-establishing the channel. Should

[1] Tandler, Forssner, and Ager, quoted by L. E. Barrington-Ward, *Abdominal Surgery of Children*, 1928, London.

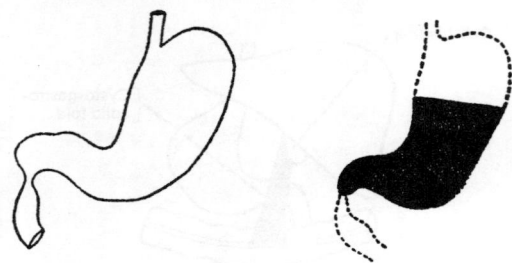

Fig. 381.—Diagrammatic representation of stenosis at junction of midgut and foregut. The right-hand figure represents X-ray appearances after ingestion of barium.

development be arrested before vacuolation occurs the intestine remains a solid cord. If development stops before the breaking down is complete, septa occur. Either of these two abnormalities produces complete obstruction. Bodian et al.[1] draw attention to the fact that mongolism occurs in 1 in 3 cases of intrinsic obstruction of the duodenum in the newborn and ascribe the failure to recognize this association to the fact that most children with duodenal stenosis or atresia die during the neonatal period when mongolism is apt to be overlooked.

Congenital Cyst of the Common Bile-duct: This is a rare condition, occurring nine times as often in girls as in boys. A large cyst lies between the layers of the lesser omentum. Into this the hepatic and cystic ducts open, and the common bile-duct leaves it. Only the supraduodenal part of the common bile-duct is affected by the condition. There is never complete obstruction to the outflow of bile into the duodenum. It has been suggested that the condition is due to some valvular obstruction in the common bile-duct at the junction of the supra- and retroduodenal portions, arising out of deficient peritoneal fixation of the duodenum (Morley[2]) (*Fig.* 382).

Accessory Bile-duct and Duodenal Diverticulum: It is thought that where the bud grows out from the junction of the fore- and midgut to form the liver, more than one process grows out from the gut, or the single outgrowth subdivides into others. These accessory outgrowths disappear as a rule. One of the accessory outgrowths (*Fig.* 382) may:

PERSIST IN ITS UPPER HALF: Forming an *accessory bile-duct*. This usually extends from liver to gall-bladder. In the operation of removal of the gall-bladder such a duct may be unknowingly divided. This results in leakage of bile into the peritoneal cavity.

[1] Bodian, M., White, L. L. R., Carter, C. O., and Louw, J. H., *Br. med. J.*, 1952, 1, 75.
[2] Quoted by L. E. Barrington-Ward, *Abdominal Surgery of Children*, 1928, 158. London.

THE ANATOMY OF CONGENITAL ERRORS 389

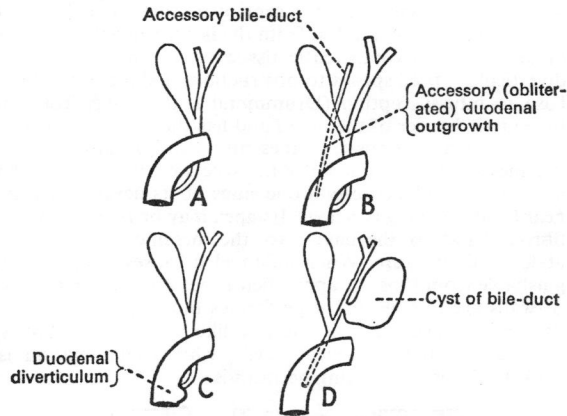

Fig. 382.—Diagrammatic representation of: A, Normal bile-ducts. B, Accessory bile-duct—persistence of upper third of accessory duodenal outgrowth. C, Duodenal diverticulum—persistence of lower part of accessory duodenal outgrowth. D, Congenital cyst of common bile-duct.

This possibility is one of the arguments in favour of drainage of the peritoneal cavity after cholecystectomy.

PERSIST IN ITS PROXIMAL HALF: This is the explanation of the occasional occurrence of *diverticulum of the second part of the duodenum*. The diverticulum protrudes from the posteromedial aspect of the second part of the duodenum, near the opening of the bile-duct. It is therefore retroperitoneal. For this reason the surgeon is chary of removing it in those cases where it causes symptoms, as there is no peritoneum there to protect the suture line in the duodenum which results from the removal of the diverticulum.

XIII. MECKEL'S DIVERTICULUM

The midgut communicates at an early developmental stage with the yolk-sac. This communication is the vitello-intestinal duct, also called the omphalomesenteric duct. Keith defines Meckel's diverticulum as the persistence of the intra-abdominal part of the vitello-intestinal duct. Normally it entirely disappears. Vestiges of it may persist (*Fig.* 383). They are:

1. **Patent Meckel's Diverticulum:** The duct entirely fails to close, small-intestine contents being discharged at the umbilicus.
2. **Meckel's Diverticulum:** The duct closes at its umbilical end but remains open at the intestinal end. This condition of Meckel's

diverticulum occurs in 2 per cent of persons. The diverticulum is 2 in. long and is found 2 ft. from the ileocaecal valve. In 2 per cent of cases accessory pancreatic tissue occurs in the vestige. A long diverticulum predisposes to obstruction; a short one with a broad base to intussusception (Drummond[1]). It springs from the antimesenteric border of the ileum and has the lumen of the small gut. It may or may not possess a mesentery; such mesentery arises from the mesentery of the small gut. Accessory pancreatic tissue may occur in its wall because at one stage of its development it is very near the developing pancreas. Its apex may be free, or attached by a fibrous band to the navel, to the mesentery, or to any intra-abdominal structure. When inflamed it causes symptoms indistinguishable from those of appendicitis, but more dangerous because:
a. It walls are thinner and it perforates more easily.
b. It is not tucked away to one side like the appendix but is in the middle of the peritoneal cavity where inflammation is more likely to spread, causing peritonitis.

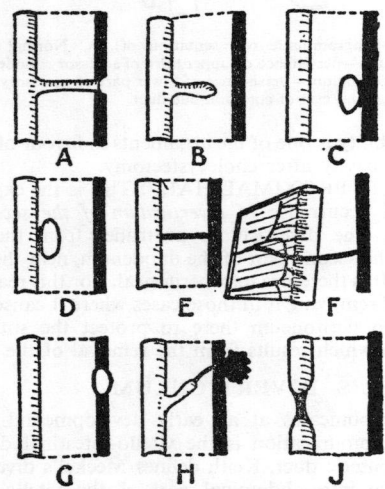

Fig. 383.—Meckel's diverticulum and its vestiges. A, Patent Meckel's diverticulum. B, Meckel's diverticulum. C, Enterotoma. D, Enterocystocele. E, Fibrous remnant of Meckel's diverticulum. F, Remnant of vitelline vessels. G, Cyst of umbilicus. H, Adenoid tumour of vitelline-duct origin coexisting with Meckel's diverticulum and attached to it by a fibrous cord. J, Obliteration of lumen of gut at region of attachment of vitello-intestinal duct.

[1] Quoted by L. E. Barrington-Ward, *Abdominal Surgery of Children*, 1928, 227. London.

Areas of mucous membrane like that of the stomach with acid-secreting properties are found in Meckel's diverticulum in 12 per cent of cases. The diverticulum then acts as a small stomach. Therefore peptic ulcer with its associated dangers of perforation and haemorrhage may be found in this remnant, leading to much distress to both the person affected and the surgeon who is confronted with the diagnosis of so difficult a case. The explanation given is that Meckel's diverticulum, being vestigial, is liable to metaplasia of its tissues, and the small-gut type of epithelium becomes changed to resemble that of the stomach. Dowse[1] states that such heterotopic gastric mucosa may occur at the neck of the diverticulum. Removal, to be adequate, should therefore include a portion of the adjacent ileum so that ectopic tissue is not left behind as would be the case if the diverticulum were amputated and treated like an appendix stump.

There are certain other interesting facts[2] in connexion with this vestige:
a. It is constantly present in some birds.
b. It may be found on any part of the midgut.
c. It may appear to be intramesenteric; such a situation is not developmental, but due to the tube being buried by inflammatory adhesions.
d. When a mesentery exists it contains an artery, the continuation of the superior mesenteric, from which its blood-supply is derived.
e. If no mesentery exists, the blood-supply comes from the vessels of the related part of the small gut.
f. Giant Meckel's diverticula do occur. Such a structure may serve as an abdominal 'sink', grow to be a yard long, and of proportionate girth, and fill the abdomen so greatly that its removal would be hazardous.
g. Meckel's diverticulum may give rise to the following pathological accidents:
  i. Intestinal obstruction.
  ii. Acute inflammation of the diverticulum.
  iii. Chronic inflammation of the diverticulum with concretions.
  iv. Tumours.
  v. Intussusception.
  vi. Peptic ulcer, causing haemorrhage or perforation.

The term 'Littre's hernia' is applied to one which contains Meckel's diverticulum (1700). Although originally applied only if the diverticulum was the sole content of the hernial sac, customary usage is to give the name to any hernia in which the vestige is found. It has been reported in inguinal, umbilical, ventral, femoral, sciatic, and lumbar herniae.

---

[1] Dowse, J. L. A., *Br. J. Surg.*, 1961, **48**, 392.
[2] These are taken from Barrington-Ward's *Abdominal Surgery of Children*.

3. **Enterotomata:** The duct closes at both ends but remains patent in the middle. This may cause cysts behind the navel called enterotomata.
4. The duct remains open at its umbilical end and appears as a raspberry red tumour at the umbilicus because it becomes turned inside out by intra-abdominal pressure.
5. The duct entirely disappears but a fibrous band remains. This represents the remains of the vessels of the duct (vitelline) and passes from the umbilicus to some part of the mesentery or to the small gut. Its importance is:
   a. It may act as a band under which a loop of gut may be compressed so causing obstruction.
   b. It may be attached to some branch of the mesenteric artery. If it be pulled on in abdominal operations it may tear the blood-vessel to which it is attached and cause fatal haemorrhage. John Frazer quotes a case of the kind.[1]

XIV. CONGENITAL DEFORMITIES OF THE RECTUM AND ANUS

The understanding and treatment of congenital malformations of the rectum and anus has been advanced by the formulation of several new concepts which have come from the writings of Browne[2] and his followers, notably Stephens.[3] These are:
   a. The name imperforate anus is a poor generic term to apply to these conditions. The great majority have an opening somewhere.
   b. The misuse of the term 'fistula' which is often applied to anal anomalies.
   c. The introduction of the concepts of (i) ectopia or failure of migration of the anus and (ii) excessive fusion of the lateral genital folds causing the covered anus.
   d. The importance of distinguishing anomalies of the anal canal from those of the rectum.

No embryological theory explains all these congenital aberrations. A view which is widely held is that the rectum is developed from the entodermal cloaca and the anal canal from the ectodermal cloaca. The hindgut is continuous with the entodermal cloaca which becomes divided into an anterior urogenital portion and a posterior rectal one by the downgrowths of the urorectal septum from above and the folds of Rathke from the sides (*Fig.* 384). Failure of these events to occur causes:
1. DEFORMITIES OF THE RECTUM: According to Stephens, the failure of the downgrowth from above and ingrowths from the sides results in rectal agenesis, the terminal rectum ending in

---

[1] *The Surgery of Childhood*, 1926, 2, 799. London.
[2] Browne, D., 'Congenital Deformities of the Anus and Rectum', *Archs Dis. Childh.*, 1955, 30, 42.
[3] Stephens, F. D., *Aust. N. Z. J. Surg.*, 1953, 22, 161, and 23, 9.

THE ANATOMY OF CONGENITAL ERRORS

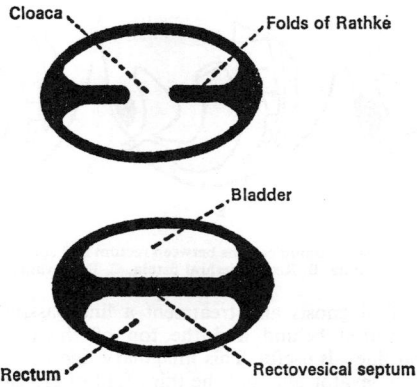

Fig. 384.—Showing development of rectovesical septum by ingrowth of folds of Rathke.

fistulous formation with the bladder in relation to the ureteric orifices in the male. In the female a fistulous opening may also occur in the region of the trigone. There may be no fistula with a high blind termination of the rectum. Externally there is no sign of the anal pit or merely a dimple (*Fig.* 385).

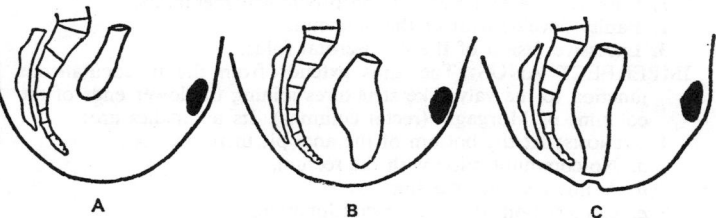

Fig. 385.—Types of imperforate anus. A, Failure of development of rectum. B, Rectum is normal but no proctodeum has formed. C, Cloacal or anal membrane has failed to rupture.

2. If the lateral mesodermal ingrowths fail to appear, there results in the male a recto-urethral fistula, the opening being regularly situated at the level of the verumontanum in the prostatic urethra. In the female the arrival of the Müllerian ducts complicates the situation and rectovaginal or rectovestibular fistula may occur (*Fig.* 386).

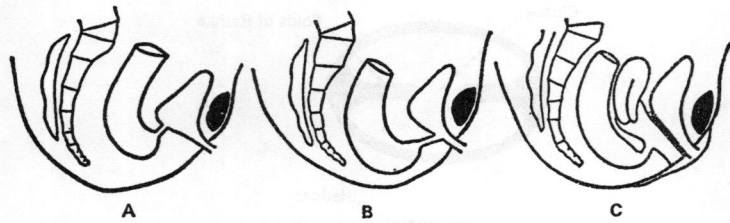

Fig. 386.—Abnormal communications between rectum and some other tube. A, Rectovesical fistula. B, Recto-urethral fistula. C, Rectovaginal fistula.

For purposes of diagnosis and treatment a line passing through the sacrococcygeal junction behind and the top of the pubis in front—the pubococcygeal line—is useful. This imaginary line passes through the verumontanum, the levator ani, and the third fold of Houston and serves to divide anal from rectal deformities. When the rectum (as shown by radiography) ends above this line then the development of the levator ani is impaired and the anal sphincteric apparatus may be vestigial. When the rectum descends below this line then the levator and its puborectalis sling are probably normal and some degree of continence is assured. Boys are much oftener affected than girls. The condition is usually associated with faulty anal development and vestigial sphincters.

DEFORMITIES OF THE ANUS: These abnormalities result from:
1. Imperfect development of the proctodeal membrane.
2. Faulty development of the perineum, or
3. Excessive fusion of the labioscrotal folds.

IMPERFECT ANUS: The anus extends from the mucocutaneous junction to the valve-like structures joining the lower ends of the columns of Morgagni (rectal columns). Its anomalies are:
1. STENOSIS: At the bottom of the anal pit there may be:
   a. No communication with the rectum.
   b. A microscopic opening.
   c. Constriction of the anorectal junction.
   d. Persistence of the proctodeal membrane.

Comment:
   The anus of the newborn should admit the little finger. Stenosis if left untreated leads to colon inertia. Microscopic anus may only be detectable by the presence of a 'fly speck' of meconium on the skin when carefully looked for. There is an efficient sphincteric mechanism. Persistence of the proctodeal membrane is a rarity. All degrees of narrowing may occur between complete occlusion or a barely perceptible opening and a well-formed but narrowed canal.

THE ANATOMY OF CONGENITAL ERRORS

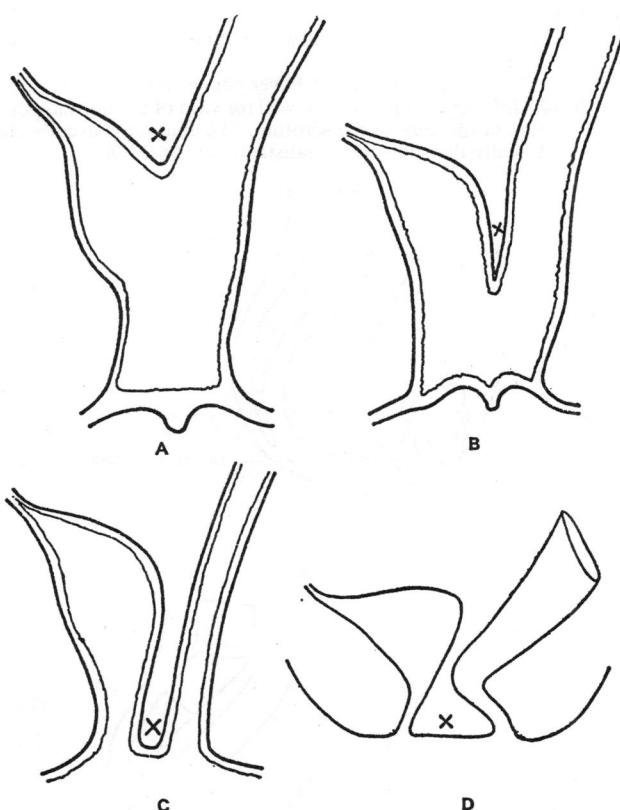

Fig. 387.—The figures demonstrate the development of the perineum by the proliferation of mesoderm and the downgrowth of the urorectal septum dividing the entodermal cloaca into the urogenital and rectal cavities. A, The entodermal cloaca. The urorectal septum is indicated by the X. B, The subdivision continues. C, The division is complete. D, The mesodermal proliferation has developed the perineum and pushed the rectum backwards. (*After Stephens.*)

2. ECTOPIA: The anal and the urogenital membranes are originally adjacent (*Fig.* 387). Mesodermal proliferation forms the perineum which separates the former from the latter. Thus the anus migrates backward. Failure to do so causes:

396 A SYNOPSIS OF SURGICAL ANATOMY

In the Female:
   a. The shotgun perineum where anus and vaginal openings are adjacent.
   b. The anus opens into the lower part of the vagina.

In the Male: The ectopic anus is well forward of the normal position, e.g., at the base of the scrotum. The anal pit is usually absent. Usually the sphincter is satisfactory (*Fig.* 388).

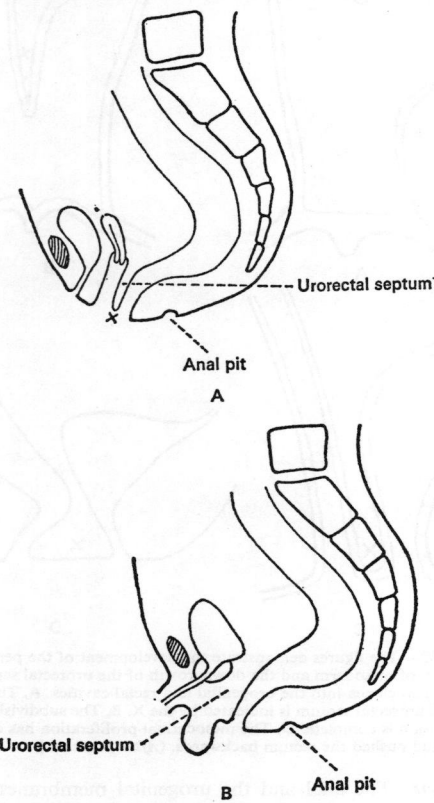

Fig. 388.—A, Ectopic anus in the female—shotgun perineum (X). B, Ectopic anus in the male. (*By courtesy of Muir, the Editor and Publishers of 'Recent Advances in Surgery'*, 4th Edition.)

THE ANATOMY OF CONGENITAL ERRORS 397

Comment:

Adequate sphincteric control is present. As some degree of stenosis usually coexists, the first principle of treatment is to secure adequate function by dilatation. No surgery may be necessary, and if it is, it is best left till the child is older. A grave error would be to look on these conditions as fistulae which they are not.

3. THE COVERED ANUS: The inner genital folds fuse from before backwards. Excessive fusion causes the covered anus. The true anus may be in the normal or ectopic situation. There is no anal opening visible. Boys are more frequently affected than girls.

In the female the vulval opening is unduly short. The anus opens at the fourchette, or the vestibule also may be occluded so that the anus, vagina, and urethra all open beneath the clitoris.

In the male the opening may be in the perineum, base of scrotum, or even reach the coronal sulcus of the penis. Rarely the track may extend forward at a deeper level and open into the bulb of the urethra. There may be an associated atypical hypospadias.

The sphincteric mechanism is satisfactory.

XV. CONGENITAL ABNORMALITIES OF THE URINARY ORGANS

Development of the Kidneys and Ureters: The kidney is formed in the pelvic region and *ascends to the loin*. The testis is formed in the loin and *descends to the scrotum*. The kidney has a double origin: (1) The glomerulus and proximal part of the tubule are formed from the metanephros; (2) The ureter, pelvis, and distal part of the tubule are formed by outgrowths from the Wolffian duct which itself is going to form the ureter.

The following are the *important* congenital abnormalities: (1) Congenital polycystic kidney; (2) Abnormal renal vessels; (3) Horseshoe kidney; (4) Congenital absence of one kidney; (5) Unilateral fused kidney; (6) Accessory kidneys; (7) Pelvic kidney; (8) Abnormalities of the ureter; (9) Abnormalities of the bladder; (10) Abnormalities of the urachus; (11) Congenital causes of obstruction to the outflow of urine.

1. Congenital Polycystic Kidney: Failure of fusion of the proximal and distal parts of the tubules results in this condition (*Fig.* 389). The kidney substance is riddled with cysts. These form because the fluid secreted by the glomeruli cannot find its way out owing to the fact that the two portions of the tubules have failed to join. The condition may be bilateral or unilateral. Thomson and Miles[1] cite a series of 200-odd cases in which the condition was unilateral in 40 per cent.

[1] *Manual of Surgery.*

Other groups of cases do not show such a high percentage of unilateral polycystic kidneys. Maurice Meltzer[1] has investigated statistics carefully, and concludes that unilateral polycystic kidney is unknown clinically, as the *apparently* normal kidney always becomes cystic later. Pathologically, however, many well-authenticated cases of unilateral polycystic disease are recorded. As the cysts increase in size

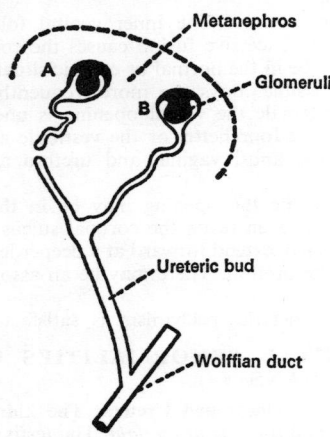

Fig. 389.—Development of kidney. A, Failure of union of metanephric and Wolffian duct elements, producing the condition which causes congenital polycystic kidney. B. Normal development.

the kidney substance is compressed, and ultimately the patient suffers from renal insufficiency, pain, haemorrhage, etc. If one-sided, the offending kidney may be removed. If both kidneys are affected, the operation devised by Rovsing may be practised, i.e., the cysts are punctured. This relieves pain and also increases renal efficiency by removing the pressure on the secreting tissue. The appearance of the pyelogram is of diagnostic value in 50 per cent of cases (Braasch[2]). The pelvis shows a characteristic broadening of the calices, with enlargement and displacement of the pelvis as a whole.

ASSOCIATED CONDITIONS: The liver, spleen, and pancreas may also be affected by the condition. The liver is the most commonly affected of these organs. The explanation is obscure. It is thought that the terminal bile capillaries become cut off from the bile-ducts

[1] *Br. J. Urol.*, 1929, 1, 55.
[2] Quoted by Binney, *Modern Urology* (edited by Hugh Cabot), 1, 691. Philadelphia.

THE ANATOMY OF CONGENITAL ERRORS

and in this way become cystic. A somewhat similar explanation is given to explain cystic disease of the pancreas. The cause of polycystic spleen is quite unknown.

2. **Horseshoe Kidney:** As the renal rudiments are ascending from the pelvic region to the loin, they normally remain entirely separate. They may, however, come in contact. Should they adhere, a horseshoe kidney may result, the two kidneys being joined by an isthmus. Though this isthmus may connect the upper poles of the kidneys (*Fig.* 390), in the vast majority of cases it connects their lower poles. This isthmus usually receives its blood-supply directly from the aorta by a special vessel. The isthmus crosses in front of the aorta and vena cava. When

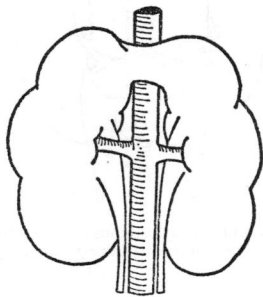

Fig. 390.—Horseshoe kidney with isthmus above.

the isthmus is large the ureters have to ascend from the renal pelvis to cross it (*Fig.* 391), and this may cause some degree of obstruction to the outflow of urine. As the fused kidney is heavy, it usually lies at a lower level than the normal kidney. The condition is usually symptomless and unsuspected, but may in very exceptional cases produce pressure on the vena cava, which is evidenced by oedema of the lower limbs. The inferior mesenteric artery may cross the isthmus when the latter is at the lower pole.

The condition may at times be diagnosed by the shape of the renal pelvis when filled with an opaque fluid by way of the ureter and X-rayed. The lower calix is directed inwards instead of outwards (*Fig.* 392).

3. **Congenital Absence of One Kidney:** This extremely important condition is fortunately rare. A kidney exists on one side. On the other side the ureter exists and opens into the bladder, the kidney being represented merely by a small nodule of tissue (*Fig.* 393, A). The importance of the condition is that if the only kidney becomes diseased, the patient has no reserve of renal tissue. The condition illustrates the fundamental

importance of determining the functional activity of both kidneys before operating on a kidney. The removal of a single kidney is disastrous.

4. **Unilateral Fused Kidney** (*Fig.* 393, B): In this condition the renal rudiments have become fused and the combined mass has passed to one side, the organ proper to that side being above, the other being below. The ureter of the displaced kidney crosses to its own side and opens into the bladder in its normal situation. Its practical importance is the same as the last.

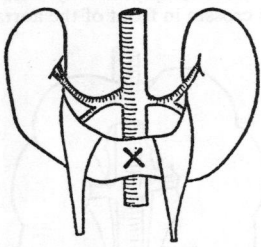

Fig. 391.—Horseshoe kidney with isthmus below. Note that isthmus (X) necessitates curving of ureters in negotiating isthmic ridge.

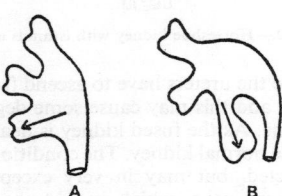

Fig. 392.—A representation of the fact that the lowest calix in a pyelogram of a normal kidney is directed outwards, whereas in a horseshoe kidney it may point downwards or inwards. A, Outline of normal pyelogram. B, Outline of pyelogram of horseshoe kidney.

5. **Accessory Kidneys:** May exist. They are of little practical importance.
6. **Pelvic Kidney** (*Fig.* 393, C): The kidney may never ascend, remaining in the pelvis, usually in the hollow of the sacrum. In this case it obtains its blood-supply from the iliac vessels. The organ may sometimes be felt per rectum or per vaginam.
7. **Abnormalities of the Ureter** (*Fig.* 394):
   a. The most common abnormality is the *bifurcation of a ureter near*

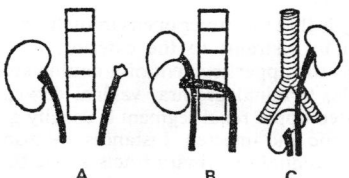

Fig. 393.—Abnormalities in development of the kidneys. A, Normal right kidney; left kidney represented by a small nodule of tissue with a normal ureter. B, Unilateral fused kidney; ureteric orifices in bladder are normal. C, Left kidney normal; right has remained pelvic.

its upper end. In this case there are two separate renal pelves which do not communicate. There is but one opening into the bladder on the affected side.

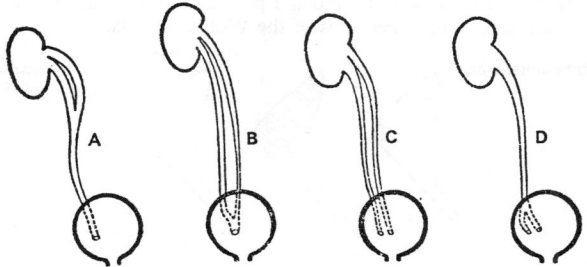

Fig. 394.—Abnormalities in development of the ureter. A, Ureter duplicated above. B, Ureter duplicated along its whole course except at opening into bladder. C, Double ureter with two vesical orifices. D, A condition which never exists. In A, B, C, the pelves are distinct from each other.

- *b.* The ureter may be double in its entire length except just at the entrance to the bladder, in which there is only one ureteric orifice appertaining to that side.
- *c.* The ureter may be double in its entire length with two separate openings into the bladder on that side. Roberts[1] points out that, for embryological reasons, the ureter which enters the bladder in the lower position drains the upper renal segment. The two ureters must therefore cross, moreover the lower frequently ends in an ectopic situation—posterior urethra, vagina, or vulva.
- *d.* Retrocaval ureter, *see* p. 543.
- *e.* Ectopic ureter: It has been pointed out by Lane[2] that the essential

[1] Roberts, J. B. M., *Br. J. Surg.*, 1960, **48**, 1.
[2] Lane, V., *Lancet*, 1962, **1**, 937.

abnormality is that the ureter opens in such a position that the urine drains without restraint to the exterior. Almost always such a ureter drains the upper segment of a double kidney and opens into the vestibule, terminal urethra, vagina, cervix, or uterine cavity. The associated upper renal segment is usually quite small and often hydronephrotic and infected. Instances are also reported in males, but enter the genital or urinary tracts above the external sphincter and are not associated with incontinence. Cystoscopically two normal ureteral orifices are seen. The treatment, if feasible, is removal of the related segment of the kidney and complete ablation of its ureter.

8. **Abnormalities of the Bladder** (*Fig.* 395): This organ has a double origin.
   a. The whole of the bladder except the base is formed from the upper (cephalic) part of the anterior (urogenital) division of the cloaca. The urachus has a similar origin.
   b. The base of the bladder and the prostatic urethra are formed from the opened-out lower ends of the Wolffian ducts.

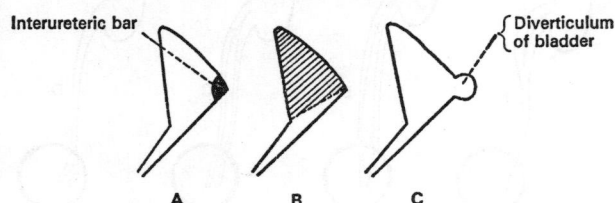

Fig. 395.—Development of bladder and diverticulum of bladder. A, Normal bladder on section, showing the interureteric bar. B, Shaded part of bladder arises from the cloaca—remainder of organ develops from the Wolffian ducts. C, Diverticulum of bladder at the common site where cloacal and Wolffian portions of the bladder meet.

These two portions join therefore along a line represented by the bar of muscle between the ureters, the interureteric bar. Like other organs which have a double origin, abnormalities may occur at the site of fusion of the two parts forming the organ. When congenital diverticula of the bladder occur, they are found somewhere along the line of the ureteric bar, namely, in close proximity to a ureteric orifice.

9. **Abnormalities of the Urachus** (*Fig.* 396): According to Cullen[1] although the allantois is continuous with the rudimentary bladder at the umbilical cord, it contributes nothing to the composition of the

---

[1] Cullen, T. S., *Embryology, Anatomy and Diseases of the Umbilicus together with Diseases of the Urachus*, 1916. Philadelphia and London: Saunders. Quoted by Hinman, F. (jun.) *Surgery Gynec. Obstet.*, 113, 605.

urachus (or bladder) which is formed from a narrowing of the apex of the bladder. It is an appendage of the bladder 2·5 cm. long at birth and 5 cm. in the adult and does not become totally obliterated. Normally it becomes a fibrous cord which may terminate at the umbilicus or extend only part of the way. Thus patency occurs in the neonatal period before development is complete whereas cysts occur in the adult.

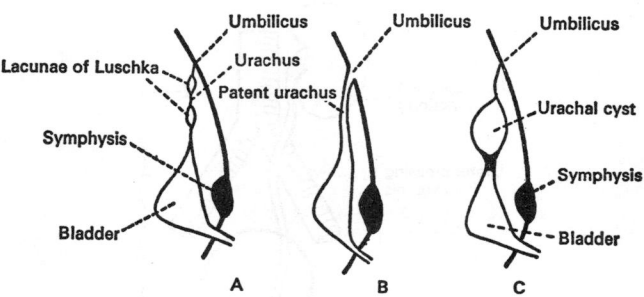

Fig. 396.—Abnormalities of the urachus. A, Lacunae of Luschka. B, Patent urachus. C, Urachal cyst.

Defective development may be responsible for:
a. PATENT URACHUS: The ligament remains open in its whole length, and when the cord falls off, urine discharges at the umbilicus. It is said that this condition is always associated with an obstruction to the outflow of urine from the bladder.
b. LACUNAE OF LUSCHKA: There may remain small cavities in the urachus. These are unsuspected during life and are only found post mortem. They are called lacunae of Luschka.
c. CYSTS OF THE URACHUS: One of these lacunae enlarges to form a cyst which may be very large. It is below the umbilicus and central in position, though the author has seen it lateral to the midline where it had gravitated because of its weight.
10. **Congenital Causes of Obstruction to the Outflow of Urine:** Narrowing of the channel or congenital valves causing obstruction may occur at the following sites (*Fig.* 397):
FROM ONE KIDNEY:
   a. At the junction of the renal pelvis with the ureter.
   b. Where the ureter crosses the brim of the pelvis.
   c. Where the ureter opens into the bladder.
FROM BOTH KIDNEYS:
   a. At the internal urethral meatus.

b. Congenital valves may occur anywhere along the urethra, especially in the prostatic and membranous parts.

c. Pin-point meatus—the opening of the glans is excessively small.

d. Extreme phimosis—the opening in the prepuce may be very small.

American urologists stress the fact that minor degrees of congenital narrowing of a ureter may and often do exist. This is commonest

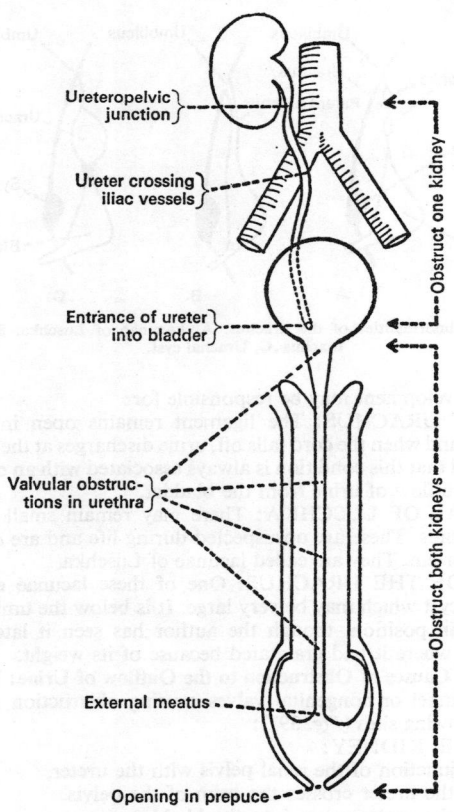

Fig. 397.—Diagram to show possible sites of congenital obstruction to flow of urine from one kidney or both.

where the ureter crosses the pelvic brim; it causes pain in the affected side but no gross disturbance of function. It is a common cause of pain in the right iliac fossa, and explains some cases of failure of appendicectomy to relieve pain in the right side.

XVI. CONGENITAL ABNORMALITIES OF THE TESTIS

Congenital Absence of the Vas Deferens: Campbell[1] explains that the testis and vasa efferentia are derived from the genital fold, whereas the vas, globus major, and body of the epididymis, seminal vesicle and ejaculatory ducts are of Wolffian origin. Thus the vas may be absent on one or both sides, or it may be double. There may be isolated renal agenesis which may affect the vesicle also. Whereas failure of the vas to develop may on occasions account for sterility, its absence does not imply testicular agenesis.

Development of the Testis: The organ is developed between the tenth and twelfth dorsal segments of the embryo. Its nerve-supply is from the tenth dorsal or thoracic segment of the cord. This accounts for the fact that in cases of injury or inflammation of the testis the patient frequently complains of pain at the level of and lateral to the umbilicus, which receives its nerve-supply from the same segment. The testis is developed on the inner side of the Wolffian body from a mesodermal ridge (the germinal ridge) covered by a specialized layer of epithelium known as the germinal epithelium, which is derived from the epithelial layer of the peritoneum. This germinal epithelium forms the actual secreting tissue of the organ, the stroma of which is derived from the mesoderm.

The epididymis is derived from the Wolffian body.

The ductus (vas) deferens is derived from the Wolffian duct.

Observe that the testis, epididymis, and ductus deferens each arises from a different structure.

Descent of the Testis: The testis, lying in the lumbar region in front of the kidney, reaches the scrotum as a result of several factors, one of which is the gubernaculum testis.

GUBERNACULUM TESTIS: John Hunter (1762) described the gubernaculum testis as a fibromuscular band attaching the testis to the bottom of the scrotum, having attained this attachment by evaginating the abdominal wall, carrying with it as its coverings into the scrotum processes from:

1. The fascia transversalis forming the internal spermatic or infundibuliform fascia.
2. The internal oblique and transversalis muscles forming the cremasteric fascia.
3. The external oblique forming the external spermatic fascia.

---

[1] Campbell, M., *Urology*, 1937, Vol. 1, 480. Philadelphia and London: Saunders.

According to Hunter the gubernaculum thus forms the inguinal canal by its passage through the abdominal wall, and its coverings are the coverings of any structure taking the same course, e.g., testis or hernia. Contracture or atrophy of the gubernaculum was considered to be the mechanism pulling the testis into the scrotum.

Backhouse and Butler[1] have shown that the gubernaculum is a purely mesenchymal column which attaches the testis to the inguinal region and floor of the scrotum. Into this structure the processus vaginalis and cremaster grow before the testis descends. On descent of the latter the mesenchymal rod swells and loses its scrotal attachment as it fails to grow in length relative to surrounding tissues. It is independent of the abdominal muscles, fasciae and fibrous tissues of the scrotum. Should such structures encroach on the gubernacular mesenchyme, the downgrowth of the processus vaginalis and cremaster muscle may be interfered with by anchoring bands (the hypothetical tails of Lockwood) resulting in ectopia testis.

The actual descent of the testis and the lengthening of the vas and testicular vessels at the appropriate time are the product of various factors in which steroid hormones and maternal gonadotrophins play an important part.

It may here be fittingly observed that the testis *descends* during its development from a lumbar to a scrotal situation, whereas the kidney *ascends* from a pelvic to a lumbar site.

CHRONOLOGY OF THE TESTICULAR DESCENT: The testis descends:

1. From loin to iliac fossa in the third month of intra-uterine life.
2. From the fourth to the seventh month it rests at the site of the internal or abdominal inguinal ring.
3. During the seventh month it is travelling through the inguinal canal.
4. In the eighth month it lies at the external or subcutaneous inguinal ring.
5. In the ninth month it enters the scrotum, reaching its base at or after birth. Scorer[2] found 4 per cent of undescended testes in full-term and 33 per cent in premature infants. Most of these reached the scrotum within three months of life; 0·7 per cent remained undescended. Descent does not occur after the infant is a year old.

FATE OF THE PROCESSUS VAGINALIS: This peritoneal diverticulum becomes occluded at two points soon after birth; first, at the internal abdominal ring; and, secondly, just above the testis, cutting off the part of the sac in relation to the testis, which is henceforward

[1] Backhouse, K. M., and Butler, H., *J. Anat.*, 1960, 94, 107.
[2] Scorer, C. G., *Br. J. Urol.*, 1955, 27, 374.

THE ANATOMY OF CONGENITAL ERRORS

known as the tunica vaginalis testis. The part of the sac between the two occlusions is the funicular process, which becomes obliterated, forming a fibrous cord, the rudiment of the processus vaginalis.

Abnormalities Resulting from Faulty Development of the Testis: These comprise some of the commonest surgical conditions: (1) Indirect inguinal hernia; (2) Hydrocele; (3) Incomplete descent of the testis; (4) Ectopia testis; (5) Polyorchidism; (6) Inversion of the testis; (7) Torsion of the testis; (8) Dislocation of the testis—not a result of faulty development, but included here for completeness.

1. INDIRECT INGUINAL HERNIA: If the processus vaginalis fails to close at the internal abdominal ring, a passage is left through which the abdominal contents may pass. Such an event may occur soon after birth or not for many years, though it is important to realize, even in the latter case, that the sac into which the hernia occurs may have existed since birth. The processus vaginalis closes a little sooner on the left than on the right, therefore hernia is commoner on the right.

TYPES OF THE HERNIA (*Fig.* 398):

   a. Vaginal or Congenital: The processus vaginalis has failed to become occluded in any part of its course. The hernia therefore descends to the base of the scrotum and the testis is behind it and may be difficult to locate. Sir Harold Stiles stressed the liability of this type of hernia to become strangulated the first time it occurs.

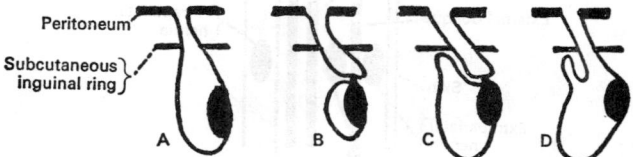

Fig. 398.—Types of indirect inguinal hernia. A, Vaginal. B, Funicular. C, Infantile. D, Encysted.

   b. Funicular: The processus is obliterated above the testis. The testis can be felt separately from the hernia, below it.
   c. Infantile: As (*b*), but a process of peritoneum of the processus vaginalis is found in front of the hernia as high up as the external ring. Therefore, at operation, a peritoneal sac is found in front of the hernial sac.
   d. Encysted: As (*a*), but a process of peritoneum lies in front of the sac up to the external ring.

   Types (*c*) and (*d*) are due to a diverticulum of the processus vaginalis being caught up at the external ring during development.

e. *Interstitial:* In this type a diverticulum of the processus vaginalis has been caught between the layers of the developing abdominal wall. The sac may be (*Fig.* 399):
   i. *Proparietal or Extraparietal* (superficial) between the superficial fascia and external oblique.
   ii. *Interparietal* (intramuscular) between the internal and external oblique muscles.
   iii. *Retroparietal or Intraparietal* (properitoneal) between the fascia transversalis and peritoneum.

This type of hernia is rare, and is usually found in association with imperfectly descended testis.

2. **HYDROCELE:** In this condition there is a collection of fluid in some part of the processus vaginalis.

TYPES OF HYDROCELE (*Fig.* 400):

a. *Vaginal:* This is a collection of fluid in the tunica vaginalis testis. It is not due to any fault of development. It is always necessary in this type to determine whether it is of the common idiopathic or primary variety, or whether it is secondary, due to some disease of the testis or epididymis.

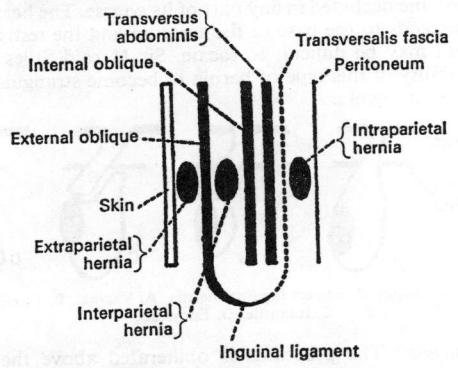

Fig. 399.—Varieties of interstitial hernia.

b. *Congenital:* This is also known as intermittent hydrocele. It is due to a tiny communication between the processus vaginalis and the peritoneal cavity, which admits of the escape of fluid into the abdominal cavity, but not of the entrance of intestine into the sac. It lessens in size on steady pressure or on lying down. It may be confused with a congenital hernia. The latter, however, reduces much more readily than the hydrocele and its reduction may be associated with a gurgle.

THE ANATOMY OF CONGENITAL ERRORS

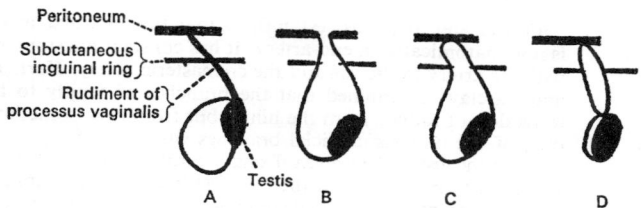

Fig. 400.—A, Vaginal hydrocele. B, Congenital hydrocele. C, Infantile hydrocele. D, Hydrocele of cord.

  c. *Infantile:* The processus vaginalis is occluded at the internal abdominal ring only.
  d. *Hydrocele of the Cord:* The funicular process fails to shrink into a fibrous cord, so that a tubular cavity results, shut off from peritoneum above and tunica vaginalis below. It becomes distended with fluid, forming one or more swellings separate from the testis.

3. INCOMPLETE DESCENT OF THE TESTIS: Cryptorchidism, i.e., absence of one testis from the scrotum, occurs in 0·1 to 0·2 per cent of all young adults (E. P. Alyea[1]).
   TYPES OF INCOMPLETE DESCENT: The testis may become arrested at any point along its long journey from lumbar region to bed of scrotum. The incompletely descended testis may be:
   a. *Lumbar:* Entire failure of descent.
   b. *Iliac:* Partial descent. The testis may be felt lying at the entrance of the inguinal canal.
   c. *Inguinal:* The testis is in the canal.
   d. *At the External Ring:* The testis frequently comes to rest just outside the external inguinal ring.
   e. *Scrotal:* The testis is in the upper part of the scrotum.
   Practicability of 'bringing down' the Testis: Generally the ductus deferens is amply long enough to extend to the testis in the scrotum. It is therefore the mesoblastic elements of the cord which are shortened, i.e., coverings of cord and vessels of testis. These have usually to be divided before the testis can be placed in the scrotum, and even then there is often a tendency to retraction. Good ultimate results are obtained in about 50 per cent of cases, and it is well to warn the parents that atrophy of the gland may occur. Many authorities consider that the chances of effective spermatogenesis after the testis is brought down are remote.

[1] *Surgery Gynec. Obstet.*, 1929, Nov. 600.

Fowler and Stephens[1] established that the testicular artery is not anatomically an end-artery. It has constant anastomoses with the artery to the vas and the cremasteric artery. Harrison and Barclay[2] determined that the branches of supply to the testis do not radiate from the hilum but from two (sometimes one) of the major superficial branches which ramify over the body of the testis. They give off small spiral vessels which enter the testis to supply it, and then double back to the periphery. The two parent vessels may lie together constituting a hazard in fixing the testis by suture. Thus the ultimate branches of the testicular artery are anatomically end-arteries. No anastomotic

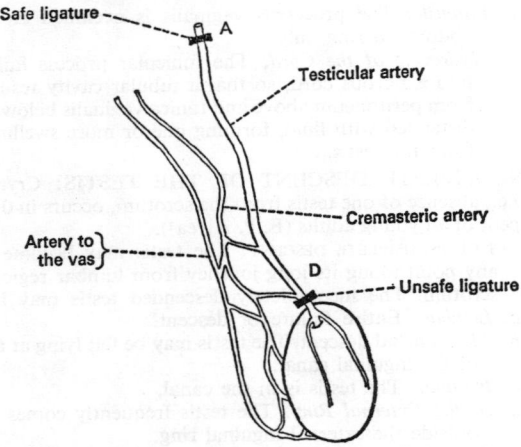

Fig. 401.—The anastomoses of the testicular artery. Ligature of testicular artery at A conserves the blood-supply to the testis. Ligature at D imperils this supply. (*By courtesy of Fowler and Stephens and the 'Australian & New Zealand Journal of Surgery'.*)

vessels enter the substance of the testis directly from either the head or tail of the epididymis. Any anastomotic supply to the testis can reach it only by way of the main testicular artery or its major superficial arteries near the testis. These facts are applicable to cases of imperfect descent of the testis.

The anastomoses referred to above take place proximal

---

[1] Fowler, R., jun., and Stephens, F. D., *Aust. N.Z.J.Surg.*, 1959, 29, 92.
[2] Harrison, R. G., and Barclay, A. E., *Br. J. Urol.*, 1948, 20, 57. Quoted by Fowler and Stephens.

to the testis. In cases of undescended testis and cryptorchids, the mesoblastic contents of the cord may be congenitally short, and it becomes necessary to divide them in order to bring the testis into the scrotum. Thus the testicular artery may have to be divided, and this section should be as high as possible to ensure the collateral arterial supply from the arteries to the vas and the cremaster. The cases which should be chosen for this procedure are those with a long loop vas (*Fig.* 401).

In addition, the testis receives an anastomotic blood-supply from the scrotal arteries, branches of the internal pudendal arteries. In two-thirds of persons these are sufficient to maintain viability. In recurrent inguinal herniae, if necessary, the cord can therefore be cut in the inguinal canal to achieve better closure of the canal, and provided the testis is not removed from its bed it will remain viable in two-thirds of the cases, although there may be temporary pain, swelling and fever.[1]

4. ECTOPIA TESTIS: Ectopia testis implies that the organ has deviated from the normal line of its descent. The ectopic testis is always one which has successfully completed its intra-abdominal descent; moreover it has negotiated the inguinal canal and external ring.

VARIETIES OF ECTOPIA TESTIS: Anchoring bands may displace the testis into the following situations, viz.: (*a*) Superficial inguinal (or interstitial); (*b*) Pubopenile; (*c*) Perineal; (*d*) Crural or femoral.

a. *Superficial Inguinal Ectopia:* This is the commonest type (W. B. Coley[2]). The testis lies lateral to the external ring, somewhere between this opening and the anterior superior iliac spine. Frequently it is just above and lateral to the ring. The testis lies in the plane between the aponeurosis of the external oblique and the deep layer of the superficial fascia (fascia of Scarpa).

b. *Pubopenile Ectopia:* This is very rare. The testis rests in front of the pubis at the root of the penis, or on the dorsum of the penis.

c. *Perineal Ectopia:* The testis is in the superficial perineal pouch, i.e., under the fascia of Colles and between it and the superficial perineal muscles. Clinically there is a lump in front of the anus to one side of the midline.

d. *Crural or Femoral Ectopia:* The testis is at the root of the thigh somewhere in the neighbourhood of the fossa ovalis (saphenous opening), which is 3·7 cm. below and lateral to the pubic spine.

[1] Harrison, J. H., *Am. J. Surg.*, 1971, **121**, 631.
[2] *Ann. Surg.*, 1908, **48**, 321.

It is worthy of note that:
  i. The ectopic, unlike the incompletely descended testis, is usually fully developed.
  ii. The ectopic testis is usually accompanied by an oblique inguinal hernia.
  iii. The ectopic testis may be divorced from the epididymis, which may lie, e.g., in the scrotum.
  iv. Ectopia and incomplete descent have been grouped together under the generic term 'imperfect descent' (Eccles).
  v. Imperfect descent of the testis shows an hereditary tendency.
  vi. A diagnosis of imperfect descent must not be hastily made in childhood and infancy as, though the scrotum is often empty, the testis may merely be temporarily absent owing to the irritability of the cremaster muscle.
  vii. The writer has brought forward evidence to show that abnormal fascial pockets and ridges exist sufficiently often in the inguinal region to explain the condition of imperfect descent on anatomical grounds without invoking the aid of hypothetical gubernacular 'tails'.[1]

5. MONORCHIDISM: It is important to distinguish between concealment of and developmental absence of a testicle. The former has a malignant potential which the latter has not. When the testis is absent the vas is usually present as they develop from different structures. The diagnosis is made by exploring the extraperitoneal tissues of the iliac fossa, locating the vas, and tracing it to its termination.

6. POLYORCHIDISM:[2] This condition is so rare as to be of the nature of a surgical curiosity. It is of interest because of the diagnostic problems it may present and because of the liability of one of the testes to undergo recurrent attacks of torsion. There are three possible variants of the condition:
   a. Duplication of the testis with a single epididymis and vas.
   b. Duplication with a separate epididymis and vas to each testis.
   c. Pseudo-duplication.

   Fig. 402 explains how two testes may be associated with a single epididymis and vas. Either the undifferentiated sex gland divides into two, or tubules persist which should normally disappear, thus forming a second gland. Should duplication be associated with two epididymides and vasa then the developmental error must involve a more extensive splitting of the anlage of testis, epididymis, and vas. The testis which has the stronger gubernacular attachment will occupy the lower position in the scrotum. Pseudo-duplication

---

[1] A. Lee McGregor, 'The Third Inguinal Ring', *Surgery Gynec. Obstet.*, 1929, Sept., 273.
[2] With acknowledgements to R. Hodgson Boggon, *Br. J. Surg.*, 1933, 20, 630.

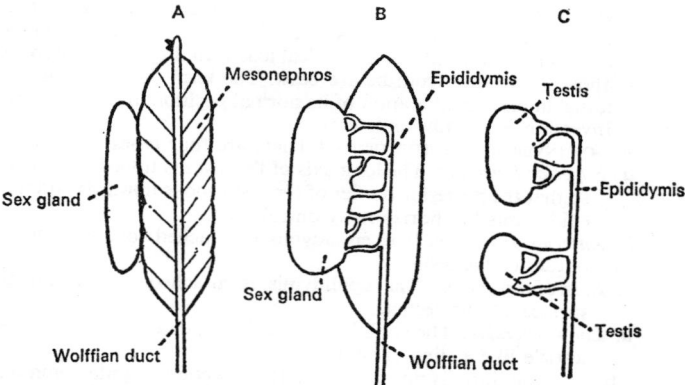

Fig. 402.—Diagrammatic representation of the genesis of polyorchidism. A, The undifferentiated sex gland. B, A further stage of development—the testis, vasa efferentia, epididymis, and ductus deferens can be distinguished. C, Owing to failure of atrophy of the anterior tubules two testes are formed. (*From the 'British Journal of Surgery'.*)

implies that both testes lie in one half of the scrotum, the other half being empty.

Only 12 cases of polyorchidism have been recorded; 9 of these were left-sided. The condition is apt to be mistaken for a spermatocele, or a hydrocele of the cord, particularly as one of the testes may be devoid of testicular sensation. Spermatogenesis has been found in half the cases.

7. INVERSION OF THE TESTIS: This is an interesting departure from the normal of congenital origin.

THE NORMAL POSITION OF THE TESTIS: The organ is suspended in the scrotum, attached above, below, and behind to the epididymis,

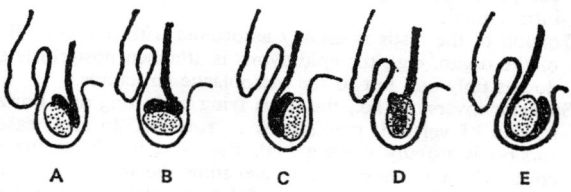

Fig. 403.—Inversion of testis. A, Testis normally orientated. B, Superior inversion. C, Anterior inversion. D, Lateral inversion. E, Loop inversion. (*After Campbell.*)

which in turn is blended with the ductus deferens and the vessels and nerves going to the testis and epididymis. It is thus held in a relatively fixed position, its vertical axis inclining obliquely from above down and from before back. The term 'inversion of the testis' implies an alteration of its normal position in the scrotum. Inversion is usually unilateral.

TYPES OF INVERSION OF THE TESTIS:[1] There are four types (*Fig.* 403):

   a. Superior Inversion: The long axis of the testis is tipped forwards, so that the posterior border of the testis looks upwards and the epididymis lies horizontally on this border.
   b. Anterior Inversion: The epididymis is attached to the anterior border of the testis.
   c. Lateral Inversion: The epididymis is attached to the lateral surface of the testicle.
   d. Loop Inversion: The epididymis and ductus deferens encircle the testicle like a sling (Testut).

The first condition is not uncommon; the second is quite common if anyone troubles to find it; the remaining two conditions are rare. Anterior inversion is of practical importance in the operation of 'tapping' or withdrawing the fluid from a hydrocele. The testis is normally posterior to the fluid and the needle is entered in front. In anterior inversion the testis is in front of the fluid and a needle entered anteriorly may damage the organ.

8. TORSION OF THE TESTIS: The term is synonymous with torsion of the spermatic cord. In this condition the testis undergoes rotation round a vertical axis, and its blood-supply is partly or wholly cut off. In the latter event gangrene of the organ occurs. The following facts are noteworthy:

   a. Torsion frequently affects an imperfectly descended testis as the organ is improperly fixed.
   b. Torsion is sometimes found associated with lengthening of the peritoneal fold (mesorchium) attaching the testis to the epididymis, a condition predisposing to twisting. In such cases the testis is completely surrounded by the tunica vaginalis and the torsion is intravaginal.
   c. Torsion of the testis is usually associated with imperfect fixation of the organ, e.g., the epididymis is attached posteriorly to the ductus only and not to the mesoblastic structures.
   d. Superior inversion, i.e., the testis lying with long axis horizontal instead of vertical, predisposes to rotation. In such cases the torsion is usually extravaginal, the twist involving the whole cord, which is shortened so elevating the testis higher in the scrotum. This elevation is a useful diagnostic point in torsion of the testis.

[1] W. F. Campbell, *Surgical Anatomy*, 1908, 537. Philadelphia.

e. It is obvious from the foregoing that in cases of torsion there is always imperfect fixation of the organ.

f. Torsion of the testis is associated with dimpling of the skin of the scrotum because of shortening of the coverings of the cord (external, cremasteric, and internal spermatic fasciae) which blend with the scrotal septum and raphe. This scrotal dimpling may be of diagnostic value in testicular torsion.[1]

9. DISLOCATION OF THE TESTIS:[2] This implies that the testis which was originally in the scrotum has been driven into an abnormal position as the result of external violence. The following facts are noteworthy:

a. The condition is excessively rare.

b. The situation taken up by the dislocated organ depends on three factors: (i) Anatomical abnormalities in the size, etc., of the testis; (ii) Obstruction at the scrotal neck or in the inguinal or perineal region; (iii) The direction and force of the external violence—this is much the most important factor.

c. The force producing the dislocation is usually something of the nature of a wheel passing over the lower abdomen and scrotum, e.g., run-over accident.

d. Immediately after the accident there is usually too much swelling to detect the dislocation. When the swelling subsides the diagnosis is easily made.

e. Reposition of the testis usually requires operation, though in four cases this was effected by manipulation.

f. In all but two cases the tunica vaginalis was intact and the epididymis accompanied the testis. In these two cases the epididymis was torn loose from the testis.

g. There are three types of dislocation (*Fig.* 404):

  i. *The Internal Dislocation Group:* The testis is forced through the external abdominal ring and may come to lie in one of three possible situations; (α) In the abdomen; (β) In the inguinal canal; (γ) In the femoral canal.

  Dislocation of this type is not possible in the normal, as the testis is too large to traverse the external ring. It is essential, therefore, that the testis be abnormally small or the ring unusually large. No case of abdominal or femoral dislocation is known, yet the theoretical possibility exists.

  ii. *The Superficial Dislocation Group:* This is the commonest type. The testis does not pass through the external abdominal ring, but comes to lie somewhere under the deep layer of

---

[1] Ger, R., *Surgery*, 1969, 66, 907.
[2] This account is taken from 'Dislocation of the Testis', by Edwin P. Alyea, *Surgery Gynec. Obstet.*, 1929, Nov., 606.

superficial fascia. The possible positions are precisely the same as those which the congenital ectopic testis may occupy, i.e.: (α) Superficial inguinal type—relatively the commonest; (β) Pubic and penile type—relatively common; (γ) Perineal type—rare; (δ) Crural type—exceedingly rare.

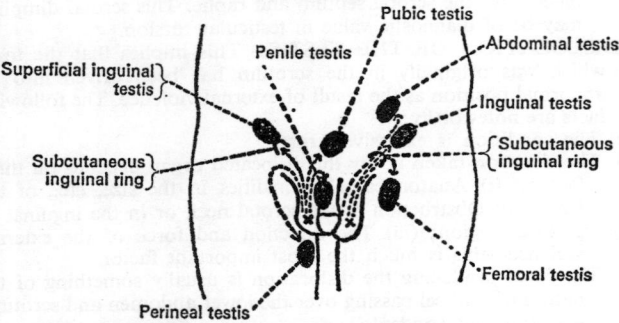

Fig. 404.—Shows the various positions which the testis may occupy when dislocated. The superficial types of dislocation are figured on the reader's left; on the right is illustrated the internal dislocation group. X denotes the normal position of the testis.

iii. *Compound Dislocation:* The skin is burst by the accident and the testis forced through the skin.

XVII. VESTIGIAL STRUCTURES IN CONNEXION WITH THE GENITAL ORGANS

In the Male:

ANATOMICAL BASIS OF SPERMATOCELES: A spermatocele, also called encysted hydrocele of the testis, is a cystic enlargement occurring behind the testicle in close relationship to the epididymis. It may occur as a single cyst or multiple ones may exist. Whereas it is considered by some that they are due to the obstruction of the normal efferent ducts from the testis, others consider that they take origin from developmental remnants which may be found near the epididymis. These are all Wolffian remnants. Probably spermatoceles may arise in either way.

The structures from which spermatoceles may arise (*Fig.* 405) are:

1. PARADIDYMIS: This, according to Toldt, consists of two structures, an upper and a lower.

   UPPER PARADIDYMIS OR ORGAN OF GIRALDÈS: This is composed of several tiny blind tubules lying in the lower end of the spermatic cord above the globus major of the epididymis but very near to it. It is always in front of the pampiniform plexus. It is not always present, and as a rule disappears in early childhood.

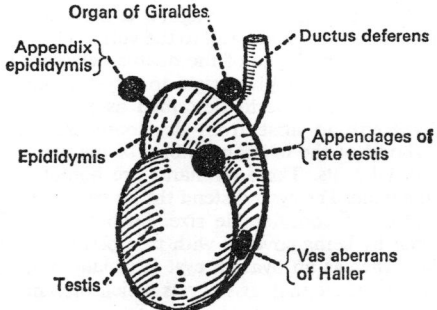

Fig. 405.—Vestigial structures which may give origin to spermatoceles.

LOWER PARADIDYMIS: This is a coiled tubule which lies behind the globus major of the epididymis.
2. VAS ABERRANS OF HALLER: This is a blind tube which lies between the tail of the epididymis and the commencement of the vas. Several of these tubules may exist.
3. APPENDAGES OF THE RETE TESTIS: These are blind tubes extending between the rete testis and the globus major of the epididymis.
4. APPENDIX EPIDIDYMIS OR STALKED HYDATID (Hydatid of Morgagni): Sits on the upper pole of the globus major of the epididymis, or on the testis. There may be two. It may be a vestige of the Müllerian duct.

Any of these vestigial structures may become distended to form a spermatocele. It will be obvious from the situations of the remnants that such a cyst will be behind the testis, and may occur in relation to any part of the epididymis.

In the Female (*Fig.* 406):
1. PAROVARIUM OR EPOOPHORON: This vestigial structure is situated between the layers of that part of the broad ligament which lies between the ovary and uterine (Fallopian) tube. It is the homologue of the male epididymis and ductus deferens, being developed from part of the Wolffian body and the Wolffian duct. It is poorly developed in the child, and reaches its highest development in middle life. The structure is made up of a horizontal tube lying below and parallel with the uterine tube. This is joined by a

number of vertical tubules which begin in blind extremities near the hilum of the ovary. The outer end of the main tube may divide into a number of tubules which are called Kobelt's tubes. The inner end of the main tube runs towards the uterus in the broad ligament reaching the upper end of the vagina. It may sometimes continue down in the anterior vaginal wall to the vulva. This tube is Gartner's duct, being the homologue of the ductus deferens. The main tube or the smaller ones may give origin to a cyst which is usually quite small. These cysts, hitherto described as parovarian, have been shown by Keith to arise from developmental remnants in the neighbourhood of the ovarian fimbria of the uterine tube and are called fimbrial cysts. These remnants are homologues of the rete testis in the male. The cysts distend the layers of the broad ligament and are often of considerable size. Such a cyst differs from an ovarian cyst by being covered with true peritoneum and by being unilocular, whereas an ovarian cyst is usually multilocular. From Gartner's duct there may arise cysts which present as cysts of the vaginal wall.

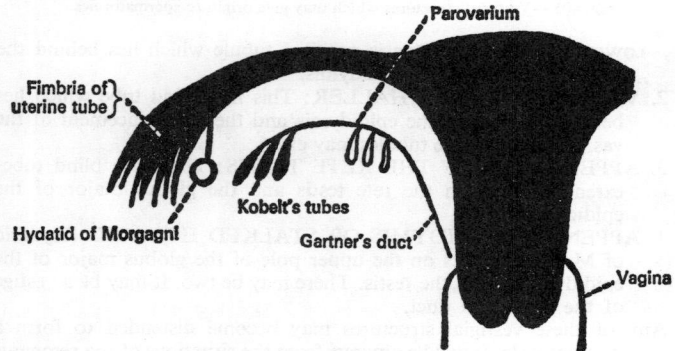

Fig. 406.—Vestigial tubules in broad ligament.

2. **HYDATID OF MORGAGNI:** This is a small cyst hanging by a stalk from the fimbriated end of the uterine tube. It is a Wolffian derivative. Cases have been described where it has caused acute abdominal symptoms by twisting round its stalk, thus undergoing strangulation.
3. **SKENE'S DUCTS:** The female urethra is surrounded with numerous racemose glands which open by small orifices on the urethral wall. Just within the meatus is an exceptionally large pair of these ducts called Skene's ducts. They frequently harbour gonococci after the

THE ANATOMY OF CONGENITAL ERRORS 419

disease has been eradicated elsewhere. These peri-urethral glands are regarded as the homologue of the prostate.

XVIII. HYPOSPADIAS

In this condition the development of the urethra is interfered with and it exists as a gutter instead of as a canal. The condition occurs almost entirely in the male.

The external genitalia are developed as follows (*Fig.* 407). There appears in the lower part of the front of the embryo an eminence—the *genital tubercle;* and below it two other eminences—the *genital swellings*—soon appear. There is a groove on the under-surface of the *genital tubercle*. This is the indifferent sexual stage of the embryo from which either male or female may develop.

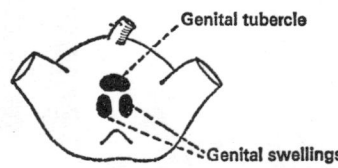

Fig. 407.—Earliest stage in development of external genitals.

- *Further Development in the Male:* The genital tubercle enlarges greatly to form the penis. The edges of the groove on its under-surface join together from behind forwards to form the urethra. Faulty fusion of the edges of the groove causes hypospadias. The genital swellings become fused together in the midline to form the scrotum.
- *Further Development in the Female:* The genital tubercle remains small, the groove on its under-surface disappears, and the clitoris results. The genital swellings take on rapid growth, and, remaining separate, form the labia.
- **Types of Hypospadias:** (1) Balanic; (2) Penile; (3) Perineoscrotal. In all types of hypospadias the prepuce is deformed, forming a triangular hood on the dorsum of the penis.
  - BALANIC (*Fig.* 408): The urethra ends at the base of the glans penis. The glans is often grooved on its under-surface.
  - PENILE (*Fig.* 409): The urethra ends anywhere between the base of the glans and the front of the scrotum. Extending forward from its orifice is a gutter on the under-surface of the penis.
  - In both these types the fault is a partial failure of fusion of the lips of the groove on the under-surface of the genital tubercle.
  - PERINEOSCROTAL: The lips of the groove on the under-surface of the genital tubercle entirely fail to fuse and the genital swellings remain separate. In other words, the individual has remained in the

420 A SYNOPSIS OF SURGICAL ANATOMY

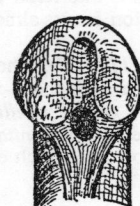

Fig. 408.—Balanic type hypospadias.

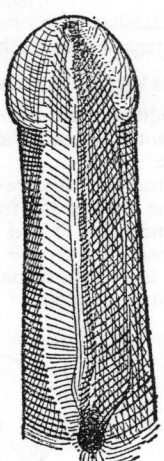

Fig. 409.—Penile type of hypospadias.

indifferent sexual stage. These persons are often brought up as females, as the genitalia resemble those of the female more than of the male. The penis is very small and not traversed by the urethra. The urethra exists as an opening between the separated halves of the scrotum. Only by doing a rectal examination and determining the presence of the uterus and ovaries can the sex be determined—a procedure by no means as easy as it sounds. Laparotomy is often necessary.

XIX. EXTROVERSION OF THE BLADDER AND EPISPADIAS

Extroversion of the Bladder: This is a condition where:
1. The anterior wall of the bladder is missing, so that its posterior wall appears as a raw area on the lower abdominal wall in which the ureteric orifices are seen. This red area is bounded above by an imperfect umbilicus, shaped like a crescent (*Fig.* 410).
2. The prostatic urethra is seen below the bladder, as its front wall is missing. The ejaculatory ducts are seen to open here.
3. The pubes remain separate so that no symphysis exists (*Fig.* 411).
4. The prostate and seminal vesicles are absent.
5. The penis opens out to form a gutter on its dorsal surface.
6. The scrotum is imperfectly formed.

THE ANATOMY OF CONGENITAL ERRORS

Extroversion is always accompanied by a gutter on the dorsal surface of the penis.

The developmental explanation of these maldevelopments is obscure, and like other imperfectly understood conditions the explanations advanced are not very easy to understand. Veilleton's account (quoted by McFarland[1]) is as follows: The openings into bowel behind and urogenital organs in front are excavated by a special plate of tissue at the lower end of the embryo. This plate is called the anal plate; its function is to disappear. Thus by the disappearance of its posterior part the proctodeum is formed, which is the excavation into the hindgut which forms the anus. The disappearance of its anterior part forms the openings into the vagina and bladder. According to Veilleton, in extroversion the anal plate extends excessively far forward—right up to the umbilicus, in fact. Now, as the function of this membrane is to disappear, its disappearance leaves a gap right up to the umbilicus, so that the front wall of the bladder is absent.

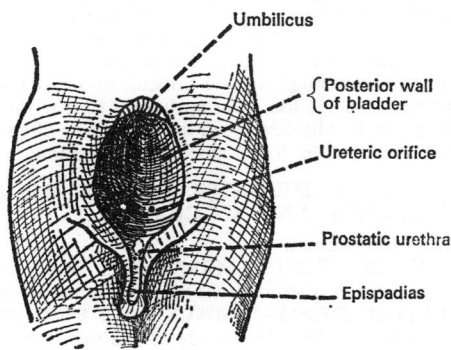

Fig. 410.—Extroversion of the bladder.

Epispadias: The anal plate does not extend so far foward, but only far enough to prevent the two halves of the genital tubercle from completely joining to form one. The result is that the penis is opened out along its middle, and the urethra forms a dorsal gutter. Like hypospadias, the condition may be of varying degree: (1) Balanic; (2) Penile; (3) Penopubic.

BALANIC: The urethra ends on the dorsum of the penis at the base of the glans, which is opened out by a gutter.

---

[1] *Surgical Pathology*, 1926, 33. London.

422 A SYNOPSIS OF SURGICAL ANATOMY

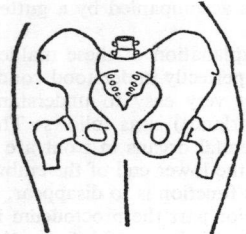

Fig. 411.—Showing the gap between the two halves of the pelvis which occurs in cases of extroversion of bladder.

PENILE: The urethral canal ends in the region of the symphysis: the penis is opened out by a dorsal gutter.

PENOPUBIC: The urethra is represented by a gutter in its entire length, the defect extending into the bladder. It passes under the symphysis, and a finger can be passed into the bladder along the gutter. The muscles controlling urination are deficient, so that the urine cannot be held but drips away.

Minor degrees of extroversion may be difficult to distinguish from severe cases of epispadias. It has been aptly said that if in such cases the symphysis pubis is fully developed the case is one of epispadias. If the two pubes are separate, it is a case of extroversion.

XX. CONGENITAL DEFECTS IN THE REGION OF THE SACRUM AND COCCYX

Posterior (Behind the Sacrum):

1. PERSISTENCE OF THE EMBRYONAL TAIL: A tail exists at the second month of embryonal life. It may persist at birth.
2. CONGENITAL DERMAL SINUS AND PILONIDAL SINUS: Developmentally the neural folds of the skin fuse in the midline of the back to close off the neural groove and form the neural tube. This fusion may be faulty, resulting in congenital dimples, pits, or sinuses which may occur anywhere from the occiput to the coccyx. These sinuses are lined by squamous epithelium and there may or may not be hair follicles and sebaceous glands in the wall. The hairs found in the sinuses are usually loose, having been sucked into the sinuses by the movements of the buttocks, and may play an important role in the causation of the infection.

Occasionally these sinuses may communicate with the dura and could thus allow organisms to gain access to the meninges and produce meningitis.[1] Such sinuses are usually situated over the

[1] Cardell, B. S., and Laurence, B., *Br. med. J.*, 1951, 2, 1558.

THE ANATOMY OF CONGENITAL ERRORS 423

sacrum or higher and have other associated abnormalities such as pigmentation or a capillary haemangioma round the external opening or a dermoid cyst or spina bifida at its inner end.

The common *pilonidal sinus* in the sacrococcygeal region is a variant of this condition. When infection occurs an abscess forms and may rupture to one or other side of the midline although the original sinus is always in the midline.

However, some cases of sacrococcygeal pilonidal sinuses are acquired conditions resulting from indriven hairs and similar sinuses are found at the umbilicus, over the pubis, and in barbers' hands.

INTERDIGITAL SINUSES OF BARBERS' HANDS: It has long been known that barbers are commonly afflicted with sinuses in the clefts between the fingers (*Fig.* 412). These usually occur between the index and middle, or middle and ring fingers of the right hand. They are the result of short portions of stiff hairs which are, by trauma, forced into the skin much as a short thorn might be.

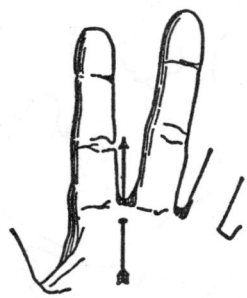

Fig. 412.—An interdigital sinus.

They cause an inflammatory reaction and other hairs find their way into the sinus. Epithelium grows in and lines the sinus and skin glands may form in its wall. It never occurs in barbers attending to females.

3 SPINA BIFIDA: Ordinary spina bifida may occur here.
4. SPINA BIFIDA OCCULTA may occur here.
5. SACRAL PARASITE: A large mass of tissue may occur here at birth. This is a 'sacral parasite' or a teratoma of the sacrum. It is due to the fact that there may be attached to the body at this site a twin which has not progressed beyond a jumble of tissues of different kinds.

Anterior (in Front of the Sacrum):
1. ANTERIOR SPINA BIFIDA: This condition may give rise to anterior sacral meningocele—a cystic tumour lying in the hollow of the sacrum.
2. DERMOID CYSTS or teratomatous formations of uncertain origin may occur in the sacral hollow.

XXI. WEBBED FINGERS (*Syndactylism*)

The hand is originally a flapper-like broadening of the end of the limb. The fingers become separated by four vertical grooves (*Fig.* 413). These grooves deepen until the flapper becomes separated into five parts which form the thumb and fingers. The thumb is the first to separate, and the fingers separate at their distal ends first. Failure of separation may take place between two or more adjacent processes. This failure may be partial or complete. If partial, two adjacent digits will be united by a web of skin at their bases; if complete, two or more adjacent digits are united in their entire length. As the thumb is the first to separate, it is never webbed.

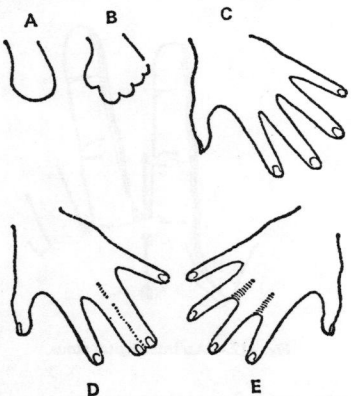

Fig. 413.—Origin of webbed fingers. A, B, C, Stages in development of hand and fingers. D, Syndactylism—complete. E, Syndactylism—partial.

XXII. SEQUESTRATION DERMOIDS

Wherever two ectodermal surfaces join together during development, there may occur a burying or sequestration of portions of ectoderm. A remnant of this kind may grow and form a tumour. This is called a sequestration dermoid. Such a growth has the following characteristics:
1. It occurs in the course of the line of developmental fusion of two ectodermal surfaces.

THE ANATOMY OF CONGENITAL ERRORS

2. Its contents are pultaceous or putty-like owing to the collection of cast-off cells from the cyst lining which fill the tumour and by the accumulation of which it grows.
3. It often contains hair, which is always the colour of the hair of the owner. This hair is formed by the hair follicles which develop in the wall of the buried ectoderm.

Such a tumour is most difficult to distinguish from a sebaceous cyst, as the latter also contains cheesy matter, cast-off cells, and hair. The only certain method of distinction lies in the histological examination of the cyst walls. In the dermoid there are found in the wall derivatives of the skin, such as sweat-glands and hair follicles, which are not found in sebaceous cysts. Of prime importance—the papillary layer of the skin is found in the wall of the dermoid, but not in that of the sebaceous cyst.

Sequestration dermoids may be found:
1. Along the lines of fusion of the face.
2. Along the line of embryonal concrescence (Bland-Sutton[1]), that is to say, the line along which the two halves of the body join. This line extends from the root of the nose, over the top of the head, down the midline of the back, through the perineum, up over the raphe of the scrotum and along the middle of the ventral and dorsal surfaces of the penis, up the front of the body to the middle of the margin of the lower lip. The line is exactly central in its whole length.

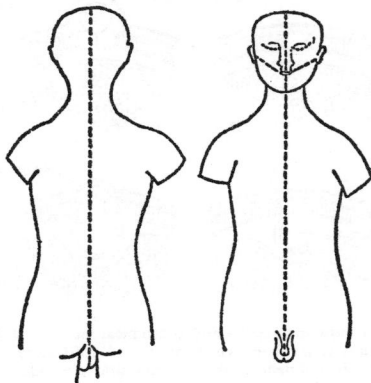

Fig. 414.—To show line of 'embryonal concrescence' and fusion lines of the face.

[1] *Tumours, Innocent and Malignant*, 1917, 524. London.

Dermoids in the Line of Embryonal Concrescence (*Fig.* 414):

DERMOIDS OF THE SKULL: These may occur anywhere along the midline of the scalp. They may occur at either angle of the orbit, being then due to faulty development of the facial processes. The former group will alone be considered here.

Scalp dermoids have peculiar characteristics:
1. They are situated in the midline.
2. They may grow to enormous proportions.
3. They often rest in an excavated area in the bony cranium.
4. They are usually attached to the dura by a fibrous stalk which passes through the suture line or even through an opening in the bone. Such an opening always has smooth regular margins.
5. They may lie:
    a. Entirely superficial to the bone.
    b. Entirely within the skull, between bone and dura.
    c. Partly within and partly without the skull.

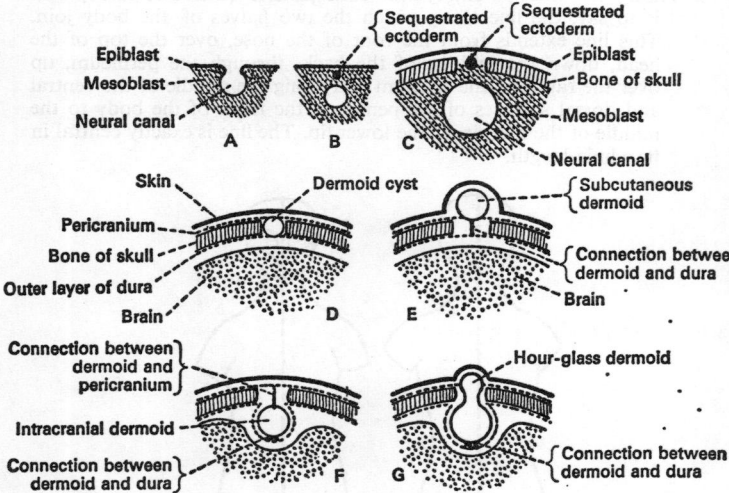

Fig. 415.—To show the genesis and anatomical features of dermoids of the skull. A, The neural canal from which brain and cord arise. B, Sequestrated ectoderm between skin and neural tube. C, Sequestrated ectoderm surrounded by developing skull bones. D, The sequestrated ectoderm becomes cystic, forming a dermoid cyst. E, Dermoid of skull superficial to the bone—note attachment to dura. F, Dermoid within the skull—note attachment to pericranium and dura. G, Dermoid partly within and partly without the skull—note attachment to dura and pericranium.

THE ANATOMY OF CONGENITAL ERRORS 427

This variable situation is accounted for by a consideration of the development of the vault of the skull (*Fig.* 415):
  i. The neural groove closes to form the neural canal from which will develop the cord and the brain.
  ii. A portion of ectoderm is buried between the surface of the body and the underlying neural tube, in cases where a dermoid is going to develop.
  iii. The mesoderm grows in between the surface and the neural tube.
  iv. The mesoderm will form the bones of the vault, also the dura mater.
  v. The sequestered portion of ectoderm is enveloped by the developing bones.
  vi. The sequestered ectoderm is therefore attached to the dura and may develop mostly deep to the bone or superficial to the bone, always retaining its dural attachment.

DERMOIDS OF THE BACK: May occur:
  1. Superficial to the vertebral arches—between them and the skin.
  2. Deep to the vertebral arches, actually within the vertebral canal, for reasons similar to those which obtain in cases of dermoids inside the skull. Such tumours may cause nerve symptons by pressing on the spinal cord. The sacrum is the commonest site of the back to be affected.

DERMOIDS OF THE PERINEUM: May occur along central raphe of perineum or scrotum, or along midline of penis.

DERMOIDS OF THE ABDOMEN: May occur: (1) Just beneath the skin; or (2) Deep to the abdominal wall.

DERMOIDS OF THE THORAX: May be found: (1) Under the skin over the sternum; (2) Under the sternum itself within the mediastinum, above or in front of the heart (*Fig.* 416).

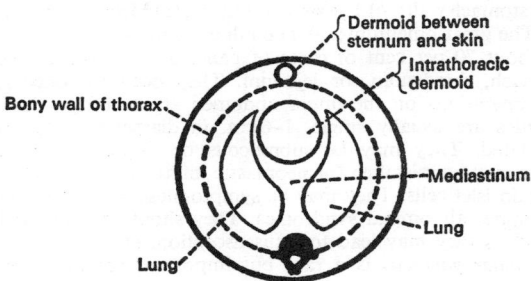

Fig. 416.—Showing two types of dermoids of the thorax.

DERMOIDS OF THE MEDIASTINUM: Two explanations have been given to account for these cysts:
1. That dermoids of the superior mediastinum arise from remnants of the branchial arches which have been carried downwards by the descent of the heart during development.
2. That dermoids of the superior or inferior mediastinum result from inclusions of ectoderm sequestrated there by the closure of the two halves of the thorax along the midventral line (Bland-Sutton). The occasional existence of bifid sternum in these cases lends support to this view.

Such tumours are often tridermal teratomata, though they may be simple dermoid cysts arising like typical sequestration dermoids from a single embryonic layer (Ekehorn[1]).

DERMOIDS OF THE FLOOR OF THE MOUTH: Dermoids may be found situated behind the symphysis menti, in the floor of the mouth, having been cut off from the skin by the developing symphysis. They are exactly *central* in position, which distinguishes them from ranula, which is a much commoner tumour situated to *one side of the midline*.

XXIII. TISSUE DISLOCATION

In the complicated process of development tissue may be displaced (dislocated) or reduplicated.

Sequestration Dermoids: May be caused by the persistence of ectodermal vestiges.

Accessory Organs: A portion of the primitive rudiment of an organ may be displaced:
1. THYROID: Accessory thyroid tissue may occur in: (*a*) The tongue; (*b*) The midline of the neck above the normal situation of the thyroid gland.
2. PANCREAS: Accessory pancreatic tissue may be found in: (*a*) The stomach wall; (*b*) The small intestine; (*c*) Meckel's diverticulum; (*d*) The great omentum; (*e*) The hilum of the spleen.

About 70 per cent of cases of pancreatic heterotopia occur in stomach, duodenum, or jejunum. They occurred once in each 500 operations on the upper abdomen at the Mayo Clinic. The nodules are usually single, 1–6 cm. in diameter, yellowish, and lobulated. They may be submucous or intramuscular and the latter may be mistaken for neoplastic infiltration. About one-third contain islet cells. They may be symptomless or present as one of the upper abdominal syndromes. They should be removed when found as they may lead to intussusception, etc.

Annular pancreas is a rare but important condition in which

---

[1] Quoted by Carrick Robertson and R. E. Bevan Brown, *Br. J. Surg.*, 1929, 17, 201.

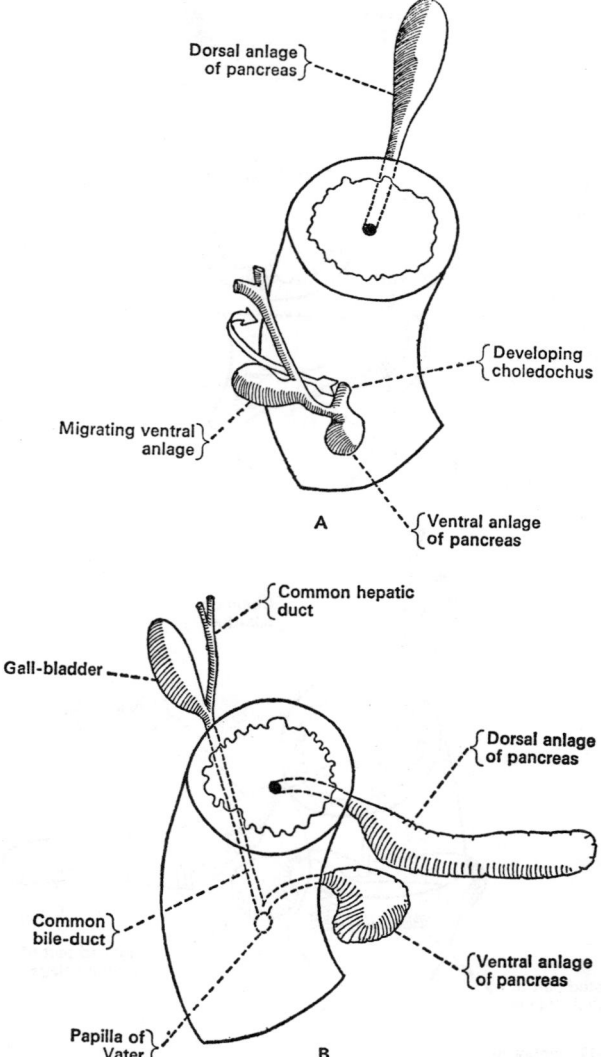

Fig. 417.—A, Normal development of the pancreas. The close association of the developing choledochus and ventral anlage of the pancreas is seen on the front of the duodenum. The arrow indicates the migration of the pancreas to the right and posteriorly together with the bile-duct and gall-bladder. The dorsal anlage and duct of Santorini are seen proximally. B, Migration of the ventral anlage of the pancreas is complete.

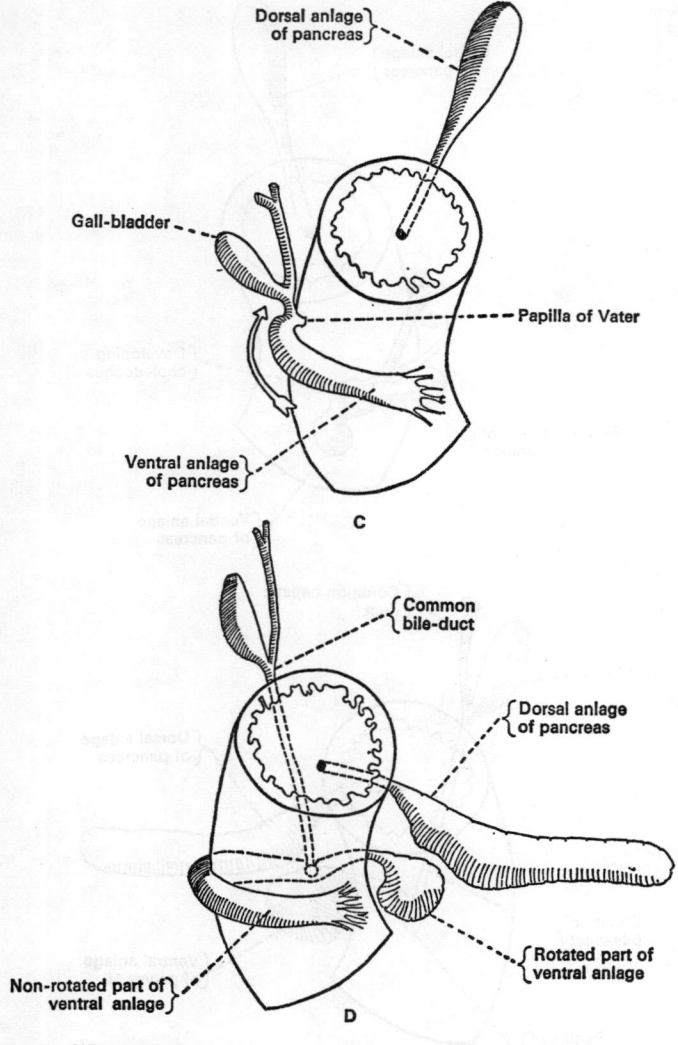

Fig. 417, continued.
C, Maldevelopment of ventral anlage of pancreas which has retained its primitive attachment to the front of the duodenum. The arrow indicates the migration of the choledochus dragging the adherent ventral anlage with it. D, The ring made by the maldevelopment of the ventral anlage of the pancreas is complete, i.e., annular pancreas. (*Designed and drawn by Dr. E. A. Thomas.*)

a ring of pancreatic tissue surrounds a part of the descending portion of the duodenum.

Explanation: The pancreas is formed by two anlage—dorsal and ventral. The dorsal one grows into the dorsal mesoduodenum. Its duct system enters directly into the duodenum—the accessory pancreatic duct (Santorini). This anlage ultimately forms the body, tail, and ventral aspect of the head of the pancreas. The ventral outgrowth is intimately attached to the developing choledochus and primitive gut. It migrates to the right (*Fig.* 417) and then dorsally, ultimately forming the dorsal part of the head and the uncinate process of the pancreas. Its duct forms the proximal part of the main pancreatic duct (Wirsung), maintaining its opening into the choledochus, and links up with branches of the dorsal duct in the body and tail (*Fig.* 418).

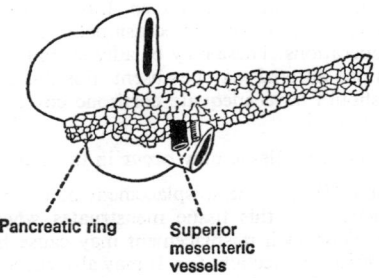

Fig. 418.—Annular pancreas.

If the ventral pouch fails to migrate around the right side of the gut, it retains its attachments both to the choledochus and to the ventral wall of the primitive gut. The origin of the choledochus has moved posteriorly consequent on the migration of the duodenum to the right. The ductal system formed by the ventral anlage thus almost completely encircles the primitive gut and may constrict this tube. This explains the not infrequent association of annular pancreas with stenosis of the second part of the duodenum. This condition occurs in one case in four. This stricture is thus the result of faulty development of the ventral pouch and is not merely an associated independent anomaly. An understanding of the development explains why, if no duodenal stricture exists, annular pancreas produces no symptoms. It is also apparent that division of the pancreatic ring incurs the serious risk of cutting through a large pancreatic duct. Thus the principle of treatment is not to interfere with the annular pancreas itself.

The obstruction is relieved by a Roux Y anastomosis of upper jejunum to duodenum above the constriction.

3. LIVER: Accessory liver tissue is sometimes found in the left triangular ligament of the liver (*see* p. 85).

4. SPLEEN: The existence of more than one spleen is the commonest anomaly of the organ. They are found in 11 per cent of autopsies (Adami). They vary in size from a pea to a walnut, and may be multiple. They are found: (*a*) Near the hilum; (*b*) In the mesentery or omentum; (*c*) In the tail of the pancreas; (*d*) On the wall of the bowel (Gray).

5. ADRENAL TISSUE: Accessory adrenal tissue is found in 22 per cent of post-mortems. It may occur in: (*a*) The kidney; (*b*) The testis; (*c*) The spermatic cord; (*d*) The epididymis; (*e*) Scattered almost anywhere in the abdomen. Little yellowish bodies the size of a pin's head or larger are occasionally found in the cord during hernia operations. These may be adrenal rudiments. In 10 per cent of cases one adrenal may be absent. For this reason all adrenalectomies should have adequate cortisone cover before, during, and after operation.

6. OVARY: Ovarian tissue may occur in the broad ligament.

7. ENDOMETRIUM: The misplacement of endometrial tissue is of great interest, as this tissue menstruates when the uterus menstruates. Thus such misplacement may cause haemorrhage which is very difficult to account for. It may also cause tumour formation. Accessory endometrial tissue may be found in : (*a*) The rectovaginal septum—here it causes a rare and interesting tumour which is called adenomyoma of the rectovaginal septum; (*b*) The uterine tube; (*c*) The hilum of the ovary (chocolate cysts); (*d*) The uterosacral ligament; (*e*) The pelvic colon.

It must be mentioned that endometriomata (misplaced uterine mucosa) are considered by most authorities to be due not to developmental error but to 'retrograde menstruation', i.e., discharge of menstrual products up through the tubes into the peritoneal cavity, where islets of mucosa may be grafted and form intraperitoneal tumours.

8. MULTIPLE RUDIMENTS: Owing to persistence of more than one rudiment, several accessory organs may occur. Thus arises the condition where numerous accessory spleens are found in the peritoneal cavity. It may happen in a disease which is usually cured by splenectomy, e.g., acholuric jaundice, that the symptoms persist after the removal of the spleen because of the existence of accessory spleens.

THE ANATOMY OF CONGENITAL ERRORS

XXIV. DIVERTICULA

A diverticulum is a small offshoot or sidetrack from a hollow viscus. In origin it may be developmental or pathological.

Characteristics (*Fig.* 419):

1. The walls of the congenital diverticulum are usually, though not always, formed of all the coats of the parent viscus, including therefore a complete muscle coat. The contents of the diverticulum can thus be expelled and debris is not likely to collect in it.
2. The pathological or acquired diverticulum does not as a rule possess a complete muscle coat. It may be covered by a few muscle fibres, which are, however, insufficient to empty it completely. It is therefore apt to become the site of stagnation of the substances which pass into it.

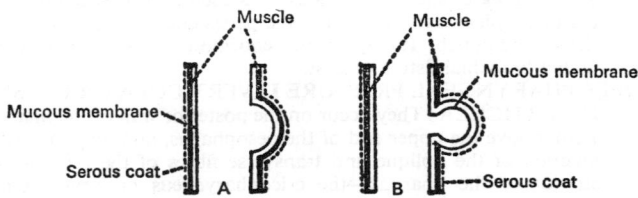

Fig. 419.—The classic distinctions between congenital and acquired diverticula. A, Congenital diverticulum: note that its wall contains all the coats of the parent viscus and the neck is wide. B, Acquired diverticulum: little or no muscle in wall; neck narrow.

3. The communication between a true or developmental diverticulum and its parent viscus is as large as the lumen of the diverticulum.
4. In a false or pathological diverticulum the communication is usually considerably smaller than the lumen of the diverticulum, so that the isthmus is very liable to become obstructed.
5. From the above facts it is obvious that in general a congenital diverticulum is not very liable to accident and may never give rise to symptoms indicative of its existence.
6. The pathological diverticulum is a constant menace to its owner, and may herald its presence by becoming obstructed, distended, or perforated.

Sites of Diverticula: (1) Pharynx; (2) Oesophagus; (3) Trachea; (4) Alimentary canal; (5) Bladder; (6) Urethra.

Diverticula of the Pharynx[1] (*Fig.* 420):

CONGENITAL CENTRALLY PLACED ANTERIOR DIVERTICULA: For example, these may occur at the base of the tongue. They are very rare.

[1] Classification is that of William Hill, *Br. med. J.*, 1926, 2, 1163.

434 A SYNOPSIS OF SURGICAL ANATOMY

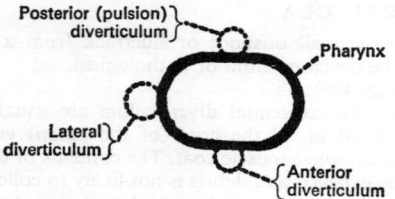

Fig. 420.—The situations of pharyngeal diverticula.

CONGENITAL LATERAL POSTFAUCIAL DIVERTICULA: These arise from the persistence of the visceral pouches of the embryo. The opening of such a diverticulum is usually behind the tonsil on the palatopharyngeal fold. It is the persistence of the inner end of the second pouch. It may become enormous. It is often associated with a branchial fistula or cyst.

DEEP PHARYNGEAL PRESSURE DIVERTICULA OR PULSION DIVERTICULA: They occur on the posterior wall of the pharynx, 1 cm. above the upper end of the oesophagus, and originate at the junction of the oblique and transverse fibres of the inferior constrictor of the pharynx—the cricopharyngeus of laryngologists.

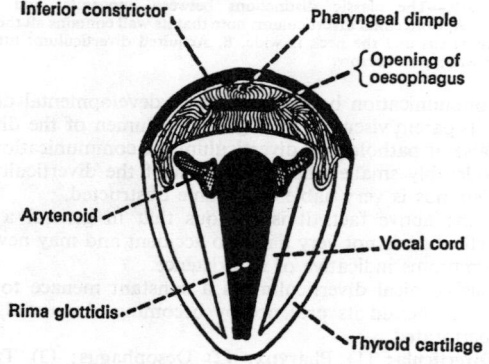

Fig. 421.—The pharyngeal dimple.

There is normally a slight gap between these two sets of muscle-fibres which is called Killian's dehiscence.[1] At this site there is often an indication of a depression. This is the 'pharyngeal dimple'

[1] Killian, G. *Ann. des Mal. de l'Oreille*, 1908, **34**, July, 11.

THE ANATOMY OF CONGENITAL ERRORS 435

(*Fig.* 421). Excessive enlargement of this recess results in pharyngeal diverticulum, the so-called 'pulsion diverticulum'. It is the commonest variety of herniation through the wall of the pharynx.

The inferior constrictor consists of a lower transverse muscle which is sphincteric and an upper oblique propulsive muscle. Incoordination of the action of these muscles may result in spasm of the sphincteric part while the propulsive part continues acting, resulting in such an increase of pressure in the laryngopharynx that the mucous membrane is eventually forced through as a pouch between the two parts of the inferior constrictor.

ORIFICE: The opening into the pouch is transverse and about an inch in length. It is situated exactly in the midline of the back of the pharynx just above the upper end of the oesophagus.

WALLS: These consist of: (1) Mucous membrane; (2) Submucous tissue; (3) A fibrous layer derived from the aponeurosis of the pharynx. Observe that there is no muscle in the wall.

Lahey[1] clarifies the clinical picture in his masterly manner: The diverticulum passes through three stages (*Fig.* 422):

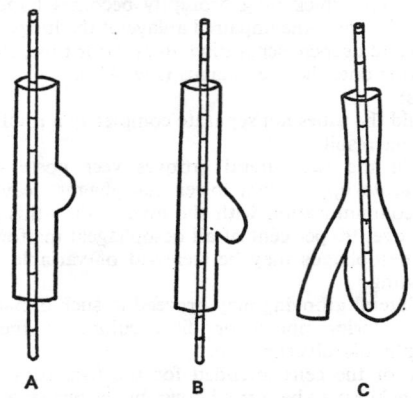

Fig. 422.—The development of a pharyngeal diverticulum. A, The bulge. B, The pouch. C, The bag. Notice the danger associated with the passage of an instrument in type C. (*After Lahey.*)

1. There is merely a bulge on the posterior pharyngeal wall and no symptoms result unless hawking from the lodgement of a food particle in the sac.
2. A definite pouch is formed. The opening is posterior. The

[1] Frank H. Lahey, *Ann. Surg.*, 1946, **124**, 617.

pouch moves with the oesophagus in swallowing. The posterior relation is the unyielding vertebral column. The pouch is thus subjected to movement and massage which, as the sac contains liquid and air, cause noises at table, very embarrassing to the sufferer, as they are audible and attract attention and comment. Moreover, during the night movement may cause expulsion of the contents of the diverticulum, resulting in an irritating and disturbing cough. Aspiration of the contents of the sac may cause lung abscess.

3. The pouch has become large. In addition to the symptoms described above definite obstruction to swallowing occurs, and the nutrition of the patient suffers severely.

Diverticula of the Oesophagus:

1. CONGENITAL DIVERTICULA of the oesophagus or trachea[1] may result from aberrations of the development of these organs which are so closely related embryologically. Very early in fetal life a thickening appears in the ventral wall of the entodermal tube (future pharynx and oesophagus) just caudal to the pharyngeal pouches. This thickening promptly becomes larger and rounded at its caudal end—the unpaired anlage of the lungs. Lateral grooves develop and deepen, separating an anterior tube, the trachea, from a posterior one, the oseophagus (*Fig.* 423).

    ANOMALIES:

    a. Should the tubes not separate completely a tracheo-oesophageal fistula results.

    b. Should the two lateral grooves veer posteriorly, they may separate upper from lower oesophagus, leaving the trachea in communication with the lower tube—this group accounts for over 90 per cent of all oesophageal malformations.

    c. The oesophagus may be stenosed or variable lengths may be missing.

    d. The lateral grooving may proceed in such a manner as to leave an anterior pouch or diverticulum of the oesophagus— epiphrenic diverticulum.

    e. Some of the cells intended for the formation of trachea and bronchus may be carried down by the growing oesophagus and form supernumerary bronchi and even lung tissue (*Fig.* 424).

    A diverticulum of the trachea—tracheocele—may occur if such a supernumerary bronchus retains a communication with the trachea.

2. TRACTION DIVERTICULUM: This is caused by the breaking down of diseased lymph-glands lying near the oseophagus (*Fig.* 425). Fibrosis occurs, and the consequent retraction of the resulting scar

---

[1] This section is based on 'Malformations of the Oesophagus, Small Intestine and Biliary Tract', by Dr. W. H. Snyder, jun., *Surg. Clins N. Am.*, 1959, 39, 1151.

THE ANATOMY OF CONGENITAL ERRORS

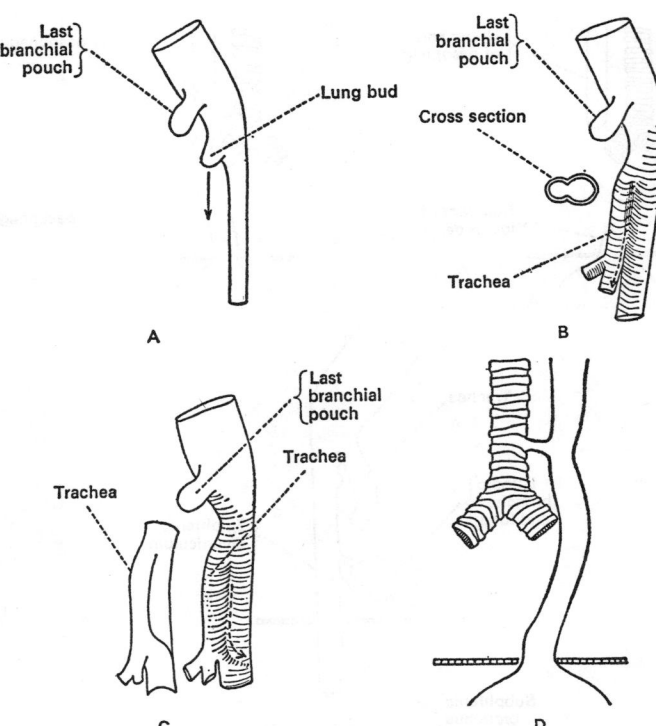

Fig. 423.—A, The lung bud develops from the anterior wall of the pharynx and oesophagus. It grows downward (arrow) to form a ridge. B, Lateral grooves develop separating trachea from oesophagus. These grooves move anteriorly below as shown by the arrow. C, The separating grooves have moved posteriorly (arrow) separating upper from lower oesophagus, leaving trachea in fistulous communication with lower oesophagus. The upper part of the oesophagus ends blindly as shown in the inset. D, Incomplete separation of trachea and oesophagus resulting in a fistula. (*By courtesy of R. Snyder, the Editor and Publishers of 'Surgical Clinics of North America'.*)

tissue pulls on the oseophagus, forming a pouch. It is a true diverticulum in the sense that its walls are composed of all the coats of the oesophagus, but it is not congenital.

3. LEUGART'S POUCH: There is a fibrous band known as Leugart's ledge passing from the left bronchus to the side of a vertebra. The

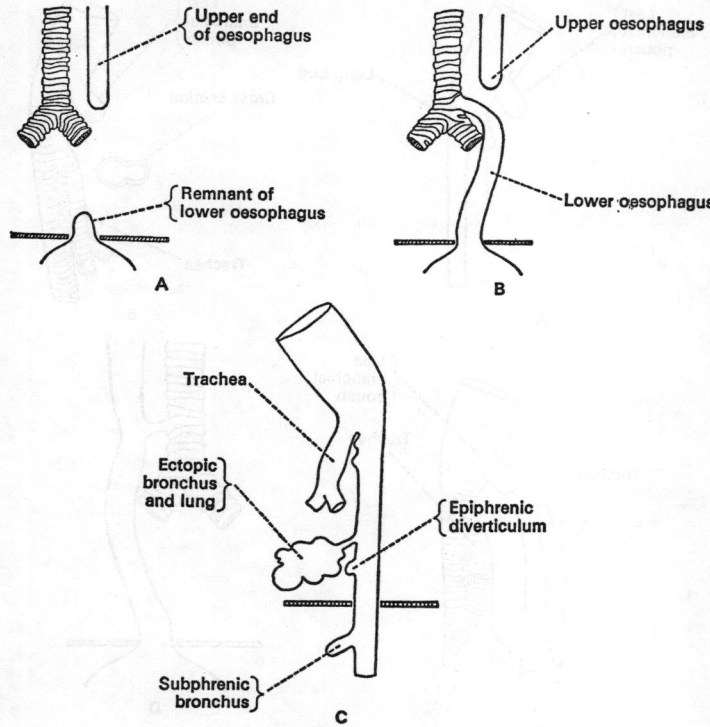

Fig. 424.—A, A portion of the oesophagus is missing. B, There is an oesophageal fistula and the upper part ends blindly. C, The diagram shows ectopic lung tissue and bronchi, also an oesophageal diverticulum. (*By courtesy of R. Snyder, the Editor and Publishers of 'Surgical Clinics of North America.'*)

oesophagus crosses this ledge. The wall of the oesophagus may prolapse over the ledge and give rise to a small diverticulum.

Diverticula of the Trachea: Diverticula of the trachea are of extreme rarity. Like diverticula elsewhere, they may be: (1) Acquired; (2) Congenital. Before considering these, there are further facts about the development and structure of the trachea which must be known in order to appreciate the method of formation of tracheoceles.

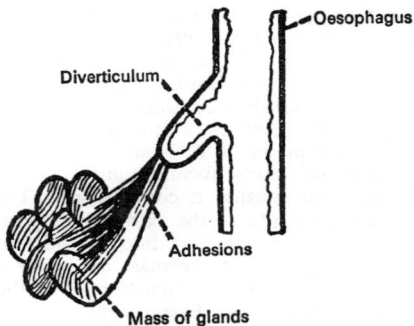

Fig. 425.—Traction diverticulum of oesophagus.

1. In the human embryo each main bronchus gives off three primary buds to form the lungs.
2. Each of the three buds on the right develops into one of the lobes of the lung.
3. Opinion differs as to what happens to the uppermost of the three buds on the left. Some authorities consider that the upper left lobe is developed from the upper two buds. Aeby,[1] also Flint,[2] think that the upper left bud normally disappears, appearing, however, in rudimentary form in rare cases, as an accessory bronchus, or rudimentary third stem bronchus.
4. The cartilaginous rings of trachea and bronchi form each two-thirds of a circle. The gap between the two ends of the ring is occupied by the transverse fibres of the unstriped trachealis muscle. There are muscle strips, therefore, completing the cartilaginous rings, and between each two adjacent strips is a potential weak area,[3] covered, however, externally by the longitudinal fibres of the trachealis, and internally by mucous and submucous coats of the trachea.
5. W. Stirling[4] states that the acini of the tracheal mucous glands lie external to the trachealis muscle so that the ducts of the glands must pierce the muscle to reach the bronchial lumen.

ACQUIRED DIVERTICULA: The great majority of tracheoceles come under this denomination, and are due to respiratory disease. They are small hernial protrusions of the mucous membrane (Bland-Sutton[5]). They vary in size from a pigeon's egg to a small

---

[1] Aeby, *Bronchialbaum der Säugethiere und der Menschen*, 1880, quoted by Stibbe.
[2] Flint, J. M., *Am. J. Anat.*, 1906, 6, 1.
[3] Muller, W. S., *Anat. Record*, 7, No. 11, 373, quoted by Stibbe.
[4] Stirling, W., *J. Anat.*, 17, 204, quoted by Stibbe.
[5] *Tumours, Innocent and Malignant*, 1917, 716. London.

orange. Some are lined with mucous membrane and are of the nature of pulsion or pressure diverticula, others are due to actual bursting of the mucosa and have no mucous lining. Rokitansky considered them due to catarrh of the trachea or chronic bronchial or pulmonary disease. Gruber[1] considers them to be retention cysts of the mucous glands. They are of little clinical interest. As a rule they produce no symptoms (J. E. Newcomb).[2]

A diverticulum may rarely form a tumour of the neck above the clavicle (resonant because it contains gas). The absence of symptoms is due no doubt to the extremely important fact that the opening from the diverticulum into the trachea is relatively large so that the contents of the mass are easily evacuated by changes of posture or pressure, stagnation being thus prevented.

CONGENITAL DIVERTICULA: Exceedingly rare. E. P. Stibbe's[3] case was due, in his opinion, to the persistence of Aeby's supernumerary bronchus (upper left bronchial bud). He stresses the fact that the opening into the posterior wall of the trachea was very minute, barely admitting a medium-sized pin. This type of tracheocele might conceivably produce symptoms due to stagnation and decomposition of the contents of the cyst. An interesting point in the case quoted was that the tumour, though arising from the back of the air-passage, had made its way to the front of this tube, lying between it and the aortic arch quite near the thyroid, for an adenoma of which it might easily have been mistaken. It was connected to the trachea by a tenuous hollow stalk.

Diverticula of the Gut: Diverticula of the alimentary canal occur in the following order of frequency: (*a*) Colon; (*b*) Meckel; (*c*) Duodenum; (*d*) Pharynx and oesophagus; (*e*) Stomach; (*f*) Jejunum. They may be: (1) Congenital; or (2) Acquired.

1. CONGENITAL DIVERTICULA AND ENTEROGENOUS CYSTS:[4] Cysts whose walls reproduce the structure of the gut, whether found in the wall of the gut, attached to the gut, or more or less remote from the gut, must have been derived from the gut. They are enterogenous cysts and originated as diverticula in the following way. Lewis has shown that in the developing gut there are many bud-like projections from the mucous membrane, which projections contain a cavity communicating with the lumen of the gut. These tiny diverticula usually cause no disturbance in the course of the muscle-fibres. It would seem that they occur normally during the course of development (*Fig.* 426). If they fail to disappear

---

[1] *Anat. Mem. Berlin*, quoted by Stibbe.
[2] *Trans. Am. lar. Ass.*, 1906, 251, quoted by Sir St. Clair Thomson.
[3] 'True Congenital Diverticulum of the Trachea', *J. Anat.*, 1929, 14, 62.
[4] For much of the matter of this subdivision the author is indebted to the illuminating article by Arthur Evans, *Br. J. Surg.*, 1929, 17, 34.

THE ANATOMY OF CONGENITAL ERRORS

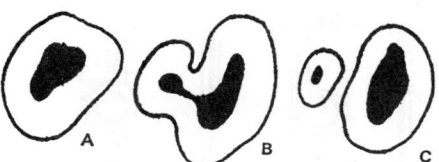

Fig. 426.—Cross-section of epithelial tube of intestine, showing development of diverticula and cysts. A, Cross-section of embryonal gut. B, Section showing a diverticulum. C, Section showing a severed diverticulum, i.e., a cyst. (*Modified from Arthur Evans.*)

they may persist as one of the following two conditions: (*a*) Congenital diverticula; (*b*) Congenital enterogenous cysts.

a. CONGENITAL DIVERTICULA: Although congenital diverticula are said to occur in any part of the gut from the oesophagus to the pelvic colon they are rare. Meckel's diverticulum (described on p. 389) is a type by itself. Another distinctive type is the 'giant diverticulum', really a reduplication of a part of small or large gut.

b. CONGENITAL ENTEROGENOUS CYSTS: Each of these arises as a diverticulum, the lumen of which is later cut off from that of the alimentary canal, thus forming a closed cavity or cyst. Such a cyst may be, in relation to the gut wall: (1) Submucous; (2) Intermuscular; (3) Subserous.

A subserous cyst may: (1) Lose its attachment to the gut and be found between the layers of the mesentery more or less remote from the parent gut (mesenteric cyst); (2) Become invaginated into the lumen of the gut.

The ileocaecal region is a favourite site for enterogenous cysts, which are sometimes called 'ileocaecal cysts'. The diagram from Evans shows the varieties which have been met with (*Fig.* 427).

Harvard Baker[1] thus describes other varieties of mesenteric cysts of congenital origin:

a. Lymphangiomatous (cf. cystic hygroma of neck).

b. Mesocolic: resulting from failure of fusion of adjacent layers of peritoneum during fetal rotation of the gut.

c. Urogenital in origin due to sequestration from the mesonephros or other parts of the urogenital system which may migrate into: (i) mesentery and form mesenteric cysts, or into (ii) broad ligament giving rise to parovarian cysts.

Malformations may affect any part of the alimentary canal from pharynx to anus. Many different names and explanations are applied to them. Ladd and Gross[2] simplified the matter of classification

---

[1] Harvard Baker, A., *Br. J. Surg.*, 1961, 48, 534.
[2] Ladd, W. E., and Gross, R. E., *Surgery Gynec. Obstet*, 1940, 70, 295.

442 A SYNOPSIS OF SURGICAL ANATOMY

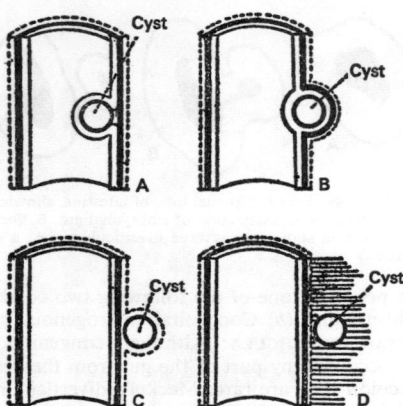

Fig. 427.—Enterogenous cysts. A, Submucosal. B, Intermuscular. C, Subperitoneal. D, Intramesenteric. (*After Arthur Evans.*)

by grouping them together as duplications of the alimentary tract. They defined these as spherical or hollow structures which possess a coat of smooth muscle, a lining of mucous membrane similar to that of some part of the alimentary canal (although not necessarily adjacent to it), and having an intimate attachment to some part of this tube. Such diverticula or duplications of the small gut may be found in the chest or abdomen, and these together with the conditions described under (*a*) and (*b*) above are all included in the term 'duplications'. Eighty per cent do not communicate with the lumen of the bowel. Eighty-two per cent declare their presence within the first 3 years of life. The blood-supply is the same as that of the parent gut, therefore the cyst cannot be enucleated without damaging the blood-supply of this bowel. Resection with the corresponding portion of the gut is therefore always necessary.

2. **ACQUIRED DIVERTICULA**: According to Edwards[1] whose account is largely followed here, the vast majority of intestinal diverticula are acquired, because of the similarity in structure whether in small or large bowel, the fact that small and large gut may be affected simultaneously, and because no antecedent pathological changes can be found in the bowel wall. The common aetiological factor is considered to be abnormal and incoordinated contraction of the bowel wall. There are two types of acquired diverticula: Primary; Secondary.

[1] Edwards, C. E., *British Surgical Practice*, 1948, Vol. 3, 256. London: Butterworth.

THE ANATOMY OF CONGENITAL ERRORS 443

Primary Diverticula are all of the nature of hernial protrusions along weak areas in the bowel wall where the feeding arteries enter. In the case of the duodenum this is along the concave border and in the jejunum the protrusions occur on the mesenteric border. Here two vessels enter close together (*Fig.* 428). If tension in the bowel lumen rises high enough, the mucous membrane is forced

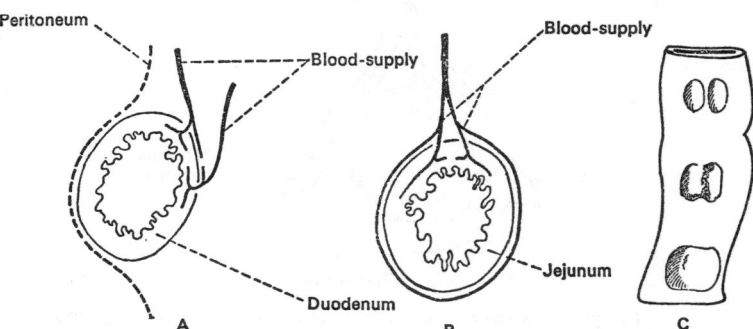

Fig. 428.—A, The blood-supply of the duodenum. B, The blood-supply of the jejunum. C, Coalescence of diverticula. (*Re-drawn from Edwards in 'British Surgical Practice'*.)

out as a pouch, one along each of the two vessels. In time as the protrusions enlarge they coalesce and form one pouch which is situated between the leaves of the mesentery. In the colon the vascular disposition is different. The artery enters at the mesenteric border and divides into two vessels which pass partly round the bowel and enter between two taenia to ramify in the submucosa. It is at these sites that colonic diverticula develop. As they protrude on the mesenteric side of each of the lateral taenia they tend to pass into the appendices epiploicae, each of which receives a feeding artery from the entering vessel before it pierces the circular muscle. These pouches are therefore widely separated, do not tend to fuse, and do not enter the mesocolon (*Fig.* 429).

These diverticula of the bowel share the following characteristics: They are flask-shaped with narrow necks. The wall consists of little besides mucosa, submucosa, and very little if any muscle tissue. They have difficulty in emptying themselves, stagnation occurs, and a train of complications follows. They are affections of middle age and after. Diverticula may affect any part of the duodenum. They are invariably situated on the side of the blood-supply, i.e., the concavity. A Vaterine diverticulum is related to the ampulla. They rarely cause symptoms, only 3 per cent requiring surgery. A large percentage are covered entirely by pancreatic tissue making their removal hazardous.

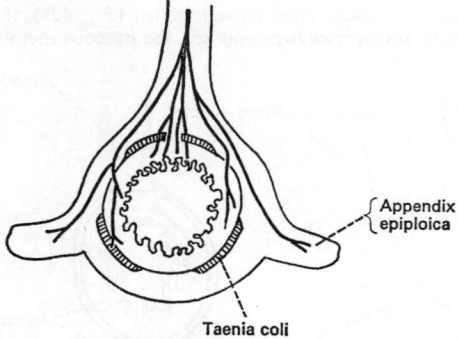

Fig. 429.—The figure shows three blood-vessels entering the colon. The central one perforates a taenia which protects the gap. The others have no such protection and the mucosa may, under certain circumstances, prolapse at their points of entry and initiate diverticula.

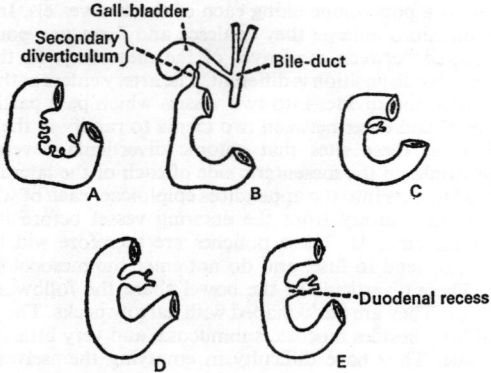

Fig. 430.—Diverticula of duodenum. A, Primary diverticula. B, Secondary diverticulum. C, Normal ampulla of Vater. D, Vaterine diverticulum due to dilatation of ampulla. E, Vaterine diverticulum—the ampulla lies at the apex of a duodenal recess (diverticulum).

The colon is by far the commonest site of acquired diverticula and 85 per cent of these occur in the pelvic colon (sigmoid). Twenty per cent become the site of diverticulitis. They do not predispose to malignancy. If cancer affects a part of the bowel containing diverticula, it is coincidental.

Secondary Diverticula: They occur only in the first part of the duodenum. They are due to chronic duodenal ulcers or to the traction of adhesions (*Fig.* 430). An ulcer causes such a pouch either by destroying a part of the gut wall, in which case the wall is formed by fibrous tissue, or by distorting the bowel so that a part of the wall forms a recess. In this case the diverticular wall is the same as that of the gut. Adhesions, e.g., of the gall-bladder to the first part of the duodenum, may pull out a funnel-shaped diverticulum which is part of the gut wall. It is a surgical axiom that adhesions between the duodenum and that part of the gall-bladder known as Hartmann's pouch must be treated with respect, as they may contain a diverticulum from the gut.

Diverticula of the Appendix: Though occasionally congenital, this is usually an acquired condition. A. J. Gardham[1] states: 'One or frequently more diverticula are found as a result of destruction of small areas of the muscle coat of the appendix by interstitial abscesses in the course of an attack of appendicitis. This destruction of muscle is probably a frequent event, but in the majority of cases the mucous membrane is involved in the destructive process, and the result is the ordinary "perforated appendix". If the mucous membrane is not destroyed a diverticulum results.' (Because the mucosa is unprotected by muscle at the site where the interstitial abscess was situated.)

The fate of such a diverticulum is of great interest. The possibilities are:
1. In the majority of cases repeated attacks of inflammation of the diverticulum lead either to its perforation with abscess formation, or to removal of the appendix.
2. In the minority of cases the inflammation dies down sufficiently to allow perforation of the diverticulum to occur without leading to abscess formation. These are the cases which ultimately develop pseudomyxoma peritonei. This is a curious ill-understood condition in which the belly is filled with jelly-like material. It arises as stated above, or more commonly from the rupture of a variety of pseudomucinous ovarian cyst. The jelly may go on forming even though the causative appendix or ovary is removed.

Diverticula of the Bladder: These may be : (1) Congenital; or (2) Acquired.
1. CONGENITAL DIVERTICULA: The bladder with the exception of the base is developed from the upper part of the cloaca. The base

[1] 'Diverticulosis of the Appendix and Pseudomyxoma Peritonei', *Br. J. Surg.*, 1928, 16, 65

is formed from the lower ends of the Wolffian ducts. The line of fusion is marked by the interureteric bar of muscle. Along this line and at the apex there may be a congenital weakness of the bladder wall which gradually yields, resulting in the occurrence of a diverticulum (Blum). Such are usually single, and occur almost solely in males (*See Fig.* 395, p. 402).

2. ACQUIRED DIVERTICULA: These occur very commonly in cases of obstruction to the outflow of urine from the bladder. The inner muscle coat of the bladder consists of an incomplete layer. Bands of muscle run in various directions, intersecting each other. Thus small depressions of the mucous membrane occur normally in the empty bladder between the muscular trabeculae. In cases of obstruction the trabeculae hypertrophy and become more prominent and the recesses become deeper and may ultimately form diverticula in which stagnation and infection occur. Such acquired diverticula are always multiple.

Urethral Diverticula[1] (*Fig.* 431): These may be congenital or acquired.

PROSTATIC URETHRA:

CONGENITAL DIVERTICULA: It has been shown that the congenital diverticulum of the prostatic urethra is due to the gradual distension of the utriculus prostaticus (sinus pocularis) which is

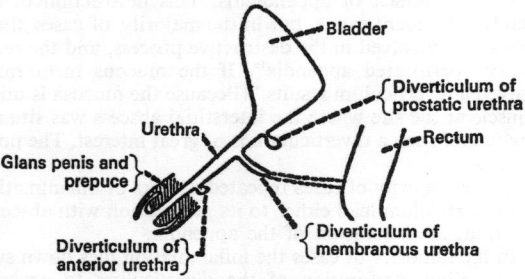

Fig. 431.—Diverticula of urethra.

normally present. A small stone lodged in this recess may slowly increase from accessions to its size deposited by the urine passing over it. In this way a large cavity may be formed communicating with the urethra.

ACQUIRED DIVERTICULA: These may be due to the persistence of the cavities of abscesses or cysts which have ruptured into the urethra.

MEMBRANOUS URETHRA: Diverticula of any kind are extremely rare. In a case of recto-urethral fistula of congenital origin which

[1] Based on 'Urethral Diverticula', by T. B. Mouat, *Br. J. Surg.*, 1928, 16, 51.

came under the writer's care there was a membranous tube connecting the rectum with the membranous urethra. This tube was occluded to cure the fistula. The part of the tube left in communication with the membranous urethra in this case is a diverticulum of the urethra of congenital origin (*Fig.* 431).

ANTERIOR URETHRA:
  CONGENITAL DIVERTICULA: These are rare, but do occur. They may be due to faulty fusion of the two skin folds which fuse in the midline of the floor of the urethra to form this channel.
  ACQUIRED DIVERTICULA: Here, as elsewhere in the urethra, acquired diverticula are much commoner than congenital ones. The acquired diverticula usually occur as the result of operations or injuries or abscesses affecting the urethra.

XXV. ARTERIAL ENTRAPMENTS

Popliteal Artery Entrapment: The popliteal artery may deviate medially from its normal course and pass deep to the femoral origin of the medial head of the gastrocnemius which may arise from a more lateral situation than usual (*Fig.* 432). This causes constriction of the

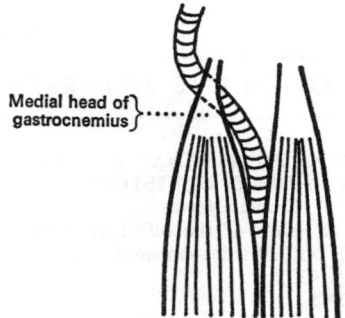

Fig. 432.—Popliteal artery passing deep to the medial head of the gastrocnemius muscle.

artery which can lead to secondary thrombosis. The condition results in disappearance of ankle pulses when the knee is forcibly extended and on arteriography the vessel is deviated medially. It may be bilateral.[1]

Compression of the Coeliac Artery by the Median Arcuate Ligament: The coeliac artery usually arises from the front of the aorta at the level of

[1] Harris, J. D., and Jepson, R. P., *Surgery*, 1971, 69, 246.

the upper third of the first lumbar vertebra and the median arcuate ligament crosses over the aorta immediately above this site. In 33 per cent of people the origin of the coeliac artery is at or above the median arcuate ligament.[1]

Occasionally the coeliac artery is compressed by the ligament, either because the artery arises from the aorta at a higher level, or more usually because the ligament crosses over the aorta at a lower level. This may result in chronic ischaemia of the abdominal viscera with postprandial pain and an epigastric bruit.

The superior mesenteric artery arises from the aorta not more than 1·5 cm. caudal to the coeliac artery and may sometimes also be affected by median arcuate ligament compression.[2]

The site of origin of the coeliac artery is inconsistent because of its cervical origin with a variable degree of descent during development. An abnormally high origin above the lower third of the 12th thoracic vertebra is frequently associated with the entrapment syndrome. The coeliac artery arises at a higher level in women than in men and the entrapment syndrome is more common in women.

Chapter XXX

THE ANATOMY OF NERVE INJURIES

I. THE ANATOMICAL AND PHYSIOLOGICAL LOSS RESULTING FROM NERVE DIVISION[3]

Cranial Nerves

First Nerve (Olfactory): A lesion of the olfactory nerves on one side results in loss of smell on that side—anosmia.

Second Nerve (Optic) (*Fig.* 433):
 1. CORTICAL LESION:
     a. Homonymous crossed hemianopia (loss of opposite visual fields).
     b. Eye reflexes normal.
 2. LESION OF OPTIC TRACT:
     a. Homonymous crossed hemianopia.
     b. Pupil reflex from opposite visual fields lost (hemiopic pupillary reaction—Wernicke).

---

[1] Lindner, H. H., and Kemprud, E., *Archs Surg.*, 1971, 103, 600.
[2] Curl, J. H., Thompson, N. W., and Stanley, J. C., *Ann. Surg.*, 1971, 173, 314.
[3] The writer would express his indebtedness in preparing this section to: (1) *Operations on Peripheral Nerves*, Sir Harold J. Stiles and M. F. Forrester Brown, 1922. London. (2) *The Clinical Form of Nerve Lesions*, A. Benisty, 1928. London. (Military Medical Manuals.)

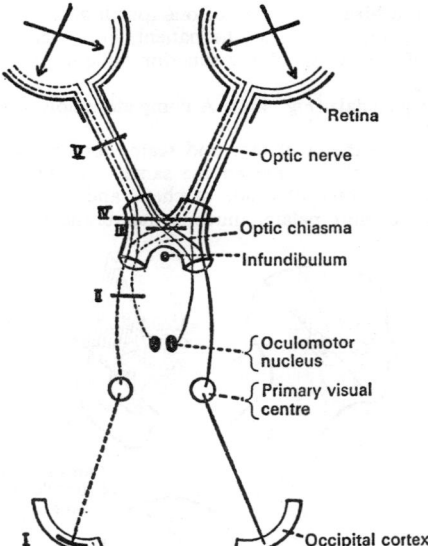

Fig. 433.—Situations of injuries of optic nerve and its central connexions. I, Cortical lesion; II, Lesion of optic tract; III Partial lesion of chiasma; IV, Complete lesion of chiasma; V. Complete lesion of one optic nerve. (*After Quervain.*)

3. PARTIAL LESION OF CHIASMA: Most often produced by a pituitary tumour: results in loss of both temporal visual fields (bitemporal hemianopia).
4. COMPLETE LESION OF CHIASMA: Blindness in both eyes and complete loss of pupillary reflexes.
5. COMPLETE LESION OF ONE OPTIC NERVE:
    a. Unilateral blindness.
    b. Loss of reflexes on that side.
    c. Loss of consensual reaction on healthy side.

Third Nerve (Oculomotor): A lesion of one third nerve results in:
  1. Drooping of upper lid (ptosis) with inability to open the eye.
  2. The pupil is fixed in a state of dilatation (uncontrolled sympathetic action).
  3. The eyeball is turned outwards and downwards (action of external rectus and superior oblique).

450 A SYNOPSIS OF SURGICAL ANATOMY

Fourth Nerve (Trochlear): A lesion of one fourth nerve: Nothing appears to be wrong on looking at the patient, but when he looks in the direction of the action of the superior oblique (down and out) he sees double.

Fifth Nerve (Trigeminal) (*Fig.* 434): A complete lesion of one fifth nerve results in:

1. Extensive anaesthesia of face and scalp, conjunctiva, and anterior two-thirds of the tongue on the same side, gums of both jaws, mucous membrane of inside of cheek and lips and hard palate and part of soft palate, mucous membrane of nose. This loss

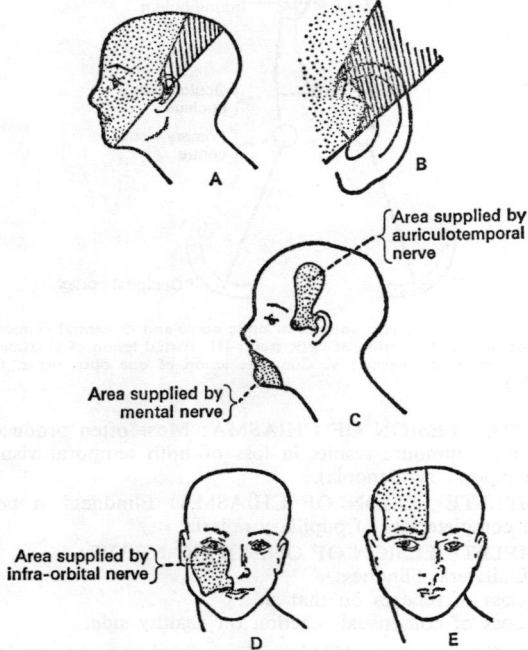

Fig. 434.—The sensory loss resulting from alcohol injection of the entire fifth cranial nerve or its divisions. A, Complete anaesthesia of fifth nerve. B, Sensory loss of the pinna in paralysis of fifth nerve. C, Sensory loss when mandibular nerve is paralysed. D, Sensory loss resulting from paralysis of maxillary nerve. E, Sensory loss from paralysis of ophthalmic division of fifth nerve. Dotted areas represent complete anaesthesia; hatched areas are partially insensitive to pin prick and light touch. (*After Wilfred Harris.*)

extends exactly to the midline, so that the patient in drinking feels as though the cup were broken.
2. Muscles of mastication on one side are paralysed (excluding the buccinator which is supplied by the seventh nerve).

FIRST DIVISION ONLY: If this nerve is divided, the loss is entirely sensory.

SECOND DIVISION ONLY: If this nerve be divided, the loss is entirely sensory.

THIRD DIVISION ONLY: Paralysis of the muscles of mastication and sensory loss.

The trigeminal nerve (not the facial) mediates deep sensibility from the face.

Sixth Nerve (Abducens): Paralysis of the external rectus of that side, resulting in a turning in of the eyeball and inability to move it out beyond the mid-point.

Seventh Nerve (Facial) (*Fig.* 435): It has been stated that the sensory root of the facial nerve (nervus intermedius) carries the fibres subserving the sensation of deep pressure from the face. Recent work goes to show that the fifth nerve conveys this type of sensibility and that the facial nerve takes no part in its conduction.

Geniculate neuralgia is the term applied to a neuralgia affecting the sensory portion of the facial nerve. It involves the deeper structure of the face and is characterized by pain in the deep posterior orbital, palatal, and nasal regions with pain in the face associated with pain in the ear. Authorities are uncertain that involvement of the sensory root of the facial nerve (Wrisberg) is the sole cause of this pain or whether the glossopharyngeal nerve is also concerned and where surgery is resorted to, both these nerves are usually divided.

1. CORTICAL LESION:
   a. Total paralysis of lower part of face on the opposite side.
   b. Partial paralysis of the upper part of the face on the opposite side.
   The upper part of the face is supplied from both sides of the cortex of the brain, so that if one cortex be injured, the upper half of the face still gets a supply from the other cortex, the paralysis being partial.
   c. Taste and salivary fibres normal.
   d. Corneal reflex retained.
   e. Stapedius not paralysed.
   f. No reaction of degeneration.
2. LESION OF INTERNAL CAPSULE: Symptoms as above, but movements of expression retained.
3. LESION AT ENTRANCE OF NERVE INTO INTERNAL AUDITORY MEATUS (e.g., in fractured skull):
   a. Paralysis of all the motor functions of the nerve. Taste fibres unaffected.

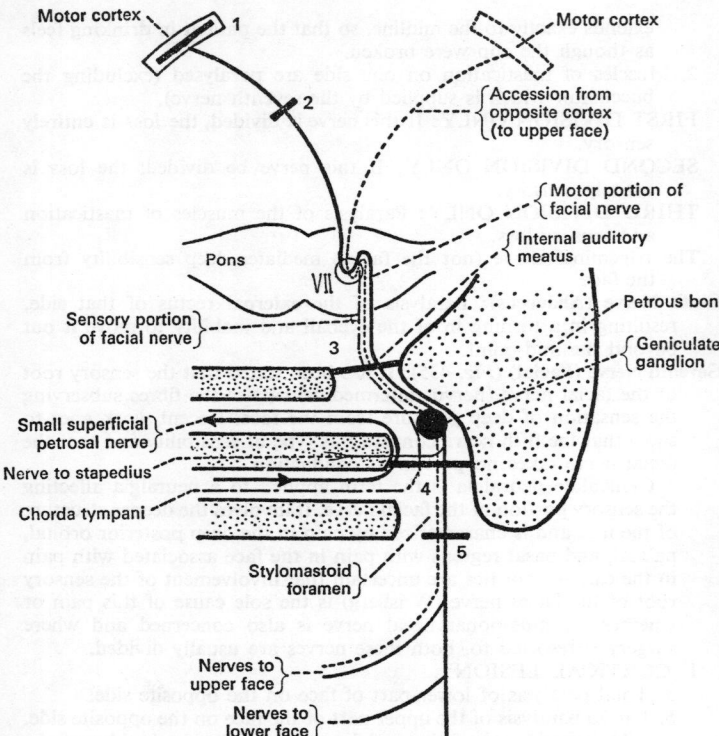

Fig. 435.—Quervain's diagram of the course of the facial nerve.

Lesion at 1: Cortical lesion. Crossed facial paralysis, complete for lower and partial for upper face. Taste and salivary fibres normal, corneal reflex retained, stapedius not paralysed. No reaction of degeneration.

Lesion at 2: Lesion of internal capsule. Same symptoms but movements of expression retained.

Lesion at 3: Lesion at internal auditory meatus. Paralysis of all motor and salivary fibres on same side. Stapedius paralysed, causing hyperacusis. Corneal reflex lost. Taste fibres unaffected. Expression and associated movements paralysed. Pronounced reaction of degeneration.

Lesion at 4: Lesion in petrous bone below geniculate ganglion. Complete motor paralysis same side. Salivary and taste fibres paralysed. Expression and associated movements paralysed. Corneal reflex lost. Reaction of degeneration. No hyperacusis, as lesion below offshoot to stapedius.

Lesion at 5: Lesion at stylomastoid foramen. Same symptoms, but taste and salivary fibres unaffected.

THE ANATOMY OF NERVE INJURIES 453

  b. Stapedius paralysed. This produces hyperacusis (ringing in ears).
  c. Corneal reflex lost.
  d. Movements of expression lost.
  e. Pronounced reaction of degeneration.
4. LESION IN BONE BELOW OFFSHOOT OF THE NERVE TO THE STAPEDIUS: Same symptoms but no hyperacusis. Taste fibres are paralysed from the anterior two-thirds of the tongue.
5. LESION AT THE STYLOMASTOID FORAMEN: The same symptoms as in (4) except that taste fibres are unaffected.

FACIAL NERVE IN RELATION TO THE PAROTID GLAND: Enucleation of parotid tumours is a common practice. It is frequently followed by recurrence of the tumour. The procedure is usually inadequate and is dictated by fear of injury to the facial nerve. It is now realized that part or the whole of the parotid gland may be removed without damage to this nerve. The concept that the branches of the nerve divide the gland into superficial and deep lobes is not generally acceptable, but all are agreed that the gland is divisible by the nerve into a suprafacial and a subfacial plane

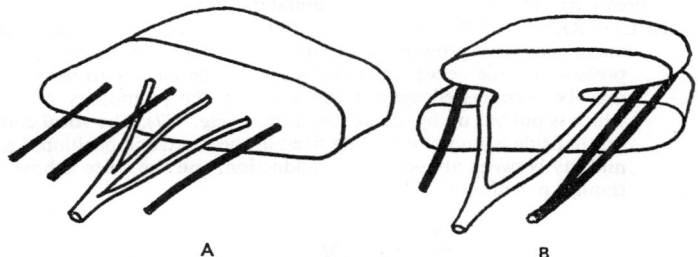

Fig. 436.—A, The facial nerve branches and a plexus of veins divides the parotid gland into a suprafacial and a subfacial plane—acceptable viewpoint. B, Unacceptable view of division of the parotid into two lobes.

(Patey) (*Fig.* 436). Parotid tumours should be removed by an anatomical dissection. The nerve is followed forwards or its terminal branches are traced back. The former is the better procedure. It entails exposing the trunk of the facial nerve at its emergence from the stylomastoid foramen; there is about 1 cm. of nerve-trunk before it enters the parotid and another centimetre before it divides into its temporofacial and cervicofacial divisions. It and its branches are followed into the parotid gland and the plane of cleavage developed between the superficial and deep portions of the gland. Thus the suprafacial portion alone, or together with part of the subfacial parotid, is removed, or a total parotidectomy is done according to the needs of the case. The nerve is under observation throughout. The presence of malignancy does not necessarily demand the sacrifice of the whole nerve.

HERPES IN A SEVENTH NERVE LESION: Affects the posterior surface of the external auditory meatus and posterior wall of inner surface of external auditory meatus and perhaps posterior half of tympanic membrane. This area is thought to be supplied by two nerves, the auricular branch of the vagus and the nervus intermedius (sensory part of seventh nerve).

Eighth Nerve (Auditory): Complete deafness on same side, also loss of equilibrium and rotary giddiness.

Ninth Nerve (Glossopharyngeal): Anaesthesia at back of tongue (posterior third), also of the pharynx.

Tenth Nerve (Vagus): Whole trunk (Syndrome of Avellis): Unilateral paralysis of the palate and larynx and anaesthesia of larynx on that side. Loss of sensation of hunger and thirst may occur. If both vagi are paralysed, there is tachycardia from paralysis of cardio-inhibitory nerves which are vagal, also slowness and irregularity of breathing. These do not occur in unilateral paralysis.

RECURRENT LARYNGEAL NERVE: Paralysis may occur in aneurysm, new growth of thyroid, by direct involvement of or pressure on the nerve; in mitral stenosis[1] the left recurrent nerve may be compressed against the aorta by the pulmonary artery, which is pushed up by the dilated auricle (*Fig.* 437). The vocal cord on that side is immobile, being fixed in the cadaveric position, i.e., midway between abduction and adduction, and the voice is hoarse though not absent.

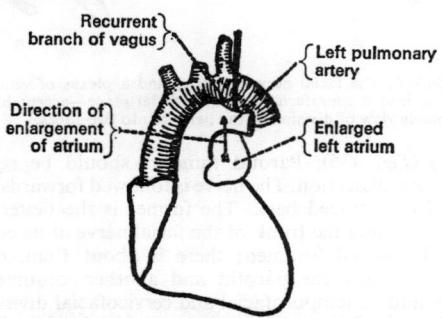

Fig. 437.—Demonstrating how a dilated left atrium may cause paralysis of left vocal cord through pressing left pulmonary artery against recurrent nerve.

[1] Frischaner, *Wien. klin. Wschr.*, 1905, Dec., 28.

THE ANATOMY OF NERVE INJURIES

BOTH RECURRENTS: The vocal cords are motionless and speech is impossible.

Eleventh Nerve (Spinal Accessory): The sternomastoid is paralysed. Paralysis of the trapezius varies according to how much of it is supplied by the third and fourth cervical nerves. The outline of the neck is altered, as the levator scapulae becomes subcutaneous and the curve of the neck is flattened. The scapula is displaced down, and its vertebral border is displaced out and is imperfectly approximated to the midline when the shoulders are braced back.

Twelfth Nerve (Hypoglossal): The corresponding half of the tongue becomes atrophied and wrinkled, and when the tongue is protruded the healthy side causes the tip to deviate towards the paralysed side.

Spinal Nerves

Before considering nerve lesions of the upper limb the reader will find it helpful to observe that:

Abduction at the shoulder is dependent on	C. 5
Adduction at the shoulder is dependent on	C. 6, 7
Flexion of the elbow is dependent on	C. 5, 6
Extension of the elbow is dependent on	C. 7, 8
Extension of wrist and fingers is dependent on	C. 6, 7
Flexion of wrist and fingers is dependent on	C. 8, T. 1

Fifth and Sixth Cervical Nerves:

1. ERB-DUCHENNE PARALYSIS: Is the commonest type of nerve injury occurring at birth, the so-called upper-arm type of birth palsy. It is produced by forcible widening of the angle between the head and the shoulder such as may be caused by traction on the arm at birth, or falling on the shoulder in later life.

   The injury occurs usually at the site where the fifth and sixth cervical nerves had joined to form the upper trunk of the brachial plexus. This is known as Erb's point. At this spot six nerves are grouped together: The fifth and sixth roots, the anterior and posterior branches of the upper trunk, and the suprascapular and subclavius nerves which are branches of this trunk (*Fig.* 438, I, and *Fig.* 152, p. 163).

   EXTENT OF THE PARALYSIS:

   a. Paralysis of:
   - Deltoid
   - Supraspinatus
   - Infraspinatus
   } Abductors and lateral rotators of shoulder

   - Biceps
   - Brachialis
   - Brachioradialis
   } Flexors of elbow

   b. Weakness of:
   - Teres major
   - Pectoralis major
   - Latissimus dorsi
   - Subscapularis
   } Adductors and medial rotators of shoulder

c. Very slight involvement of: Pronator teres
Supinator
Flexors of wrist
Thenar muscles

CLINICAL APPEARANCE: The arm hangs at the side in an attitude of internal rotation with the forearm pronated and with flexed fingers and wrist—the 'porter's tip' hand. Abduction and external rotation at the shoulder are lost, so too are flexion and supination of the forearm. Sherren states that when occurring in later life there is always a sensory loss accompanying this lesion. It takes the form of dulling of sensation over the lower part of the deltoid and arm and perhaps the forearm, with possibly a very small area of total anaesthesia in this region.

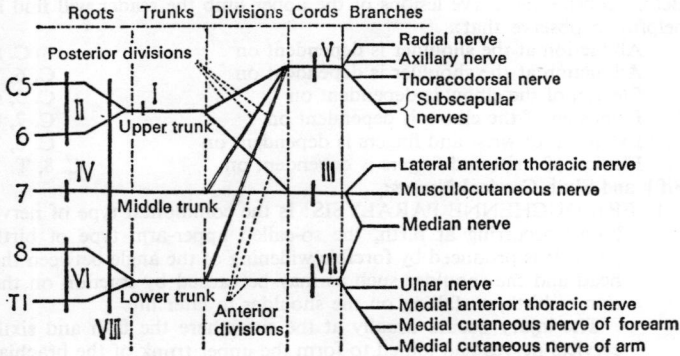

Fig. 438.—Diagram of brachial plexus to illustrate sites of lesions enumerated in the text. The dotted lines divide the plexus into roots, trunks, division, cords and branches. I, Lesion of C. 5, 6 at Erb's point; II, Lesion of roots of C. 5, 6; III, Lesion of outer cord; IV, Lesion of C. 7; V, Lesion of posterior cord; VI, Lesion of roots of C. 8 and T. 1; VII, Lesion of inner cord; VIII, Lesion of whole plexus.

2. LESION OF THE ROOTS OF THE FIFTH AND SIXTH NERVES (*Fig.* 438, II): If the nerves are damaged above their point of union to form the upper trunk of the plexus, there is also—
   a. Paralysis of the rhomboids (supplied by the dorsalis scapulae nerve from C. 5).
   b. Paralysis of most of the serratus anterior (supplied by the long thoracic nerve (Bell) from C. 5, 6, and 7).
A lesion of the *outer cord* differs from that of the 5th and 6th at Erb's point in that in the former: (*a*) There is no involvement of the shoulder muscles or brachioradialis; (*b*) There is complete

paralysis of the pronator teres and radial flexors of the wrist (*Fig.* 438, III).

Seventh Cervical Nerve: A lesion of this nerve produces:
1. Paralysis of the coracobrachialis, which is not involved with the biceps in Erb's paralysis.
2. Paralysis of all the radial nerve distribution except the brachioradialis (*Fig.* 438, IV).

Posterior Cord of Brachial Plexus (C. 5, 6, 7, and 8): Produces paralysis of:
1. Deltoid and teres muscles.
2. Latissimus dorsi, subscapularis, and brachioradialis.
3. Extensors of: (*a*) Elbow—triceps and anconeus; (*b*) Wrist—extensores carpi radialis longus and brevis, and extensor carpi ulnaris; (*c*) Fingers—extensores digitorum communis, digiti minimi, indicis proprius, pollicis longus, pollicis brevis, and abductor pollicis longus (*Fig.* 438, V).

It will be noted that the axillary and radial nerves, which are components of the posterior cord, are the two great extensor nerves of the upper limb.

Eighth Cervical and First Thoracic Nerves: A lesion of these nerve-roots causes:
1. Paralysis of the intrinsic muscles of the hand.
2. Paralysis of the flexors of the digits (*Fig.* 438, VI).

In contrast with this, a lesion of the *inner cord* causes paralysis of the flexor carpi ulnaris in addition to the paralyses resulting from a lesion of C. 8 and T. 1 roots (*Fig.* 438, VII).

Combined Lesions of the Median and Ulnar Nerves: Cause paralysis of: (1) Intrinsic muscles of the hand; (2) Flexor carpi ulnaris; (3) All the flexors of the digits; (4) The pronators; (5) All the flexors of the wrist.

A scheme represents this as follows:

$$\left.\begin{array}{l}\left.\begin{array}{l}\text{Paralysis of intrinsics of hand}\\ \text{Paralysis of flexors of digits}\end{array}\right\} \text{C.8, T.1} \\ \text{Flexor carpi ulnaris} \\ \text{Pronators} \\ \text{All flexors of wrist}\end{array}\right\} \text{Inner cord} \left.\begin{array}{l}\\ \\ \end{array}\right\} \begin{array}{l}\text{Combined}\\ \text{median and}\\ \text{ulnar}\end{array}$$

SENSORY LOSS:
1. Total anaesthesia over all the ulnar area and in the two terminal phalanges of the middle and index fingers.
2. The thumb, outer half of the palm of the hand, and sometimes the palmar aspect of the proximal phalanges of the second and third fingers remain sensitive to a very deep prick. This sensibility is accounted for by the probable assistance given by the fibres of the superficial branch of the radial and lateral cutaneous nerves of the forearm.
3. All the median area may be completely anaesthetic.

4. Sense of position, deep sensibility, bone sense, and stereognostic sense are lost in the areas mentioned (A. Benisty[1]).

Klumpke's Paralysis: The lower-arm type of birth palsy. The motor loss is the same as that resulting from injury to C. 8 and T. 1 roots, as these are the roots affected by Klumpke's paralysis. There is anaesthesia along the inner side of the forearm, hand, and little finger—claw-hand results. There is in most cases paralysis of the cervical sympathetic.

Whole Brachial Plexus Type of Paralysis: Features:
1. Total flaccid paralysis of the upper limb with wasting and degeneration of the muscles.
2. Complete anaesthesia of the hand, forearm, and lower part of arm (*Fig.* 438, VIII).

In this accident the first thoracic nerve-root of the plexus is liable to be torn close to the cord. As a result the fibres going via this root and the cervical sympathetic to supply the pupil are torn, resulting in contracted pupil and slight ptosis (Wilfred Harris[2]). The presence of contracted pupil on the side of the injury is taken by surgeons to denote the fact that the nerve-roots have been avulsed from the cord where suture is impossible. This sign, therefore, indicates the futility of attempting operation in an injury of this nature.

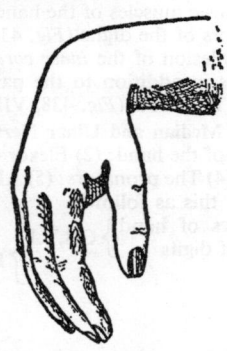

Fig. 439.—Drop-wrist resulting from radial-nerve palsy.

Radial Nerve: Complete division of nerve before branching causes:
MOTOR: Paralysis of:
1. Extensors of elbow, wrist, knuckles, and all joints of thumb.
2. Supinator and brachioradialis (chiefly a flexor of the elbow).

The motor loss causes a typical drop-wrist (*Fig.* 439).

[1] *Clinical Forms of Nerve Lesions*, 1918, 109. London.
[2] *Neuritis and Neuralgia*, 1926. London.

SENSORY: The cutaneous sensibility (to wool and prick) is lost over the dorsum of the second and third metacarpals and corresponding proximal phalanges. At its maximum this extends over the whole dorsum of the thumb and almost to the tips of index and middle fingers. At its minimum it is reduced to the index knuckle (*Fig.* 440).

The muscles affected show loss of pain and muscle sense. Joint sense is usually unaffected. The reason why the sensory loss is so slight is because of the overlapping of adjacent sensory areas

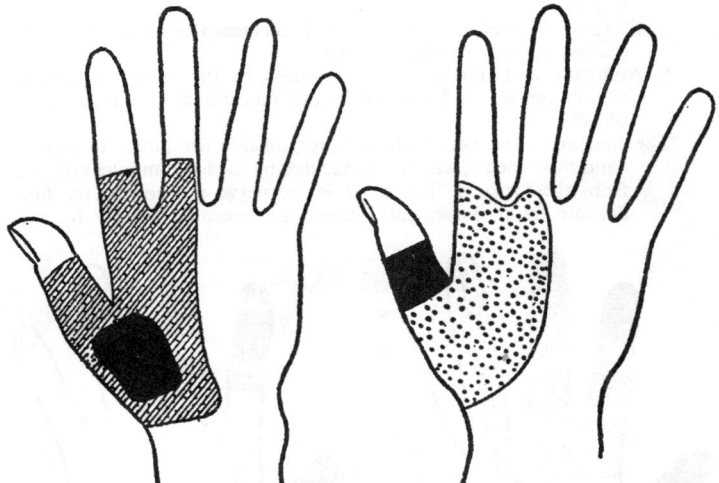

Fig. 440. — Two common types of sensory loss on dorsum in cases of complete division of radial nerve. (*Modified from Benisty.*)
Black area Complete anaesthesia except to deep pricking, which often feels like touch.
Shaded area Slight loss to touch, heat, and cold.
Dotted area Marked anaesthesia to prick, slight anaesthesia to touch, heat, and cold.

supplied by other cutaneous nerves. These are the dorsal and lateral cutaneous nerves of the forearm. When one of these nerves, or the sensory branch of the radial nerve (superficial branch of the radial), is divided in the forearm, there is usually no sensory loss to be detected because of this overlapping of skin territories. Two of the nerves must usually be divided before anaesthesia results. Division of the radial nerve in the axilla causes an area of sensory loss because it supplies two of the three nerves mentioned, viz., the dorsal cutaneous nerve of the forearm and the superficial branch of the radial nerve.

Median Nerve: Complete severance causes:

MOTOR: Paralysis of:

1. The pronators.
2. The radial flexor of the wrist.
3. Flexors of all the proximal interphalangeal joints.
4. Flexors of the terminal joints of the thumb and index and middle fingers.
5. Flexors of the first and second metacarpophalangeal joints (including flexor pollicis brevis).
6. Abductor and opponens pollicis—loss of the power to rotate thumb opposite index finger for the 'pincer action' in picking up objects.

The median is the nerve which is responsible for powerful coarse hand movements, which are executed by the long muscles coming from the forearm. The ulnar is the nerve responsible for fine delicate hand movements, which are executed mainly by the

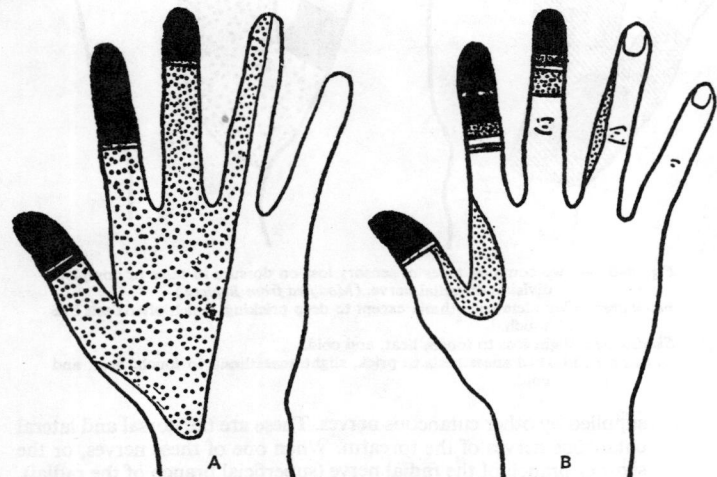

Fig. 441.—Anaesthesia resulting from complete division of median nerve. A, Palmar. B, Dorsal. (*After Stiles.*)
Black area, Anaesthesia to deep pressure and pain.
Dotted area, Anaesthesia to wool and prick.
White lines, Loss of joint sense.

THE ANATOMY OF NERVE INJURIES

intrinsic small muscles of the hand. C. 6 and 7 are the vital sensory posterior nerve-roots in the median nerve distribution.

SENSORY:

MUSCLE PAIN is lost in the above muscles.

ANAESTHESIA TO PRESSURE is evident at the ends of the thumb, index, and middle fingers.

JOINT SENSE is lost in interphalangeal joints of index, and last joints of thumb and middle finger.

CUTANEOUS: This is seen at a glance in the diagrams (*Fig.* 441).

TROPHIC CHANGES are very prominent in cases of damage to the median nerve. They are most marked in the terminal phalanx of the index finger.

Ulnar Nerve: Complete division causes:

MOTOR: Paralysis of:

1. Ulnar flexor of wrist (flexor carpi ulnaris).
2. Flexors of terminal phalanges of the ring and little fingers, i.e., profundus digitorum.
3. Muscles of the hypothenar eminence, i.e., abductor, flexor, and opponens digiti minimi.
4. Adductor pollicis.
5. Palmaris brevis.
6. All the interossei and inner two lumbricals. This loss results in a mild degree of clawing of the hand in which the first phalanges of the fingers are extended and the second and third flexed. It is not a true claw-hand (*Fig.* 442).

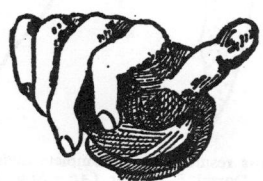

Fig. 442.—The position of fingers in paralysis of ulnar nerve—so-called 'ulnar claw-hand'.

SENSORY:

DEEP:

1. Muscle pain—lost in all above muscles.
2. Joint sense—lost in all joints of little finger and interphalangeal joints of ring finger.
3. Pressure sense—lost on ulnar border of hand and whole of little finger.

CUTANEOUS: Light touch, prick, and temperature lost over area as shown in *Fig.* 443.

ANOMALOUS NERVE-SUPPLY TO THE MUSCLES OF THE HAND

Rowntree[1] found that in 20 per cent of cases there was some anomaly in the nerve-supply of the intrinsic muscles of the hand. Every gradation occurred from complete ulnar to complete median innervation.

The flexor brevis pollicis usually has a supply from each of these nerves. The first (or first and second) dorsal interosseous muscle may be supplied by the median nerve. An important point made by

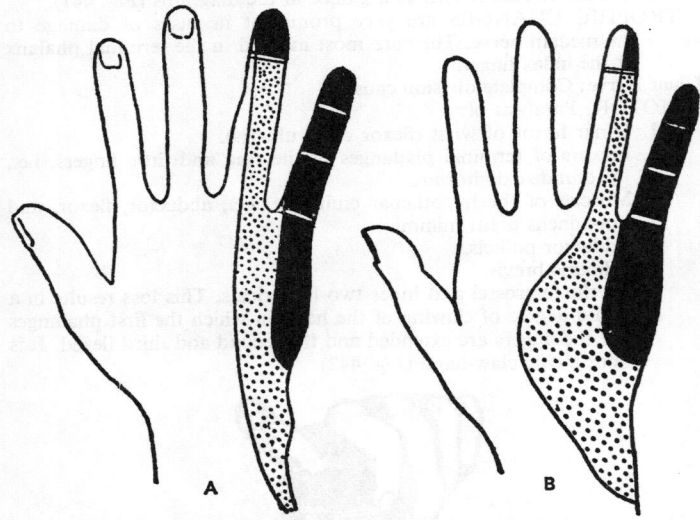

Fig. 443.—Sensory loss resulting from complete division of ulnar nerve. A, Dorsal. B, Palmar. (*After Stiles.*)
Black area, Anaesthesia to deep pressure and pain.
Dotted area, Anaesthesia to wool and prick.
White lines, Loss of joint sense.

this investigator was that a nerve, such as the ulnar, may carry the supply to hand muscles while above the elbow whereas, in the hand, these muscles receive their supply from the median. Therefore he stresses the importance of respecting communications between nerves.

CLAW-HAND (*Fig.* 444): A combined median and ulnar lesion at the elbow causes a true claw-hand of severe type. This results in

---

[1] Rowntree, T., *J. Bone Jt Surg.*, 1949, 31B, 505.

hyperextended wrist and metacarpophalangeal joints and flexion of interphalangeal joints. The same type of clawing is produced by a lesion of the inner cord of the brachial plexus and by Klumpke's paralysis. Duchenne clarifies the point that the position taken up by the hand is the result of paralysis of the interosseous and lumbrical muscles.

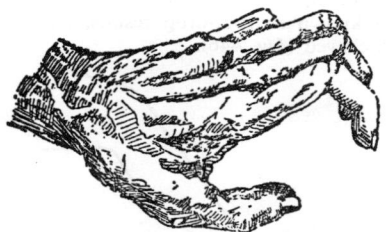

Fig. 444.—Claw-hand.

OPTIMUM POSITION OF THE HAND: This is the position the hand assumes when it rests on a table completely relaxed. The finger tips just fail to touch the palm and the wrist is extended midway between the plane of the forearm and full extension (*Fig.* 445). This is the position in which the wrist-joint should be splinted after most of the injuries in the neighbourhood, e.g., Colles's

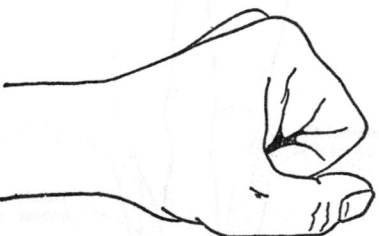

Fig. 445.—The optimum position of the hand.

fracture. It is a mistake to fix the wrist in full extension which may lead to impairment of movement subsequently, especially in older people, due to the formation of adhesions between tendons and sheaths. Exceptionally, in hemiplegics for example, an almost useless hand may take up the accoucheur's position, with tips of thumb and forefingers in contact with each other. There may be just enough useful finger movement to enable such a hand to pick up or hold an object. Endeavours to improve function may not only fail but may sacrifice such function as did exist.

Sciatic Nerve: Severance of the nerve at its origin causes:

MOTOR: Paralysis of:
1. All the hamstrings, i.e., all flexors of the knee, except sartorius.
2. All leg muscles.
3. All foot muscles.

A condition known as foot-drop results, and ultimately the toes become clawed (*Fig.* 446).

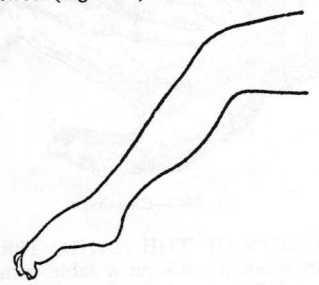

Fig. 446.—Position of foot in paralysis of sciatic nerve.

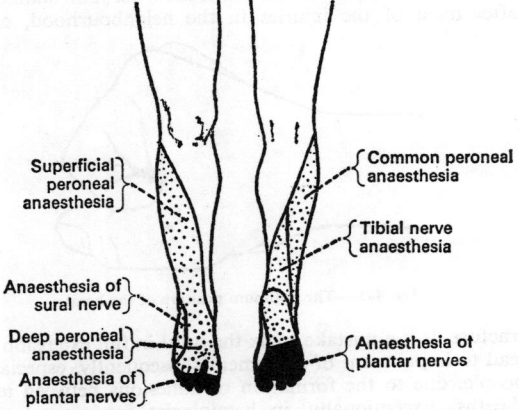

Fig. 447.—Sensory loss in complete division of sciatic nerve. Joint sense is lost in ankle and all the foot joints. (*After Stiles.*)
Black area, Anaesthesia to deep pressure and pain.
Dotted area, Anaesthesia to wool and prick.

SENSORY:
DEEP: Loss of joint sense in ankle and all foot and toe joints.
Loss to pressure beyond the metatarsal heads.
Loss of muscle pain in all the paralysed muscles.
CUTANEOUS: As in diagram (*Fig.* 447).
TROPHIC ULCERS: Occur especially on points subjected to pressure, i.e., heel and balls of toes.

Tibial Nerve: Division of this nerve results in:
MOTOR: Paralysis of:
LEG: Popliteus, soleus, gastrocnemius, tibialis posterior, flexor digitorum longus, flexor hallucis longus.
FOOT: All the muscles of the foot excepting only the extensor digitorum brevis.
If this nerve is divided the foot is held dorsiflexed at the ankle and everted, and the tendo Achillis prominence is lost. No movement for lowering the foot can be made. Severe disability results. The sole is paralysed and the patient cannot stand on his toes.
SENSORY:
CUTANEOUS: Sensibility is lost on the plantar surface of the toes and on the dorsal aspect of their last phalanges.

Peroneal Nerve: Severance of the nerve causes:
MOTOR: Paralysis of: Peroneus longus and brevis, tibialis anterior, extensor digitorum longus, extensor hallucis longus, peroneus tertius, extensor brevis digitorum.
There is foot-drop, i.e., the ankle is fully plantar-flexed and cannot be dorsiflexed. The foot is adducted and inverted. The second and third phalanges can, however, be extended by the interossei, which are supplied through the tibial nerve.
SENSORY:
CUTANEOUS: There is sensory loss on the dorsum of the foot and on the outer surface of the leg (*Fig.* 448).

An interesting type of ischaemic palsy may affect the peroneal nerve. It occurs in obliterative vascular lesions affecting the femoral and popliteal arteries. Usually the motor functions are impaired in excess of the sensory and the prognosis is good. Ferguson and Liversedge[1] quote Sunderland[2] to the effect that in ischaemic palsies of this type the tibial nerve is never affected as it receives a liberal supply of vasa nervorum from the gluteal vessels, profunda perforating branches, and still additional vessels in the popliteal space and calf, whereas the peroneal nerve receives only one nutrient vessel in the popliteal space.

After suture of the sciatic nerve or its main branches, the long-term functional results are much better when the tibial

[1] Ferguson, F. R., and Liversedge, L. A., *Br. med. J.*, 1954, Aug., 7.
[2] Sunderland, S., *Archs Neurol. Psychiat.*, Chicago, 1945, 54, 283.

nerve is affected than when the peroneal is the nerve involved. In more than four-fifths of the former and only about one-third of the latter are such results obtained.

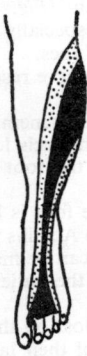

Fig. 448.—Sensory loss in division of common peroneal nerve. (*After Benisty.*)
  Black area, Complete anaesthesia.
  Dotted area, Slight sensory loss to touch, heat, and cold.

Cervical Sympathetic: Section of this nerve-trunk causes:
1. Some dropping of the upper lid—ptosis. The cervical sympathetic supplies one-third of the levator palpebrae superioris.
2. Contraction of the pupil.
3. Recession of the eyeball—enophthalmos—because of paralysis of the orbital muscle of Müller which lies on the floor of the orbit and which is responsible for keeping the eyeball forward. It is supplied by the sympathetic.
4. Sweating only occurs on the non-affected side of the face.

Phrenic Nerve: Division of this nerve in the neck may cause paralysis of one half of the diaphragm. In some cases a considerable part of the nerve runs with the nerve to the subclavius and joins the main trunk of the phrenic in the thorax. In such cases division of the phrenic may leave the action of the same side of the diaphragm relatively unimpaired (*see* p. 164).

The paralysing of one side of the diaphragm is effected surgically in cases where it is desired to collapse the lower lobe of the lung (e.g., bronchiectasis). If the diaphragm is out of action on one side, it rises to its highest position and the lower lobe of the lung does not expand in respiration. To be certain of destroying the whole nerve it is exposed in the neck and forcibly pulled upon. It then tears at its diaphragmatic end. This is the operation of phrenic exairesis or avulsion.

II. RELAXATION OF NERVES

When a portion of a nerve-trunk is missing, whether from a gunshot wound or from a tumour necessitating the removal of part of the nerve,

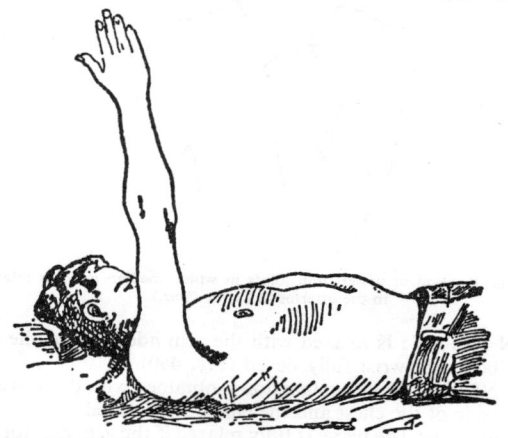

Fig. 449.—Position of upper limb which gives fullest relaxation of branches of brachial plexus in the axilla. (*After Platt.*)

it is necessary to sew the two ends together. If much of the nerve is missing it is necessary to resort to various expedients to effect approximation of the two ends. These expedients are: (1) Relaxation by posture; (2) Relaxation by transplantation; (3) Approximation in stages. All these means may fail to secure approximation in a very extensive gap. The surgeon must then bridge it by using as grafts portions of other nerves, or by sewing both ends into an adjacent nerve, hoping that the sheath of this nerve will act as a guide to the growing axis cylinders. The outlook for recovery of function in either case is very bad. If the nerve to be joined is a very important one in a limb, the gap may be lessened by removing a part of the limb bone.

Relaxation by Posture:

BRACHIAL PLEXUS: The nerves of the plexus are relaxed by approximating the head to the shoulder on the affected side. This position may be maintained after the operation by adhesive strapping or plaster-of-Paris.

468 A SYNOPSIS OF SURGICAL ANATOMY

BRANCHES OF THE PLEXUS IN THE AXILLA: The nerves are best relaxed with the arm flexed to a right angle, i.e., brought into a position of forward elevation until at right angles to the operating table (Platt[1]) (*Fig.* 450).

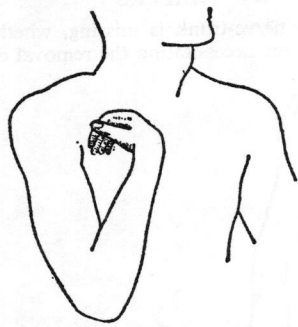

Fig. 450.—Position of upper limb joints in which median nerve is relaxed to the uttermost. (*After Platt.*)

MEDIAN NERVE: Is relaxed with the arm adducted to the side and the elbow and wrist fully flexed (*Fig.* 450).

RADIAL NERVE: Fullest relaxation is obtained with the arm adducted to the side of the chest and the elbow fully flexed.

ULNAR NERVE: The nerve is fully relaxed if the arm and forearm are put in the 'reversed position' (Platt[2]). The arm is brought into forward flexion at the shoulder-joint, i.e., vertical to the plane of the table, and the wrist and elbow are flexed.

SCIATIC NERVE: The greatest relaxation is obtained with the hip hyperextended and the knee fully flexed (*Fig.* 451).

PERONEAL AND TIBIAL NERVE (external and internal popliteal): As for the sciatic.

Transplantation of Nerves: This is a means of securing additional relaxation. It is also a valuable means of obtaining a new bed for a nerve if its old one has become unsuitable for any reason. The method is only applicable to two nerves—the radial and ulnar.

RADIAL NERVE: The nerve is brought from the back of the arm to the front of the limb, being placed in a muscular tunnel in the brachialis (*Fig.* 452). It will be apparent that the procedure is only possible in cases where the nerve is divided, whether from injury or removal of a tumour.

---

[1] *Modern Operative Surgery,* 1924 1, 339. London.
[2] Ibid., 352.

THE ANATOMY OF NERVE INJURIES

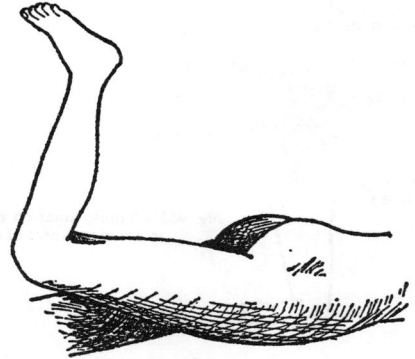

Fig. 451.—Position of lower limb joints in which sciatic nerve is relaxed to the full.

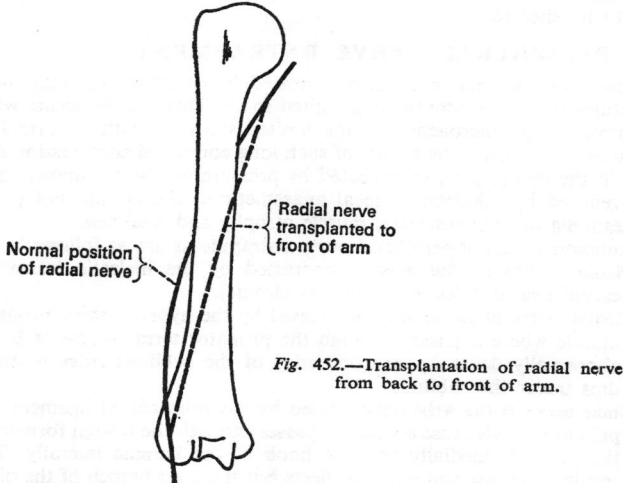

Fig. 452.—Transplantation of radial nerve from back to front of arm.

ULNAR NERVE: This nerve may be transposed intact, by exposing it in its groove at the back of the elbow and simply bringing it forward round the internal epicondyle and placing it in a groove in the flexor muscle mass (*Fig.* 453).

470 A SYNOPSIS OF SURGICAL ANATOMY

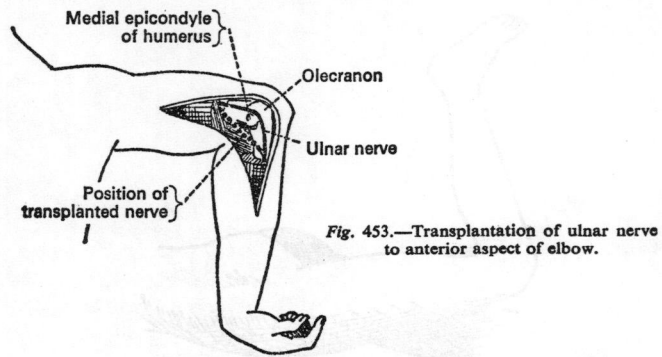

Fig. 453.—Transplantation of ulnar nerve to anterior aspect of elbow.

Approximation in Stages: The two ends are approximated as much as possible and fixed by sutures exerting tension on the nerves. At a later date there may be sufficient 'slack' to enable complete apposition to be effected.

III. PERIPHERAL NERVE ENTRAPMENT

Peripheral nerves may become compressed by neighbouring anatomical structures in areas where there is limited space. This usually occurs when abnormal tissue encroaches on the limited space or with abnormal or excessive movement. The results of such long continued compression are: pain in the dermatome, exacerbated by pressure on the entrapment site, and relieved by injection of local anaesthetic at the entrapment point, paraesthesia or hypoaesthesia, muscle atrophy and weakness.

Common points of peripheral nerve entrapments are as follows:[1]

1. **Median nerve at the wrist**, compressed by the inelastic transverse carpal ligament (carpal tunnel syndrome).
2. **Median nerve at the elbow** compressed by the hypertrophied pronator muscle where it passes through the pronator teres muscle or by an abnormally dense aponeurotic edge of the sublimis ridge where it dips under the sublimis.
3. **Ulnar nerve at the wrist**, compressed by the volar carpal ligament and palmaris brevis muscle where it passes through the trough formed by the pisiform medially and the hook of the hamate laterally. This results in motor and sensory effects but the deep branch of the ulnar nerve may be compressed as it pierces the adductor digiti minimi with exclusively motor effects.
4. **Ulnar nerve at the elbow** compressed in the cubital tunnel against the

[1] Thompson, W. A. L., and Kopell, H. P., *N. Engl. J. Med.*, 1959, 260, 1261.

posterior aspect of the medial epicondyle of the humerus in cases of cubitus valgus or by external compression when a patient is on the operating table, in bed, or in an armchair.
5. **Posterior interosseous nerve** may be compressed just distal to the elbow where it goes beneath the aponeurotic bridge of the extensor carpi radialis brevis or as it penetrates the supinator muscle. This is a motor nerve and compression results in deep poorly localized pain in the lateral part of the elbow aggravated by rotation and extension of the wrist.
6. **Suprascapular nerve at the shoulder** may be kinked by the edges of the suprascapular notch in forward protrusion of the shoulder girdle with the arm in adduction. It is a motor nerve and compression results in a deep, poorly localized pain at the posterior aspect of the shoulder and later muscle atrophy may be seen.
7. **Lateral cutaneous nerve of the thigh**[1] compressed as it goes beneath or through the inguinal ligament medial to the anterior superior iliac spine when in the recumbent position resulting in pain and paraesthesia down the lateral aspect of the thigh, relieved by hip flexion (meralgia paraesthetica).
8. **Ileo-inguinal nerve**[2] compressed by muscle action as it pierces the transversus abdominis or internal oblique muscle near the anterior superior iliac spine to produce pain in the groin, upper medial thigh, scrotum or labium majus, relieved by flexing the hip.
9. **Obturator nerve** compressed in the obturator canal by osteomyelitis or an obturator hernia, with resultant pain over the medial part of the thigh and knee and later with weakness of the adductor muscles.
10. **Peroneal nerve at the knee** compressed by the peroneus longus muscle at the neck of the fibula to produce pain on the lateral aspect of the leg and dorsum of the foot.
11. **Anterior tibial nerve at the ankle** compressed by the extensor retinaculum, producing pain in the big toe.
12. **Saphenous nerve in the thigh** compressed where it perforates the deep fascia which forms the roof of Hunter's Canal, causing pain in the medial aspect of the leg and ankle.
13. **Posterior tibial nerve at the ankle** compressed by the flexor retinaculum behind the medial malleolus when sitting in a squatting position, causing pain in the sole of the foot (tarsal tunnel syndrome).

---

[1] Ghent, W. R., *Can. med. Ass. J.*, 1961, 85, 871.
[2] Ghent, W. R., *Ileo-inguinal Entrapment Syndrome. Current Diagnosis*, (Ed. Conn, H. F., Clohecy, R. J. and Conn, R. B.) 1966. Philadelphia: Saunders.

Chapter XXXI

BODILY HABITUS

THERE are four great types of bodily habitus: (1) Hypersthenic; (2) Sthenic; (3) Hyposthenic; and (4) Asthenic. Because of the marked contrast, the first and last types will be first considered.

Hypersthenic Type (*Fig.* 454): These constitute 5 per cent of individuals. Characteristics:

1. Massive, powerful physique; great weight; heavy bony framework.
2. The thorax is wide and deep, but short from above down; as a result the lungs are relatively short but very wide at their bases, though they narrow sharply towards the apices, which project but little above the clavicles.
3. The heart is transverse in position—the transverse heart.
4. The subcostal angle is very wide, and the xiphoid process is broad and large (*Fig.* 454).

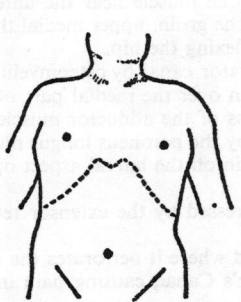

Fig. 454.—Bodily habitus. The shape of the hypersthenic type. (*After Mills.*)

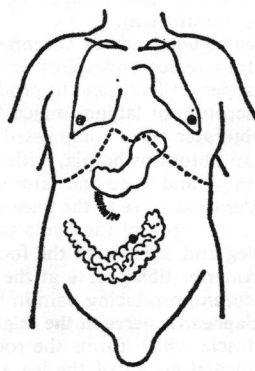

Fig. 455.—Bodily habitus. Position of viscera in hypersthenic type. (*After Mills.*)

5. The abdomen is very capacious in its upper part, being wider and more roomy than the lower part.
6. The stomach and alimentary canal are high in position (*Fig.* 455). The pylorus is the lowest part of the stomach, which has great motility and marked tonus.
7. The colon is high in position; the transverse colon *is* transverse.

BODILY HABITUS

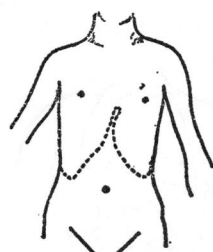
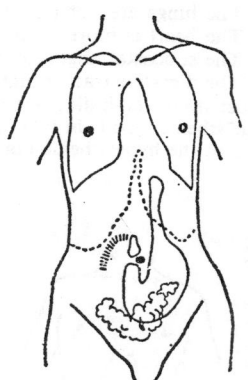

Fig. 456.—Bodily habitus. Configuration of asthenic type. (*After Mills.*)

Fig. 457—Bodily habitus. Position of viscera in asthenic type. (*After Mills.*)

Asthenic Type (*Fig.* 456): Constitutes 12 per cent of individuals. This type differs in every particular from the previous one.
1. The physique is slender and frail. The bony framework is light.
2. The thorax is long and narrow.
3. The lungs are long and slender, being wider above than below and extending well above the clavicles.
4. The heart has its long axis parallel to the long axis of the body—the vertical heart.
5. The subcostal angle is very narrow and the xiphoid process cannot as a rule be felt.
6. The abdomen is of characteristic shape. It is narrow above but widens considerably below.
7. The pelvis is very wide and capacious.
8. The gastro-intestinal tract is very low in position (*Fig.* 457).
9. The stomach is atonic, the great curvature depends much lower than the pylorus and may be in the pelvis.
10. The colon is long, with a capacious caecum which is very low, being often in the pelvis.
11. The transverse colon is *not* transverse but drops very low between its two extremities.

Sthenic Type (*Fig.* 458): Constitutes 48 per cent of persons.
   Characteristics:
1. Body weight is considerable, and bony framework rather heavy.
2. The thorax is inclined to be short and deep.

3. The lungs are not long and tend to be wider below.
4. The heart is more transverse than longitudinal.
5. The subcostal angle forms a right angle.
6. The digestive tract is high and active (*Fig.* 459).

Most stout well-built persons belong to this type.

The sthenic type is in general characterized by similar features to those of the hypersthenic but these features are not so accentuated.

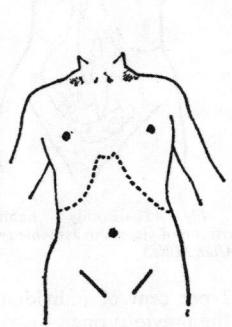

Fig. 458.—Bodily habitus. Configuration of sthenic type. (*After Mills.*)

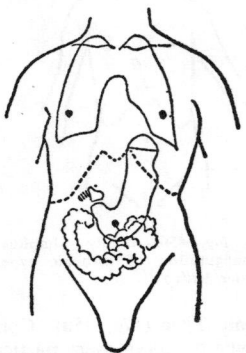

Fig. 459—Bodily habitus. Position of viscera in sthenic type. (*After Mills.*)

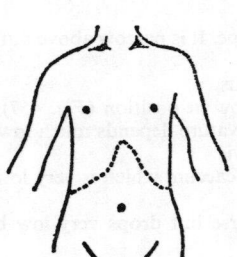

Fig. 460.—Bodily habitus. Configuration of hyposthenic type. (*After Mills.*)

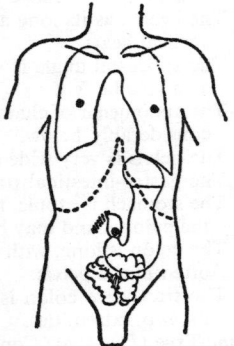

Fig. 461.—Bodily habitus. Position of viscera in hyposthenic type. (*After Mills.*)

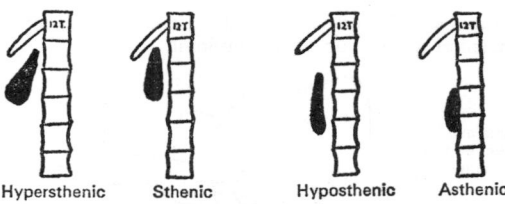

Fig. 462.—Position of gall-bladder in different types of habitus as shown by cholecystography. (*After Davies.*)

Hyposthenic Type (*Fig.* 460): Constitutes 35 per cent of persons. The Venus de Milo belongs to this type. The visceral characteristics are those of the asthenic in less marked degree, lacking the extremely low position. The lungs are intermediate in proportions. The heart is 'pendant'. The tonus is not brisk, and motility is slow rather than rapid. The other characteristics are those of the asthenic in less pronounced degree (*Fig.* 461).

Gall-Bladder Position in Relation to Bodily Habitus (*Fig.* 462[1]): Francis Davies[2] has shown that, comparing the hypersthenic and sthenic with the hyposthenic and asthenic types, the gall-bladder in the former:
1. Lies at a higher level and at a greater distance from the midline.
2. Empties more quickly.
3. Moves more with respiration.

Chapter XXXII

ANATOMICAL ANGLES. STIFF JOINTS

I. ANATOMICAL ANGLES

Femur:
UPPER END: The neck of the femur makes an angle with the shaft of about 130° (vertical neck-shaft angle), being a little less in the adult than in the child. The neck of the femur is directed upwards, inwards, and forwards, the angulation forwards being 12° (this is also called the declination angle—*Fig.* 463). Any considerable alteration of these angles results in deformity and disability. The

[1] These shadows of the gall-bladder were obtained by X-rays after a dye had been given which is excreted in the bile and gives a shadow with X-rays when in the gall-bladder.
[2] 'Normal Cholecystography', *Br. med. J.*, 1927, June 25 1138.

conditions which affect the angles are coxa vara, coxa valga, and congenital dislocation of the hip-joint.

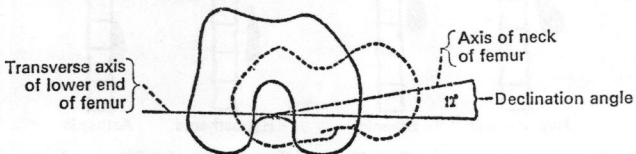

Fig. 463.—The forward or declination angle of the femur. (*After Scudder.*)

COXA VARA (*Fig.* 464): In this condition both the vertical and the forward neck-shaft angles are altered. The vertical angle is reduced, it may be to less than a right angle, and the head is bent back, reducing the forward or declination angle. The condition is caused by a disproportion between the neck of the femur and the strain (body-weight) which is put on it. This disproportion may be congenital or acquired, e.g., by injury or disease. It is obvious that in coxa vara the lesion may be:
1. At the epiphysial junction of the head and neck, e.g., slipping of the epiphysis—epiphysial coxa vara.
2. In the neck of the femur, e.g., bending—cervical coxa vara. Cervical coxa vara can only occur before the age of four years. At this age the neck becomes completely ossified, having been cartilaginous previously. Once ossified, it is sufficiently strong to bear the body-weight without bending.

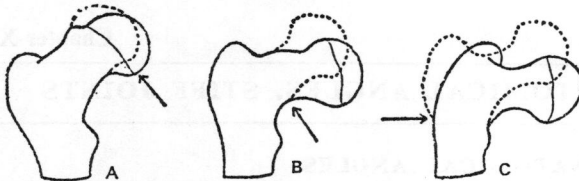

Fig. 464.—Coxa vara. The dotted lines represent the normal. The arrows indicate the site of the origin of the deformity. A, Epiphysial type. B, Cervical type. C, Bending of the shaft of the femur.

3. Bending of the shaft of the femur just below the great trochanter. This may occur in rickets or because of the softening of the bone from disease within it, e.g., cysts.

As a result of the alteration in the relation of the neck to the shaft of the bone there results: (1) Deformity; (2) Interference with function.

1. *Deformity:*
    a. The great trochanter is raised, being higher than on the normal side; as a result it is unduly prominent.
    b. The limb is not held in the normal position in walking, etc., but is adducted and rotated out, so that the toes look outwards.
2. *Interference with Function:* The movement of abduction is diminished, as there is less room between the trochanter and the dorsum ilii, on account of the raising of the trochanter. The patient may limp because of the shortening of the distance between the head and the lower end of the femur. As a result of the shortening on one side the spine is tilted to maintain the body erect; this is scoliosis. If both sides are affected, the limbs may be crossed in walking because of the adduction deformity which exists; this is scissors gait.

SLIPPING OF THE UPPER FEMORAL EPIPHYSIS[1]: This is a condition which is worthy of special mention. The affection is one of older childhood and adolescence and is unilateral, whereas the cervical type is often bilateral. The main interest in the aetiology centres round the fact that it is not severe *direct* violence which initiates the slipping of the head, but mild *indirect* trauma, e.g., the repetition of some frequently performed act such as jumping off a bicycle. Once the slipping has begun the body-weight will tend to increase it. There are several factors which have a bearing on the aetiology of the condition:

1. The periosteum around the neck of the femur becomes thinner during adolescence, thus depriving the epiphysis of the head of support.

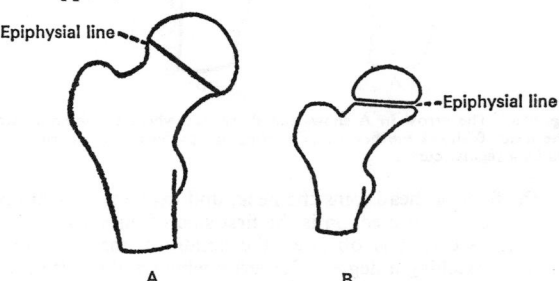

Fig. 465.—To show the plane of the epiphysial line of the femoral head in A, Adult. B, Child.

---

[1] For some of the subjoined facts I am indebted to E. N. Wardle, *Br. J. Surg.*, 1933, 21, 313.

2. The plane of the epiphysial line is horizontal in childhood but begins to get more vertical after the age of ten years. A glance at *Fig.* 465 will show how the epiphysial line is subjected to strain only when it changes from the horizontal to the oblique.
3. A separated epiphysis is universally a fracture separation —i.e., a portion of the metaphysis is separated with the epiphysis. In slipped upper femoral epiphysis there exists a pure separation with no fracture of the metaphysis.
4. The type of injury resulting in the deformity suggests a tearing of blood-vessels with associated hyperaemia. Lerich and Policard[1] have shown that hyperaemia is associated with decalcification. It is this deprivation of lime salts which, when subjected to the constant shearing force of the body-weight, results in the slipping of the head.
5. Endocrine disturbances have been invoked to explain those cases where the lesion is only one of several epiphyses involved.

Trethowan[2] indicated the great importance of the sharp projection normally present in a radiograph where the upper border of

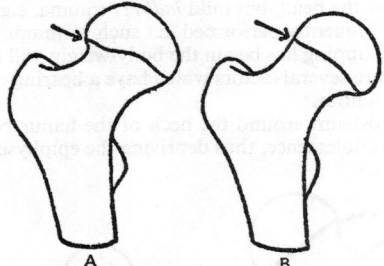

Fig. 466.—The arrow in A shows the sharp rise where the femoral neck joins the head. B shows the first stage of slipping epiphysis. The sharp rise is replaced by a regular curve.

the femoral head joins the neck, and explains how disappearance of this projection is the first sign of slipping, and that if weight-bearing is obviated the condition may be prevented from reaching a degree of severity which will result in lifelong disability (*Fig.* 466).

COXA VALGA: This is a much rarer condition than the preceding. Here the vertical neck-shaft angle is increased, either congenitally

---

[1] Leriche and Policard, *Pathological Physiology of Bone.*
[2] W. H. Trethowan, *Choyce's System of Surgery,* 1932.

ANATOMICAL ANGLES. STIFF JOINTS

or as the result of injury. The distance between the crest of the ilium and the trochanter major is increased. The limb is held in a position of abduction and external rotation.

CONGENITAL DISLOCATION OF THE HEAD OF THE FEMUR: In this condition the child is born with the head of the femur outside its socket, resting usually on the dorsum ilii behind the acetabulum. This condition is associated with important changes in the upper end of the femur:

1. The neck of the femur is short.
2. Coxa vara often exists.
3. The forward or declination angle is considerably increased, being anything from 30° to 90° instead of the normal 12°.

The result of this is that in a radiograph of the joint with the toes looking forward, no neck of the femur can be seen, the epiphysis appearing to sit on the top of the vertical shaft (*Fig.* 467). If,

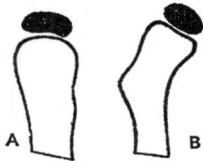

Fig. 467.—Radiographs of upper end of femur in congenital dislocation of hip-joint. A, Schematic representation of upper end of femur with toes directed forwards; the neck of the bone is not seen. B, With the foot rotated in as far as possible; the neck is seen.

however, the limb now be rotated fully inward so that the toe look inwards at a right angle, and another plate be taken, the neck will be seen.

SHAFT: This important weight-bearing bone has normally a forward and outward curvature of its shaft. It is of great moment to remember this in fractures of the bone, so that the normal angulation may be restored, otherwise deformity and wrong transmission of weight result.

LOWER END:

KNOCK-KNEE (GENU VALGUM): The normal inclination of the femora is such that each makes an angle of about 172° with the bones below the knee. This angle is open outwards. The leg bones are exactly vertical. This angle depends on the width of the pelvis, i.e., distance between the acetabula. As the distance is greater in the female, the outer angle between the femur and tibia is less in the female, as in the male the femoral shafts more nearly approach the vertical (*Fig.* 468). As the bony surfaces taking part in the knee-joint are exactly horizontal, it follows that the medial condyle of the femur must project farther down than the lateral (when the femur is held vertically). If this projection of the condyle is increased, then it pushes the inner condyle of the tibia down, and as a result the shaft of the tibia can no longer remain vertical but is pushed out, so that the inner aspect of the knee

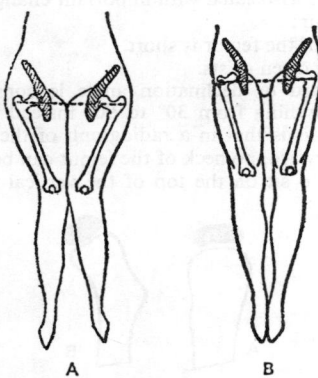

Fig. 468.—To show the natural tendency to knock-knee in women owing to the greater obliquity of the femora. A, Female. B, Male.

is unduly prominent—knock-knee (*Fig.* 469). This condition is usually due to rickets, and is thought to be due to excessive formation of bone at the inner side of the lower portion of the diaphysis, this being responsible for the further downward projection of the inner femoral condyle (*Fig.* 469, A). It is of the first importance to realize that in rickety knock-knee the only part of the inner condyle which projects too far distally is its lower or distal surface; the posterior surface is unaffected; therefore if the knee be flexed the deformity disappears (*Fig.* 470).

BOW-KNEE (GENU VARUM): In this condition, the reverse of knock-knee, the lower limb forms an arc with the concavity inwards. The external condyle of the femur projects too far distally. The condition is easily confused with bow-leg, in which deformity the knee-joint is normal, the tibia being curved between the knee and ankle. The conditions are distinguished by dropping a vertical line from the head of the femur (just medial to the femoral artery) to the ground with the patient standing erect. In genu varum this line falls inside the knee, in bow-leg it passes through the centre of the knee-joint (*Fig.* 471).

ANATOMICAL ANGLES. STIFF JOINTS 481

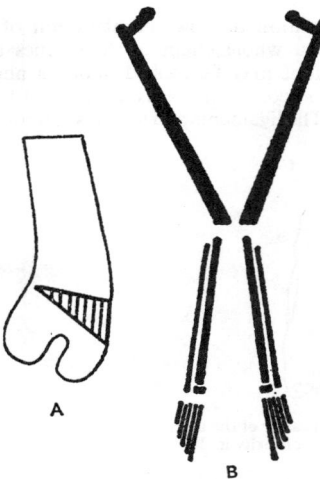

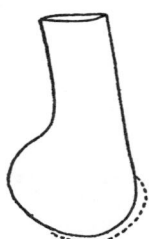

Fig. 469.—A, Showing overgrowth of bone at the inner end of the diaphysis which is the direct cause of the knock-knee. B, Knock-knee.

Fig. 470.—Demonstrating the fact that the fault of the lower end of the femur resulting in rickety knock-knee affects only the inferior part of the bone, as shown by the dotted line. In flexion, therefore, the deformity disappears, as the posterior part of the epiphysis is normal.

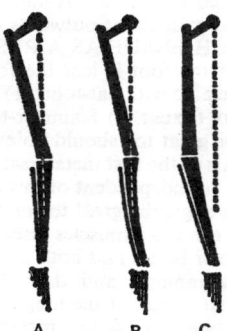

Fig. 471.—A, Normal alignment of lower limb bones. B, Bow-leg. C, Bow-knee. The dotted line is a vertical from head of femur to the ground.

482 A SYNOPSIS OF SURGICAL ANATOMY

Flat-foot: This is an excellent illustration of how the alteration of an anatomical angle may produce a whole chain of deformities and disabilities. The arches of the foot may be looked upon as angles which are concave downwards and convex upwards. In flat-foot these angles become straightened out. The ligaments and tendons supporting

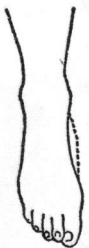

Fig. 472.—To show how the concavity of the inner border of a normal foot becomes a convexity in flat-foot.

the arch become inefficient, and the head of the talus is no more supported and drops. It forces its way between the internal malleolus and the tubercle of the scaphoid, with the result that the fore-foot is deflected laterally and into valgus. Thus it comes about that the inner border of the foot, which should normally show a slight concavity, is replaced by a convexity (*Fig.* 472). A vertical line dropped from the patella along the crest of the tibia should pass normally through the second intermetatarsal space. In flat-foot it passes internal to this space, showing the displacement outwards of the fore-foot.

DISABILITIES WHICH ENSUE AS A RESULT OF FLAT-FOOT: When the arch of the foot is lost the following conditions often follow or are associated with flat-foot: (1) Hallux valgus; (2) Hallux rigidus; (3) Hallux flexus; (4) Hammer-toe.

HALLUX VALGUS: The great toe should point straight forwards in line with the long axis of the first metatarsal bone. When the fore-foot is displaced out or independent of this the great toe may be bent laterally. As the angle the great toe makes with the metatarsus is then abnormal, the small muscles inserted to the outer side of its base (half of flexor brevis and both adductors) are now acting at a mechanical advantage, and they pull the great toe farther laterally. The line of pull of the long extensor of the toe, instead of being along the line of the first metatarsal and the big toe, now acts along a line external to that, and still further increases the deformity (*Fig.* 473). The normal angle of the great toe once upset, the muscles and tendons increase the deformity.

ANATOMICAL ANGLES. STIFF JOINTS

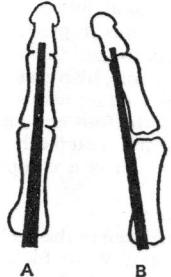

Fig. 473.—Showing how the tendon of the extensor hallucis longus acts as a bowstring increasing the deformity of hallux valgus once the phalanges are deviated laterally. A, Normal alignment. B, Alignment in hallux valgus.

HALLUX RIGIDUS: In this condition the great toe is in a line with the first metatarsal, but cannot be extended beyond the horizontal. Normally, the extensor hallucis longus acts over an angle in extending the toe and is at a mechanical advantage. When the foot arch has dropped, this angle disappears and the extensor is at a mechanical disadvantage (*Fig.* 474). This is a factor (though not the only one) in the production of hallux rigidus.

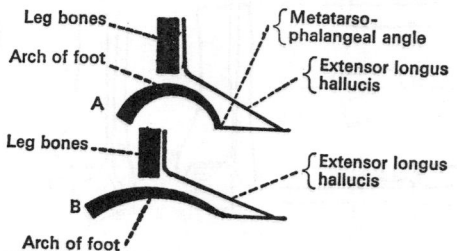

Fig. 474.—A, Showing how the extensor hallucis longus acts normally across the metatarsophalangeal angle. B, The angle is obliterated by flat-foot; the extensor is at a disadvantage predisposing to hallux rigidus.

HALLUX FLEXUS: The great toe may be permanently flexed towards the sole owing to the flexors being at a mechanical advantage.

HAMMER-TOE: Owing to the displacement of the great toe outwards the other toes are cramped for room, and as a result one of the toes, usually the second, is displaced forwards. It is acutely flexed at the first interphalangeal joint and extended or flexed at

484 A SYNOPSIS OF SURGICAL ANATOMY

the second interphalangeal joint. The bones forming the first interphalangeal joint form a prominence which the footwear presses on, causing a corn, and the point of the last phalanx may press against the boot sole, also resulting in a corn.

Club-foot: In congenital talipes equinovarus, the normal alignment of the fore-foot to the rest of the foot and leg is disturbed. The muscles acting on the inner side are at a great mechanical advantage and greatly increase the deformity, which is a complex one, consisting of the following components:
1. Adduction of the fore-foot.
2. Varus of the fore-foot and often of the heel also, i.e., rotation inwards round the longitudinal axis of the foot.
3. Equinus, i.e., pulling up of the heel.
4. Rotation of the tibia inwards. This may be so severe that the whole foot is rotated inwards through 90°, so that instead of the long axis of the foot being directed forward, it is in the coronal plane of the body, and the one foot must be lifted over the other in walking.

Horizontal Joint Lines: The joint lines are horizontal at the wrist, knee, and ankle. In dealing with fractures which may affect the direction of these joint lines the first surgical principle to be observed is to maintain

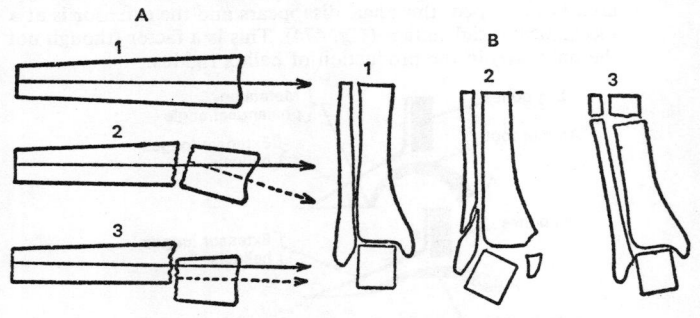

Fig. 475.—To show the importance of restoring the horizontal joint line at the wrist and ankle.

A, *Wrist:* 1, Represents the lower half of the radius, the arrow indicating the long axis of the bone; the joint line is transverse to this axis. 2, Shows a fracture, the distal fragment being rotated back; the joint line is no more horizontal. 3, Shows a fracture with dorsal displacement of the distal fragment, but no rotation. The joint line is still transverse; if unreduced this displacement will not cause so serious a disability as that which will result from (2), because of the direction of the joint line.

B, *Ankle:* 1, The lower leg and talus; the joint line is horizontal. 2, Pott's fracture; the upper surface of the talus is no more horizontal. Faulty weight-bearing results. 3, Fracture of both bones with inward displacement of the distal fragment; the ankle-joint is no more horizontal.

ANATOMICAL ANGLES. STIFF JOINTS

the horizontal direction of the articulation. Failure to observe this rule will result in disability which may be progressive. At the wrist weakness of the hand will ensue. In the lower limb the results are still more serious because of the alteration of the line of weight transmission—e.g., if the normal horizontal plane of the ankle-joint is disturbed, not only will the ankle suffer, but also the knee, hip, and even the lower spinal joints will be affected by osteoarthritis (*Fig.* 475). This explains Trethowan's dictum that if manipulation of a Pott's fracture does not secure perfect anatomical restoration of the ankle-joint, the treatment becomes a 'mere matter of carpentry' to attain this end.

Calcaneal Angle: The calcaneus is fractured more often than any other tarsal bone, being comparable in this respect with the navicular or scaphoid in the carpus. The treatment of crush fractures with displacement is a difficult problem, because it is important to restore the normal obliquity of so important a weight-bearing bone. Normally this bone is set at an angle so that only its tuberosity comes in contact with the ground. In fractures due to falls on the heels the bone may be crumpled so that its long axis is horizontal instead of being oblique.

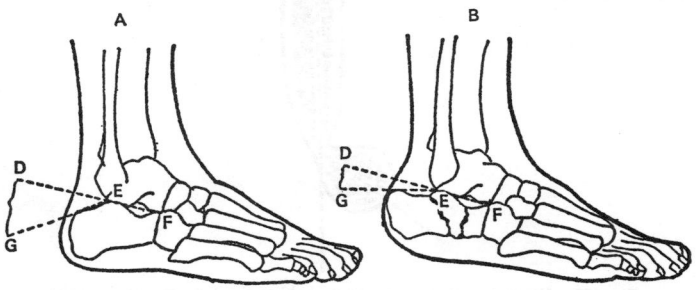

Fig. 476.—To show the calcaneal angle. A, The line DEF touches the highest point of the bone and its anterior extremity; GE touches the posterior extremity and the highest point; the resultant angle is the calcaneal angle DEG; it is 30°. B, The calcaneus has been crushed; the bone lies more horizontally; the calcaneal angle is reduced.

As a guide in reducing such a fracture the calcaneal angle is useful. This angle is normally 30°, and the method of its determination is shown in *Fig.* 476.

Elbow: In extension the forearm bones make an angle with the humerus, resulting in an arc which is convex inwards. This is the 'carrying angle', and is due to the inner condyle of the humerus being set obliquely so that the axis of the elbow-joint is transverse between the radius and the humerus but oblique between the ulna and the humerus (*Fig.* 477).

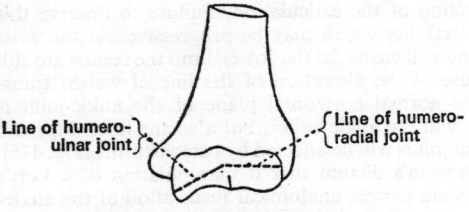

Fig. 477.—Demonstrating the obliquity of humero-ulnar joint in comparison with transverse humero-radial joint. It is this obliquity which pushes the ulna laterally, producing the carrying angle.

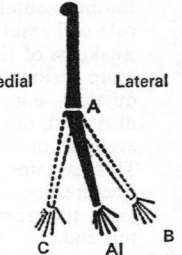

Fig. 478.—A AI, The normal carrying angle; AB, Increase of carrying angle—cubitus valgus; AC, The opposite condition—cubitus varus.

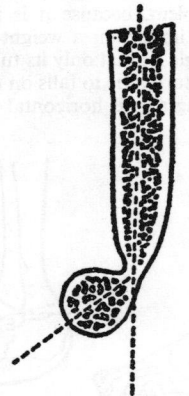

Fig. 479.—Vertical section of the lower half of the humerus to show the angle made by the long axes of shaft and capitulum.

The angle is 10° to 15° in extension, and disappears on full flexion.

The inner lip of the trochlea is a ridge which is much deeper distally than anteriorly, so that the ulna (with the forearm) is deflected laterally in full extension by this ridge, the deflexion disappearing in flexion as the ridge becomes less distinct.

The angle may be disturbed by fractures of the lower end of the humerus or by rupture of the collateral ligaments, which act as stays to the bones.

If the carrying angle is increased the condition of cubitus valgus results. If it is obliterated the condition of cubitus varus ensues (*Fig. 478*).

Lower Humeral Angle: The lower articular end of the humerus is set at an angle to the shaft of the bone. The angle is 60°. It is of great importance to restore this angle in the setting of fractures of the condyles or fractures which cross the bone immediately above the articular cartilage, such as diacondylar fractures and separations of the lower epiphysis. So, too, in estimating the position in cases of supracondylar fractures, the angle must be restored. The angle is estimated best in a lateral radiograph of the elbow region and shown in *Fig.* 479.

II. THE OPTIMUM ATTITUDE FOR STIFF JOINTS

In cases where the bones taking part in an articulation are likely to adhere together as the result of disease, or are to be fixed together by the surgeon's

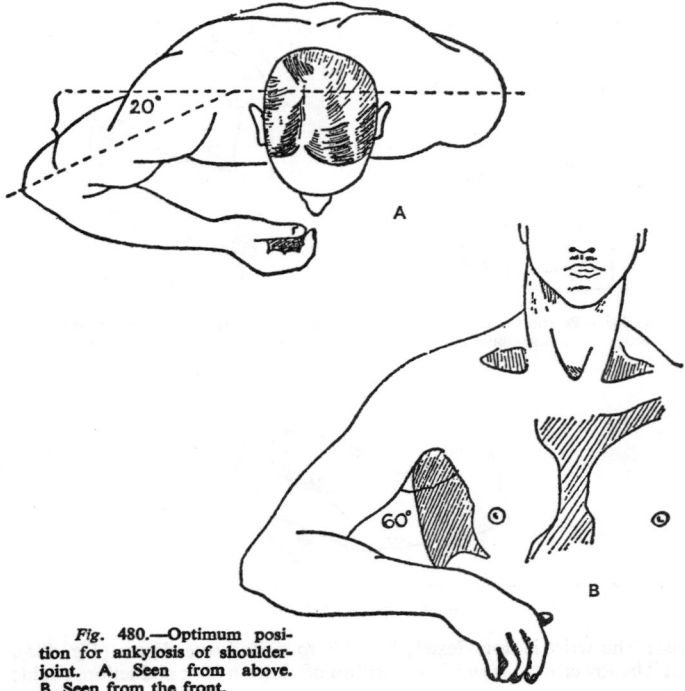

Fig. 480.—Optimum position for ankylosis of shoulder-joint. A, Seen from above. B, Seen from the front.

efforts, it is of the first importance to put the bones in that position which will be of the greatest use and least hindrance to the patient. This is the 'optimum position', and is definite for every limb joint.

Shoulder: 45° to 90° abduction. 20° flexion in front of the coronal plane (*Fig.* 480). The younger the patient, the greater the abduction angle made at the shoulder-joint. In the position of partial abduction the arm may be brought to the side by movements of the scapula on the chest wall; the younger the patient, the more free this movement.

Elbow: If one elbow is fixed it is best that it be at a right-angle (*Fig.* 481). If both elbows are fixed, the right is put at an angle slightly less than a right-angle and the left at an angle more than a right-angle. The right hand can then be brought to the mouth (*Fig.* 482). The left hand can be used for cutting up food and can also reach the trouser pocket. In all cases the forearm is put in a position midway between pronation and supination.

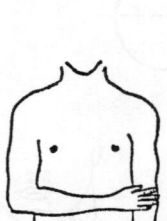

Fig. 481.—Position of choice for ankylosis of the elbow-joint.

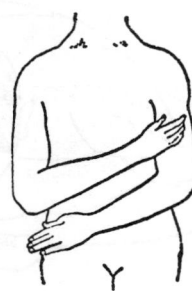

Fig. 482.—Positions of elbows when both require to be ankylosed.

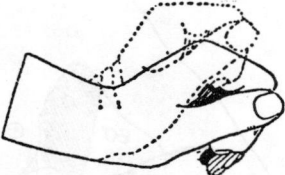

Fig. 483.—Optimum attitude for ankylosis of wrist-joint. The dotted hand is too fully extended.

Wrist: The wrist is dorsiflexed, *but only to a moderate degree* (*Fig.* 483).
Hip: The lower limb is put in a position of: flexion 30°; abduction, slight;

ANATOMICAL ANGLES. STIFF JOINTS

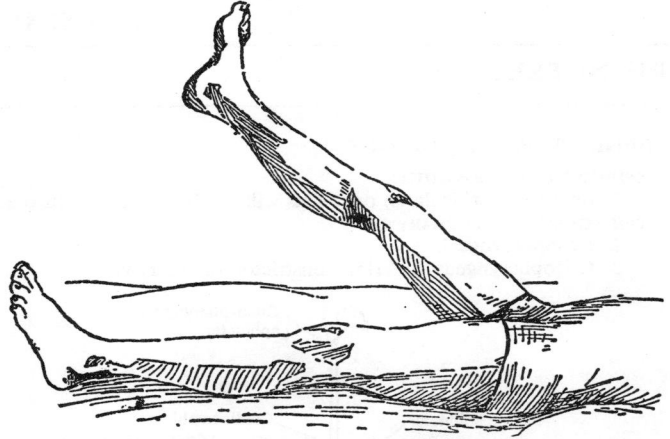

Fig. 484.—Optimum position for ankylosis of hip-joint. The limb can be brought on the couch if the patient arches the lumbar spine.

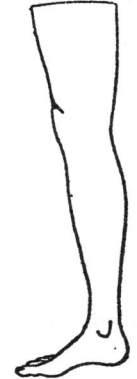

Fig. 485.—Optimum attitude for ankylosis of knee-joint.

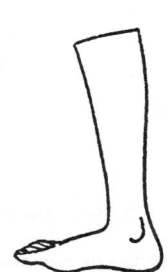

Fig. 486.—Optimum attitude for ankylosis of ankle-joint.

lateral rotation, slight (*Fig.* 484). This enables the patient to sit and to walk better than if the limb were quite extended.

Knee: Full extension. Some surgeons prefer very slight flexion (*Fig.* 485).

Ankle: Dorsiflexed a little more than a right-angle (*Fig.* 486).

Chapter XXXIII

SPHINCTERS

I. SPHINCTERS OF THE GUT

SPHINCTER OF THE MOUTH:
  1. Sphincter (orbicularis) oris. This will not be considered further.

SPHINCTERS OF THE PHARYNX:
  2. Nasopharyngeal.
  3. Cricopharyngeus (inferior constrictor of pharynx).

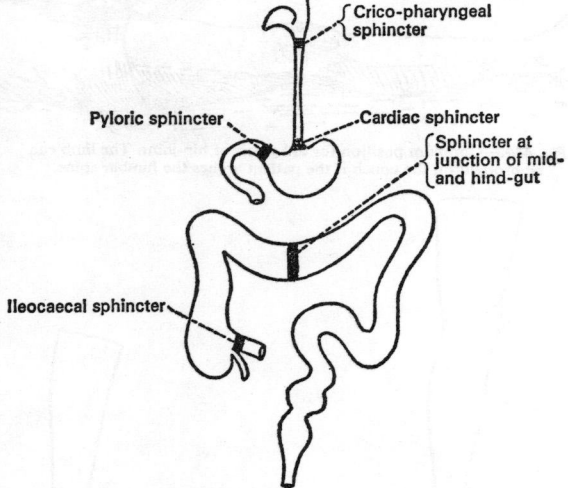

Fig. 487.—Sphincters of the alimentary canal. (*After Keith.*)

SPHINCTERS OF THE STOMACH:
  4. Cardiac.
  5. Pyloric.

SPHINCTERS OF THE SMALL INTESTINE:
  6. Duodenojejunal flexure.
  7. Ileocaecal valve.

SPHINCTERS OF THE LARGE INTESTINE:
  8. Valve of Gerlach.

9. Transverse colic.
10. Internal sphincter ani.
11. External sphincter ani.

Nasopharyngeal Sphincter:[1] This sphincter or valve is made up by the soft palate and the superior constrictor of the pharynx. It consists, therefore, of two parts: (1) Palatal; (2) Pharyngeal.

PALATAL PART: This consists of two groups of muscles with opposing functions:

GROUP 1: The abductors consist of the palatopharyngei, palatoglossi, and tensores of the palate. They open the valve.

GROUP 2: The adductors consist of the levatores palati. They close the valve.

PHARYNGEAL PART: The superior constrictor of the pharynx. A part of this muscle has a sphincteric action. This part is called:

THE RIDGE OF PASSAVANT: In 1896 Passavant described a specialized part of the superior constrictor of the pharynx. It takes origin from the palatal aponeurosis and extends round the pharynx. Passavant considered that the transverse ridge formed on the back and sides of the pharynx when this muscle contracts was an essential factor in shutting off the naso- from the oropharynx in swallowing. It has been shown, however, that the ridge is not always present. It can be seen in some cases of cleft palate. X-rays have, moreover, demonstrated that during speech the soft palate makes contact with the posterior wall of the pharynx a centimetre or two above the level of the ridge. In swallowing, the ridge plays little if any part.

Cricopharyngeus or Inferior Constrictor of the Pharynx: The inferior constrictor muscle consists of two parts, a lower transverse part and an upper oblique portion. The lower transverse fibres arise from the cricoid and pass horizontally backward round the pharynx to be inserted into a median raphe at the back of this tube. Its function is to prevent regurgitation of the oesophageal contents into the pharynx. The upper oblique fibres arise from the cricoid and thyroid cartilages, and encircle the hypopharynx, ending in the median raphe. In the act of swallowing the upper (oblique) part of this muscle propels the contents downwards and the lower (transverse) part relaxes to allow the contents to pass into the oesophagus. Incoordination of this action, with failure of the cricopharyngeus to relax, will result in increased pressure in the pharynx with the production of a pharyngeal diverticulum.

The Oesophagogastric Junction:[2] Normally gastric contents cannot regurgitate into the oesophagus because of the mechanism at the

---

[1] The account of this sphincter is taken from 'Cleft Palate', by W. E. M. Wardill, *Br. J. Surg.*, 1928, 16, 128.
[2] Muller Botha, G. S., *The Gastro-Oesophageal Junction*, 1962. London: Churchill.

cardia preventing this. Continence of the cardia depends on muscular and mucosal factors which operate together.

The inferior oesophageal sphincter is not apparent on dissection but there is a functional sphincter, as seen on pressure recordings, at the level where the oesophagus traverses the hiatus in the diaphragm. The diaphragm may add additional external support to the sphincter during straining, but the so-called 'pinch-cock' effect of the diaphragm is of secondary importance. On radiographs this inferior sphincter is shown as an empty segment where the oesophagus goes through the diaphragm.

The inferior oesophageal sphincter alone would probably not prevent reflux, but it is supported by mucosal folds at the cardia which plug the orifice to make a water-tight seal. These mucosal folds are not passive but are controlled by the muscularis mucosae and the inferior oesophageal sphincter which draw them together and keep them in close apposition.

THE OESOPHAGEAL HIATUS: The oesophageal hiatus in the diaphragm lies anterior to the aorta and is in the right crus in 55 per cent of cases while in the remainder the left crus of the diaphragm plays a variable part in the formation of the hiatus. The width of the hiatus varies between 1·8 and 2·5 cm.

THE NERVE-SUPPLY OF THE OESOPHAGUS:[1] The vagi are the motor nerves to the oesophagus. In the body of the oesophagus there are only cholinergic receptors and vagal stimulation results in contraction. In the inferior oesophageal sphincter there are both cholinergic and adrenergic receptors, but innervation is largely adrenergic and vagal stimulation results in relaxation of the sphincter.

Afferent visceral pain impulses pass along the sympathetic nerves which are closely related to the somatic sensory fibres of the phrenic and intercostal nerves in the posterior horn of the spinal cord. Afferent impulses from the oesophagus may thus 'overflow' into adjacent somatic neurones in the posterior horn to give pain referred to the neck, arm, chest, or back. Some pain fibres must be carried in the vagus nerves because occasionally oesophageal pain is referred to the ear, presumably via the auricular branch of the vagus (*Fig.* 130, p. 139).

Achalasia:[2] In this condition there is failure of the inferior oesophageal sphincter to relax during deglutition and an absence of co-ordinated peristalsis in the body of the oesophagus, resulting in an obstruction at the cardia. By means of electron microscopy Wallerian degeneration is seen in the vagus nerve, the oesophageal smooth muscle shows changes of denervation, there is a reduction in the number of cells

[1] Ellis, F. G., Kauntze, R., and Trounce, J. R., *Br. J. Surg.*, 1960, 47, 466.
[2] Cassella, R. R., Brown, A. L., Sayre, G. P., and Ellis, F. H., *Ann. Surg.*, 1964, 160, 474.

in the dorsal motor nucleus of the vagus nerve, and in most cases (especially those of long standing) there is degeneration or even absence of myenteric ganglion cells. These findings support the theory that this disease primarily affects the extrinsic neural structures (either the dorsal motor nucleus or the vagus nerve) and that the oesophageal changes are secondary.

DIFFUSE SPASM OF THE OESOPHAGUS: There is a neuromuscular incoordination of the lower two-thirds of the oesophagus in response to deglutition, resulting in simultaneous diffuse contraction of the oesophagus from the aortic arch downwards. This causes intermittent dysphagia and retrosternal pain. The sites of contraction are constant and this later results in hypertrophy of the circular muscle and diverticula between the areas of hypertrophy.

Pyloric Sphincter: Torgersen[1] has described the circular muscle of the pyloric canal as a triangular-shaped muscle in the position of an inverted V with the apex at the pyloric end of the lesser curvature and the two limbs spreading out towards the greater curvature. This specialized circular muscle extends along the greater curvature for about 5 cm., but is bunched up on the lesser curvature to form a thick mass about 2 cm. long (muscle torus). The right edge of this muscle is thickened to form the pylorus.

On the outside of this circular muscle there is the longitudinal muscle which partly extends over the pylorus to be continuous with the longitudinal muscle of the duodenum and is partly inserted into the circular muscle at the pylorus and the submucosa in the area.

These circular and longitudinal muscles form a functional entity, contracting concentrically to form the emptying mechanism of the stomach. The narrow lumen of the distal limb of the circular muscle acts as a filter resulting in regurgitation of solid material back into the stomach, so slowing down gastric emptying. At the end of this concentric contraction the canal is shortened and closed, thus preventing regurgitation of duodenal contents during duodenal contractions.

This specialized muscle may become abnormal:

1. Hypertrophic pyloric stenosis in the infant. There is hypertrophy of the circular muscle presenting with pyloric obstruction from the second week of life. Medical measures may overcome this obstruction but division of the hypertrophied muscle (the Ramstedt operation) may be necessary.
2. Spasm and secondary hypertrophy following other gastro-intestinal disorders, e.g., peptic ulcer, hiatus hernia, cholelithiasis, and appendicitis.
3. Primary hypertrophic pyloric stenosis in the adult due to ineffectual contractions of the circular muscle as a result of a deficiency of the longitudinal muscle.

[1] Torgersen, J., *Acta radiol.*, 1942, Suppl. XLV.

The Ileocaecal Junction:[1] The ileum projects into the lumen of the caecum as an oval-shaped slit-like opening lying horizontally with upper and lower lips which coalesce at the sides and are prolonged on to the caecal wall as frenula. The lips of the valve contain a muscle layer which is the continuation of the muscle layers of the ileum and the colon which have fused. This projection may be unusually large due to fatty infiltration and may then be seen on a barium meal or enema when it must be differentiated from an abnormal filling defect. If abnormally enlarged, as in children with abundant lymphoid tissue in the mucosa and submucosa, the valve may be the start of an intussusception.

The ileocaecal junction has two functions: (1) It mechanically prevents reflux from the colon into the ileum. When the colon is distended the lips are tautened and the resultant firm apposition prevents regurgitation. In cases of large-bowel obstruction the competent ileocaecal valve will result in a closed-loop obstruction between it and the obstruction distally, and by admitting the entry of ileal contents but not allowing regurgitation the tension in the caecum rises enormously. Tension gangrene and rupture of the caecum may result. On barium enemata the majority of ileocaecal valves permit regurgitation but this is not an indication of the true state of affairs under physiological conditions when the pressure rises much more gradually. (2) It regulates the transit of ileal contents into the caecum by true sphincter action. The sphincter resists the progress of ileal contents into the caecum, but when food is taken the terminal ileum empties its accumulated contents into the caecum.

The Caecocolic Sphincter:[2] The muscle in the frenula of the ileocaecal valve may represent the caecocolic sphincter of lower animals because in man there is a muscular contraction at this site during colonic mass peristalsis, which carries away the contents of the colon but leaves behind the contents present in the caecum.

II. THE CHOLEDOCHODUODENAL MECHANISM

The Anatomy of the Pancreatic Ducts: According to Millbourn[3] the pancreatic duct (Wirsung), which is developed from the ventral pancreas, is the sole or main excretory channel in 90 per cent of cases, and the accessory pancreatic duct (Santorini), developed from the dorsal pancreas, in 10 per cent. The pancreatic duct generally enters the bile-duct at its distal end before its termination at the ampulla of Vater and only exceptionally (5 per cent) together with the bile-duct at the common papilla of Vater. From this papilla the duct first runs dorsally into the pancreas parallel to the common duct up

---
[1] Fleischner, F. G., and Bernstein, C., *Radiology*, 1950, 54, 43.
[2] Oppenheimer, A., *Radiology*, 1940, 34, 545.
[3] Millbourn, E., *Acta anat.*, 1950, 9, 1.

towards the cranial part of the head of the pancreas. Thence it bends more or less at right-angles into the body and tail. With the pancreatic duct as the main or sole excretory channel, the accessory duct is present in 50 per cent of cases. Its duodenal opening is on the lesser papilla which is constantly oro-ventral to the main papilla.

In 40 per cent of cases this duct is open and in 10 per cent blind; in half of the former group the accessory duct is of sufficient calibre to substitute for a blocked main duct. The accessory duct pursues a horizontal course across the pancreas (*Fig.* 488). Millbourn[1] states that the range of individual variations in the calibre of the main pancreatic duct varies from 1·0 to 7·0 mm., the average being 3·1 mm. These figures were determined by operative cholangiography. The post-mortem dimensions are in general 1 mm. greater. The calibre increases as age advances. The accessory pancreatic duct lies nearer the pylorus and is nearer the surface than the main duct. It is thus more likely than the main duct to injury in operations such as gastrectomy. Such trauma may precipitate acute pancreatitis as a postoperative complication.

The Anatomy of Pancreatitis: The intramural part of the common bile-duct is surrounded by a thickening of the longitudinal and circular muscle of the duodenal wall—the sphincter of Oddi (1887). This occlusive structure is a definite muscle layer which can act independently of the general duodenal musculature. It is controlled by a local nerve net and central nervous control seems unlikely (Sherlock).

Many factors can cause it to contract, e.g., perforated peptic ulcers, and morphine and most analgesics have the same effect. In 95 per cent of cases the main pancreatic duct opens into the distal end of the common bile-duct. This duct is dilated at its distal end and this dilatation bulges into the duodenal wall forming the ampulla of Vater (1720). The pancreatic duct enters the ampulla in the thickness of the duodenal wall at the circumferential position of 5 o'clock.

The nature of the choledochoduodenal mechanism has a profound influence on pathological conditions affecting the gall-bladder and pancreas. It is generally agreed that reflux of bile into the pancreatic duct is an important factor, though not the only one, in the genesis of pancreatitis. Contrariwise reflux of pancreatic ferments into the gall-bladder may cause acute cholecystitis (Flexner). One of the complications of acute pancreatitis is obstruction of the pancreatic ducts which in turn is an important factor in the genesis of chronic pancreatitis.

'The Double Channel': Some authorities (Doubilet and Mulholland)[2] contend that the anatomicophysiological arrangements at the site of the sphincter are such that a 'common channel' may be formed not

[1] Millbourn, E., *Acta chir. scand.*, 1959, 118, 286.
[2] Doubilet, H., and Mulholland, J. R., *Surgery Gynec. Obstet.*, 1948, 86, 295.

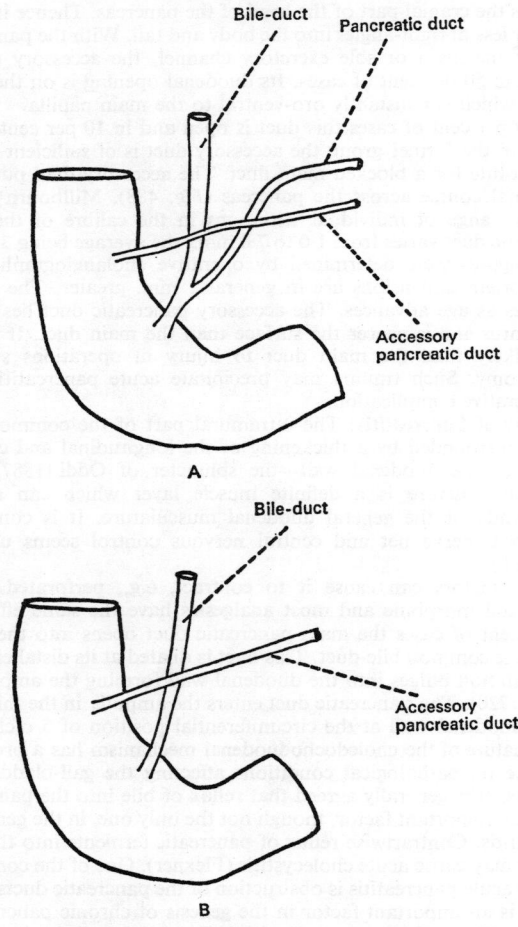

Fig. 488.—The anatomy of the pancreatic ducts. A, The usual arrangement—90 per cent of cases. B, The accessory pancreatic duct is the only excretory channel in 10 per cent of cases. C, (opposite page) The bile-duct and pancreatic duct have separate openings into the duodenum. (*By courtesy of Millbourn and 'Acta Anatomica'.*)

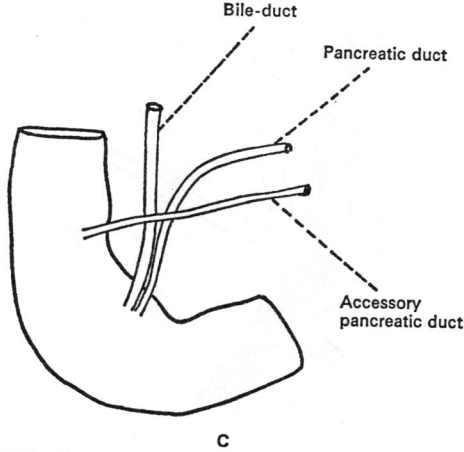

Fig. 488 (continued).

only by stenosis of the opening but also by a mere spasm of the sphincter, resulting in stagnation and mixing of the bile and pancreatic secretions. Other authorities consider that stenosis at the papilla of Vater is the important factor in producing a 'common channel' (*Fig.* 489).

Stenosis may follow inflammation of the papillary area (Odditis) or trauma consequent on the passage of gall-stones or previous operative instrumentation. According to Smith,[1] in the pathogenesis of pancreatitis, bile reflux is a very important factor, but only one of several. The pancreatic ductal pressure is higher than that in the bile-duct. Pancreatic fluid thus normally enters the latter. If for any reason these fluids cannot enter the duodenum freely, stagnation occurs. Should the pressure gradient become reversed, bile must enter the pancreatic duct and acute pancreatitis follows. As a result of such an attack the permeability of the pancreatic ducts is increased which renders the organ more vulnerable to bile reflux—chronic pancreatitis.

It is pertinent to remark that the pancreas has no true capsule such as that of the kidney or spleen. It is covered by a thin layer of connective tissue which contains fat in the obese. It is readily understandable that trauma, or obstructed pancreatic secretions, may rupture this tenuous peri-pancreatic tissue, resulting in the spilling of secretions or the formation of pseudo-cysts.

Smith, R., *Recent Advances in Surgery*, 5th ed., 1959, 390. London: Churchill.

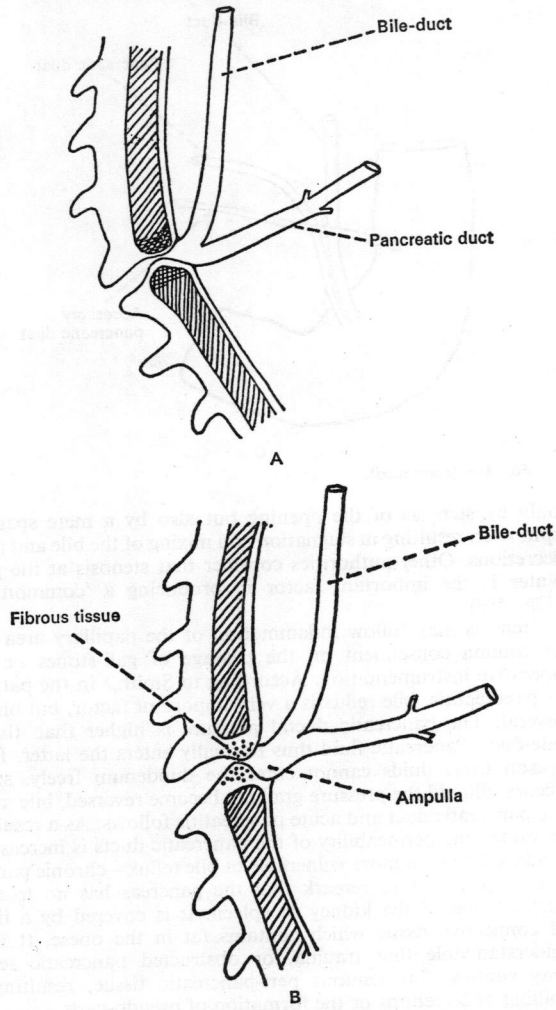

Fig. 489.—A common channel for bile and pancreatic secretions is produced in A by spasm of the sphincter of Oddi. In B it is produced by fibrosis causing stenosis.

III. SPHINCTERS OF THE URINARY TRACT

Junction of the Renal Pelvis with the Ureter: No actual sphincter exists here, yet it is at this point that peristaltic waves commence to travel down the ureter. In some cases the neuromuscular co-ordination may be impaired, leading to an inability of the urine to leave the kidney pelvis, thus resulting in hydronephrosis.[1] This is a further example of achalasia.

Sphincters of the Bladder: There are two of these, internal and external, i.e., the sphincter vesicae at the neck of the bladder and the sphincter urethrae membranaceae. These muscles govern the outflow of urine from the bladder. The internal sphincter is destroyed in the operation of prostatectomy. The urinary control is, however, unimpaired if the external sphincter is left intact.

Chapter XXXIV

THE RELATIONSHIPS OF THE VASCULAR PATTERN TO SURGERY

I. THE BLOOD-SUPPLY OF THE SPINAL CORD

In preparing this section the writer has been guided by the exhaustive review on *Neurologic Complications of Aortic Surgery*, by Adams and van Geertruyden.[2]

All parts of the aorta have been removed by operation. Neurological complications following such surgery are uncommon but very important as they may result in permanent damage of a crippling nature. It becomes then of great consequence to understand the mechanism of these happenings so as to try to forestall them. This means a knowledge of the blood-supply of the cord. This is the one organ on which the effects of vascular occlusion are imperfectly understood.

Blood-supply to the Cord in the Fetus:

SEGMENTATION: There are as many spinal arteries as there are nerves and spinal segments (*Fig.* 490).

Blood-supply to the Cord after Birth:

DESEGMENTATION: During subsequent evolution of the human embryo, changes of considerable significance occur by the processes of desegmentation, regression, and progression in the radicular spinal arteries. Many of these vessels disappear entirely leaving a

---

[1] Treves and Keith, *Surgical Applied Anatomy*, 456.
[2] Adams, H. D., and van Geertruyden, H. H., *Ann. Surg.*, 1956, 144, 514. Philadelphia: Lippincott. (*By courtesy of the authors, and the Editor and Publishers of 'Annals of Surgery.'*)

relatively few but variable number to supply the cord. Thus certain vessels regress and others progress by an increase in size proportionate to the length of cord they supply. The phenomenon of regression and progression is furthest advanced in the lower third of the thoracic and entire lumbosacral cord. These vessels are called radicular arteries. The only constant spinal vessels are the uppermost two anterior and posterior segmental branches from the vertebral arteries. A variable number of radicular arteries are supplied from the vertebrals, the upper two intercostal branches of the costocervical trunk, the aortic intercostals and the lumbar arteries. Each of these vessels enters a spinal foramen to supply branches to the cord.

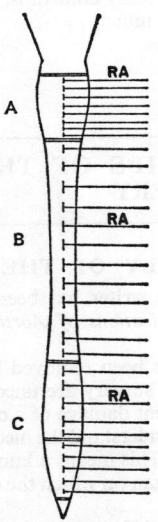

Fig. 490.—Phylogenetic development of the vascular system of the spinal cord in its initial stage where each segment receives an individual radicular artery (RA) (rabbit). A, B, C represent the three divisions of the cord. (*By courtesy of Adams and van Geertruyden, the Editor and Publishers of 'Annals of Surgery'.*)

The cervical cord, supplied through the vertebral and costocervical branches of the subclavian arteries, has a generous blood-supply and has not suffered neurological damage from aortic surgery. When ischaemic cord lesions do follow such procedures, they invariably involve the lumbosacral cord, with or without involvement of the thoracic portion of the cord. Thus knowledge of the definitive features of the vascular supply to the cord is pertinent to the surgeon.

Kadyi (1889) found that the blood-supply is equal to all parts of the cord. Only about a quarter of the nerve-roots are accompanied by significant spinal arteries. The average number of anterior radicular arteries is eight. The largest of these, the arteria radicularis magna, usually arises from the right or left first lumbar artery at the level of the interspace between the 1st and 2nd lumbar vertebrae. It may, however, come off anywhere between the 9th thoracic and the 4th lumbar segment. It always supplies the distal quarter of the cord.

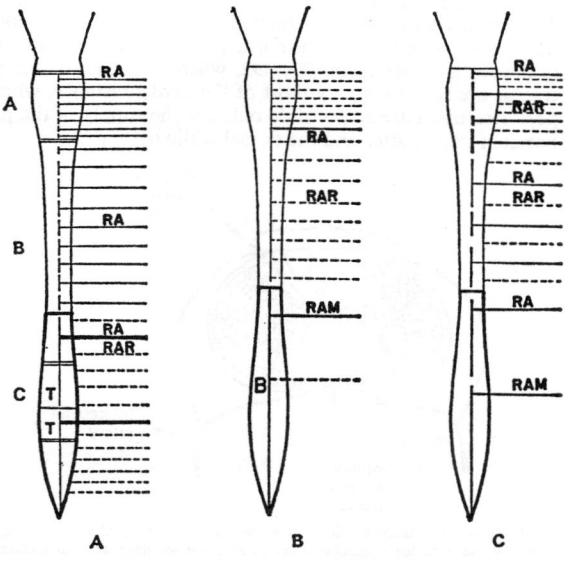

Fig. 491.—A, A succeeding stage of phylogenetic development. In the lower thorax and lumbosacral areas most of the segmental arteries have regressed (RAR) leaving two radicular arteries. The tractus arteriorsus anterior (T) is being formed by fusion of ascending and descending branches of the primitive segmental radicular arteries (RA). B, Type 1 of a final phylogenetic pattern. Desegmentation (RAR) has advanced leaving only a high radicular artery (RA) and the arteria radicularis magna (RAM). The well-developed tractus arteriosus anterior (B) supplies the lower third of the cord. C, Type 2 of a final phylogenetic pattern. Radicular arteries (RA) persist at all levels. The two lower important arteries (RA and RAM) remain. The tractus arteriosus anterior is less well developed. (*By courtesy of Adams and van Geertruyden, the Editor and Publishers of 'Annals of Surgery'.*)

Amongst the many possible variations two well-defined patterns of supply occur:

If the great radicular artery has a high origin then there is a small number of important radicular arteries.

If the great radicular is low there are numerous small radicular arteries (*Fig.* 491).

The anterior arterial tract lies on the front of the cord. It is the only spinal vessel which carries a blood-supply along the entire length of the cord. It is formed by anastomosing cranial and caudal branches of the radicular vessels. It is a most important vascular pathway. The two posterior arterial tracts are formed in a similar manner from the posterior branches of the spinal arteries. These tracts are much more tenuous and are continuous only in the upper and lower parts of the cord. The relative importance of these pathways is apparent in *Fig.* 492, where branches of the anterior tractus are seen to supply most of the cord substance, whereas the posterior tracti are responsible only for the supply of the posterior horns of grey matter and the dorsal white matter.

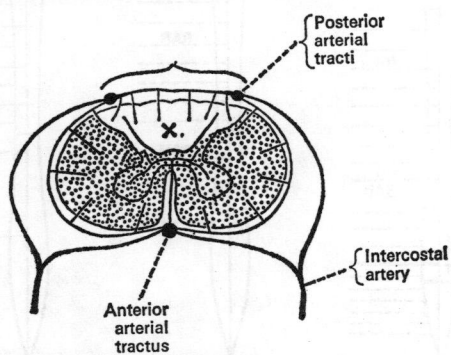

Fig. 492.—The diagram illustrates the large area of the cord (stippled) supplied by the anterior radicular arteries and the anterior arterial tractus and the small part which is dependent on the posterior vessels (X). (*By courtesy of Adams and van Geertruyden, the Editor and Publishers of 'Annals of Surgery'*.)

Applications:

1. THE COLLATERAL CIRCULATION OF THE CORD: In the fetal condition with a spinal artery to each cord segment there is little anastomosis between adjacent segments. So, too, in the fully developed vascular arrangements, the more radicular arteries there are, the less well developed is the anterior spinal tract.

   In general then, the pattern of relatively few large radicular arteries is associated with a large anterior anastomotic pathway —the tractus anterior—which ensures a good collateral in case radicular arteries are occluded.

The subclavian arteries may supply half of the cord if the cord receives no upper radicular artery from the aorta. If the branches to the cord from the subclavians are cut off, ischaemic damage may occur to the upper thoracic and lower cervical cord. The upper cervical cord is protected by the excellent anastomosis between the vertebrals through the basilar.

2. **HOW NEUROLOGICAL DAMAGE IS PRODUCED BY SURGERY:** Two features characterize the arterial supply to the cord—the wide variations which occur and the small number and

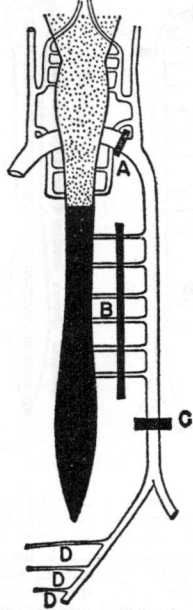

Fig. 493.—Neurological damage which may follow occlusion of the aorta or intercostal arteries. Blocking the aorta at A may cause damage to the spinal cord and peripheral nerves. Section of intercostal arteries (B) may interfere with the vascular supply to the cord. Infrarenal occlusion (C) may interfere with the blood-supply of the peripheral nerves (D) owing to diminution of the blood current via branches of the aorta. (*By courtesy of Adams and van Geertruyden, the Editor and Publishers of 'Annals of Surgery'.*)

size of the vessels supplying this vital structure. The blood-supply of the thoracic and lumbar parts of the cord is therefore precarious.

The tissues vary in their resistance to ischaemia, the grey matter being most sensitive and the tissues becoming more resistant towards the periphery. Thus the peripheral nerves will tolerate deprivation of blood-supply for a longer period than the cord. Yet, though both may be damaged by ischaemia, the cord will suffer

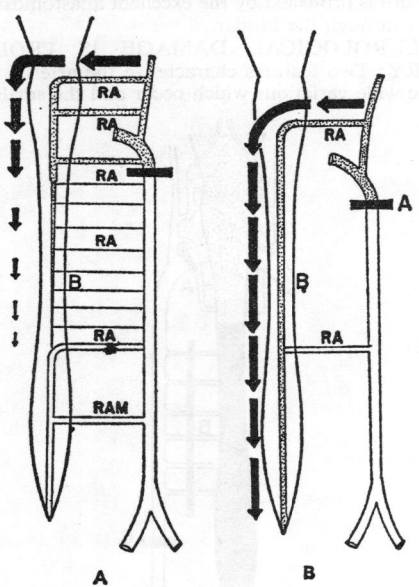

Fig. 494.—A, There are many radicular arteries (RA and RAM) in this type of cord supply. The tractus arteriosus anterior (B) is therefore poorly developed. Occlusion of the aorta just beyond the left subclavian endangers the vitality of the cord, as shown by the diminishing arrows. B, In this type of cord supply there are but two radicular arteries (RA). The anterior spinal anastomotic vessel B is adequate for the supply of the cord when the aorta is interrupted at A, as indicated by the sturdy arrows. (*By courtesy of Adams and van Geertruyden, the Editor and Publishers of 'Annals of Surgery'.*)

first, and a distinction as to which is the affected system may be difficult to make. Thus the time of aortic occlusion is a factor. According to Adams and van Geertruyden the length of time during which the spinal cord can withstand vascular occlusion is 18 minutes.

RELATIONSHIPS OF VASCULAR PATTERN 505

The age of the patient is an additional factor—young tissues withstanding ischaemia better than those of older persons, many of whom have damaged vessels.

Aortic occlusion does not cut off all the blood-supply to the area below. The blood-supply drops to about a quarter because of collateral supply. Many cases of saddle emboli of the aorta or ligature of that vessel below the renals are not followed by neurological damage or gangrene.

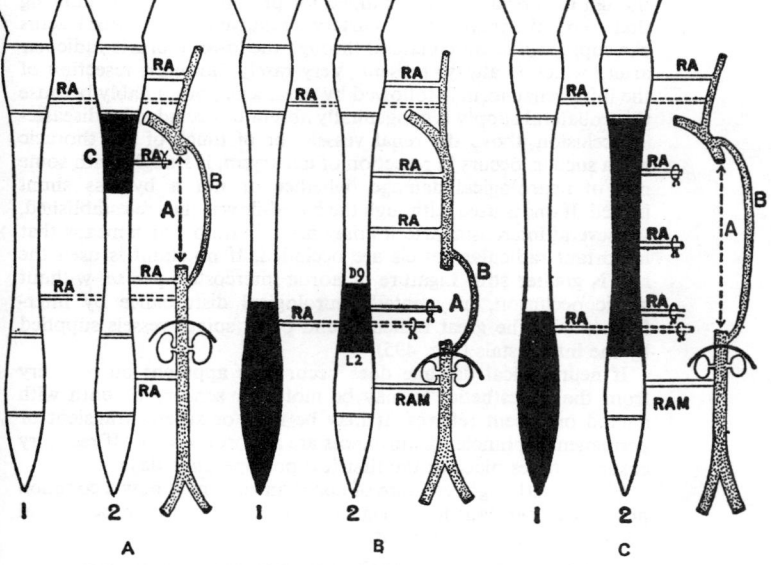

Fig. 495.—A, In 1, suprarenal aortic resection (A) using a shunt (B) will not damage the cord because there are two large radicular arteries (RA) and therefore a well-developed anterior arterial tractus. In 2 the identical procedure may damage the cord, as shown by the black area (C), because of the poorly developed anterior arterial tractus consequent on the presence of numerous small radicular arteries. B, Resection of the lower thoracic aorta (A) using a shunt (B) may damage the cord because in 1 one of the two radicular arteries (RA) is occluded, and in 2 a radicular artery (RA) is occluded and the tractus arteriosus anterior is poorly developed. The lower part of the cord escapes because the arteria radicularis magna (RAM) is undamaged. C, Resection of the thoracic aorta distal to the subclavian will in 1 produce the same cord damage as in B1. In 2 the cord damage will be more extensive than in B2 because more radicular arteries have been affected. (*By courtesy of Adams and van Geertruyden, the Editor and Publishers of 'Annals of Surgery'.*)

Neurological damage may be produced in several ways:

By aortic occlusion: the higher the block the greater the danger. The safe period for aortic occlusion at the level of origin of the left subclavian artery is 50–60 min., whereas below the renals it is double that length of time. A high aortic block not only diminishes the blood-supply to distal tissues, including peripheral nerves, but also cuts off the intercostal and lumbar blood-supply to the radicular arteries. On the other hand, neurological damage does not follow resection of aneurysms, with grafting, below the renal vessels, even though the aorta may be clamped for prolonged periods, showing that even if the great radicular artery is removed, the anterior tractus can supply sufficient collateral through the lower thoracic radicular artery which is always present. Very rarely, however, resection of the infra-renal aorta is followed by paraplegia, presumably because this collateral supply is congenitally absent or occluded by disease.[1]

Occlusion above the renal vessels, or of much of the thoracic aorta such as occurs in resection of aneurysm, is fraught with some risk of neurological damage, whether or not a by-pass shunt is used. If one is used, although the blood-flow is thus re-established, yet several intercostal arteries may need division which means that important radicular vessels are occluded. If no shunt is used the risk is greater still. Ligature of aortic intercostals *per se*, without aortic occlusion, may entail neurological disturbance by interference with the great radicular and other spinal vessels supplied by the intercostals (*Fig.* 495).

If neurological damage does occur it is apparent on recovery from the anaesthetic. It may be motor or sensory or both with altered or absent reflexes. It may be mild or severe, transient or permanent. Sphincter disturbances are almost constant. If recovery ensues it takes place in the first few postoperative days.

Finally, although resection of aortic aneurysms is now a common procedure, permanent damage to the spinal cord or peripheral nerves is an infrequent event.

II. THE SURGICAL ANATOMY OF THE HEART AND GREAT VESSELS

1. The Heart

In the preparation of this section the writer is indebted to the work of Brock.[2]

The heart is a modified blood-vessel which is specialized to form a muscular pump. Its development is complex and imperfections in the process are common. Some are not amenable to surgical correction, others are.

---

[1] Coupland, G. A. E., and Reeve, T. S., *Surgery*, 1968, **64**, 878
[2] Brock, R. C., '75th Bradshaw Lecture. The Present Position of Cardiac Surgery', *Ann. R. Coll. Surg.*, 1958, Vol. 23(4), 213.

Atrial Septal Defects: The development of the interauricular septum is so complex that its imperfect closure is the commonest cardiac defect and occurs in about 25 per cent of persons. It is commoner in females. The fistulae are not functionally significant unless their total area exceeds 0·75 sq. cm. They may be single or multiple and situated high, low, or central on the atrial partition. They may be 4 cm. or more in diameter with a gap of 20 sq. cm.; in fact a common auricular chamber may exist. The effect is to produce a shunt from left to right. No cyanosis exists as the blood shunted has been through the lungs. The amount of blood so diverted may amount to many litres a minute. Thus much more blood flows through the right side of the heart than through the left. As long as the resistance in the pulmonary circuit does not rise appreciably, the pressures in the right side of the heart and the pulmonary artery are normal or nearly so. When this resistance becomes considerable there is damming back of blood, pressures in the auricles become equalized and there ultimately occurs a reversal of flow in the shunt leading to eventual death. In some of these cases the shunt may be closed by operation.

Congenital Pulmonary Stenosis: In the second month of fetal life the bulbus cordis—the original fourth chamber of the developing heart—becomes incorporated into the third or ventricular chamber, thus becoming the infundibulum of the right ventricle. Keith[1] says that the importance of recognizing the bulbus cordis as a separate constituent of the heart wall lies in the fact that 95 per cent of congenital malformations of the heart are the result of its imperfect transformation to form the infundibulum of the right ventricle. In nearly every case of congenital stenosis of the pulmonary orifice there is a cavity of variable size under the malformed valves—the remains of the bulbus cordis.

In half the cases the pulmonary stenosis is the only cardiac abnormality, i.e., the 'pure type'. The remaining cases are associated with other defects such as interauricular or interventricular septal defects.

Several anatomical types occur. Fortunately from the surgical viewpoint the commonest type is a defective pulmonary valve—the cusps not being separate but represented by a dome-shaped structure with a small hole in the centre. The obstruction may be in the valve ring or in the infundibulum. In the latter case there may be a shelf-like structure at varying distances below the valve, or the infundibulum may be funnel-shaped or a diaphragm may partly block it. There is usually an infundibular chamber of varying size between the shelf and the valve (bulbus cordis). The valvular and infundibular types may coexist. The pulmonary vessels are usually smaller than normal and the blood-pressure in them is subnormal. The right ventricle responds to the increased work load by hypertrophy and ultimately by dilatation.

[1] Keith, A., *Human Embryology and Morphology*, 5th ed., 1933, 368. London: Arnold.

508 A SYNOPSIS OF SURGICAL ANATOMY

These conditions can in many cases be bettered by surgery as pioneered and carried out by Brock.

Tetralogy of Fallot: This is the commonest cause of the cyanotic states due to cardiac abnormalities. It forms 75 per cent of all cases of cyanotic congenital heart disease. The conditions embraced by the title are:

1. Pulmonary stenosis.
2. Overriding of the aorta.
3. An interventricular septal defect.
4. Hypertrophy of the right ventricle.

There is always some dextro-position of the aorta, which comes to override the defect in the upper part of the interventricular septum, thus communicating with both ventricles. Though Fallot's description dates from 1888, it was not until 1947 that Taussig's[1] brilliant interpretation of the pathological physiology of the condition rendered possible remedial measures such as the Taussig–Blalock shunt. The

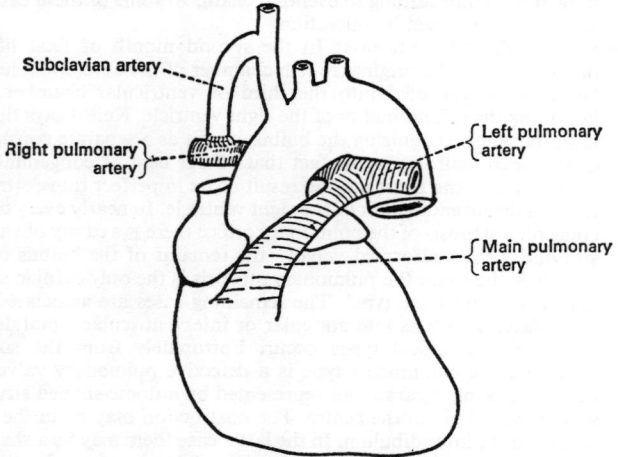

Fig. 496.—The Blalock operation for 'blue babies'.

cyanotic state is due to (*a*) the mixture of arterial and venous blood carried to the lungs by the aorta which overrides both ventricles, and to (*b*) insufficient blood entering the lungs because of the pulmonary stenosis, the latter usually being of the infundibular type. The pulmonary artery and its branches are smaller than normal and may be too small

[1] Taussig, H. B., *J. thorac. Surg.*, 1947, 16, 241.

to carry a shunt. There may be associated defects such as interauricular septal defects, patent ductus, etc.

As a result of obstruction the right ventricle hypertrophies and may ultimately be thicker than the left. In course of time, as Gross[1] points out, collateral pathways develop to take more blood to the lungs. These are:
1. The bronchial vessels through their numerous communications with the pulmonary arteries.
2. Small subpleural vessels which occur in great numbers round the hila of the lungs.
3. Systemic vessels grow into the lungs across the bridge supplied when the lung becomes adherent to the chest wall.

The Taussig–Blalock or Pott's operations are based on the principle of getting more oxygen into the blood by diverting some of the impure aortic output into the lungs by shunts of varying kinds, such as direct anastomosis of the aorta to the pulmonary artery, or turning down the subclavian artery and anastomosing it to the left pulmonary artery (*Fig.* 496). The results are admirable, but should anything happen to occlude the shunt, the patient's end-condition is worse than before operation; furthermore the patent septum is always a potential danger because of emboli from the right side of the heart passing straight through into the systemic circulation causing brain abscess. Thus these operations do nothing to relieve the basic pathology. The procedure now finding favour conforms to surgical principle by relieving the obstruction and closing the fistula. Open heart surgery makes this possible in many cases.

Acquired Cardiac Defects: Brock[2] points out that obstruction at the mitral valve can be surgically relieved in 70 per cent of cases. In properly selected ones the mortality is less than 5 per cent. He stresses the fact that the left ventricle is the most important muscular organ in the body, and that in aortic stenosis the pressure in the ventricle (determined by percutaneous puncture) may be 300 mm. Hg whilst that in the brachial artery is normal. The obstruction admits of relief in cases where it is indicated.

ACCESS TO THE CHEST: Discussing standard exposures to the thorax, Brock condemns trapdoor incisions or the sacrifice of a healthy rib. Wide exposure is obtained—the patient lying on the opposite side—by an inframammary incision along the whole length of the 5th rib, cutting across latissimus, separating the serratus anterior from the bone, retracting the scapula forwards, separating the periosteum from its lower border, and opening the

---
[1] Gross, R. E., *The Surgery of Infancy and Childhood*, 1953, 886. Philadelphia and London: Saunders.

[2] Brock, R. C., '75th Bradshaw Lecture. The Present Position of Cardiac Surgery', *Ann. R. Coll. Surg.*, 1958, Vol. 23(4), 213.

chest through the rib bed. For operations on the heart the patient lies supine and an inframammary incision is made along the 4th rib on one or both sides depending on the exposure required. The sternum is divided transversely or by the step method, e.g., the chest is opened through the 3rd rib bed on one side and the 4th on the other. The incisions give good exposure and do not cause deformity or disability (*Fig.* 497). Should wider mediastinal exposure be required the total midline vertical division of the sternum advised by Milian may be used.

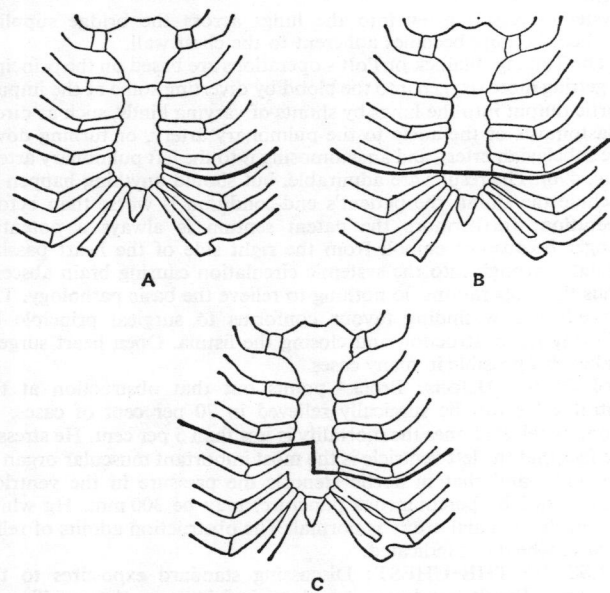

Fig. 497.—Incisions giving access to the heart. A, Incision for dealing with cardiac arrest. B, Incision in the fourth intercostal spaces dividing the sternum. C, Step cut incision.

2. Congenital Anomalies of the Great Vessels

The embryological events which result in anomalies of the arch of the aorta and its great vessels occur at the end of the branchial stage of development of the central vascular system (6th week). The diagram (*Fig.* 498) shows the aortic sac, the ventral and dorsal aortae, and five of the original six aortic arches, the fifth being short-lived. The fourth arches, so important in the development of the future arch of the aorta, are shown black in the figure. The pulmonary arteries develop from the sixth pair of arches. The paired dorsal aortae have completed the aortic vascular ring below by fusing to form the descending aorta at about the level of the eighth to ninth segments. From the paired dorsal aortae and the descending aorta arise intersegmental arteries destined for the supply of the cord and developing somites. Many of these vessels disappear in whole or in part. The third to eighth arise from the paired dorsal aortae. The first aortic intercostal artery is the intersegmental artery of the tenth segment.

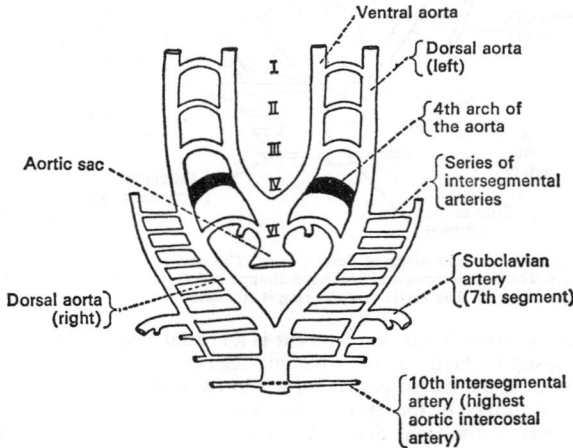

Fig. 498.—The aortic arch complex of the human embryo, after a modification of Rathke's original schema (1858). Because of their significance the fourth aortic arches are shown in black. (*This and the succeeding diagrams of aortic arch anomalies are used by courtesy of Barry and the Editor of the 'Anatomical Record', re-drawn and modified by Thomas.*)

Fig. 499 is a diagrammatic representation of a later stage of development, the paired dorsal aortae still forming a vascular ring. The first, second, and fifth arches have disappeared as have many of the segmental arteries.

The normality or otherwise of the final stage of development (8th week) of the aortic arch system depends largely on the fate of the eighth segment of the right paired dorsal aorta.

In the description of aortic arch anomalies the writer has been guided by Barry.[1]

[1] Barry, A., *Anat. Rec.*, 1951, 111, 221.

512 A SYNOPSIS OF SURGICAL ANATOMY

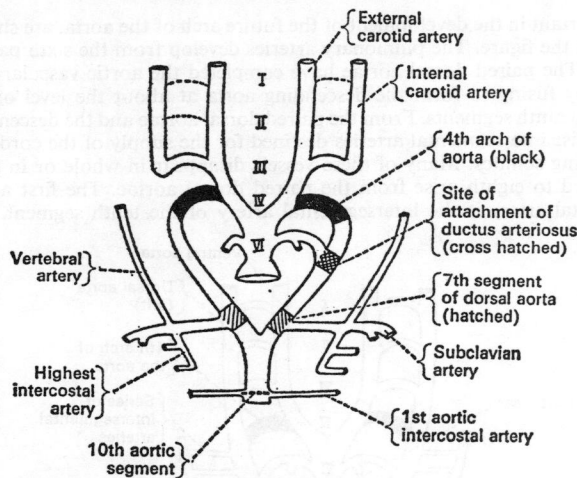

Fig. 499.—A later stage of development. The aortic arches are shown by numbers. The first, second, and fifth have disappeared as have many of the intersegmental arteries. The aortic vascular ring is still complete.

Subclavian Arteries: Their development is a crucial embryological factor. The vessel to the limb bud is the intersegmental artery of the seventh segment of the paired dorsal aorta. On the right side the subclavian artery is formed by the right fourth aortic arch, the third to the seventh segments of the right dorsal aorta together with the right seventh intersegmental artery. Several factors combine to enable the subclavian to attain its final position. One of these is the disappearance of the eighth segment of the right dorsal aorta. The vascular ring is broken (*Fig.* 500). On the left side the subclavian artery is formed entirely by the intersegmental artery of the seventh segment of the left dorsal aorta.

ABERRANT RIGHT SUBCLAVIAN ARTERY: Occasionally the right subclavian arises from the right eighth intersegmental artery. It thus comes about that when the development of the aortic arch system is complete this aberrant vessel is the last branch of the arch of the aorta and must extend to the right to reach the right upper limb. What has occurred is that, though the seventh intersegmental artery of the right dorsal aorta assists the anomalous eighth to form the subclavian, the vascular ring must be broken to enable the aberrant vessel to attain its final situation on the arch. The arc of the ring which regresses is some part or all of that section of it

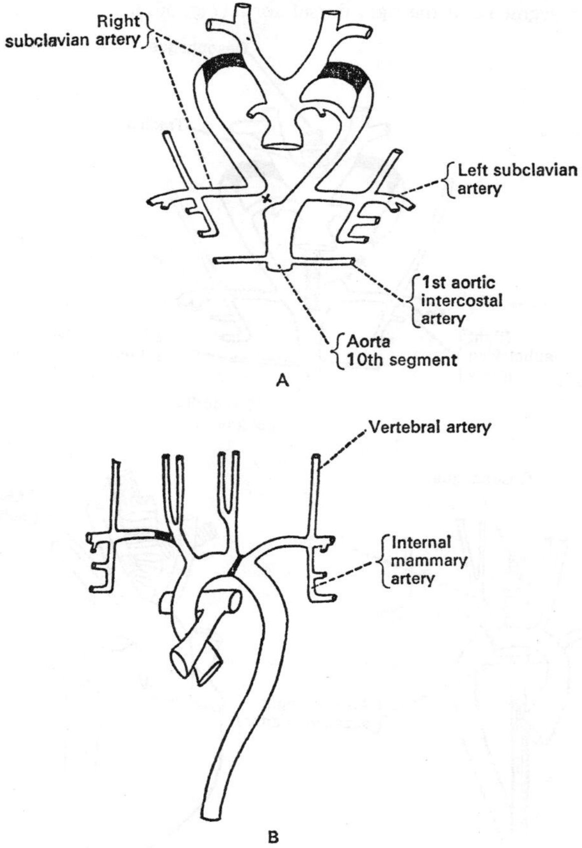

Fig. 500.—A, The diagram shows that the eighth segment of the right dorsal aorta has degenerated (X) breaking the vascular ring. Note that the right subclavian artery is formed by the right aortic arch, the third to the seventh segments of the right dorsal aorta, and the seventh intersegmental artery, whereas the left subclavian artery is formed by the left seventh intersegmental artery only. The fourth aortic arch is black. B, The development of the subclavian arteries is complete. The fourth aortic arch is black.

formed by the right fourth aortic arch and the third to the seventh segments of the right dorsal aorta (*Fig.* 501).

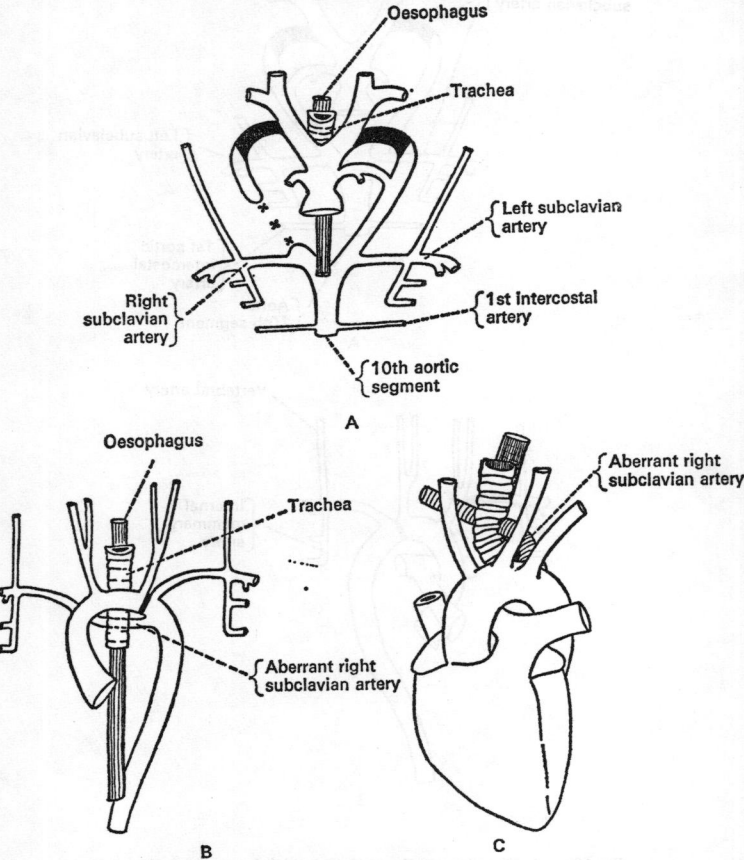

Fig. 501.—Aberrant right subclavian artery. A, The eighth segment of the right dorsal aorta has persisted. The vascular ring is broken higher up (XXX). The right subclavian artery is the last branch of the permanent arch of the aorta. The primitive fourth arches of the aorta are shown in black. B, Final position of aberrant right subclavian artery. C, Aberrant right subclavian artery from an actual case.

DYSPHAGIA LUSORIA (Bayford, 1761): *Lusus naturae* implies a freak of nature. This condition may result from the presence of an aberrant right subclavian artery. In the fully developed state this artery must cross the midline to get to the right side of the neck. It usually passes (*a*) behind the oesophagus in 85 per cent, but may (*b*) go between it and the trachea or (*c*) in front of both. On X-ray the oesophagus is seen to be indented at the level of the 3rd or 4th thoracic vertebra.

The condition does not always cause symptoms. When it does the child swallows slowly and with difficulty and perhaps has pain. The symptoms are relieved by dividing the aberrant vessel. Modern surgical treatment was initiated by the brilliant report of Gross.[1]

Aortic Arch: The innominate artery arises from the right horn of the aortic sac (the dilatation of the cephalic part of the truncus arteriosus). The ascending aorta develops from the truncus. The part of the arch of the

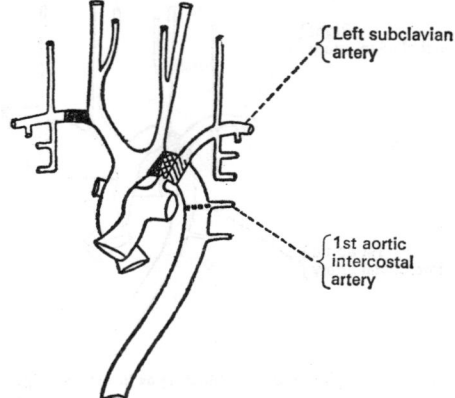

Fig. 502.—The component parts of the arch of the aorta distal to the origin of the left common carotid. Black, fourth aortic arch. Cross-hatched, third to sixth segments of left dorsal aorta. Hatched, seventh segment of left dorsal aorta. From there to the dotted line across the aorta (tenth segment) the arch is formed by the eighth and ninth segments of the left dorsal aorta.

aorta between the innominate artery and the left common carotid derives from the left horn of the aortic sac. The small part of the arch between the left common carotid and subclavian is made up partly by the left fourth aortic arch, and partly by the third to the seventh segments of the left dorsal aorta. The eighth to the tenth segments of

[1] Gross, R. E., *New Engl. J. Med.*, 1945, 233, 586.

the left dorsal aorta complete the formation of the aorta up to the junction of the paired dorsal aortae to form the descending aorta. It is apparent from the foregoing that though the fourth aortic arch participates in the formation of the arch of the aorta, it contributes but a small part of it (*Fig.* 502).

ANOMALIES OF THE AORTIC ARCH SYSTEM:

RIGHT AORTIC ARCH: In birds it is the right half of the aortic vascular ring which persists. This may occur in human beings. This right aortic arch may connect with the descending aorta on the left or continue on the right throughout its entire length. The three large branches of the arch are the mirror image of the normal—they are the left innominate, the right common carotid, and the right subclavian. The circulation is not basically altered by the condition and there is no extra strain on the heart. It coexists with the tetralogy of Fallot in 20 per cent of cases (*Fig.* 503).

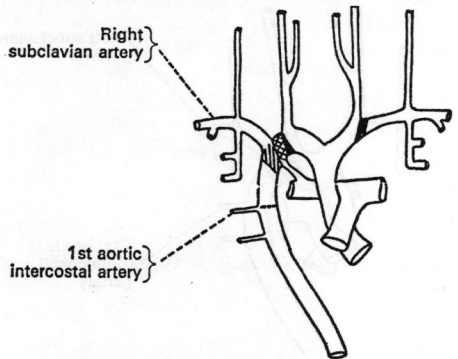

Fig. 503.—Right aortic arch. Shading as in previous figure.

CERVICAL AORTIC ARCH: This is a rare developmental anomaly which is important because the arch of the aorta lies well up in the right side of the neck and may be mistaken for aneurysm of the right common carotid artery. It is distinguished from the latter by the fact that it is present in infancy. Furthermore, if such an arch is compressed (a procedure that may be necessary for diagnosis during operation), the femoral pulses will be obliterated, which will not be the case in aneurysm of the common carotid. Its causation is undecided. Harley[1] mentions two possibilities: (*a*) the heart has failed to descend, or (*b*) the arch (being on the

[1] Harley, H. R. S., *Br. J. Surg.*, 1959, **46**, 200.

RELATIONSHIPS OF VASCULAR PATTERN 517

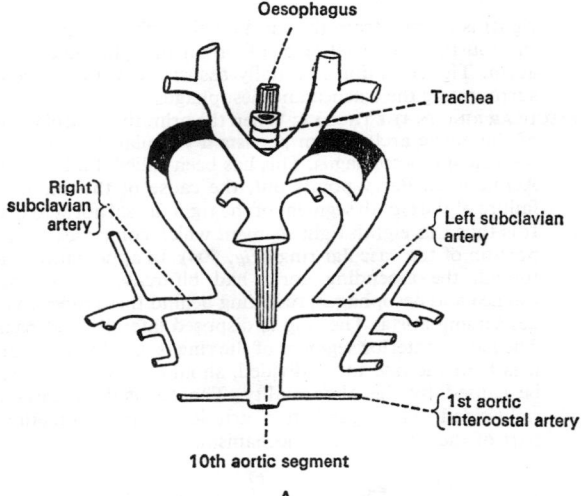
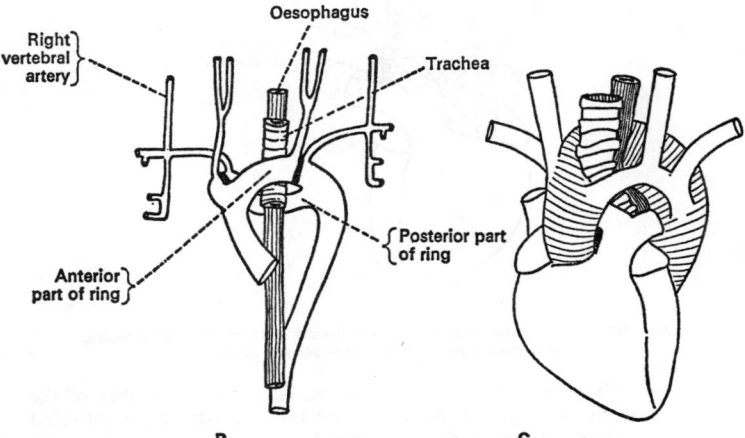

Fig. 504.—Persistence of the vascular ring in the thorax. A, The primitive vascular ring. B, Persistence of the vascular ring—so-called 'double aortic arch'. The ring embraces oesophagus and trachea. C, The vascular ring in an actual case.

right) is formed from the third aortic arch and not from part of the fourth—the usual level of origin in right-sided arch of the aorta. The condition is usually associated with a vascular ring surrounding the trachea and oesophagus.

VASCULAR RING IN THE THORAX: When the primitive vascular symmetry of the aortic arch system persists a vascular ring surrounds the trachea and oesophagus. This has been called double aortic arch. Actually, as Barry points out, the cause of the anomaly is the failure of the eighth segment of the right dorsal aorta to disappear. It is thus this eighth right segment which comprises the posterior portion of the vascular ring (*Fig.* 504). In appearance it looks as though the ascending aorta had bifurcated to surround the trachea and oesophagus, reuniting behind these tubes to form the descending aorta. The ring is disposed laterally and backwards. The left or anterior segment of the ring is usually the smaller, and it is then the one to be divided, should compression symptoms be caused by the abnormality. The descending aorta may be right-sided. The ligamentum arteriosum may sometimes be a part of the compressing mechanism.

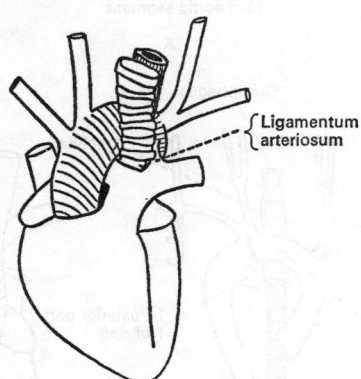

Fig. 505.—The ligamentum arteriosum forms part of the compressing mechanism on trachea or oesophagus or both.

There are numerous possible variations of anomalies of the aortic arch system. An important one consists of a right-sided arch of the aorta with a left ligamentum arteriosum. This happens when the right fourth aortic arch forms the arch of the aorta (the left aortic arch precursors regressing). Such a vessel passes down on the right of the trachea and oesophagus. The ligamentum arteriosum connects the pulmonary artery with the upper part of the descending aorta. If this ligament is in front of and to the right of the trachea all is well. More often it passes to the left of the trachea and round the oesophagus. Thus a ring is completed embracing trachea and oesophagus. There may be room for these structures or serious compression symptoms may arise. In infants extreme tracheal obstruction and consequent lung infection may be fatal within a year or two of birth. In adults dysphagia is the commoner symptom (*Fig.* 505). The obstruction is relieved by dividing the ligamentum arteriosum.

Part of the arch of the aorta may be absent. This is a rarity, but may be compatible with life. It is usually associated with patency of the ductus arteriosus and of the interauricular septum.

Other anomalies occur affecting the innominate or the left common carotid artery. If the innominate is more to the left than usual, or the left common carotid is more to the right, the trachea may be compressed. Gross treats these cases by dislocating the offending vessel forward and fixing it to the sternum, thus liberating the trachea.

DUCTUS ARTERIOSUS: Reference to *Fig.* 499 shows that the ductus arteriosus represents the distal portion of the sixth left aortic arch. At birth it is about 1·25 cm. in length and about the diameter of a

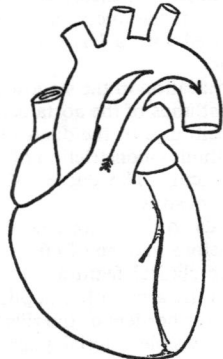

Fig. 506.—Patent ductus arteriosus.

goose quill. In early fetal life it forms the continuation of the pulmonary artery, and opens into the aorta just beyond the origin of the left subclavian artery. It conducts most of the blood from the right ventricle into the aorta. With the enlargement of the branches of the pulmonary artery, the ductus becomes chiefly connected to the left pulmonary artery. It is completely closed functionally between the fourth to tenth days. The closure is not organically complete until the end of the second month. It becomes the ligamentum arteriosum which connects the left pulmonary artery to the arch of the aorta (*Fig.* 505).

PATENT DUCTUS ARTERIOSUS: The ductus arteriosus may remain patent. Though this may be, it is not usually, associated with other cardiac defects. It occurs much more commonly in girls (70 per cent) than in boys. The condition is similar to an arteriovenous fistula. This shunt produces little if any evidence of cardiac embarrassment, but the patient is exposed to the risks of retarded development, overwork of the heart, and bacterial infection. Gross,[1] the pioneer in closure of the patent ductus, advises its surgical division in all cases. The mortality is under half per cent and the results of surgery are most satisfactory (*Fig.* 506).

COARCTATION OF THE AORTA: The condition occurs about once in 1500 post-mortems. Boys are affected twice as often as girls. Intracardiac abnormalities frequently coexist. Though this condition may affect any part of the aorta, 98 per cent of coarctations affect the first part of the descending aorta just beyond the arch. Whether the condition develops before or after birth is unknown, as is the cause. One theory is that the abnormality is due to hyper-involution of the ductus arteriosus, as the condition is sometimes associated with a large patent ductus. The theory is not always tenable.

There is much variation in the stenosis. There may be a diffuse narrowing of the isthmus of the aorta between the left subclavian and the point of entrance of the ductus arteriosus, or there may be a localized—isthmic—constriction of the aorta, just above the entrance of the ductus. The degree of narrowing varies from slight to complete obstruction.

Coarctation leads to disabling complications. Three-quarters of the cases die before the age of 40 (Abbott) (*Fig.* 507).

The outstanding clinical features of the condition are raised arterial pressure in the arm with a popliteal pressure below this, grooving of the lower borders of the ribs by enlarging intercostal arteries, and often visible arterial pulsation on the back. It is therefore necessary to determine the popliteal blood-pressure in all cases of hypertension lest coarctation of the aorta be overlooked.

---

[1] Gross, R. E., *The Surgery of Infancy and Childhood*, 1953, 806. Philadelphia and London: Saunders.

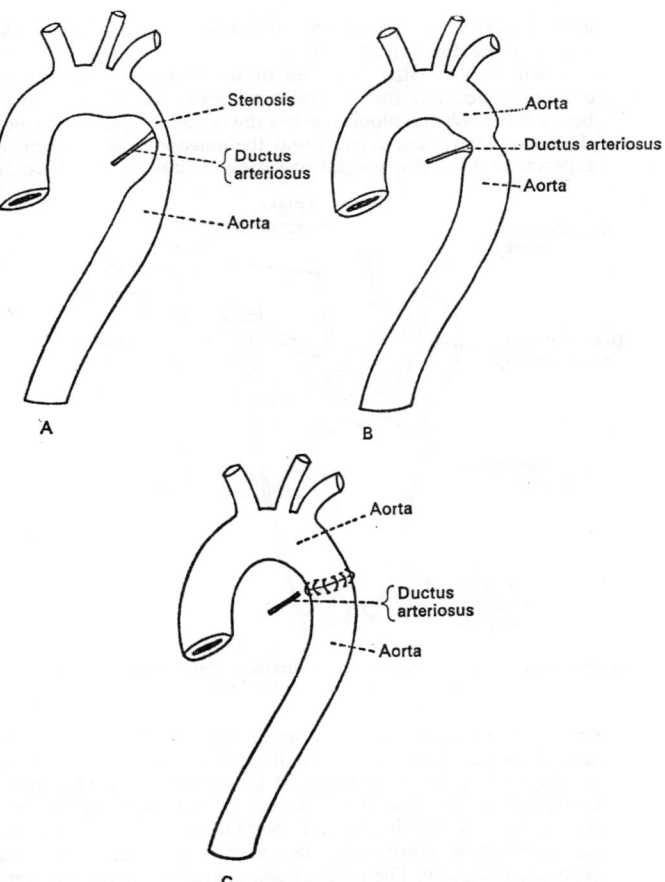

Fig. 507.—A, Infantile type of coarctation. B, Adult type of coarctation. C, The stenosed area has been excised and an end-to-end union performed.

COLLATERAL CIRCULATION: Maude Abbott[1] points out that in the isthmic type of coarctation the vascular changes only occur in the vicinity of the narrowing itself, and that from the mid-thoracic

[1]Abbott, M. E., *Am. Heart J.*, 1928, 3, 574.

aorta onwards the circulatory pattern is preserved. This is well shown in the diagram (*Fig.* 508).

It will be seen that branches of the subclavian arteries are entirely responsible for the collateral above the block, whereas below the block the blood reaches the descending aorta through the aortic intercostal arteries and the anastomoses between the superior and inferior epigastric vessels. Clinically this becomes

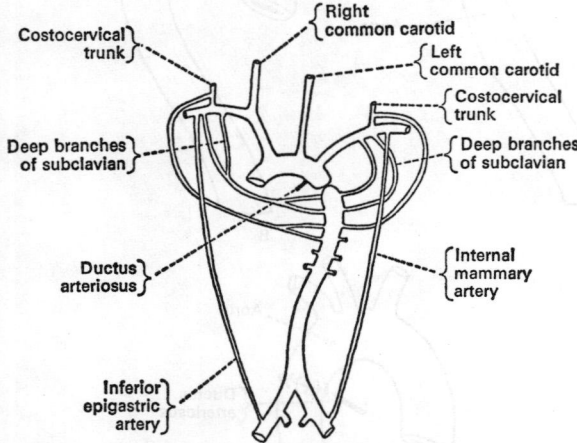

Fig. 508.—The collateral circulation in coarctation of the aorta. (*Re-drawn from Taussig who gives credit to King.*[1])

evident in teen ages or later. Pulsation may be seen and felt above and below the clavicles, in the axillae, in the anterior intercostal spaces, and in the epigastrium. It is specially noticeable in the upper half of the back. It is best seen in spare subjects but these signs may be absent in cases of coarctation. Vessels such as the intercostals are enormously distended and tortuous. Surgical exposure is bloody. The anterior spinal artery (tractus anterior), which is in the circuit of the collateral, may be so enlarged as to produce pressure on the spinal cord.

Many authorities (Crafoord, Gross) believe that most cases of coarctation should be operated on, chiefly to relieve the hypertension. Excision of the stenosed segment and reconstruction of the aorta, with or without grafting, can be carried out with a

[1] King, J. T. jun., *Archs intern. Med.*, 1926, 38, 69.

small mortality and a complete cure of the hypertension in the great majority of cases.

Congenital anomalies may affect any of the four valves of the heart. The number or size of the cusps may vary and may result in incompetence, stenosis, or even atresia. Dextrocardia—in which the heart lies on the right side and the apex points to the right—is the result of primary reversal of the primitive cardiac loop. The heart and large vessels are reversed as in a mirror image. Dextrocardia may affect the heart only or be one feature of total transposition of the viscera, i.e., situs inversus.

III. THE BLOOD-VESSELS OF THE LIVER

The writer wishes to express his indebtedness in preparing this section to Child.[1]

The vessels serving the liver may be divided into:

1. Vessels at the lower hilum.
2. Vascular arrangements in the liver.
3. Vessels at the upper hilum.
4. Collateral arrangements of the liver.

1. **Vessels at the Lower Hilum:** These are the portal vein and hepatic artery.

   THE PORTAL VEIN is formed in front of the head and behind the neck of the pancreas by the union of the superior mesenteric and splenic veins. This union occurs at the level of the 2nd lumbar vertebra. The vessel is 5–7·5 cm. long and passes up and to the right in the gastrohepatic (lesser) omentum, to enter the hilum of the liver, where it immediately divides into its right and left branches. Its main tributaries are the coronary (left gastric), pyloric, cystic, and pancreaticoduodenal veins. It carries 75 per cent of the blood entering the liver.

   VARIATIONS (Child): In contrast to the hepatic artery, the portal vein is singularly free of anomalies. Such as do occur are rare but of surgical importance: (*a*) The portal vein may empty directly into the inferior vena cava; (*b*) The vein, its formative vessels and tributaries, may lie anterior to the pancreas and duodenum; (*c*) The pulmonary veins join the portal; (*d*) Congenital stricture of the vein may occur (*Fig.* 509).

   Comment:

   In the early embryo the vitelline veins anastomose together across the ventral and dorsal sides of the developing duodenum. The ventral part of this venous plexus usually disappears, the dorsal section forming the portal vein.

---

[1] Child, C. G., *The Hepatic Circulation and Portal Hypertension*, 1954. Philadelphia and London: Saunders.

524 A SYNOPSIS OF SURGICAL ANATOMY

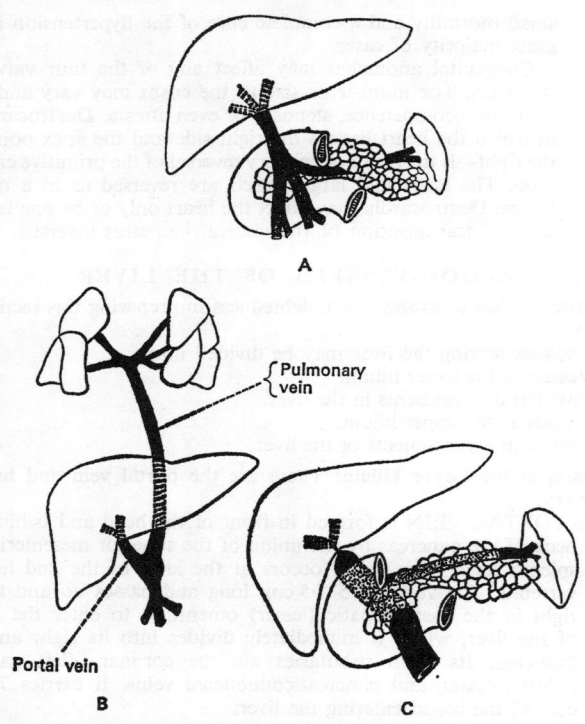

Fig. 509.—Anomalies of the portal vein. A, The vein and its tributaries lie anterior to the duodenum. B, The pulmonary vein joins the portal. C, Congenital stricture of the portal vein. (*By courtesy of Child.*)

If these conditions are reversed a preduodenal portal vein results. Several cases have been described where duodenal obstruction occurred because of this malposition.

THE HEPATIC ARTERY: This vessel first pursues a horizontal course and then bends sharply at right-angles to run upwards in the lesser omentum to the left of the bile-duct. It has been compared to the bend on a badly driven nail (*Fig.* 510).

The frequent variations of the vessel or its branches are in sharp contrast to the stable anatomy of the portal vein. In over 90 per cent of cases this vessel arises from the coeliac axis.

RELATIONSHIPS OF VASCULAR PATTERN

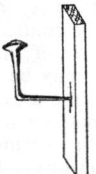

Fig. 510.—The course of the hepatic artery represented by a badly driven nail.

It may come from the superior mesenteric or from the aorta directly. The vessel divides near the liver into right and left branches which supply the respective lobes. One or other of these vessels may arise anomalously, e.g., from superior mesenteric, aorta, or left gastric. Such vessels may have unusual relationships in the right free border of the lesser omentum and present hazards in cholecystectomy (p. 82). Accessory right or left hepatic arteries may occur. In ligature of the left gastric artery in gastrectomy it is wise to look for a large vessel which this artery sometimes supplies to the liver. This may be an accessory left hepatic artery, alternatively it may be the only artery of supply to the left lobe.

The common hepatic artery gives off the gastroduodenal, right gastric, and cystic arteries. It is occasionally the site of aneurysm. Should this condition affect the vessel before the origin of the gastroduodenal branch, proximal ligature of the common hepatic would not injure the liver as an efficient collateral would build up

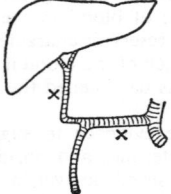

Fig. 511.—Ligature of the common hepatic artery at the top X would cut off the blood-supply of the liver. Interruption of the vessel at the other X would not endanger the liver which would be protected by the collateral supply through the gastroduodenal artery, etc.

through the gastroduodenal and right gastric arteries. Should the aneurysm arise in the distal part of the hepatic then proximal ligature would cut off the blood-supply to the liver (*Fig.* 511).

Pringle's manœuvre: The vessels in the free border of the lesser omentum may be controlled by compression between the thumb and index finger of the left hand. The measure is an emergency one which may be useful in cases of injury to one of the large vessels in the area. It is safe for 30 minutes if the blood-pressure is normal, but in the presence of shock the pressure should be released each 15 minutes.

2. **Vascular Arrangements in the Liver:** The vasculature of the liver is so complex that Mann stated that the story of the circulation of the liver is buried under its own literature.

The capacity of the hepatic system of veins is twice that of the portal veins, whilst the latter system is more voluminous than the hepatic arteries and bile-ducts. The portal venous system is unique in that it begins and ends in capillaries. The liver may be visualized as a mass of blood in which innumerable plates of liver cells are suspended, each being a single cell in thickness. The central veins are the terminal collecting tubules of the hepatic veins. Each may be looked on as the axis of a hepatic unit, which, though poorly demarcated, is called the lobule. The central vein receives the blood from the sinusoids. These cavities are larger than capillaries and communicate through innumerable interstices with neighbouring sinusoids. They also pour blood directly into larger branches of the hepatic veins. The portal radicle communicates with the sinusoid only at its tip. The hepatic artery supplies nourishment to the portal spaces. It also communicates with the smaller branches of the portal vein and with the sinusoids. All the blood-vessels to, from, and in the liver are devoid of valves. There is evidence to suggest that the terminal veins of the venous system of the liver have elaborate sphincteric mechanisms which are under drug, hormonal, and nervous control. Therefore the volume of blood in the liver may be regulated. The organ is thus a blood reservoir characterized by such intermittence of its circulation that much of the blood it contains may be momentarily inactive. In fact Gross has likened the liver to a sponge of blood.

Comment:

1. There is little evidence to suggest that the normal shunts between hepatic arterioles and portal venules become sufficiently opened up in cirrhosis of the liver to constitute an important factor in portal hypertension. The rationale for ligature of the hepatic artery is thus invalid.

2. Portal obstruction and its surgical relief are dealt with on p. 528.

3. **Vessels at the Upper Hilum:** Rodney Smith has applied this apt term to the site on the upper surface of the liver where the hepatic veins emerge. These vessels consist of the right and left hepatic veins, the former being the larger. There is also a middle hepatic vein, variable

in size, which sometimes joins one of the larger veins. It is important as it drains a strip of both right and left lobes of the liver.

In addition there are inconstant smaller veins which may enter the vena cava anywhere in its post-hepatic course.

The hepatic veins are almost sessile where they enter the vena cava. They are large and dangerous structures to deal with in partial hepatectomy. So much is this the case that it has been advised that they be secured in the liver by dissection to expose them.

The hepatic veins are rarely anomalous. In azygos continuation of the inferior vena cava, the hepatic veins may enter the right auricle directly.

OUTFLOW BLOCK: Obstruction to the venous drainage from the liver is seen in conditions such as thrombophlebitis, pressure from tumours, or portal hypertension. This is the cause of ascites, the composition of which is approximately the same as that of liver lymph.

4. **Collateral Arrangements of the Liver**: Obstruction of the portal vein is dealt with on p. 528, and of the hepatic artery on p. 558.

HEMI-HEPATECTOMY: The right or left halves of the liver may be removed for certain tumours, e.g., various types of hepatoma. After the skin the liver is the commonest site of haemangioma. The operation is rendered feasible by two facts. The first is that embryologically and functionally the liver is divisible into two portions of approximately equal weight. The line of division (the principal plane of Rex—1888) runs from the inferior vena cava to the tip of the gall-bladder, passing obliquely across the surface of the liver about 2·5 cm. to the right of the falciform ligament. This division leaves the quadrate and half of the caudate lobe as part of the left half of the liver. Each half has its own artery, vein, and bile-duct. The small branches of the arteries and veins of the two sides do not communicate at any point (though Legall did describe a small arteriolar anastomosis across the plane in 1923). The one-time idea that there were two portal streams in the liver has been abandoned. The other reason rendering hemi-hepatectomy possible is that three-quarter removal of the organ is compatible with normal life (*Fig.* 512)—a remarkable observation by virtue of the fact that the liver is responsible for at least 250 known physiochemical processes.[1] The human liver is sterile, therefore the problem of infection does not arise.

Whereas the left lobe may be removed through a vertical abdominal incision, with possible removal of the xiphisternum, removal of the right lobe requires a thoraco-abdominal exposure, extending the whole length of the 8th intercostal space to the umbilicus. The diaphragm is divided up to the vena cava. The liver is rotated into the thorax and the right hepatic artery, right branch of the portal

---

[1] Pack, G. T., and Molander, D. W., *Archs Surg.*, 1960, 80, 685.

vein, and right hepatic duct are secured and divided. The peritoneal attachments of the liver are cut. Finally the right hepatic vein is severed. The liver is sectioned with a blunt instrument, such as the handle of a knife, and vessels tied as they are exposed.

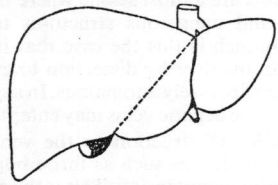

Fig. 512.—The right and left lobes of the liver are divided into separate functional units by the dotted line.

Two years after removal of the right lobe of the liver the organ was found to be fully as large as a normal intact liver. This is a true compensatory regenerative hyperplasia.[1]

PORTAL OBSTRUCTION:[2] Herrick showed that in the normal liver rise of portal pressure was 1 mm. for every 40 mm. of pressure in the hepatic artery, but in the cirrhotic liver the portal pressure rose to 1 mm. for every 6 mm. of arterial pressure. The portal system lies between two capillary beds. The portal vein carries three-quarters of the blood entering the liver. The normal portal pressure (11–15 cm. water) is higher than the systemic venous pressure (about zero) because portal blood must be forced through the second capillary bed—the liver sinusoids. The venous hypertension which characterizes cirrhosis of the liver is largely due to obstruction of the hepatic venous radicles. They are less protected than those of the portal system and are compressed by regenerating nodules of liver tissue and fibrosis. It is this post-sinusoidal compression also which is such an important factor in the development of ascites. Other factors causing portal hypertension are (*a*) the great increase in calibre of communications between portal and hepatic veins which now become venous shunts, and (*b*) the formation of arteriovenous shunts between portal radicles and hepatic arterioles consequent on great development of normal small intercommunications.

Patients with portal block are divisible into (1) those with intrahepatic block and (2) those with extrahepatic block. In the first group fall the cirrhoses. In the second group are:

[1] Islami, A. H., Pack, G. T., Schwartz, M. K., and Smith, E. R., *Ann. Surg.,* 1959, **150,** 90.

[2] In the preparation of this subsection tribute is paid to the article by A. O. Whipple, published as the E. Starr Judd lecture, *Ibid.,* 1945, **122,** 449.

a. Fibrotic processes:
  i. An extension into the portal vein of the fibrotic process which takes place at birth in the umbilical vein and the ductus venosus as they empty into the left portal vein.
  ii. Thrombosis of the portal vein or a main tributary by trauma, inflammation, or outside pressure.
b. Cavernomatous transformations: The replacement of the portal vein or its formative vessels by a cavernomatous mass of small tortuous vessels of uncertain aetiology ascribed variously to canalization of an organized thrombus or neoplasia.

Collateral channels enlarge in the endeavour to by-pass the cirrhotic liver and carry the obstructed portal blood to the systemic circulation. These channels are the anastomoses normally existent between portal and systemic circulations and are usually quite inadequate to relieve the back-pressure (*see* p. 320). On the other hand, they add both to the hazards of the disease—witness oesophageal varices—and to the risks of surgery which is attended with severe and trying haemorrhage in operations for these conditions. Obstruction to the portal return, whether intra- or extrahepatic, produces enlargement of the spleen with the likelihood of attacks of severe haemorrhage such as that due to rupture of an oesophageal varix. If the obstruction is in the liver that organ will be cirrhotic, if the block is extrahepatic the liver will be normal. In intrahepatic obstruction the collateral circulation is taking blood from the obstructed liver into the systemic circulation. In extrahepatic portal obstruction, however, the blood is trying to circumvent the block and flow towards the liver. The channels are small, consisting of veins in the ligaments of the liver, venae comites of the portal vein and hepatic artery, and veins around the umbilicus which convey blood to the liver via the veins of the round ligament.

Diaphragmatic veins also take a share in the collateral. If the block is severe then blood may also be shunted away from the liver by the usual porto-systemic channels. It is noteworthy that the absence of valves in the portal system of veins enables blood to flow in either direction and the operation of shunting is based on this fact. Treatment for portal bed block has not been a successful field of medical enterprise and for many years surgeons have exercised ingenuity to combat the disease.

Blakemore and Lord[1] have thrown a strong ray of light on a dark corner by devising a practical method of diverting the portal into the systemic circulation—Eck fistula.

The idea is an old one but these workers rendered it practical by perfecting the technique for anastomosing the portal vein to the

---

[1] Blakemore, A. H., and Lord, J. W., jun., *J. Am. med. Ass.*, 1945, 127, No. 12, 685; *Ibid.*, 1945, No. 13, 748.

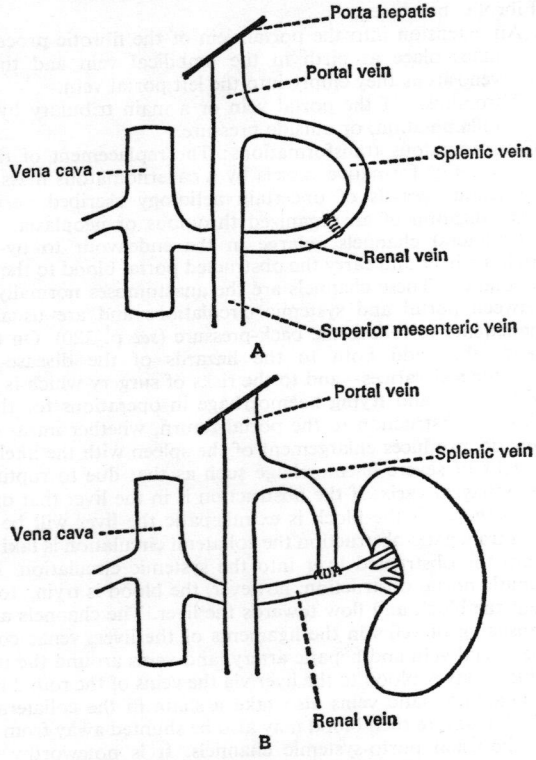

Fig. 513.—(For legend, see below)

inferior vena cava. The procedure is one requiring consummate skill, a trained team, and all the adjuncts of modern surgery, but it has established its place in therapy. Any large portal vessel may be joined to a large systemic vein. The splenic has been joined to the left renal end to end, necessitating removal of the spleen and kidney. The splenic has been joined to the renal end to side, preserving the kidney. The superior mesenteric, proximal end, has been implanted into the inferior vena cava. The portal vein, distal end, has been implanted into the inferior vena cava. This is the procedure of choice. The proximal end of the portal vein is ligatured (*Fig.* 513).

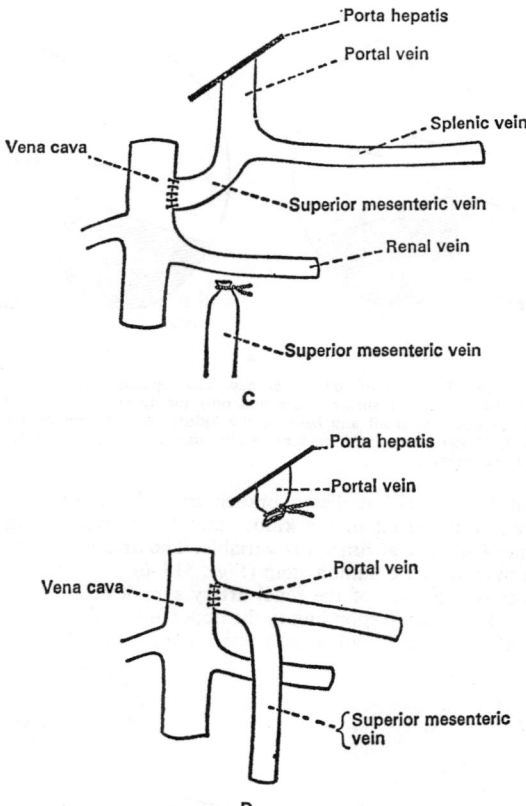

Fig. 513.—Types of portal shunts. The diagrams are explained in the text.

IV. A. BLOOD-SUPPLY OF THE KIDNEY

Graves[1] has demonstrated that the kidney has a segmental arterial supply with minor variations. He divides the organ into apical, upper, middle, lower, and posterior segments, of which only the first and last embrace both anterior and posterior portions of the kidney (*Fig.* 514). The renal artery divides into anterior and posterior divisions.

[1] Graves, F. T., *Br. J. Surg.*, 1954, 42, 132.

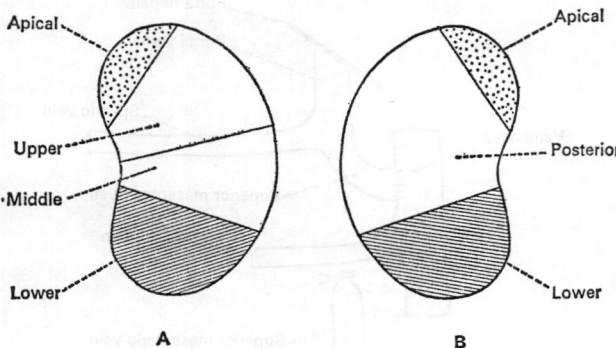

Fig. 514.—Diagram of the left kidney. The segments conforming to the arterial distribution are shown. Note that only the apical and lower segments appear on both the front and back of the kidney. A, Anterior aspect of left kidney. B, Posterior aspect of left kidney. (*By courtesy of Graves and the 'British Journal of Surgery'.*)

The anterior vessel supplies a branch to each of the four segments represented on the front of the kidney and are correspondingly named. The origin of the apical branch is variable. The arteries to two adjacent segments may have a common stem (*Figs.* 515–6).

The posterior branch of the renal artery supplies a large area on the back of the kidney corresponding to the upper and middle segments of the front of the viscus. It is called the posterior segment (*Fig.* 515 B).

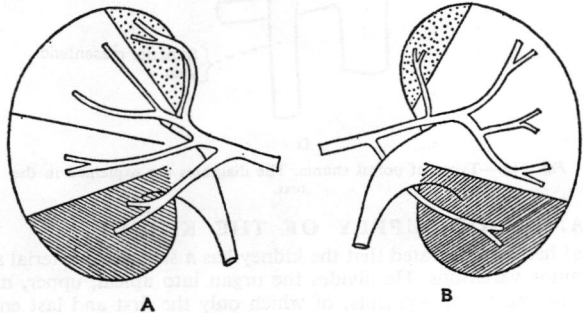

Fig. 515.—A diagram of the right kidney showing the arterial supply to the segments. A, Anterior view of right kidney. B, Posterior view of right kidney. (*By courtesy of Graves and the 'British Journal of Surgery'.*)

The fact that the major calices also have some constancy of pattern makes it possible to carry out segmental resections of the kidney. The blood-supply of the lower segment lends itself best to such a local resection, though the procedure is also carried out with other segments. Although there is no collateral circulation between the segments of the kidney there is free intercommunication of all veins.

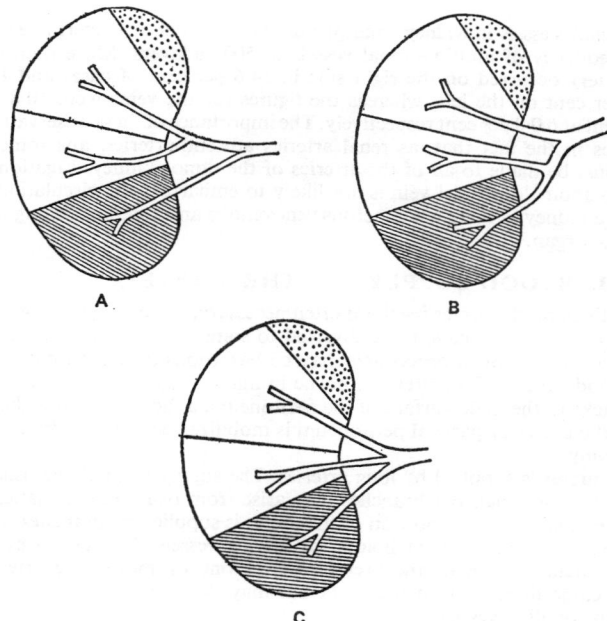

Fig. 516.—Diagram showing, in the right kidney, the variations of the upper, middle, and lower segment arteries from the anterior divisions of the renal artery. A, Type 1. B, Type 2. C, Type 3. (*By courtesy of Graves and the 'British Journal of Surgery'*.)

The blood-supply to the kidney is interrupted temporarily in operations such as anastomosis of the splenic to the renal artery beyond a stenosis which is causing hypertension. The safe length of time depends on the normality or otherwise of the kidney and should not exceed 30 min. (Poutasse).

ABERRANT RENAL ARTERIES: Graves[1] points out that aberrant renal arteries are not accessory vessels, as generally supposed, but are normal segmental arteries whose origin is more proximal than usual. This is an important observation, as division of a vessel of this kind will produce renal ischaemia in the same way as occurs when a segmental renal artery is tied. He ascribes the presence of such vessels to persistence of mesonephric arteries which normally disappear.

The Renal Vessels in Kidney Transplantation: Smith et al.[2] determined the frequency of multiple renal vessels in 500 cadavers. More than one artery occurred on the right side in 14·6 per cent of cases and 19·4 per cent on the left, whereas the figures for the veins were 10·8 per cent and 0·8 per cent respectively. The importance of these observations lies in the fact that, as renal arteries are end-arteries, anastomoses must be made to all of the arteries of the donor kidney. Ligation of an anomalous renal vein is not likely to embarrass the circulation of the kidney as there are generous venovenous anastomoses throughout the organ.

IV. B. BLOOD-SUPPLY OF THE URETER[3]

Operations on the ureter itself are often necessary. On other occasions the urinary stream may have to be diverted to some part of the bowel or to the skin surface. Such procedures may be hazardous unless the nature of the blood-supply of the ureter is borne in mind. This tube is 25 cm. long and sticks to the undersurface of the peritoneum, a fact to be remembered when the posterior parietal peritoneum is mobilized as in the operation of colectomy.

The ureter is supplied by long arteries. The supply from above usually comes via the renal, but branches may arise from ovarian, spermatic, or colic vessels. The pelvic portion of the ureter is supplied by branches from the vesical, middle haemorrhoidal, or uterine vessels. In most cases the intermediate portion of the ureter receives one or more long arteries. These come directly from the aorta but may derive from the testicular, ovarian, or iliac vessels.

These three sets of long vessels lie near the peritoneum and give branches to it. They divide into ascending and descending vessels which run in the adventitial covering of the ureter where they anastomose and form a plexus which sends fine twigs into the wall of the duct (*Fig.* 517). In 10 per cent of cases the intermediate portion of the ureter receives only minute twigs from peritoneal vessels. In 2 per cent of cases there are several long arteries

---

[1] Graves, F. T., *J. Anat.*, 1956, 90, 553.
[2] Smith, G. T., Calne, R. Y., Murray, J. E., and Dammin, G. T., *Surgery Gynec. Obstet.*, 1962, 115, 682.
[3] This account is based on the work of Daniel, O., and Shackman, R., *Br. J. Urol.*, 1952, 24, 334.

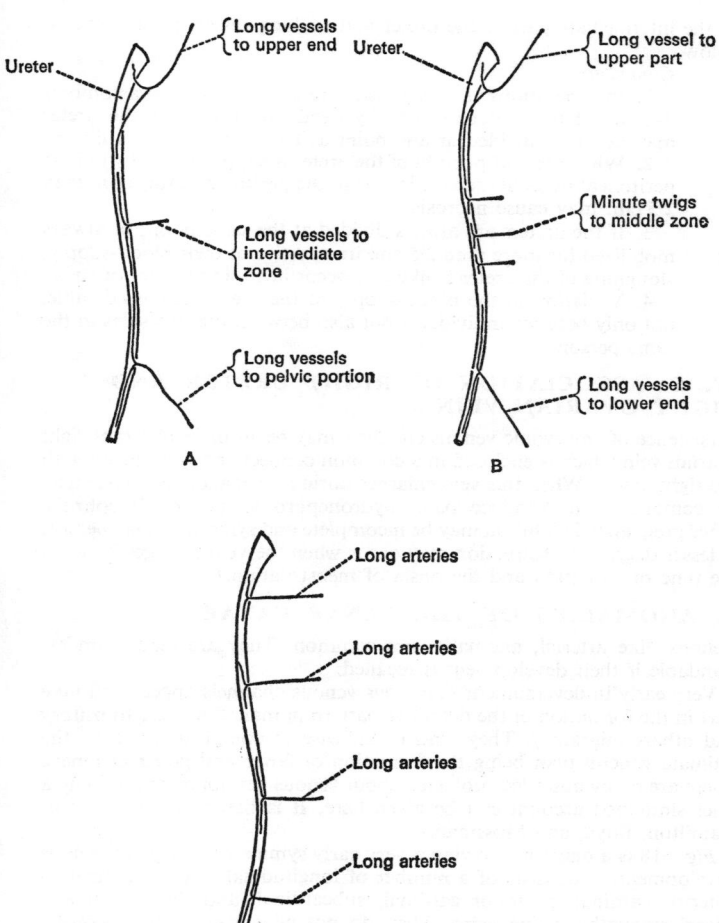

Fig. 517.—The blood-supply of the ureter. A, The usual type of vascularization by three sets of long vessels. B, The intermediate zone is supplied only by minute vascular twigs. C, The diagram shows several long arteries to the intermediate zone, but none from above or below. (*After Daniel and Shackman, 'British Journal of Urology'*.)

to the intermediate part of the ureter and no long vessels from above or below.

Comments:

1. In operations to establish uretero-intestinal anastomoses 5–6 cm. of the ureter are usually freed. In most cases the ureter may be safely divided at any point as the blood-supply is liberal.

2. When the mid-portion of the ureter is supplied only by minute peritoneal twigs, its separation from the peritoneum for more than 2·5 cm. may cause necrosis.

3. If the ureters are always divided at the same point, or always mobilized for more than 2·5 cm. irrespective of their blood-supply, sloughing of the ureter is likely to occur in 10–15 per cent of cases.

4. Variation in the blood-supply of the ureters is considerable, not only between individuals but also between the two sides in the same person.

IV. C. ASSOCIATION OF RIGHT URETER AND RIGHT OVARIAN VEIN

Persistence of embryonic venous channels may result in an aberrant right ovarian vein which is enclosed in a common connective tissue sheath with the right ureter. When this vein enlarges during pregnancy the ureter may be compressed to produce pain, hydronephrosis, and pyelonephritis. After pregnancy involution may be incomplete and symptoms may persist. A lesser degree of obstruction may occur when the vein enlarges between the time of ovulation and the onset of menstruation.[1]

V. ANOMALIES OF THE VENAE CAVAE

Venous, like arterial, anomalies are common. They are readily understandable if their development is recalled.

Very early in development numerous venous channels appear and take part in the formation of the definitive pattern in man. Some are transitory and others migratory. They tend to increase in complexity at first, the ultimate general plan being the formation of fewer and larger channels. There are many unsettled problems about venous development and only a brief simplified account can be given here. It is based on the work of Hamilton, Boyd, and Mossman.[2]

Fig. 518 is a diagram showing a very early symmetrical stage of venous development. It consists of a number of longitudinal venous channels—anterior cardinal, posterior cardinal, subcardinal, and the medial and lateral sympathetic line veins. They do not all appear simultaneously. It is apparent that preponderant final pathways could develop on either or both sides and that numerous variations could occur, e.g., the lower ends

---

[1] Derrick, F. C., Rosenblum, R. R., and Lynch, K. M., *J. Urol.*, 1967, 97, 633.

[2] Hamilton, W. J., Boyd, J. D., and Mossman, H. W., *Human Embryology*, 1946, Ch. 9. Cambridge: Heffer.

RELATIONSHIPS OF VASCULAR PATTERN 537

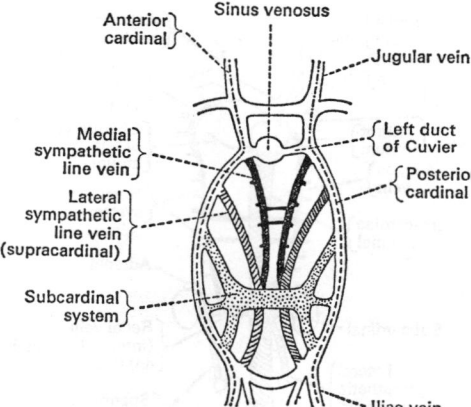

Fig. 518.—The early symmetrical stage of development of the veins, showing several systems of longitudinal channels. The same shadings and markings of vessels are used in this and the next two diagrams for ease of identification. (*Constructed by Thomas from Hamilton, Boyd, and Mossman.*)

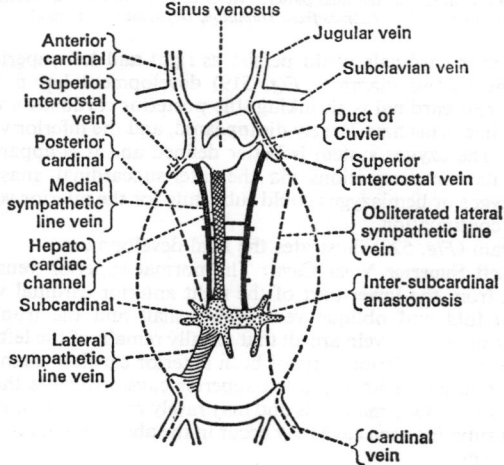

Fig. 519.—A later stage of development. More definitive patterns are appearing such as the vena cava and azygos systems. Refer to *Fig. 518*. (*Constructed by Thomas from Hamilton, Boyd, and Mossman.*)

538 A SYNOPSIS OF SURGICAL ANATOMY

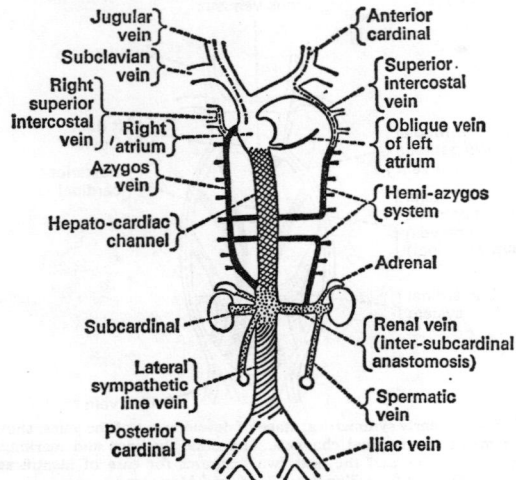

Fig. 520.—Diagram of the final pattern. Refer to *Fig.* 518 for identification. (*Constructed by Thomas from Hamilton, Boyd, and Mossman.*)

of both anterior cardinals could persist as right and left superior venae cavae. In the second diagram (*Fig.* 519) development has progressed. The left anterior cardinal is shrinking, the posterior cardinals and lateral sympathetic line veins have largely disappeared, and the inferior vena cava has formed. The azygos system is better defined and it is apparent that, because of its communications via the inter-subcardinal anastomoses, either the azygos or hemiazygos could substitute for the inferior vena cava, i.e., azygos continuation.

The diagram (*Fig.* 520) illustrates the final development.

Persistent Left Superior Vena Cava: The normal superior vena cava is derived from the lower part of the right anterior cardinal vein. The vestigial fold and oblique vein of Marshall and the trunk of the superior intercostal vein are all that usually remain of the left superior vena cava. The inferior parts of both anterior cardinal channels may persist resulting in right and left superior cavae which is the normal state in some lower mammals and may rarely occur in man. Part or all of a left superior vena cava may occur in the absence of its counterpart on the right.

In most cases there are no associated developmental defects and the condition does not impair health or longevity. In a minority of cases there are associated cardiovascular anomalies such as septal defects, etc.

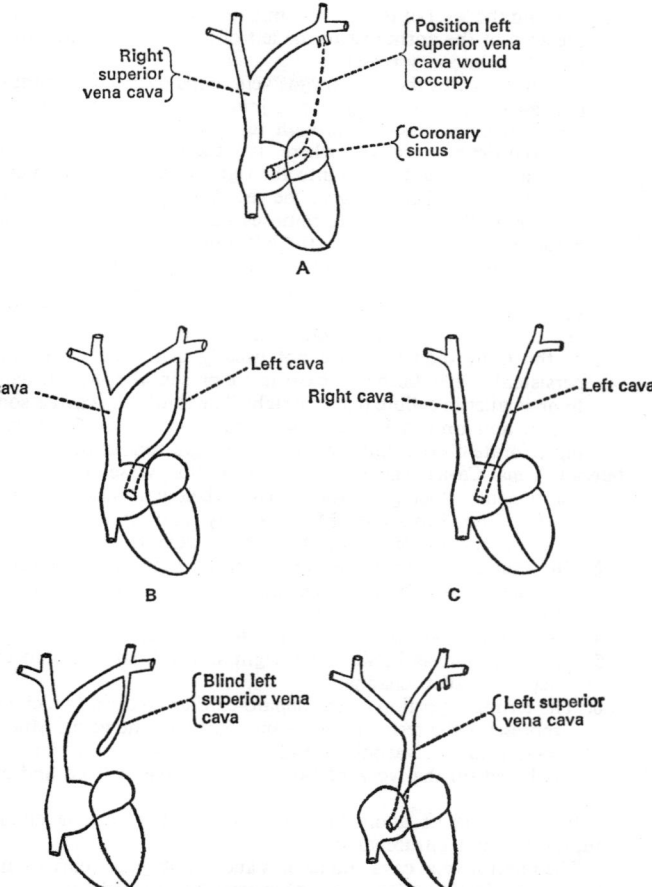

Fig. 521.—Anomalies of the superior vena cava. A, Normal right superior vena cava. B, Right and left venae cavae are shown with cross anastomosis. C, Right and left venae cavae. No cross anastomosis. D, A blind segment of the left superior vena cava is present. It can empty into the right vessel. E, Left superior vena cava. (*Re-drawn by courtesy of Winter and the Editor of 'Angiology'*.)

From the level of the left innominate vein the vessel descends across the arch of the aorta just to the left of the left vagus, and in front of the left pulmonary vessels.

In many cases the hemiazygos vein loops over the bronchus just as the azygos does on the right, and joins the vessel. The vena cava then turns medially, passing through the pericardium into the posterior atrioventricular groove, where it becomes continuous with the coronary sinus and opens into the right atrium. It may enter the left atrium. In open heart surgery the vessel is important whether it enters the right or left atrium. Anastomoses may or may not exist between the cavae in the position where the left innominate vein should be. This anastomosis is significant in cases where the left vena cava is only partially persistent and its caudal portion ends blindly. Rarely the vessel may receive all or part of the pulmonary venous drainage. The anastomosis conveys the blood into the right vena cava. The features of the right vena cava are not usually disturbed when the left is persistent. When both venae cavae are present the left is usually equal to or smaller in calibre than the right. The right vena cava is sometimes absent and only a left superior vena cava exists. Occasionally an imperforate fibrous cord represents the right vena cava (*Fig.* 521).

Inferior Vena Cava: The development of this vessel is complex. The components which go to form it (from below upwards) are according to Hamilton, Boyd, and Mossman[1] as follows:

1. A small portion of the right posterior cardinal vein.
2. The caudal portion of the right lateral sympathetic line vein.
3. The anastomosis between the right lateral sympathetic line vein and the right subcardinal vein.
4. The intermediate portion of the right subcardinal vein.
5. The anastomosis between the right subcardinal vein and the right hepato-cardiac channel.
6. The terminal portion of the hepato-cardiac channel (which probably represents the termination of the right vitelline vein). Much of this section on the variations and anomalies of the inferior vena cava is based on the work of Edwards[2] who has defined and classified them.

In describing its anomalies the inferior vena cava is divided into suprarenal and infrarenal parts.

The inferior vena cava and azygos and hemiazygos veins are normally in communication with each other near the renal level.

Suprarenal Anomalies: Azygos continuation of the suprarenal segment is also spoken of as absence of the inferior vena cava. In this condition the suprarenal part of the inferior vena cava is absent or rudimentary,

---

[1] Hamilton, W. J., Boyd, J. D., and Mossman, H. W., *Human Embryology*, 1946, Ch 9. Cambridge: Heffer.
[2] Edwards, E. A., *Angiology*, 1951 2, 85.

RELATIONSHIPS OF VASCULAR PATTERN 541

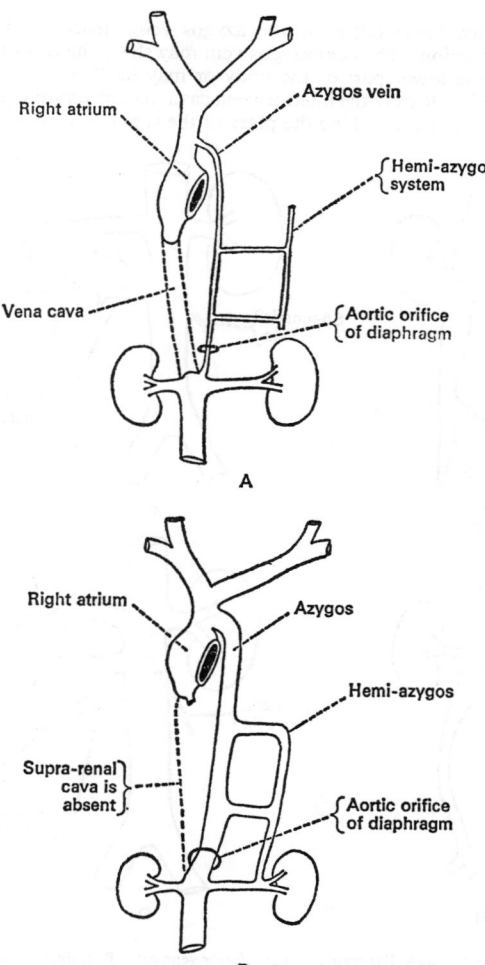

Fig. 522.—A, The azygos system assists the inferior vena cava in the drainage of the lower part of the body, i.e., normal. B, Absence of the inferior vena cava or azygos continuation.

542   A SYNOPSIS OF SURGICAL ANATOMY

its place being taken by the azygos vein, hence the term 'azygos continuation'. The hemiazygos vein may share the transport of blood from the lower part of the body or may itself be the main channel (*Fig.* 522). Rarely the inferior vena cava may be entirely left-sided, the hemiazygos vein taking the place of the suprarenal cava and draining

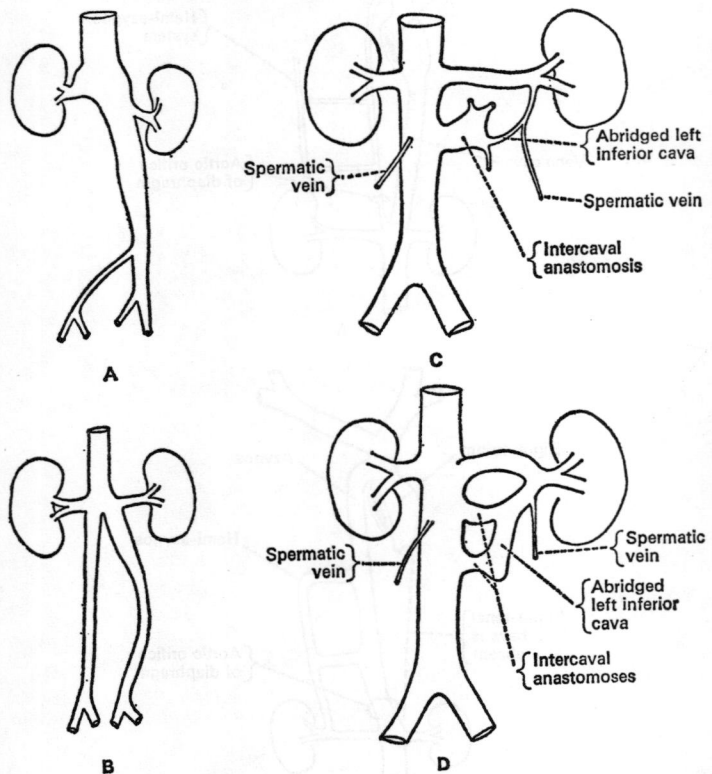

Fig. 523.—A, Diagram of a left inferior vena cava. B, A diagram of coexistent right and left inferior venae cavae. C, The diagram shows an abridged left inferior vena cava and a caval diverticulum connecting it with the right inferior cava. (*Modified from Edwards.*) D, The drawing shows intercaval anastomoses between the right vena cava and an abridged left one. (*By courtesy of Edwards and the Editor of 'Angiology'. Re-drawn.*)

into the azygos major, or exceptionally it may open into the coronary sinus. Such conditions are surgically important, e.g., anastomosis of the portal vein to the vena cava in portal hypertension may be difficult or impossible. In *situs inversus* the vena cava is on the left as the entire vascular system is transposed, as are the viscera.

Infrarenal Anomalies: This part of the vena cava may be:
 a. Left sided (not associated with *situs inversus*).
 b. Double.
 c. Abridged.
 d. Pre-ureteric.

Complete left-sided inferior vena cava may occur, there being no right cava present, or it may exist together with a right inferior vena cava. 'Abridged left inferior vena cava' is the term applied by Edwards when just a part of a left vena cava exists. Such a vessel is connected to the right inferior vena cava by the left renal vein (derived from the inter-subcardinal anastomosis) lying in its customary position in front of the aorta. In addition one or more large communications may connect the cavae behind the aorta. These are intercaval anastomoses. In this way a so-called 'venous renal collar' is formed. Diverticula of the infrarenal portion of the normally placed vena cava may occur. They may be large and are posterior to the aorta (*Fig.*523). The left kidney may ascend to its normal level retaining its primitive venous drainage so that the left renal vein is behind the aorta.

Comments:

The inferior vena cava may require ligature or division so that a knowledge of possible anomalies is valuable to the surgeon. Failure to find the infrarenal cava on the right of the aorta requires search to the left of this vessel.

Operations in the neighbourhood of the renal pedicle may disclose unusual venous arrangements of which the surgeon should be aware. The confluence of the common iliac veins may be anterior to the right common iliac artery and aorta instead of posterior as it usually is.

Collateral Circulation (*see* p. 319).

Retrocaval Ureter: This rare anomaly is readily understood by reference to the development of the inferior vena cava. The posterior cardinal veins form the iliacs and their confluence at the commencement of the inferior cava. The lower parts of their upward extensions disappear later. The right lateral sympathetic line vein forms the vena cava below the renals, and the subcardinal veins form the renal veins and a part of the vena cava above their level. The bud from the Wolffian duct grows towards the metanephros through the aperture between the posterior cardinal and the right sympathetic line veins. Normally the posterior cardinals atrophy. Exceptionally the right one may persist. In that case it forms the inferior vena cava as the supracardinals atrophy. The ureter then winds round the inferior cava instead of lying lateral to it (*Fig.* 524).

Retrocaval ureter may not cause symptoms. If it does it is during adult life. They are of an obstructive type and may result in

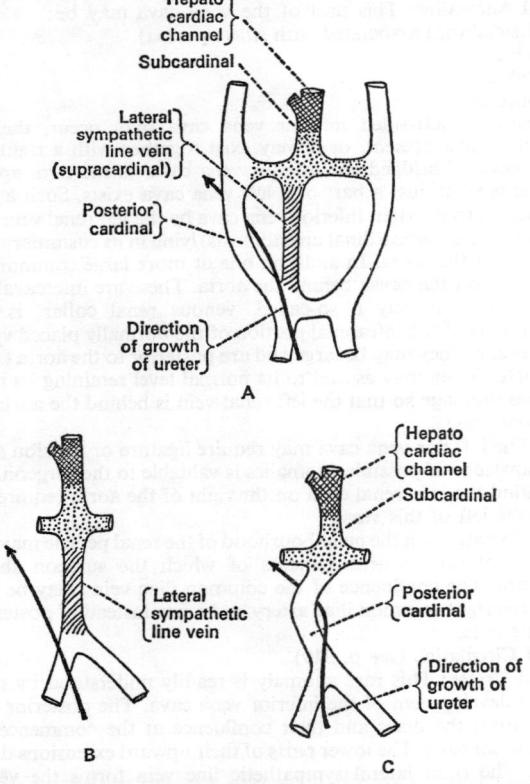

Fig. 524.—The embryogenesis of retrocaval ureter. (Compare *Figs.* 518–520.) **A,** The line of growth (arrow) of the bud from the Wolffian duct towards the metanephros is between the lateral sympathetic line vein and the posterior cardinal vein. **B,** The posterior cardinal vein has disappeared and the relationship between the ureter and future vena cava is normal. The position of the ureter is shown by the arrow. **C,** The lateral sympathetic line vein has regressed. Now the posterior cardinal forms the lower part of the inferior vena cava and lies in front of the ureter—retrocaval ureter. (*By courtesy of Moonen and van Velthoven. Modified.*)

RELATIONSHIPS OF VASCULAR PATTERN 545

hydro-nephrosis or stone formation. The condition is thus not primarily ureteric in origin. X-rays are distinctive. The lesion is dealt with by dividing the vena cava, bringing the ureter lateral, and reconstituting this great vein. Should this not be feasible the vessel ends are tied.

VI. THE BLOOD-SUPPLY OF TENDONS

Tendons, like bone, are not static structures. Their metabolic activity requires an intact vascular supply. As their collagen content degenerates it requires replacement. They have a longitudinal system of slender vessels derived from several sources. The proximal third is supplied by vessels entering from the musculotendinous junction, the distal third from vessels entering through the periosteal attachment, whereas the middle third is nourished by a specialized arrangement. Bunnell divides tendons into those which have a straight pull, which travel through paratenon, and those which pull round corners through a tendon sheath. Paratenon consists of a

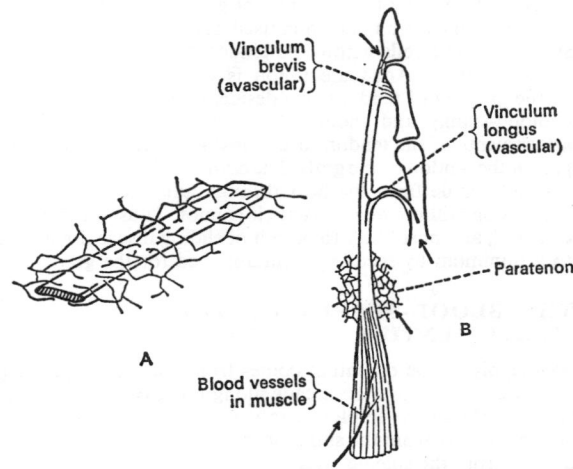

Fig. 525.—The nature of the blood-supply to tendons. A, Paratenon is shown carrying blood to the intermediate part of the tendon. B, The blood-supply of the long flexor of the fingers. The four arrows indicate the vascular mechanisms.

specialized system of loose elastic fatty tissue, attached on the one hand to the tendon, and on the other to surrounding tissues. The paratenon thus lengthens or recoils accordingly as the tendon gets longer or shorter. It carries the blood-supply to the middle portion of the tendon. This supply ends where a tendon enters a sheath. Beyond that point the flexor digitorum profundus tendons receive their blood-supply via the vessels in the vinculum longus. The vinculum brevis, which gains attachment to the tendons of the flexor sublimis, carries no blood-supply to the tendon, the final 5 cm. of which is thus dependent for its supply on the vessels entering at its bony insertion (*Fig.* 525).

Comment:

A normal tendon subjected to linear stress does not rupture. If a break occurs this is at the musculotendinous junction, the periosteal attachment, or through the belly of the muscle. If the tendon itself ruptures, it is the result of wear stress which has caused microscopic injury to the blood-vessels in the tendon, resulting in cellular death followed by collagenous disintegration and replacement by fibrous tissue. This is the explanation of rupture of the tendo Achillis or long head of biceps, etc., in young athletes.

Tendon injuries are common. When the divided tendon is sutured, it heals by the ingrowth of young connective tissue which does not come from the tendon itself but is supplied by surrounding structures. The cells within the tendon do not begin to proliferate for some days. Adequate union is dependent on blood-supply. In the grafting of tendons two desiderata are necessary for success—blood-supply and sliding. The normal blood-supply from the attachments of the tendon to the host is inadequate for the central part of the tendon or the graft. The additional blood-supply required can only come from the host through adhesions. If these are lax the tendon will move, otherwise it cannot. Thus adhesions, though essential, are most likely to permit of sliding if scar tissue is reduced to a minimum by securing a suitable bed for the graft.

VII. THE BLOOD-SUPPLY OF THE GREATER OMENTUM

The blood-supply of the omentum comes from the right and left gastro-epiploic arteries which form an arcade along the greater curvature of the stomach. The right gastro-epiploic artery arises from the gastro-duodenal artery or occasionally from the superior mesenteric artery. The left gastro-epiploic arises from the splenic artery.

The right epiploic (omental) artery (from the right gastro-epiploic artery) and the left epiploic artery (from the left gastro-epiploic artery) form an anastomotic (epiploic) arcade in the lower part of the omentum which is joined by accessory epiploic arteries (from the two gastro-epiploic arteries) and provide a rich blood-supply to the omentum (*Fig.* 526). When mobilizing the greater omentum from the greater curvature of the stomach it is therefore not necessary to preserve the gastro-epiploic arcade provided the epiploic arcade is preserved.

In 2·9 per cent of people the anastomosis between the 2 main epiploic

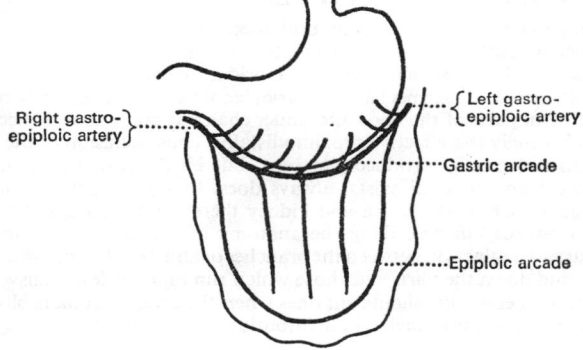

Fig. 526.—Blood-supply of the greater omentum.

arteries takes place 2–3 cm. from the gastro-epiploic arch[1] (*Fig.* 527). In such cases this epiploic arcade may be ligated during mobilization of the omentum and this may result in necrosis of part of the greater omentum if the right or left epiploic artery is also ligated.

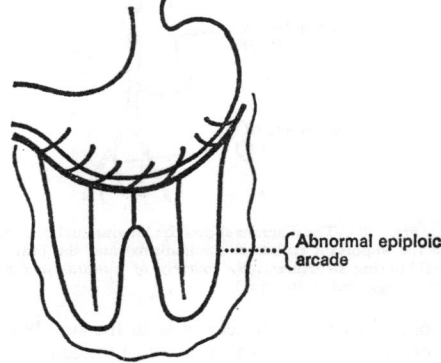

Fig. 527.—Abnormal position of epiploic arcade in the greater omentum.

[1] Alday, E. S., and Goldsmith, H. S., *Surgery Gynec. Obstet.*, 1972, 135, 103.

VIII. COLLATERAL CIRCULATIONS

The surgeon must know the natural mechanisms which operate when the vascular pathways are interrupted—the collateral circulation.

The Collateral Circulation provides a bridge to carry blood across an obstruction. This mechanism varies enormously in its efficiency in different parts of the body and under changing conditions. It becomes increasingly less effective proximodistally. Thus occlusion of the aorta does not usually produce gangrene, but blockage of the capillaries (where no collateral exists) always does. In some highly specialized organs such as the retina and kidney there is no collateral.

Edwards,[1] in describing the anatomy of the collateral pathways, makes a distinction between the branches of an arterial trunk, which run up and down the part, and those which run more or less transversely. The former are the significant ones when the arterial trunk is blocked. The others—the branches of distribution—may develop small adjacent

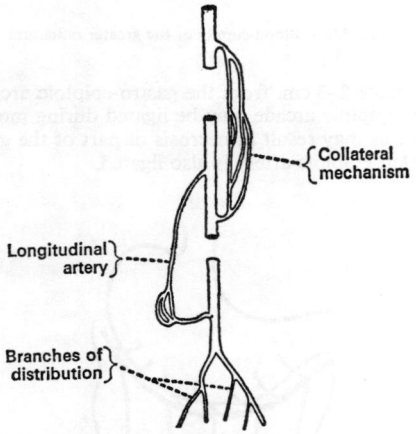

Fig. 528.—The diagram shows the longitudinal branches of an artery (which are the important collateral mechanisms) and the branches of distribution to neighbouring structures. (*By courtesy of Edwards and the Editor of 'Surgery, Gynecology, and Obstetrics'.*)

inosculations, which help little in the supply of the area beyond the block (*Fig.* 528). It is this factor of vascular disposition which makes the results of the disruption of the blood-flow in big vessels so variable. In acute war injuries in World War II, DeBakey and

[1] Edwards, E. A., *Surgery Gynec. Obstet.*, 1958, **107**, 183.

Simeone[1] reported the incidence of gangrene following interruption of main vessels as 26 per cent in the case of the brachial, 53 per cent in the femoral, and 73 per cent in the popliteal. Edwards speaks of the vulnerability of junctional zones where two or more arteries supply the part. If one is preponderant and becomes occluded, the smaller remaining one may not be able to supply the ischaemic area. This is noteworthy in the heart if there is great disparity in the coronaries.

The Venous Collateral Mechanisms are on the whole more generous than the arterial ones. The integrity of certain veins is essential because of the absence of or paucity of collaterals. Such are the retinal, the superior vena cava, and the inferior cava above the renals, the portal, and the superior mesenteric.

Either innominate may be tied as a rule with safety, so too the subclavian. The removal of one internal jugular vein is a safe procedure. It is necessary on occasions to remove the remaining internal jugular, either as a staged procedure or simultaneously.

Although all are not agreed, Schweizer and Leak[2] of the Memorial Cancer Center, New York City, after studies of the cerebrospinal fluid pressures during and after these procedures, conclude that the risk to the patient is minimal, and should not be allowed to interfere with operation if it is indicated. Batson[3] has estimated that the cross-sectional area of the vertebral venous system is greater than that of the two jugulars.

THE VENOUS COLLATERAL AFTER LIGATION OF THE INTERNAL JUGULARS: In bilateral radical clearance of lymph-glands of the neck, not only the internal jugulars but the anterior and external jugular veins will also be sacrificed. The intracranial venous sinuses which drain the brain communicate extensively with the system of emissary veins (*see* p. 296), with the veins of the orbit, and with the prevertebral venous plexuses. The intracranial venous drainage is thus assured to the exterior of the skull. Its passage to the heart, and that of the other structures in the head and neck, is by three main routes:

a. Along the visceral compartment of the neck via pterygoid and pharyngeal plexuses; tracheal, thyroid, and oesophageal veins to the vertebral and innominate veins.

b. Through the occipital and the deep cervical plexuses to the first and superior intercostal veins, the vertebral, subclavian, and uppermost intercostal veins.

c. Through the vertebral venous plexuses via their communications with the intracranial sinuses above and their drainage into vertebral, innominate, and intercostals below.

---

[1] De Bakey, M. E., and Simeone, C. F., *Ann. Surg.* 1946, **123**, 534. Quoted by Edwards.
[2] Schweizer, Olga, and Leak, G. H., *Ann. Surg.*, 1952, **136**, 948.
[3] Batson, O. V., *Proc. Fedn Am. Socs exp. Biol.*, 1944, **3**, 139. Quoted by Schweizer and Leak.

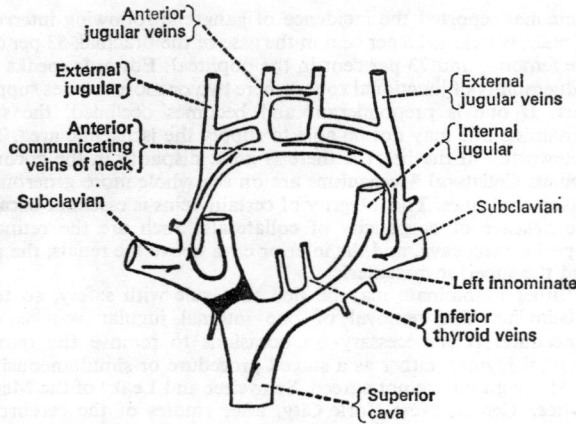

Fig. 529.—Obstruction of the right innominate vein. The arrows show the direction of the blood-flow. (*By courtesy of Barrett and the 'British Journal of Surgery'*.)

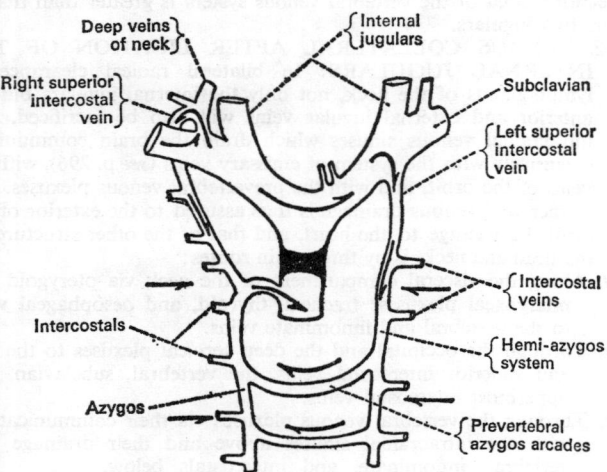

Fig. 530.—The collateral circulation when the superior vena cava is obstructed above the azygos. Arrows show direction of blood-flow. (*By courtesy of Barrett and the 'British Journal of Surgery'*.)

The collateral circulation, when the great veins of the superior mediastinum are obstructed, is described by Barrett.[1] When one of the innominate veins is obstructed the other is usually spared. It supplies a ready collateral pathway to the superior vena cava through the cross communications of the numerous veins in the anterior part of the neck (*Fig.* 529).

Obstruction of the superior vena cava above the entrance of the azygos (*Fig.* 530): the main collateral pathways are the superior intercostal veins which carry the blood to the azygos and hemiazygos systems and so to the heart. The more superficial veins, such as chest wall veins and the internal mammary, which inosculate with the inguinal veins, do not carry sufficient of the load to cause prominence of the veins on the front of the chest.

When the caval obstruction involves the azygos entry as well, then the collaterals inside and outside the chest wall carry the blood to the inferior vena cava (*Fig.* 531). There is great dilatation of the

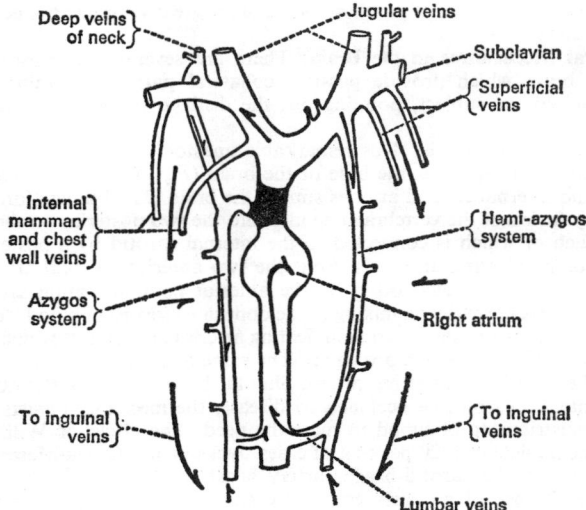

Fig. 531.—When the azygos and superior vena cava are both blocked, all blood is carried to the inferior vena cava by collaterals within and without the chest. The arrows show the rerouting of blood. The long lateral arrows denote the passage of blood from upper limbs, etc., to the veins in the inguinal region. (*By courtesy of Barrett and the 'British Journal of Surgery'.*)

[1] Barrett, N. R., *Br. J. Surg.*, 1958, 46, 207.

552 A SYNOPSIS OF SURGICAL ANATOMY

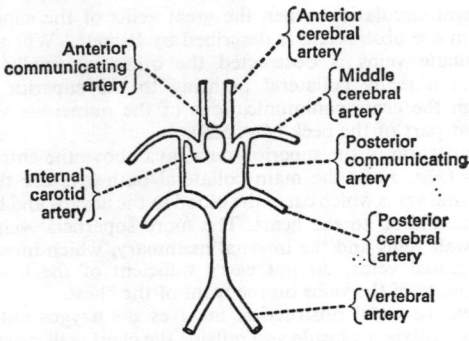

Fig. 532.—The circle of Willis.

veins of the front of the chest. None of the great veins mentioned has valves.

Collateral Mechanisms in the Brain: There are several mechanisms in the brain which provide possible collateral pathways. Brain[1] has reviewed the subject, pointing out the distinctive features of these areas:

a. The circle of Willis: This remarkable anastomosis lies in the subarachnoid space at the base of the brain (*Fig.* 532). The vertebral and internal carotid arteries supply the brain. The basilar (formed by fusion of the vertebrals) divides into the two posterior cerebrals, each of which is connected to the internal carotid by a posterior communicating artery. In front the two anterior cerebral arteries are joined to each other by the anterior communicating artery. There is normally no mixing of the opposing streams of blood which meet in the posterior communicating arteries at points at which the pressures of the two are equal. The same applies in the middle of the anterior connecting artery. Should, however, the vertebral or internal carotid be occluded by disease, the mechanism exists for redistribution of blood to meet the need. The circle of Willis is incomplete in 5–20 per cent of cases. Jackson and Garza-Mercado[2] refer to the carotid-basilar artery anastomosis. This is the rare persistence of an early embryonic channel connecting the cavernous part of the internal carotid artery with the upper third of the basilar. It is named the trigeminal artery and may be as large as the internal carotid. It passes lateral to the posterior clinoid process or through the dorsum sellae, being in close proximity to

[1] Brain, R., *S. Afr. med. J.*, 1957, 31, 1006.
[2] Jackson, I. A., and Garza-Mercado, R., *Angiography*, 1960, 11, 103.

the semilunar ganglion or fifth nerve. Its practical importance is: (i) that it may be an important collateral channel reinforcing the circle of Willis if, e.g., one of the vertebral arteries is missing; (ii) it has been considered a rare causative factor in trigeminal neuralgia; (iii) it may be misleading in the interpretation of cerebral angiograms.

b. On the surface of the brain every vessel forms anastomoses.
c. Once an artery has entered the brain no anastomoses occur.
d. In the orbit anastomoses take place between branches of the internal and external carotid arteries.

Though collateral pathways are numerous in the brain they are often inadequate.

Ligation of the common carotid artery is hazardous. There is a mortality of 25 per cent and a high degree of cerebral complications especially in old people.

Collateral Circulation in Special Areas

When a main blood-vessel is occluded, the vitality of the part supplied by the vessel depends on the efficiency of the collateral circulation. If the circulation is suddenly cut off, as by embolism or ligature, gangrene may occur. Gradual occlusion such as commonly occurs in atherosclerosis is much less likely to be followed by death of tissue. Even the abdominal aorta may obliterate slowly and produce little in the way of symptoms. Major limb arteries, which are atherosclerotic, may become further occluded during the enforced rest entailed by operation. The first indications of this may be intermittent claudication when the patient resumes his normal activities. The lesson is clear that the doctor in attendance should be aware of the state of the limb arteries prior to any operation. If gangrene occurs, its extent is remarkably constant in relation to the situation of the occlusion.

Results of Sudden Occlusion:

ABDOMINAL AORTA AT BIFURCATION: Gangrene often follows, producing symmetrical gangrene of both lower limbs up to the inguinal ligaments. Some cases of saddle emboli of the aortic bifurcation, or ligature of that vessel below the renals, are not followed by gangrene.

EXTERNAL ILIAC OR (COMMON) FEMORAL ARTERY: Gangrene almost always follows. Gangrene extends as high as mid-thigh.

SUPERFICIAL FEMORAL OR POPLITEAL ARTERY: Gangrene does not usually occur (as the profunda maintains the circulation). If it does, it extends almost to the knee-joint.

POPLITEAL AT BIFURCATION: If gangrene follows, it reaches well up the leg.

AXILLARY ARTERY: Not usually followed by gangrene. If this develops it reaches the middle of the arm.

BRACHIAL ARTERY: Not usually followed by gangrene. If this develops it reaches the junction of the middle and lower third of the forearm.

The routes taken by the blood in occlusion of main vessels are as follows:

Abdominal Aorta: The block being below the origin of the inferior mesenteric artery, the following anastomoses convey blood to the pelvis and lower limbs:

ABOVE		BELOW
1. Inferior mesenteric anastomoses	with	Visceral branches of hypogastric artery (internal iliac)
2. Lumbar arteries	with	Parietal branches of hypogastric, e.g., ilio-lumbar
3. Internal mammary	with	Inferior epigastric artery

Common Iliac Artery: Blood is conveyed to the area below the block as follows:

ABOVE		BELOW
1. Inferior mesenteric anastomoses	with	Visceral branches of hypogastric
2. Ovarian	with	Uterine and vesical arteries
3. Middle sacral	with	Lateral sacral branches of hypogastric
4. Internal mammary and lower intercostal and lumbar arteries	anastomose with	Inferior epigastric

Hypogastric (Internal Iliac) Artery: Devascularized area is supplied through:

1. The numerous communications between the two branches of the hypogastric arteries.
2. The numerous communications between the two branches of the hypogastric arteries and the inferior mesenteric artery.

It is sometimes expedient to ligature both hypogastric arteries in continuity, either as a planned procedure to diminish bleeding during the operation of abdominoperineal resection of the rectum, or as an emergency measure to control pelvic bleeding following severe trauma to the pelvis or reactionary haemorrhage consequent on hysterectomy. The procedure is not followed by adverse results due to ischaemia, as an effective collateral circulation develops between the branches of external iliac, internal mammary, and lumbar vessels proximally and their inosculations distally with the terminal branches of the divided hypogastric vessels.

RELATIONSHIPS OF VASCULAR PATTERN

External Iliac Artery: The circulation is re-established via:

ABOVE		BELOW
1. Branches of hypogastric	anastomose with	Branches of external iliac
2. Vessels of anterior abdominal wall	anastomose with	Branches of: (1) External iliac (inferior epigastric and deep circumflex iliac); (2) Femoral (superficial inferior epigastric, circumflex iliac, and external pudendal vessels)

Femoral Artery:
1. **JUST BELOW THE INGUINAL LIGAMENT:** The blood commonly reaches the limb via the branches of the hypogastric to the buttock (the gluteal arteries) and thigh (the obturator artery). The collateral circulation is therefore much less efficient than the previous one, as the block is distal to the inferior epigastric and circumflex iliac arteries.
2. **AT THE APEX OF THE FEMORAL (SCARPA'S) TRIANGLE:** Collateral circulation:

ABOVE		BELOW
1. Branches of profunda (perforating and muscular and lateral circumflex)	anastomose with	Superior articular branches of popliteal, anterior tibial recurrent (from anterior tibial)
2. Branches of hypogastric to buttock (gluteals and obturator)	anastomose with	Muscular branches of femoral and popliteal

3. **IN THE ADDUCTOR CANAL (HUNTER'S CANAL):** The collateral circulation is the same as that in the preceding paragraph.

Popliteal Artery: Collateral circulation:

ABOVE		BELOW
1. Lateral femoral circumflex, arteria genu suprema, branches of femoral	anastomose with	Anterior and posterior tibial recurrents (from anterior tibial)
2. Superior articular branches of popliteal	anastomose with	Inferior articular branches of popliteal

As the collateral circulation is poor, the surgeon prefers to ligate the femoral in the adductor canal, in which case the collateral circulation is much better.

Anterior Tibial Artery: Because of its situation this vessel presents considerable interest. Although it supplies a group of anti-gravity muscles, these are much less frequently the site of intermittent claudication than the posterior gravity-assisted group of muscles of the leg. This implies that the vascular economy of the extensor muscle group is a liberal one. The anterior tibial blood-supply is reinforced by perforating branches of both the posterior tibial and the peroneal arteries.

Despite these facts, a condition of acute ischaemic paralysis—the anterior tibial syndrome—may develop in the muscles of the anterior tibial compartment. It affects persons subjected to unaccustomed exercise, such as recruits carrying out long route marches or those indulging in violent sports such as high jumping or football (fresher's leg). The anterior tibial compartment houses the tibialis anterior, the long extensors of the toes and the peroneus tertius muscles, the anterior tibial nerve which supplies them, and the arteries mentioned above. The anterior tibial artery and its two veins enter the compartment through an orifice in a dense unyielding membrane and lie on it throughout. The space is bounded behind by this interosseous structure, in front by the deep fascia, and at its sides by bone (*Fig.* 533).

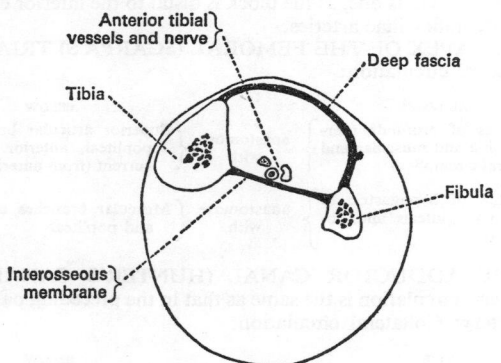

Fig. 533.—The anatomy of the anterior tibial compartment.

Trauma to or ischaemia of the muscles causes oedema leading to swelling which the osteofascial compartment cannot accommodate. Great pain occurs. The muscle suffers ischaemia. Necrosis may occur. The circulation to the limb as a whole remains unimpaired, the foot remains warm and the ankle pulses are present. As the blood-supply to the compartment is unaffected, it is thought that unaccustomed exertion leads to trauma of the muscle-fibres themselves, resulting in swelling and increased pressure within a confined space ending in ischaemic necrosis. Harman[1] has shown that the fate of a muscle deprived of its blood-supply depends, not on what happens to the main vessels of the area, but on the circulation in the muscle itself.

---

[1] Harman, J. W., *Am. J. Path.*, 1948, 24, 625, quoted in Leader in *Br. med. J.*, 1966 1, 1061.

As this syndrome may develop within a few hours it may become necessary to decompress the compartment by slitting up the deep fascia.

Innominate Artery: After occlusion of this vessel the collateral circulation is abundant. The blood reaches:
1. HEAD AND NECK: By the common carotid and vertebral of the opposite side. The external carotids communicate freely and the two vertebrals and internal carotids inosculate freely in the circle of Willis.
2. ARM: By:
   a. The intercostals, both anterior (from internal mammary) and posterior (from the aorta), communicating with the costocervical trunk (second part of the subclavian) and with the lateral thoracic, alar thoracic, and subscapular branches of the axillary. This is the intercostal anastomosis.
   b. The internal mammary (first part of the subclavian) communicates by its superior epigastric branch with the inferior epigastric (external iliac).

Common Carotid Artery: Collateral circulation is covered by:

Free communications between the arteries of the two sides both within and without the skull and by the enlargement of branches of the subclavian artery. The chief communications outside the skull are:

ABOVE		BELOW
1. Superior thyroid	anastomoses with	Inferior thyroid arteries
2. Descending branch of occipital	anastomoses with	Deep cervical artery and ascending branch of transverse cervical

The vertebral is said to take over the supply of the carotid within the skull.

Origin of the Subclavian Artery: Obstruction at the origin of the subclavian artery results in hypotension in the distal artery where the vertebral artery arises and retrograde flow of blood can occur from the brain through the vertebral artery to the subclavian artery distal to the obstruction. This results in ischaemic neurological symptoms in association with ischaemic symptoms in the affected arm (subclavian steal syndrome).

Third Part of the Subclavian Artery: Collateral circulation:

ABOVE
1. The intercostal anastomosis as above
2. The scapular anastomosis:

		BELOW
Transverse scapular artery and descending branch of transverse cervical from first part of subclavian	anastomose with	Subscapular and circumflex humeral branches of axillary

558 A SYNOPSIS OF SURGICAL ANATOMY

Brachial Artery:
1. IN ITS UPPER THIRD:

ABOVE		BELOW
Circumflex humeral and subscapular	anastomose with	Arteria profunda brachii

2. IN ITS MIDDLE THIRD: Below the origin of profunda and superior ulnar collateral arteries.

ABOVE		BELOW
Branches of profunda and superior ulnar collateral arteries	anastomose with	Inferior ulnar collateral, and radial, ulnar, and interosseous recurrent arteries

Splenic Artery: This vessel is unique inasmuch as it may be mobilized and anastomosed to renal, superior mesenteric, or hepatic arteries, when the indications exist. It is unnecessary to remove the spleen because of the collateral supply it receives through its short gastric branches.

Hepatic Artery: During the performance of a difficult operation on the bile-ducts or stomach the surgeon is rightly nervous of injuring the hepatic artery. Such an accident is always serious. The actual facts in connexion with injury to the hepatic artery are as follows:[1]
1. Twenty-eight cases have been reported, with 16 deaths.
2. Experimental evidence goes to show that because of the anastomosis of the inferior phrenic arteries with the hepatic, occlusion of the latter may be compensated for by the inferior phrenic collateral circulation. This, however, is not to be depended on.
3. Congenital arterial anomalies, such as the existence of two hepatic arteries, exist in 33·3 per cent of cases. The only blood-supply to the left lobe of the liver may have an anomalous origin, e.g., from the left gastric artery, and in tying this vessel during gastrectomy such a vessel should be looked for and protected (Rodney Smith).
4. (*a*) Ligation of the hepatic trunk before any branches are given off is not attended with any impairment of hepatic nutrition; (*b*) Ligation of the hepatic trunk before the right gastric is given off is not usually attended by ill effects; (*c*) Ligation beyond the origin of the right gastric is attended with total or severe liver necrosis unless, through disease, a collateral circulation has already developed, or an anomaly in the blood-supply to the liver is present.
5. Whereas ligation of the hepatic artery is always serious, it is not necessarily fatal. The danger of liver necrosis increases in direct proportion as the point of ligation proceeds distally.
6. Collateral circulation (*Fig.* 534):
   a. Ligation proximal to the origin of the right gastric artery: the blood reaches the liver via the left gastric and left gastro-epiploic and inferior pancreaticoduodenal arteries.

---
[1] Graham, Roscoe R., and Cannell, Douglas, *Br. J. Surg.*, 1933, 20, 566.

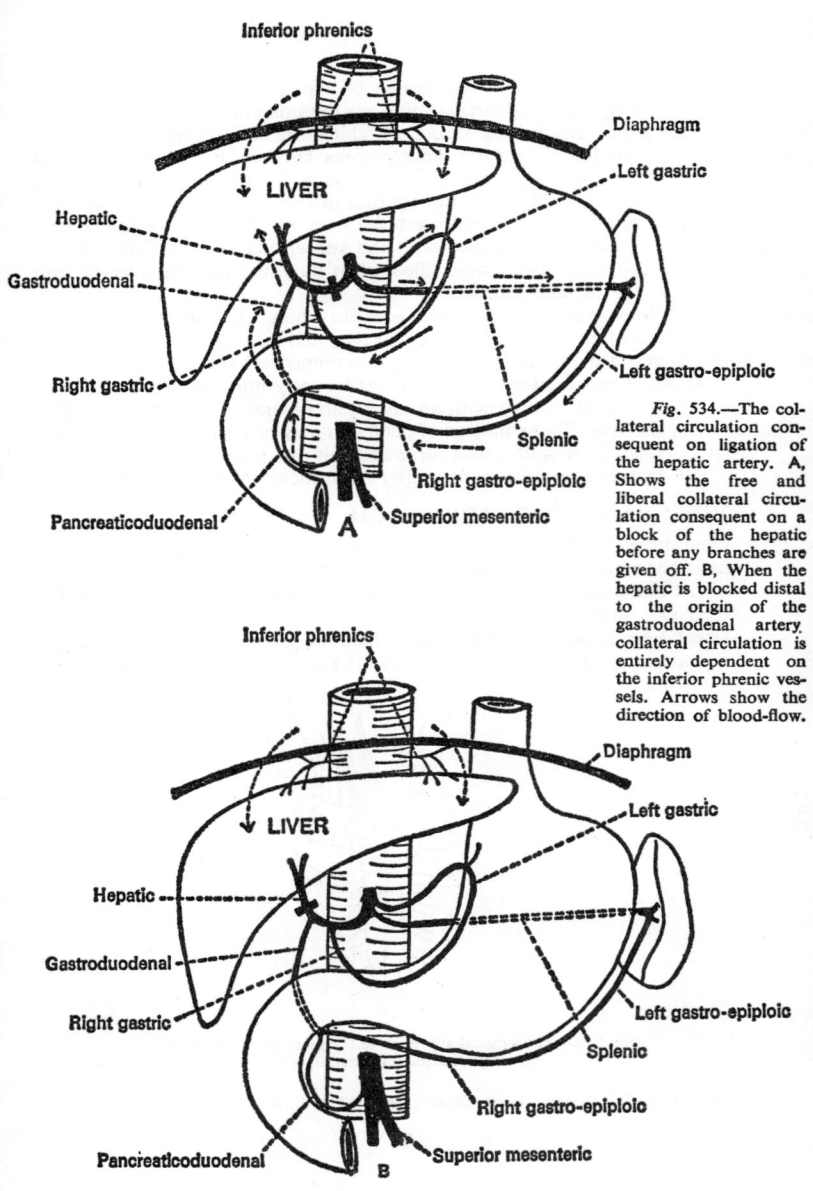

Fig. 534.—The collateral circulation consequent on ligation of the hepatic artery. A, Shows the free and liberal collateral circulation consequent on a block of the hepatic before any branches are given off. B, When the hepatic is blocked distal to the origin of the gastroduodenal artery collateral circulation is entirely dependent on the inferior phrenic vessels. Arrows show the direction of blood-flow.

b. Ligature distal to the origin of the gastroduodenal artery: the only collateral circulation is via the small inferior phrenic vessels.
   c. Segall[1] studied the vascular architecture of the liver post mortem. He found that the anastomoses between the blood-vessels in the liver were made up of vessels larger than capillaries. An emulsion injected after ligation of either the right or left hepatic artery filled the entire arterial tree. The branches of the hepatic vessels anastomosed with the subcapsular vessels. The inferior phrenic vessels were filled when an emulsion was injected into the hepatic arteries.
7. All experimental evidence goes to show that arterial blood is essential for the nutrition of the liver and that the venous blood conveyed by the portal vein cannot compensate for arterial occlusion.
8. The hepatic artery may be tied at its entry into the liver as the only means of dealing with an aneurysm of one of its branches within the liver. The exhibition of penicillin may protect the liver from necrosis. Most authorities agree that this procedure is hazardous as the factors operative in man differ from those which obtain in the dog.

VIII. VASCULAR APPROACH

Operations on the blood-vessels are carried out through the familiar incisions which are used for their display. Modern emphasis on the surgery of the blood-vessels requires a description of some of the methods used in their exposure.

Great Vessels of the Upper Mediastinum are approached by splitting the sternum in whole or in part, and if necessary extending the incision

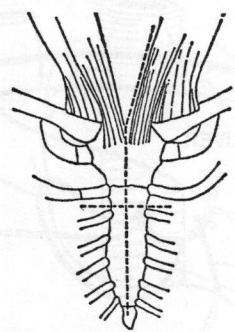

Fig. 535.—The surgical approach to the great vessels of the upper mediastinum (dotted lines).

[1] Segall, H. N., *Surgery Gynec. Obstet.*, 1923, 37, 152.

RELATIONSHIPS OF VASCULAR PATTERN 561

into an intercostal space on one or both sides. Such an exposure may be required, e.g., for cases of trauma to the great veins. If access to the neck is also necessary the incision is extended up along the anterior border of the appropriate sternomastoid muscle (*Fig.* 535).

Aneurysms of the Thoracic Aorta are approached through an appropriate rib bed or intercostal space usually on the left side.

Aneurysms of the Abdominal Aorta are usually below the renal vessels. They are dealt with through an incision extending from xiphoid process to pubis (*Fig.* 536). Should they involve the upper abdominal

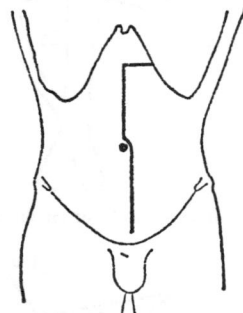

Fig. 536.—The incision for a resection of an abdominal aneurysm.

aorta, adequate access and proximal control of the aorta are obtained by combining the left thoracic approach with the abdominal one. An incision in the left paracolic gutter which allows the splenic flexure to be mobilized enables the abdominal viscera to be displaced to the right, so that the whole of the abdominal aorta is approached by the retroperitoneal route. A shunt can then be made between the thoracic and lower aorta establishing a by-pass whilst the aneurysm is excised under vascular control (*Fig* 537). Aneurysms of all parts of the aorta have been successfully replaced by prostheses.

Dissecting Aneurysms: The tunica media of arteries to muscles consists of concentric circular layers of smooth muscle. In larger vessels the muscle is gradually replaced by elastic fibres. In still bigger vessels, like the axillary or femoral, the elastic tissue takes the form of fenestrated membranes alternating with muscle. In the aorta the media is made up mostly by such discontinuous sheets of elastic structure.

Dissecting aneurysms are formed by a split in the coats of the aorta. The wall of this great vessel is nourished in two ways (Burman).[1]

---

[1] Burman, S. O., *Surgery Gynec. Obstet.*, 1960, **110**, 1. Collective review.

562 A SYNOPSIS OF SURGICAL ANATOMY

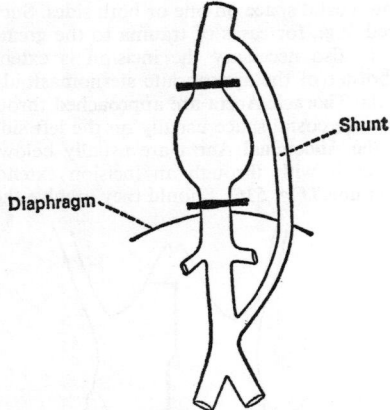

Fig. 537.—Resection of an aneurysm of the thoracic aorta using a shunt

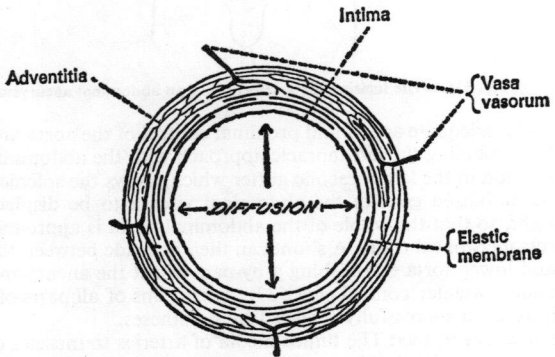

Fig. 538.—The blood-supply of the aorta.

The intima and adjacent part of the media are fed by diffusion from the central blood-current.[1] The adventitia and outer part of the media are supplied via the vasa vasorum from intercostal and other arteries which form a plexus in the adventitia (*Fig.* 538). There is thus a part of the media which will be the first to suffer should, e.g., the vasa

[1] In atherosclerotic arteries the thickened intima may become vascularized by capillary ingrowth.

vasorum fail in their function because of hypoxia or sclerosis. This leads to mucoid degeneration in the ground substance of the media which may result in the appearance of clefts in the vessel wall. Such dehiscences may occur because of congenital defects of ground

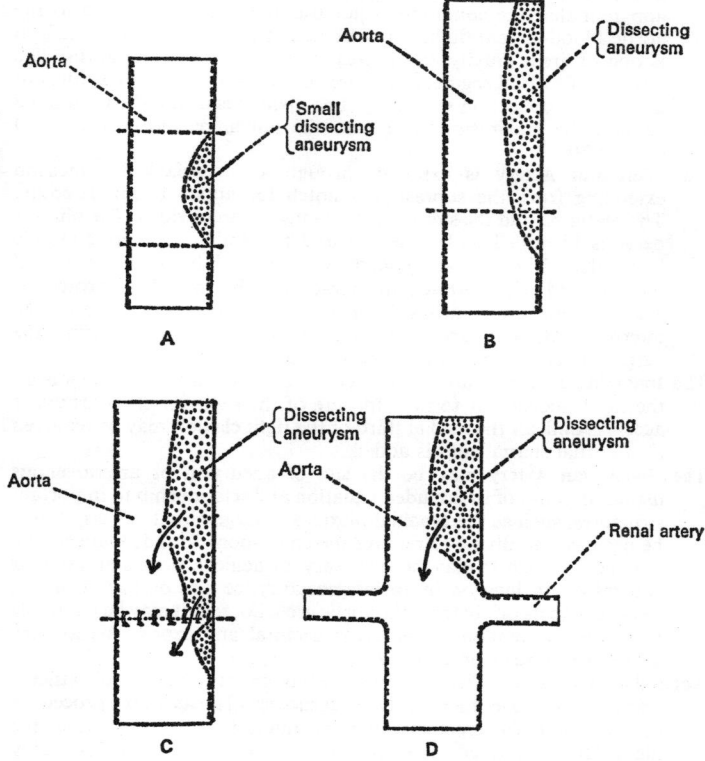

Fig. 539.—Dissecting aneurysm: A, Excision of the affected area. The resulting gap will be treated by the insertion of a graft. B, An extensive dissecting aneurysm is treated by transecting the vessel through the affected area. The upper line of division of the inner wall of the aneurysm is left open to drain into the parent vessel, which is then reconstituted. C, The operation completed. D, When the aneurysm is adjacent to an essential vessel such as the renal artery, it is treated by opening the aorta and making a window in the inner wall of the aneurysm, thus permitting pressure to be lessened by drainage into the host vessel.

substance in the vessel wall and affect young people, or they may be due to generalized degeneration of this tissue. Such clefts may be empty or contain blood. This may dissect its way between the coats of the vessel and produce a dissecting aneurysm, which, though usually in the thoracic part of the aorta, may affect any part or all of it. It is apparent that the condition is not traumatic and is not due to the aortic blood-stream finding a weakness in the intima. The condition is one of great gravity and is treated by transecting the aorta. The coats of the distal segment only are then approximated by sutures to prevent the dissection spreading. The divided ends are then re-united so that the aneurysm drains into the lumen of the parent vessel (*Fig.* 539).

The Vertebral Artery is exposed through a supraclavicular incision extending from the suprasternal notch for about 10 cm. laterally. The platysma and the sternomastoid muscles are divided. The phrenic nerve is identified and preserved and the scalenus anterior muscle is divided. The internal jugular vein is mobilized and retracted medially and on the left side the thoracic duct is exposed and protected. The vertebral artery arises from the subclavian artery opposite the internal mammary artery. Care is needed to avoid injuring the vertebral vein which may lie anterior to the artery.

The Innominate Artery can be exposed by a supraclavicular incision on the right side similar to the exposure of the right vertebral artery. If access is difficult the medial third of the right clavicle may be removed or a partial sternal split is added.

The Subclavian Artery may be the site of aneurysm or arteriovenous fistula. Because of its secluded situation and relationship to important structures, such as the brachial plexus and large blood-vessels, it may be necessary to divide or remove the collar-bone for adequate access. On the left side it may be necessary to achieve proximal vascular control by an incision in an intercostal space and occlusion of this vessel above its origin from the aortic arch. So, too, it may be advisable to divide the tendon of the great pectoral and expose the axillary artery for control or grafting.

Aorto-iliac Exposure: These vessels are commonly the site of atherosclerosis. Moreover they are the most successful areas for the procedure of thrombo-endarterectomy. It is an interesting fact that when the iliacs are obliterated, the common femoral is almost invariably patent, though it may be far from normal. These vessels lend themselves well to extraperitoneal exposure by an oblique incision such as that used for exposure of the ureter (*see* p. 761). It runs obliquely forward from the loin towards the mid-inguinal point and then curves vertically downwards in the line of the femoral artery. The external oblique is split in the direction of its fibres. Internal oblique and transversus abdominis muscles are cut across but not the falx

RELATIONSHIPS OF VASCULAR PATTERN

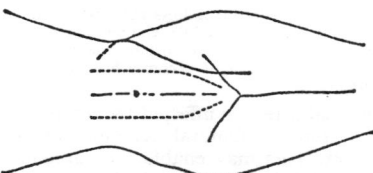

Fig. 540.—The incision for the extraperitoneal exposure of the bifurcation of the aorta and the iliac vessels, also the common femoral artery.

inguinalis (conjoint tendon). Thus, nerves are not divided. In the lower part of the incision the fascia lata is divided over the femoral vessels. The whole length of the iliacs and even the aortic bifurcation are thus exposed, including the upper femoral vessels (*Fig.* 540).

Note: The objections of surgeons to the division of muscles have largely fallen away providing the nerve-supply is not impaired. Thus the external, internal oblique, and transversus abdominis muscles may be divided a finger's breadth above the outer half of the inguinal ligament if necessary. By opening the inguinal canal, lifting the cord aside, and dividing the posterior wall of the canal (fascia transversalis), good access is obtained to the lower iliac vessels, lymph-glands in the area, the vas deferens, testicular vessels, etc. The inguinal area is not weakened by this procedure.

Popliteal Artery: This vessel is 20 cm. long. It begins at the opening in the adductor magnus as the continuation of the superficial femoral. It ends at the lower border of the popliteus muscle by dividing into the anterior and posterior tibial arteries. This corresponds in level to the lower border of the tubercle of the tibia.

Palma considers that the trauma caused by the constant pounding of this vessel against the unyielding tendon of the adductor magnus muscle, with which the vessel is in contact, may give rise to the development of slow changes in the vessel wall, causing first narrowing and then occlusion. He has advocated, in suitably selected cases, that the tendon be divided.

Boyd describes fixation of the popliteal artery to the capsule of the knee-joint by a fibrous band at the upper level of the condyles of the femur. He considers that the primary thrombosis, which sometimes occludes the popliteal artery in young people, probably results from the effects of recurring stresses (stretch strains) between the mobile part of the artery and the more fixed part.

Compare this to the result of sudden injury or violence applied to other hollow structures in relation to sites of fixation. In the aorta traumatic rupture occurs most commonly at the aortic isthmus just beyond the left subclavian origin, where the remains of the ductus arteriosus and the origin of the big vessels from the arch render this part of the aorta more fixed than the less firmly anchored descending aorta.

So, too, when rupture of the intestine follows abdominal trauma, it tends to occur where the fixed duodenum joins the mobile jejunum at the duodenojejunal flexure. Traumatic rupture of the oesophagus almost invariably occurs in its lower part before the mobile thoracic oesophagus becomes fixed by its passage through the hiatus in the diaphragm.

When the popliteal artery is affected by atherosclerosis, the distal segment, like the common femoral, remains patent in a surprising percentage of cases. This may enable the surgeon to improve the vascularity of the limb below the knee, by bringing a graft from above to the lower patent popliteal vessel.

SURGICAL APPROACH:

UPPER SEGMENT: With the patient lying prone the popliteal artery is readily approached by a vertical incision in the popliteal space. This incision should never be straight as keloid readily develops in this area. It may consist of several gentle alternating curves (the lazy S) or a ⌐ incision may be made.

The first structure encountered on dividing the strong deep fascia is the tibial nerve. The popliteal vein covers the artery behind the knee.

An alternative approach is from the medial aspect.

The patient lies supine with the thigh externally rotated and the knee flexed. The incision is made longitudinally along the lower third of the medial aspect of the thigh crossing the adductor tubercle. The deep fascia is divided in front of the sartorius muscle which is retracted posteriorly. By blunt dissection between the adductor magnus anteriorly and the hamstring muscles posteriorly, the popliteal vessels are encountered in the popliteal fossa.[1]

LOWER SEGMENT: When extensive exposure of the popliteal artery is required and particularly when a femoropopliteal graft or thrombo-endarterectomy is contemplated, the medial approach is superior. It also allows access to the saphenous vein which may be required as the graft.

The patient lies supine with the knee moderately flexed and the thigh externally rotated.

A vertical incision is made a finger's breadth behind the posterior border of the upper tibia (*Fig.* 541). The long saphenous vein and nerve are protected. The deep fascia is incised and the space exposed between the medial head of the gastrocnemius posteriorly and the tibial origin of the soleus muscle anteriorly. Blunt dissection in this space exposes the medial popliteal nerve, the popliteal vein, and the popliteal artery in this order.

If, in addition, the mid-popliteal artery requires exposure, division of the gracilis, semitendinosus, and sartorius muscles

---

[1] Henry, A. K., *Extensive Exposure*, 2nd ed., 1959. Edinburgh: Livingstone.

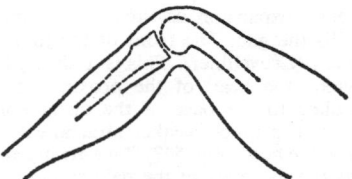

Fig. 541.—The incision for exposing the lower part of the popliteal artery.

together with the medial head of the gastrocnemius gives excellent exposure.

Operations for any purpose whatever in the popliteal area may be followed by:

a. Contracture or keloid formation in the scar. Incisions should therefore be wavy rather than straight.

b. Drop foot. The tibial nerve gets many vasa nervorum high up from the gluteals, etc., whereas the peroneal gets only one and that in the popliteal space. The latter nerve is therefore more vulnerable than the former to the effects of obliterative vascular disease or operative trauma causing drop foot. Motor are more affected than sensory fibres and the prognosis for recovery is good. In this connexion it is noteworthy that Bentley and Schlapp[1] show that when the nutrient vessels of a peripheral nerve have been occluded, the nerve may be oxygenated by diffusion from surrounding tissues.

IX. DIGITS AND DRAINAGE

Impairment of the venous drainage of the lower limb occasions so much disability, and so much attention has been devoted to it, that the problems due to defective drainage in the upper limb are in danger of being overlooked by the student.

Moberg's[2] writings on the subject are illuminating.

The Digits:

THE DIGITAL JOINTS: Knowledge of the metacarpophalangeal and interphalangeal joint anatomy is essential to the accurate diagnosis and proper handling of surgical conditions of the fingers. At the carpometacarpal joint the head of the metacarpal articulates with the first phalanx, forming a condyloid joint, allowing flexion, extension, and slight side-to-side movement. The interphalangeal are plane or hinge joints permitting flexion and extension alone. All these joints have weak capsular ligaments, defective posteriorly,

---

[1] Bentley, F. H., and Schlapp, W., *J. Physiol.*, 1943, 102, 62. Quoted by Kendall, D.
[2] Moberg, E., *Surg. Clins N. Am.*, 1960, 40, 367. The writer is indebted to this article for much of this section.

where the extensor expansion, assisted by the lumbrical interosseous component, fills the gap. The front of the joint is formed by the palmar ligament (Cruveilhier). This is a strong fibro-cartilaginous plate with which the head of the proximal bone articulates. It is firmly attached to the base of the distal bone and thins out proximally to gain a much weaker attachment to the metacarpal just proximal to the head (*Fig.* 542). This arrangement allows flexion at the joint as the thin part of the palmar ligament can buckle. If these joints are dislocated and the palmar ligament is avulsed the tear is much more likely to occur at the weak proximal attachment. It may be displaced between the bone ends and interfere with reduction. Dislocation of any finger-joint implies *ipso facto* the rupture of ligaments.

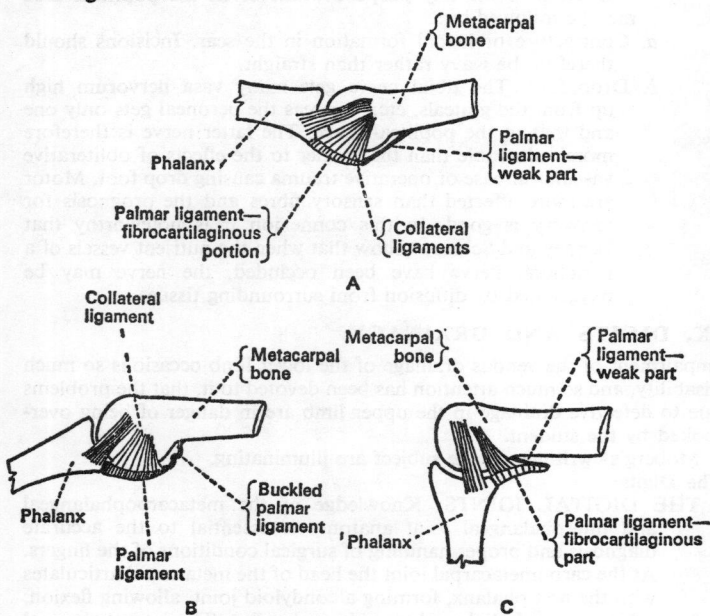

Fig. 542.—These diagrams show the anatomy of the accessory ligaments of the metacarpophalangeal joints in different positions. A, The joint is extended. The palmar ligament is tense, the collateral ligament is lax. Note the attachment of the latter structure to the former. B, The joint is semi-flexed. The thin part of the palmar ligament is buckled. The collateral ligament is lax. C, The joint is fully flexed. The palmar and collateral ligaments are tense. (*Modified from Moberg.*)

RELATIONSHIPS OF VASCULAR PATTERN 569

If a sesamoid exists at the joint it is buried in the fibrocartilaginous palmar ligament. At the sides this ligament is joined in the transverse plane by the deep transverse ligaments of the palm and in the vertical plane by the collateral ligaments. The fibrous flexor sheath is attached to the palmar ligament and the long flexors rest on it (*Fig.* 543). The joint is strengthened at the sides by the powerful collateral ligaments which run from the back of the proximal bone to the front of the distal one gaining additional attachment to the

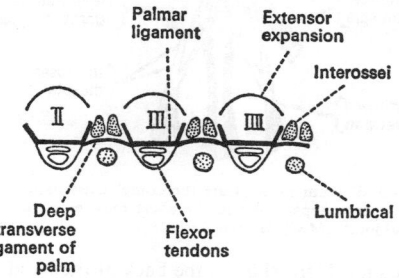

Fig. 543.—A diagram showing a transverse section of II, III, and IIII metacarpophalangeal joints to demonstrate their intimate relationships to the long and short muscles.

palmar ligament. These ligaments are lax in extension and tense in flexion. The interphalangeal joints are essentially similar in structure to the metacarpophalangeal ones.

RELATED STRUCTURES: Reference to the diagram (*Fig.* 544) shows how the musculotendinous apparatus, on which finger movement depends, is wrapped around the metacarpophalangeal joints. Much the same applies to the interphalangeal joints with appropriate changes for their location.

The loosely applied term—sprain—is gradually being replaced by more exact diagnosis. Tears of ligaments can often be diagnosed and localized and may require surgical repair. Their proper treatment implies a knowledge of how they function and what position is necessary for coaptation.

When the anatomical example given above of the disposition of tissues in the joints is taken in conjunction with the fact that this wonderful packaging applies *pari passu* to the hand as a whole, it will be appreciated that to maintain or restore meticulous functions of that member, following injury, imposes a grave burden on the surgeon. Injury implies swelling, so does repair.

The palmar fascia is so dense that interstitial fluids must pass

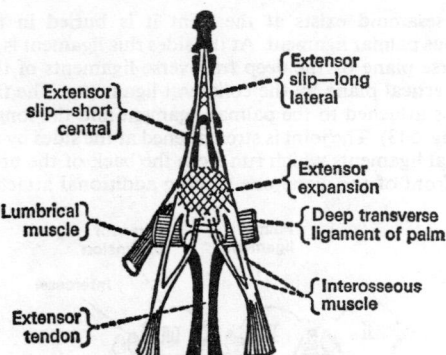

Fig. 544.—A diagram to illustrate the complicated nature of the arrangements of the extensor apparatus and the short muscles in relation to a metacarpophalangeal joint. (*Modified from Entin.*)

to the dorsum. If the skin on the back of the hand is lifted with the examiner's fingers when the digits are extended and a fist is made, it is apparent that there is no slack. Thus even swelling of the skin may impede flexion.

The Drainage: The venous return (with which lymphatic drainage is so closely allied) depends on the *vis-a-fronte* of the blood-pressure, and the *vis-a-tergo* supplied by several factors, notably muscle contraction. The feet swell during the prolonged inactivity of a journey by air. The same may occur in feet or hands in very ill patients confined to bed. The calf muscles form the venous pump in the lower limb. Use of the upper limb for any purpose entails use of the hand, which is so constructed that, whenever it is used, the pumping mechanism comes into action. The osteofascial compartments of forearm and arm comprise additional pumping relays. Breakdown of the pumping mechanism, local or widespread, necessarily follows lack of mobility. Injury to a finger, or any part of the limb, means restricted movement due to pain, swelling, splintage, etc. Exudates and tissue fluids stagnate, and though ultimately they dissipate, there may remain some deposition of proteins, and thickening of tissue, with resultant restriction of mobility. Thus splinting a finger in extension causes shortening of the collateral ligaments which means impaired flexion. Fixing the wrist in *full* extension (as opposed to the moderate extension of the position of rest) will cause adhesion of tendons to sheaths in older persons who have splints applied for a lesion perhaps not related to these tendons.

It is not yet common knowledge that the sympathetic component to a limb is necessarily also involved in injury. Pain may evoke pathological vascular reflexes which add a dire factor to the problem if local hyperalgesia occurs. Major and minor causalgias may follow. This implies further immobility and oedema. Joint and tendon functions become restricted, osteoporosis occurs, until finally the fingers, the hand, or the entire limb may become seriously damaged. This sequence of events, restricted mobility, oedema, and organization of exudates, is the cause of the frozen hand, the shoulder-hand syndrome, and the numerous minor degrees of functional impairment. It is specially noteworthy that a relatively minor or even forgotten injury may set this train of events in progress. Even distant lesions (myocardial, etc.) not primarily affecting the limb at all may act as the trigger mechanism, the common factor being the syncytial nature of the sympathetic nervous system.

THE SHOULDER-JOINT is an outstanding example of the consequences of defective drainage due to injury and disuse. It is a common site of fractures, dislocations, and lesions of the musculotendinous cuff. Most are treated with the arm at the side and the forearm on the body, in the sling position. Following operations on the breast the limb is in a similar position, and even though the patient is enjoined to 'put the hand to the back of the head', the danger to restriction of shoulder mobility is still there. Stagnation

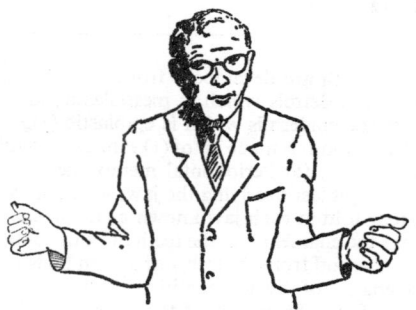

Fig. 545.—The position of the forearms which is necessary to maintain abduction at the shoulder-joint.

of periarticular fluids due to trauma and/or lack of mobility produces defective movement because the pumps have not been working.

A special factor operates at the shoulder-joint. Reference to p. 201 will serve as a reminder that the second 90° of abduction at this joint can only occur if the limb is fully rotated outwards. When the arm is at the side and the forearm across the chest it is fully rotated inwards. Organization of stagnant fluids causes contraction of periarticular ligaments and muscles (subscapularis, latissimus dorsi, pectoralis major, etc.). Restriction of external rotation and abduction ensues which is very troublesome or impossible to correct. This is always regrettable, more particularly if it follows an injury or operation not directly related to the joint, e.g., a lesion of the hand or an operation for cancer of the breast. Most, if not all, such cases could be prevented if the practitioner in charge made it a personal duty to secure full external rotation of the limb daily. This simple manœuvre is demonstrated by keeping both elbows at the side of the body with the forearms at right-angles in the transverse plane (*Fig.* 545). When freer movement becomes possible full abduction can be executed.

Failure to appreciate the inter-relationships between trauma, on the one hand, and mobility and drainage, on the other, may lead to disaster, just as a minor fracture may result in a major deformity if the principles of treatment are not observed.

Chapter XXXV

THE TEETH

Development: The teeth are developed[1] from the skin, the dentine being derived from the dermis which is mesoblastic, and the covering of enamel from the epidermis which is epiblastic (*Fig.* 546).

Constituent Parts: A tooth is made up of (1) Pulp; (2) Dentine; (3) Enamel; (4) Crusta petrosa; (5) Periodontal membrane.

ENAMEL: The epiblast overlying the jaws grows into them, forming a semicircular fold in each jaw known as the *dental shelf*. From this shelf arises the enamel of all the teeth of both dentitions. The dental shelf first gives off from its deep surface ten buds in each jaw. These form the enamel of the first dentition. Posterior to them other buds arise which form the enamel of the second dentition.

DENTINE: As each enamel bud grows downwards it becomes hollowed out and cup-shaped and meets a condensation of mesoblast which is partly surrounded by the enamel bud (*Fig.* 546). The epithelial cells comprising the bud lay down the enamel of the crown. The more superficial cells of the enamel bud do not form enamel, but persist as the cuticular membrane which covers the enamel at birth, being, however, soon worn off (Nasmyth's membrane). The

[1] This account of the development of the teeth is essentially that given by Keith, *Human Embryology and Morphology*, 3rd ed., 163.

THE TEETH 573

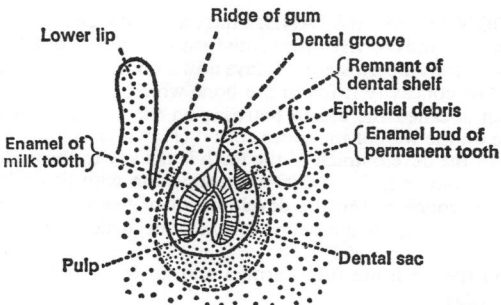

Fig. 546.—Anatomy of a developing tooth. (*After Keith.*)

condensed mesoblast within the enamel bud forms the dentine. This mesoblast lays down a very dense bone at the periphery which is the dentine or ivory, and within this is the tooth pulp. There is an aperture in the base of the dentine where the vessels and nerves enter the pulp.

DENTAL SAC: The inverted cup-shaped enamel bud becomes surrounded by a dense layer of mesoblast known as the dental sac. When the tooth erupts, it breaks its way through that part of the sac overlying the crown of the tooth.

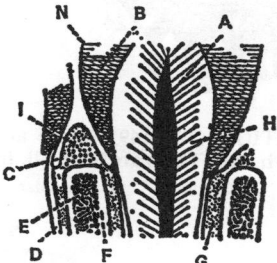

Fig. 547.—Anatomy of the tooth and its socket. A, Pulp. B, Enamel. C, Gingival trough lined by epithelium. D, Cementum which secures the ends of the fibrous bundles to the dentine. E, Cancellous bone of interdental septum. F, Lamina dura, which appears as a white line in an X-ray, and is continuous over the top of the septum in the neck socket. G, Periodontal membrane, which appears as a black line in an X-ray—it has strong fibrous bands which sling the tooth in its socket. H, Dentine. I, Interdental papilla, not visible in X-ray, greatly filling the spaces between the teeth. N, Nasmyth's membrane, an epithelial layer covering the enamel and reflected on to the gum at the termination of the enamel in the gingival trough. (*After C. Bowdler Henry, 'Lancet', 1930, March 1.*)

574 A SYNOPSIS OF SURGICAL ANATOMY

PERIODONTAL MEMBRANE: That part of the dental sac surrounding all but the crown of the tooth forms the periodontal membrane. This is really a periosteum. It lays down bone on both its surfaces—from its concavity it forms the bone which covers the dentine and which is called the crusta petrosa; on the convexity it lays down bone on the wall of the tooth socket (*Fig.* 547).

The nature of the development of the teeth is the key to the understanding of the tumours which may arise in connexion with them. Parts of the structures concerned in the development of teeth may persist, being known as the paradental debris of Malassez, which will be referred to again.

On eruption the teeth are fully formed and grow no further.

Dental Formulae:

FIRST DENTITION (*Fig.* 548): These teeth appear between the sixth and twenty-fourth months, the lower ones preceding the upper. There are twenty in all. There are no premolars, the formula being:

Incisor	Canine	Premolar	Molar
2	1	0	2

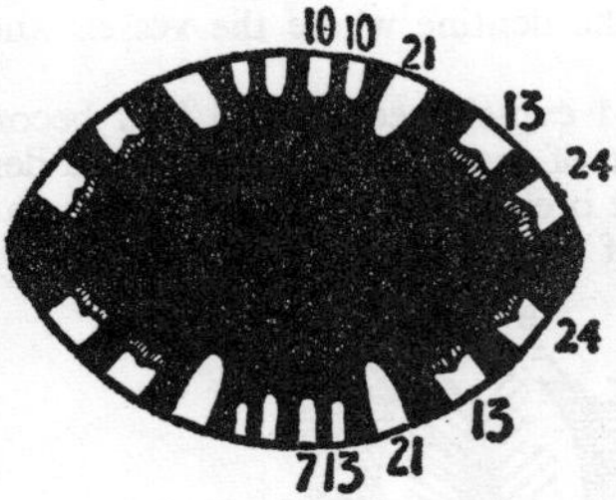

Fig. 548.—Teeth of first dentition, showing month of eruption on one side. (*After Hamilton Bailey.*)

SECOND DENTITION (*Fig.* 549): These appear between the sixth and twenty-fifth year. There are 32 in all, the formula being:

Incisor	Canine	Premolar	Molar
2	1	2	3

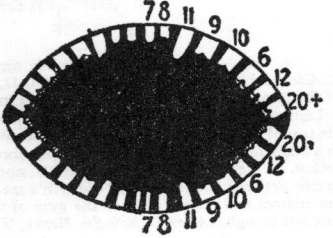

Fig. 549.—Teeth of permanent dentition, with year of eruption shown. (*After Hamilton Bailey.*)

Osteomyelitis of the Jaw: Mowlem[1] sheds valuable light on the aetiology of osteomyelitis of the jaw in relation to dental extractions. He shows that whereas this disease is met on occasions in the mandible, it is never seen in the upper jaw. The reason is dependent on the blood-supply. In the lower jaw incisor extraction may be followed by limited areas of osteomyelitis. The further back in the jaw extraction is done, the greater the possibility of more widespread bone infection, as the inferior alveolar or dental artery is in relation to the back teeth. Osteomyelitis is due to direct trauma to main vessels, or to thrombosis consequent on infection. The blood-supply to the upper jaw is segmental and vertical; it is not dependent on a single vessel, and thus trauma or infection is most unlikely to cause a cutting off of the blood-supply to the teeth.

Extraction of deciduous teeth is not followed by the risk of these grave complications, not because of a difference in the bacterial flora, but because damage to the main artery to the lower jaw is prevented by the teeth of the second dentition intervening between teeth and vessel, or because the extraction of deciduous teeth is associated with much less trauma than that attendant on the removal of permanent teeth.

Odontomes: A generic term applied to tumours arising from the parts concerned in the development of the teeth. Surrounding the roots of the teeth are numerous microscopic vestiges of the structures which give rise to teeth. This debris (*Fig.* 550) has been called the paradental

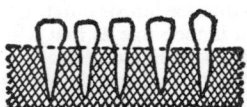

Fig. 550.—Diagrammatic representation of the paradental debris (cross-hatched).

debris (Malassez). Malassez compared the relation of this debris to the roots of the teeth with the relation of wire netting (the debris) nailed to a row of palings (the teeth). It is from these vestiges that some odontomes arise.

---

[1] *Br. med. J.*, 1944, **1**, 517.

Chapter XXXVI

THE LIMPS OF INFANTILE PARALYSIS. 'SNAPPING' JOINTS

I. THE LIMPS OF INFANTILE PARALYSIS[1]

These are the results of anatomical loss. One muscle or group of muscles may be paralysed, producing characteristic alterations in the gait of the patient. To the experienced eye the diagnosis of the anatomical loss can often be made by an observance of the gait. Nine characteristic limps are described by Jones and Lovett—those due to paralysis of the: (1) Gluteus medius; (2) Gluteus maximus; (3) Hip adductors; (4) Hip flexors; (5) Quadriceps; (6) Gastrocnemius; (7) Dorsal flexors of the foot; (8) Abdominal muscles; (9) Spinal muscles.

Gluteus Medius Limp: The function of this muscle is complicated. Its actions are:
1. To abduct the limb.
2. To tilt the pelvis to the side on which weight is being borne in walking. This gives the opposite limb room between the pelvis and the ground to move forward in taking a step.

Loss of this function causes the patient to lurch over to the affected side in bearing weight on that side. It is very like the limp produced by unilateral congenital dislocation of the hip. In this condition the patient lurches to the affected side but also somewhat forwards. In that due to a paralysed gluteus medius the limp is purely lateral, having no forward element in it. The gait is the same as that which arises from marked shortening of the leg on one side (*Fig.* 551, A). The limp can be distinguished temporarily by giving the patient a 4·5-kg. weight to carry in the hand on the affected side. This acts by changing the centre of gravity and compensates for the loss of the muscle. This limp is the most difficult of all to treat, as it cannot be disguised by any apparatus.

Gluteus Maximus Limp: When the main extensor of the thigh is paralysed the resulting walk is unsightly, as when weight is borne on the affected side, the body is suddenly jerked back and the next step with the sound limb is hurried.

Loss of the Adductors of the Hip: This does not cause a limp. The loss may be difficult to detect, but can be accentuated by asking the patient to put one foot directly in front of the other in walking. When the adductors are paralysed this can only be done by swinging the trunk round with each step.

---

[1] The information in this section is taken from Jones and Lovett's *Orthopaedic Surgery*. 1923, 452–3. London.

Hip Flexor Limp: When the iliopsoas is paralysed the limb on the affected side can only be brought forward on taking a step by twisting the body forward (*Fig.* 551, B).

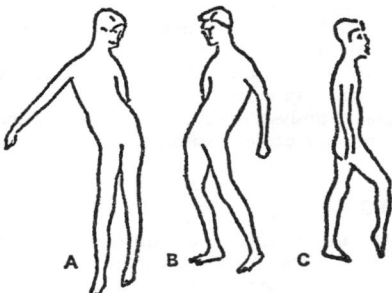
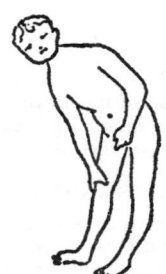

Fig. 551.—Limps. A, Gait in paralysis of gluteus medius of right side. B, Gait in paralysis of hip flexors. C, Gait in paralysis of dorsiflexors of foot. (*After Jones and Lovett.*)

Fig. 552.—Gait in quadriceps paralysis. (*After Jones and Lovett.*)

Quadriceps Limp: This huge muscle extends the knee. It is therefore one of the main muscles concerned in walking, as the ability to bear the body-weight on the knee depends on its efficiency. In going upstairs, and especially downstairs, the quadriceps plays an extremely important part. A stringent test for any muscle which is transplanted to take the place of the quadriceps is that the patient be able to walk downstairs without falling. When the muscle is paralysed the patient may be able to walk without apparatus by using one of the following manœuvres, thus preventing the knee from doubling up beneath him:
1. The thigh is kept pressed back by the patient's hand, thus preventing flexion of the knee (*Fig.* 552).
2. The thigh is hyperextended, locking the joint.
3. The patient in walking rotates the whole lower limb in or out, so that it cannot bend on bearing weight.
4. If the hamstrings are strong the patient can carry the centre of gravity forward by bending the body forward so that he walks without full extension of the knee.

Gastrocnemius Limp: In walking the heel is brought down first, the gait being clumsy with no springiness. When one side only is affected, the gait is irregular, a longer pause being made on the good than on the affected foot. If both sides are affected, the gait is waddling, the feet being bent upwards.

Loss of the Dorsiflexors of the Foot: The condition of 'drop foot' ensues (*Fig.* 551, C). The patient has to lift the foot high off the ground in walking to let the toes clear the ground.

Loss of the Abdominal Muscles: The abdominal muscles play a part in walking, producing a slight 'roll' in the act. When they are weak the patient stands or walks with flexed hips, marked lordosis, and a pot belly. With unilateral paralysis of the abdominal muscles, and especially of the quadratus lumborum, the pelvis on the affected side is dropped in taking the weight on the leg on the sound side.

Loss of the Extensors of the Spine: Paralysis or severe weakening of these muscles makes walking or sitting erect impossible, unless a support is applied to the spine.

II. 'SNAPPING' JOINTS

This is a peculiar and rare condition in which a certain movement of a joint is accompanied by an audible click. It may occur in an otherwise normal joint, or more commonly in one the seat of disease. In osteo- and rheumatoid arthritis grating sounds are common in joints; at the knee, for instance, creakings are often heard when the joint is flexed and extended. We are here only concerned with clicks in healthy joints.

Snapping Hip: F. H. Albee[1] describes two types: (1) Intra-articular type; (2) Extra-articular type.

1. INTRA-ARTICULAR TYPE: This may occur in children, otherwise normal, when the thigh is flexed and adducted, and is due to the head of the femur slipping over the upper border of the acetabulum. It is rare, and only likely to occur with flabby muscles and a lax capsule.
2. EXTRA-ARTICULAR TYPE: There are several possible causes:
   a. Friction between the gluteus maximus or fascia lata and the great trochanter. In extension the muscle or fascia into which it is inserted slips over the trochanter with an audible snap.
   b. The slipping of some other tendon over a bony prominence round the joint.

Snapping or Clicking Knee: May be due to:

1. Recurrent subluxation of mild degree owing to the tibia slipping forward or rotating outwards on the femur in extension. It is common in infants. Laxity of the capsule necessarily coexists.
2. Undue mobility of the lateral meniscus (external semilunar cartilage).
3. Slipping of the biceps, semimembranosus, or some other tendon over a bony projection—usually an exostosis.
4. Discoid lateral meniscus. This is an interesting congenital anomaly. During the very early development of the menisci, these bodies are roughly circular, and only later, when absorption of the central

[1] *Orthopedic and Reconstruction Surgery*, 1919, 449. Philadelphia.

part occurs, do they become semilunar. Should this absorption fail to occur, discoid meniscus results. The condition is found in the young, often below the age of ten years, affects the lateral meniscus, is often bilateral, and causes an audible click and a palpable jar in flexion or extension of the knee. With this there is associated pain. All these symptoms result from disharmony in the joint and are not associated with trauma. The condition is treated by excision of the affected meniscus.

Slipping Peroneus Longus: The tendon of this muscle runs down to pass behind the external malleolus. It may, owing to laxity of the peroneal retinaculum, slip out of its groove on to the outer surface of the malleolus. The condition is painful and may be accompanied by a click. It is treated by forming a bony shelf projecting back from the malleolus to prevent the tendon becoming dislocated.

Trigger Finger: This is a condition sometimes encountered in a finger where the digit cannot be extended after it has been flexed, so that on extending the closed hand the affected finger remains flexed. The patient usually pulls it straight with his other hand, the extension occurring with a sudden recoil. It is due to a localized disparity between the size of the tendon and its sheath, i.e., local enlargement of the tendon, or constriction of its sheath. The same series of events may occur on again flexing the finger. The middle and ring fingers are usually affected, though any of the others or even the thumb may be affected.

Snapping Jaw: By this is meant an audible snap in one or other temporomandibular joint on opening and closing the mouth. It is due to too free movement of the intra-articular disc or cartilage which sometimes needs removal because of the annoyance caused by the condition. It is an occasional complication which follows reduction of a dislocated jaw, being again due to too great a range of mobility of the disc consequent on the stretching of the joint ligaments.

Snapping Neck: Cases have occurred[1] where extension of the neck from a flexed position is accompanied by an audible click which is painful and occurs whenever the neck is straightened. It is due to friction between the 5th and 6th cervical spines. It is cured by removal of one of these processes.

---

[1] Lang, *Zentbl. Chir.*, 1917, No. 4, quoted by Royal Whitman, *Orthopaedic Surgery*, 1924, 233. London.

Chapter XXXVII

THE PATHOLOGY OF BONE IN TERMS OF ANATOMY

From the developmental point of view there are two types of bones: (1) Membrane bones—in which the bone develops in a membrane; (2) Cartilage bones—in which the bone is laid down in cartilage.

Anatomical Facts:

MEMBRANE BONES: These are for the most part flat bones, e.g., the bones forming the vault of the skull and face. The clavicle and mandible are also membrane bones.

CARTILAGE BONES: These are of different shapes and lengths, e.g., long, short, short long, flat, and irregular bones. All except some of the irregular bones have primary and secondary ossific centres. Cartilage bones comprise the greater part of the skeleton.

THE CONSTITUENT PARTS OF A LONG BONE BEFORE THE COMPLETION OF GROWTH (*Fig.* 553): The bone consists of:

1. The diaphysis or shaft.
2. The epiphysis, of which each long bone has at least one at either end, and often several. One of the epiphyses at each end is covered with articular cartilage, and all or part of this epiphysis is inside the capsule of the joint.

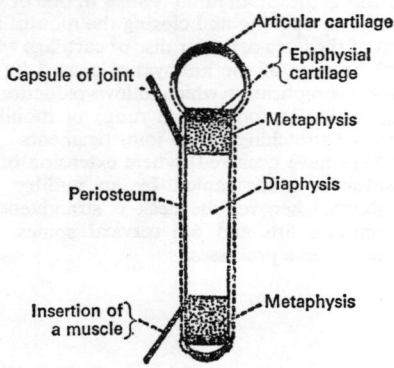

Fig. 553.—Some features of the anatomy of bone. Observe: (1) Dipping in of periosteum at epiphysial line. (2) Fusion of capsule with periosteum. (3) Attachment of the tendon of a muscle to the bone in the metaphysial region.

3. **The epiphysial cartilage**: this is a plate of cartilage intervening between the epiphysis and the end of the diaphysis. From this cartilage the growth in length of the bone occurs by additions of osseous tissue to the related parts of epiphysis and diaphysis.

4. **The metaphysis** is that part of the *diaphysis* which abuts on the epiphysial plate. It is highly vascular; it is less strong than the rest of the diaphysis.

5. **The periosteum**: this structure consists of two layers, the inner of which is tacked down to the epiphysial line, continuing on over the epiphysis to blend with the articular cartilage. The outer layer is continuous with the joint capsule. Pus deep to both layers is prevented, therefore, by the above-mentioned 'tacking down' from extending on to the epiphysis (*Fig.* 554). The periosteum is a vascular membrane assisting in the blood-supply of the bone, and is an osteogenic structure, depositing bone on the surface of the shaft and thus adding to its girth.

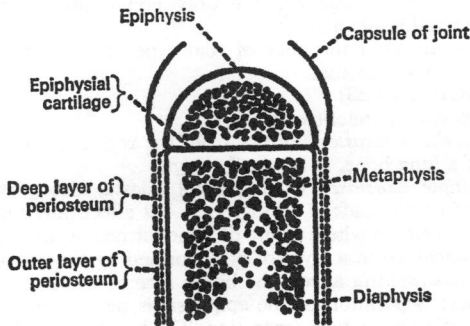

Fig. 554.—Figure showing relation of periosteum to epiphysial cartilage and capsule of the joint. Observe that pus between periosteum and bone cannot spread beyond the epiphysial cartilage because the deep layer of the periosteum blends with this structure; notice also that the outer layer of the periosteum is continuous with the capsule of the joint.

LONG BONES AFTER GROWTH IS COMPLETE: The bone consists now of a solid osseous structure with neither epiphyses, metaphyses, nor epiphysial cartilages.

Pathological Facts: Diseases of bone show a decided predilection for certain anatomical sites, and the same may be said of tumours affecting bone. So, too, some diseases attack membrane bones for choice, others select cartilage bones.

MEMBRANE BONES:

1. Although frequently complicated in shape, their ossification is for the most part simple, e.g., one or two ossific centres only, as they are protective and not weight-bearing.
2. They have very poor regenerative powers; thus the bones of the skull vault show no regenerative power, so that the defects occasioned by trauma or disease are permanent unless filled in by bone-grafting. The mandible shows, however, strong regenerative powers.
3. Association with special pathological conditions:
    a. They escape pathological change in the disease of achondroplasia.
    b. They are the only bones affected in the disease of cranio-cleido-dysostosis.
    c. They may be affected by acute pyogenic osteomyelitis though this is uncommon.
    d. They are more often affected by chronic osteomyelitis, e.g., tuberculous, and are the only bones affected by creeping periostitis (leontiasis).
    e. They are common sites of that type of bone growth known as ivory osteoma.

CARTILAGE BONES:

1. CONGENITAL BONE DISEASE:
    a. *Cancellous Exostosis* grows from the region of the metaphysis of a long bone. It is usually single.
    b. *Multiple Exostoses*, or diaphysial aclasia, also grow from the end of the shaft of a long bone, but affect only those parts of the skeleton where a core of bone formed in cartilage becomes ensheathed in a layer of bone formed by the periosteum.
    c. *Achondroplasia* affects the bones formed in cartilage.
2. TRAUMA: Separation of the epiphysis is never a pure separation but rather a fracture separation. The break occurs through that part of the metaphysis which abuts on the epiphysial cartilage. The lesion occurs in youth as a result of that form of violence which would produce a dislocation in the adult. It is of great importance to realize that the epiphysial cartilage is displaced with the epiphysis adhering to the latter, as the future growth of the bone depends on the reposition of the separated fragment in its proper situation.
3. INFECTION:
    a. Acute osteomyelitis: this is a disease of childhood. It has a marked predilection for the long bones. The part of the bone affected is the metaphysis, because of the rich blood-supply and delicate nature of the bony lamellae in this region. These considerations in the presence of mild injury to the bone and a

symptomless bacteriaemia may precipitate the formation of acute abscess of bone. Because of the unyielding nature of bone, acute inflammation spreads with great rapidity in its interior, resulting in speedy death of portions of the bone. Hence the need of urgent treatment in acute osteomyelitis. The inability of bone to expand also accounts for the great pain resulting from disease in it.

b. Chronic osteomyelitis, due to causes like tuberculosis, typhoid, etc., often chooses the metaphysis of a long bone, but has a tendency also to affect bones like ribs, os innominatum, sternum, etc.

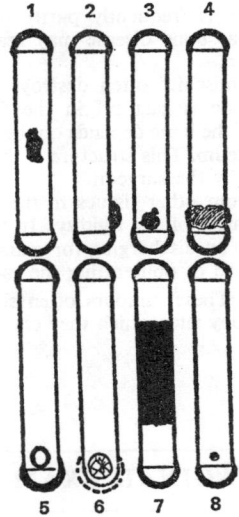

Fig. 555.—Pathology of bone in terms of anatomy. The characteristic situations of the various types of tumours of bone. The cross line is the epiphysial cartilage. 1, Metastatic carcinoma. 2, Periosteal fibrosarcoma. 3, Solitary chondroma. 4, Osteogenic sarcoma. 5, Solitary cyst of osteitis fibrosa. 6, Benign giant-cell tumour. 7, Ewing's tumour. 8, Acute osteomyelitis.

c. Tuberculous and syphilitic disease of the short long bones, metacarpals, and phalanges is located in the middle of the diaphysis instead of at the metaphysis because of the peculiarities of the blood-supply of these bones.

Tuberculosis of a vertebra begins in one of three sites:

i. In the upper or lower metaphysis of the body of the bone, i.e., just beneath the plate of cartilage in relation to the epiphysis of the upper or lower surface of the body. This is the type which affects children.
ii. Just beneath the anterior longitudinal ligament where the vessels supplying the front of the body of the bone enter it. This is the type which often affects adults.
iii. In one of the vertebral processes. This is rare.

d. The epiphysis is relatively immune to bone disease except by extension from the shaft or neighbouring joint, but osteomyelitis, especially syphilitic, sometimes attacks this part of the bone.

e. The metaphysis is frequently partly or wholly intracapsular. It follows that bone disease may readily erupt into a joint and vice versa.

f. Inflammatory mischief often destroys large parts of a bone. The dead bone is cast off in the form of sequestra. The restoration of the bone depends on the bone-forming functions of the periosteum. This structure is therefore treated with the greatest care by the surgeon.

g. Bone differs from other tissues in the body in that it cannot contract because of its rigidity. It follows that cavities in bone often go on discharging for years or for life unless some surgical method of obliterating the cavity is resorted to.

TUMOURS OF BONES: These tumours often show a remarkable constancy in the bony sites which they choose (*Fig.* 555).

Chapter XXXVIII

RECTAL AND VAGINAL EXAMINATION

The doctor may obtain information of great value by digital examination per rectum (P.R.) or per vaginam (P.V.)

Information to be gained P.R.:

IN THE MALE:
1. The external sphincter ani is felt like a roll of tissue if contracted.
2. The internal sphincter ani is felt as a narrowing of the anal canal for 2·5 cm. above the external sphincter.
3. The rectum proper is appreciated as a relatively capacious tube above (2).

ANTERIORLY:
   4. The membranous urethra is not palpable. A stone in it may be felt, so may a bougie.
   5. The bulbo-urethral (Cowper's) glands may, if enlarged as they sometimes are in gonorrhoea, be felt between the finger in the rectum and the thumb on the perineum.
   6. The prostate—its apex, lateral, and posterior lobes—may be felt. Stones in the gland may impart a gritty feeling to the examining finger as they rub against each other. Prostatic tissue separates a bougie in the prostatic urethra from the rectal finger. Should the bougie be pushed through the wall of the bulbous or membranous urethra (false passage), it is felt much more distinctly by the examining finger, being then between the prostate and the anterior rectal wall.
   7. The seminal vesicles, indistinctly felt when healthy, and lower ends of the deferent ducts are felt above the prostate when diseased.
   8. The trigone of the bladder is felt between the vesicles, particularly if the bladder is full. A stone here may possibly be felt. If the prostate is much enlarged, the finger cannot reach the bladder.
   9. Rectovesical pouch. The distance of the floor of this pouch from the anus varies according to whether the bladder is full or empty, being 7·5 cm. from the anus in the former case, and 5 cm. in the latter. It is therefore within reach of the examining finger, and a mass here formed by a tumour or a collection of fluid is palpable.

POSTERIORLY:
   10. Coccyx and sacrum—irregularities of these bones and tumours in relation to them.
   11. Lymph-glands, if enlarged, behind the rectum.

EXTERNALLY:
   12. The ischiorectal fossae.
   13. Bony wall of the true pelvis, ischial spines, and sacrotuberous ligaments.
   14. Internal iliac or hypogastric lymph-glands may be felt if enlarged.

WITHIN THE LUMEN OF THE RECTUM:
   15. Faeces or foreign bodies if present.
   16. Ballooning, i.e., great dilatation of the rectal ampulla, may be found in cases of cancer of the upper rectum.
   17. The lowest transverse fold of the rectum (valve of Houston) can sometimes be felt projecting inwards into the lumen of the bowel.

IN THE FEMALE: The bladder and urethra cannot be felt P.R. in the female. The following may be felt in addition to the appropriate items in the above list:

1. The perineal body.
2. The rectovaginal septum.
3. The cervix and external os uteri.
4. The ovaries, if they have dropped (prolapsed) into the rectovaginal pouch.
5. The uterosacral ligaments.

IN THE CHILD: There may be felt in addition:
1. Structures in the lower abdomen, e.g., pelvic colon.
2. The prostate is vestigial, and therefore even a small stone in the bladder may be felt in boys.

SPECIAL POINTS OF INTEREST:
1. The rectum of a newborn infant admits the index finger of an adult.
2. Piles are *not* palpable, unless some complication, e.g., clotting of the contained blood, makes them so.
3. The size of the os uteri during labour is now frequently determined through the rectal wall. The object of this is to avoid the necessity of making frequent vaginal examinations, with the attendant risks of infection.

Information to be gained P.V.: The condition of:
1. The vagina—abnormalities of its entrance or walls.
2. The urethra—is felt as a cord in the anterior wall, and may be rolled against the symphysis.
3. The rectum—if it contains faeces or a foreign body, or is the site of a tumour. Faeces may be indented by the vaginal finger.
4. The cervix uteri and external os. Normally the cervix slopes downwards and backwards.
5. The roof of the vagina, divided by the cervix into anterior, posterior, right and left lateral fornices.
6. The rectovaginal pouch—the finger in the posterior fornix is separated from this pouch by the thickness of the vaginal wall, pelvic fascia, peritoneum. The pouch is normally empty except for coils of gut. It may contain the uterus, prolapsed ovaries and tubes, inflammatory collections of fluid, tumours, and almost any abdominal viscus. The floor of the rectovaginal pouch varies in distance from the skin of the perineum being 5-7·5 cm. above it. In complete prolapse of the rectum the pouch lies in the rectum or prolapses through the anus.
7. The ureter, if thickened or the seat of a stone, may be rolled against the pelvic bone just before it enters the bladder.
8. The diagonal conjugate of the female pelvis is the distance between the lower border of the symphysis and the promontory of the sacrum. It is a most important measurement in determining whether the pelvis is large enough to transmit the fetal head. It is determined by endeavouring to feel the promontory of the sacrum P.V. and measuring the distance between the landmarks noted.

Bimanual Examination: This examination is conducted with one or two fingers of the right hand in the vagina and the left hand on the lower abdomen, and palpating the structures between the two hands. By this means the pelvic organs may be examined. A bimanual examination may be done in the male, the forefinger of the right hand being in the rectum. Large stones or tumours of pelvic organs may thus at times be felt.

Combination of P.R. and P.V.: In the female valuable information may be gained by examining the patient with the forefinger in the vagina and the adjoining finger in the rectum. The condition of the rectovaginal septum and the pouch of Douglas are best investigated thus. The value of this method of examination cannot be exaggerated. Time and again when a P.V. discloses no apparent pathology the combined method described will enable that additional information to be gained which will permit of the diagnosis being established.

Chapter XXXIX

ANATOMICAL BASES OF CLINICAL TESTS

Milian's Sign: Cellulitis involves the subcutaneous tissues, erysipelas affects the skin. Cellulitis of the face always stops short of the pinna because there is no subcutaneous tissue here, the skin being firmly bound to the underlying cartilage. Erysipelas, on the other hand, may extend on to the pinna. This fact is valuable in distinguishing these conditions.

Psoas Test (Ludloff): In rupture or irritation of the psoas muscle pain is produced in the psoas area when the patient lifts the heel from the bed in the *sitting* position. Other hip flexors are then out of action.

Trendelenburg's Tests: Used in testing for:

1. VARICOSE VEINS:

   ANATOMICAL FACT ON WHICH THE TEST IS BASED: The great saphenous is the longest vein in the body. The column of blood in the vein has to ascend against gravity. The pressure of this column is broken by from 10 to 20 valves in the interior of the vein. Should the vein become distended from the effects of varicosity, the valves cannot occlude the lumen. Near its entrance into the femoral there is a valve. Should this be incompetent the whole force of the blood column in the iliacs and inferior vena cava is thrust upon the long saphenous. The test is used to determine whether the valve at the upper end of the long saphenous vein is functioning efficiently.

PERFORMANCE OF THE TEST: The patient lies down, and the limb which is affected with varicose veins is elevated to empty the veins. The thumb is placed over the saphenous opening (fossa ovalis 3·8 cm. below and 3·8 cm. lateral to the pubic spine), thus occluding the upper end of the long saphenous vein, and the patient is told to rise. When he is erect the thumb is removed from the vein. If the vein fills up slowly from below, the valve at the upper end of the saphenous vein is efficient. If the vein fills up rapidly from above the moment the pressure is removed, then the valve is not efficient. In the latter case Trendelenburg's operation is indicated, i.e., removal of part or whole of the long saphenous vein. This will obviously prevent blood running down into the vein from above.

2. CONGENITAL DISLOCATION OF THE HIP: This sign was first described by Duchenne of Boulogne in 1867.

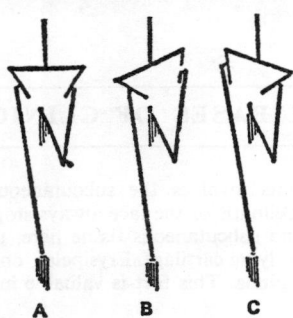

Fig. 556.—Trendelenburg's hip test. A, Normal. B, Appearance sometimes seen in coxa vara. The right is the affected side. C, Congenital dislocation of hip. The right is the affected side.

ANATOMICAL FACT ON WHICH THE TEST IS BASED: Two sets of muscles go from the os innominatum to the femur:

a. The Iliotrochanteric: These are short powerful muscles which go from the ilium to the region of the great trochanter, e.g., glutei, obturators, piriformis, quadratus femoris, etc. These are the muscles which maintain the pelvis at a horizontal level with the patient standing on one leg, *provided the head of the femur is in its socket* (and the bone intact).

b. The Iliofemoral: Long muscles going from the os innominatum to the femur, e.g., adductors and hamstrings. (These muscles do not really arise from the ilium but from the pubis and ischium.) They are not concerned with the balancing of the pelvis in standing on one limb apart from their function as stays to the joints.

PERFORMANCE OF THE TEST: The patient stands on one leg. If the hip-joint on that side is normal, the pelvis rises slightly on the opposite side as determined by the level of the anterior superior iliac spines. If the side the patient is standing on is the site of congenital dislocation of the hip, then the pelvis *sinks on the opposite side* as shown by the level of the spines (*Fig.* 556, C). As the femoral head is out of its socket in dislocation, the iliotrochanteric muscles are not powerful enough to maintain the horizontal position of the pelvis, and the opposite side may be seen to drop lower the longer the patient stands on the affected limb. This is a positive Trendelenburg.

Thomas's Hip Flexion Test:

ANATOMICAL BASIS OF THE TEST: Full flexion of the normal hip-joint with the patient recumbent brings the anterior aspect of the thigh into contact with the anterior abdominal wall and flattens out the normal lumbar curve so that the hand *cannot* be pushed through between the lumbar region of the spine and the mattress. The opposite thigh meanwhile remains in the same plane as the trunk, i.e., flat on the mattress, if the hip-joint on that side is also normal.

When a hip-joint is diseased, e.g., by tuberculosis, the thigh takes up a position of flexion. A considerable degree of flexion of the thigh may be disguised by increasing the forward bend or lordosis of the lumbar spine. The patient may then be seen lying in bed with both lower limbs resting on the mattress, thus entirely hiding the flexion deformity of the hip.

PERFORMANCE OF THE TEST: Thomas showed that this flexion may be clearly indicated by flexing the sound thigh firmly on the abdomen. This flattens out the forward bend of the lumbar spine and the affected thigh is bent up to whatever degree of true flexion exists.

In performing the test the free hand is between the spine and the mattress. As soon as the back touches the hand the pressure on the sound side is discontinued, thus preventing the misleading result which would ensue should the sacrum be tilted off the bed.

Subdeltoid Bursa Test (Dawbarn's Sign):

ANATOMICAL BASIS OF THE TEST: The acromion process is separated from the upper aspect of the shoulder-joint, and the upper half of the deltoid muscle from the surgical neck of the humerus, by a bursa—variously called the subdeltoid or the subacromial. The important point is that there is only one bursa, *which disappears entirely under the acromion when the arm is abducted to a right-angle.*

PERFORMANCE OF THE TEST: If this bursa is inflamed and pressure is applied immediately below the tip of the acromion with the arm by the side, the patient will complain of pain. If now the arm is abducted to a right-angle and pressure made in the same place, no pain will be complained of, as the inflamed bursa has receded under cover of the acromion process. This condition is said by many authors to be due to a sprain of the tendon of insertion of the supraspinatus and not to a bursitis (Bankart[1]). In either case the test is equally applicable.

Palpation of Certain Abdominal Organs:

ANATOMICAL FACT ON WHICH THE PALPATION OF KIDNEYS, SPLEEN, GALL-BLADDER, AND EDGE OF LIVER IS BASED: On inspiration these structures, which possess some mobility, are pushed down by the descent of the diaphragm, and may then come in contact with the palpating fingers.

KIDNEYS: The lower poles of normal kidneys can often be felt in the above way. If the kidney possesses abnormal mobility the whole of the organ may be felt in inspiration. In the condition known as movable kidney, or nephroptosis, the organ becomes unduly mobile. The mobility is often divided into degrees, depending on whether the whole or part of the organ is palpable, and whether it slips up again on expiration or may be retained at the lower level of its excursion by the examiner's hand. It has been stated that the normal kidney may be felt in 90 per cent of cases. This is a degree of accuracy to which few attain. Palpation is easier on the right than on the left, because the examiner usually stands on the right, and also because the right kidney is lower and moves more freely than the left. It is so unusual to palpate the left kidney that an abnormality should be suspected if the organ is felt.

SPLEEN: Is not palpable normally, and must be enlarged to twice[2] its normal size before its lower pole can be felt on inspiration. It is then felt, rather farther round to the left than one would be inclined to think, by pushing the fingers up under the left costal margin at its left extremity, the patient being on his back (Hamilton Bailey[3]). The position of the spleen is variable, for which reason McNee advises that it should always be palpated for in three positions: (1) At the left extremity of the left costal margin; (2) In the middle of the left costal margin; (3) Beneath the epigastric extremity of the left costal margin.

GALL-BLADDER: This structure may be palpated by pushing the fingers up under the right costal margin exactly where the linea

---

[1] *Manipulative Surgery*, 1932. 127. London.
[2] Though smaller degrees of enlargement may occasionally be palpable in thin subjects who relax completely.
[3] *Physical Signs in Clinical Surgery*, 1973. 242. Bristol.

semilunaris (outer border of the rectus) meets it (ninth costal cartilage). In inspiration the liver and gall-bladder descend, and the latter may come within reach of the examiner's fingers. Murphy's test is based on this fact. The sign may be tested for in two ways:
1. The patient sits up and bends forward, thus relaxing the abdominal muscles. The fingers are pushed under the costal margin at the site of the gall-gladder. If the patient now takes a deep breath, the gall-bladder impinges against the examiner's fingers, which are pressing upwards. If the organ is diseased, this pressure against it produces sharp pain and the inspiration is sharply cut off. This is a positive Murphy's sign.
2. With the patient recumbent and the left hand resting on the lower chest in such a fashion that the thumb lies in the gall-bladder angle exerting firm pressure, the patient is told to breathe deeply. If the sign is positive the patient 'catches his breath' when the inflamed gall-bladder comes within scope of the pressure of the examiner's thumb.

Rovsing's Test, or the Opposite-sided Test, in Appendicitis: If the appendix is acutely inflamed, pressure over the left iliac fossa may cause pain in the right iliac fossa. The test is based on the fact that pressure on the left side over the iliac colon displaces gas in the colon upwards and increases the pressure in the caecum, which causes pain by disturbing the inflamed appendix.

Obturator Test: If the appendix hangs over the pelvic brim it rests against the side wall of the pelvis, i.e., on the pelvic fascia and obturator internus muscle—separated from these structures by the peritoneum lining the side wall of the pelvis. If the organ becomes inflamed in this situation, the fascia may become oedematous and inflamed also. If now the obturator internus muscle is stretched by flexing and rotating the thigh inwards, the patient will complain of pain because the stretched muscle pulls on and irritates the overlying inflamed fascia and peritoneum.

Queckenstedt's Test for Spinal Block:
ANATOMICAL BASIS OF THE TEST: The contents of the cranium are packed inside the skull with great economy of space so that any increase of the contents raises the intracranial pressure, and so raises the pressure of the cerebrospinal fluid (normally 110 – 150 mm. of water). This increase is transmitted to the fluid in the spinal subarachnoid space. Compression of both internal jugular veins above the sternal ends of the clavicles dams back blood in the skull and so raises the intracranial pressure. Should a part of the spinal subarachnoid space be completely cut off above by, for example, a tumour, this increase of pressure will not be transmitted to the part of the subarachnoid space below the tumour.

PERFORMANCE OF THE TEST: With the patient lying on his side a lumbar puncture is done at the site of election (between the 3rd and 4th lumbar spines). The hollow needle is connected to a manometer. The jugular veins are compressed. If there is no rise in the pressure of the cerebrospinal fluid in the manometer on carrying out this procedure, there is a block in the subarachnoid space somewhere between the needle and the skull.

In interpreting the result of the test it is to be remembered that a normal response will ensue however much the subarachnoid space be obstructed providing there is an opening not smaller than that of the lumbar puncture needle being used.

Taylor[1] has shown that, provided an expanding spinal tumour does not obstruct the extradural as well as the intradural spinal veins, the Queckenstedt test is unreliable in detecting obstruction of the cerebrospinal fluid pathways above the level of the sixth cervical vertebra. The reason is that jugular compression distends the vertebral venous plexus as low down as the level of C.7. This increase of the venous pressure is transmitted to the theca below the obstruction, causing a rise in the C.S.F. level of the lumbar manometer.

Measurement of the Long Bones: It is sometimes of the first importance in fractures, dislocations, and disease to compare by measurement the lengths of the long bones.

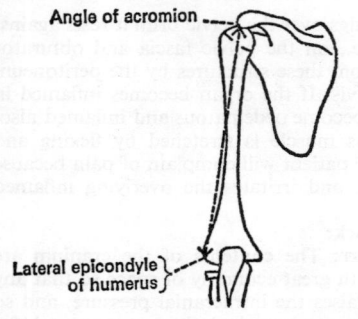

Fig. 557.—Measuring the humerus.

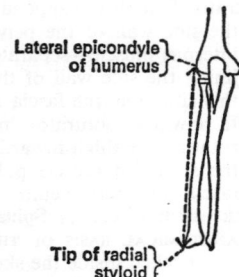

Fig. 558.—Method of determining relative lengths of the radii.

UPPER LIMBS: These measurements are taken with the arm at the side of the body and the elbow bent to a right-angle.

HUMERUS: Measure the distance from the prominent, easily felt angle of the acromion to the lateral epicondyle of the humerus (*Fig.* 557).

[1] Taylor, A. R., *Lancet*, 1960, 2, 1001.

ANATOMICAL BASES OF CLINICAL TESTS 593

RADIUS: Measure from lateral epicondyle of the humerus to the tip of styloid process of the radius (*Fig.* 558).

ULNA: Measure from the upper end of the olecranon to the head of the ulna or tip of its styloid (*Fig.* 559).

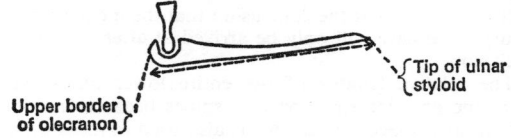

Fig. 559.—Method of measuring the ulna.

RELATIVE LEVELS OF THE RADIAL AND ULNAR STYLOIDS: Of great importance in the diagnosis of fractures of the radius. The radial styloid should project 0·6 cm. distal to the ulnar styloid.

The best method of determining the levels of the styloids of the radius and ulna is as follows (*Fig.* 560). Facing the patient, whose hand is palm downwards, the nail of one of the examiner's index fingers is pushed against the tip of the ulnar styloid. The nail of the other index is pushed against the tip of the other styloid, the examiner's index fingers being flexed at the proximal interphalangeal joints.

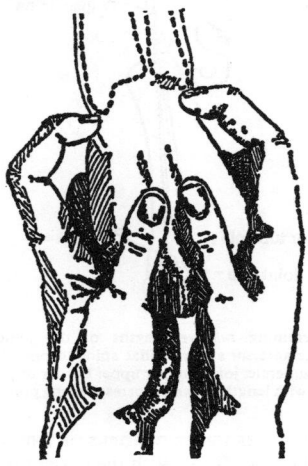

Fig. 560.—Method of palpating styloid processes of radius and ulna.

594 A SYNOPSIS OF SURGICAL ANATOMY

LOWER LIMBS: It is important to remember that the relative lengths of the lower limbs are equal in only 10 per cent of cases. The femur is more liable to inequality than the tibia. A variation of a centimetre in the comparative length of the lower limbs may therefore be looked upon as within the limits of normal. It goes without saying that the conclusion that the inequality is not due to injury or disease will only be arrived at after a careful process of exclusion.

The relative lengths of the entire lower limbs are measured from the anterior superior iliac spines because the upper end of the femur is inaccessible. This is also used in measuring the length of the femur.

LIMB LENGTH: The spines must be exactly on the same horizontal level and the lower limbs extended and symmetrically positioned. The measurement is made from the anterior superior iliac spine to the tip of the medial malleolus.

FEMUR: Measurement is made from the anterior superior iliac spine to one of the following bony points: (1) Adductor tubercle; (2) The lower limit of the medial condyle (joint line); (3) The upper border of the patella (a movable and therefore not very accurate point) (*Fig.* 561).

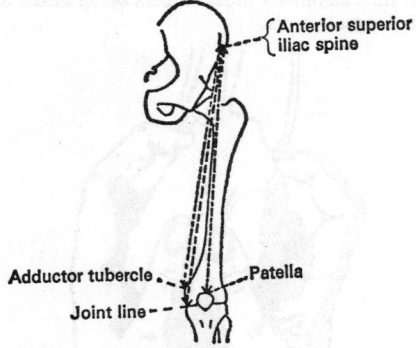

Fig. 561.—Determining *relative* lengths of the femora. Measurements may be made from the anterior superior iliac spine to one of the following bony landmarks: adductor tubercle, joint line, or upper border of patella. Measurement obtained is compared with length between corresponding points on other side.

RELATIVE HEIGHTS OF THE UPPER BORDERS OF THE GREAT TROCHANTERS: *Bryant's Triangle* (*Fig.* 562): With the patient on his back, the lower limbs parallel, and spines of ilia on the same horizontal level:

Mark out the anterior superior iliac spine; mark out the posterior superior angle of the great trochanter. Drop a vertical line from the anterior superior iliac spine. Measure

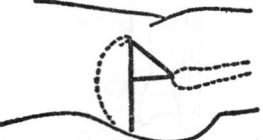

Fig. 562.—Bryant's triangle.

the shortest distance between this line to the posterior superior angle of the great trochanter. This length should be the same on both sides. If it is not, it denotes one of three things (Trethowan): (1) Dislocation of the upper end of the femur; (2) Fracture of the femoral neck; (3) Alteration of neck–shaft angle of the femur, e.g., coxa vara or valga.

Nélaton's Line: The same information may be gained by drawing a line joining the anterior superior iliac spine to the tuberosity of the ischium (*Fig. 563*). This line should touch the upper border of the great trochanter. If the trochanter is above this line, it means that one of the above three conditions exists.

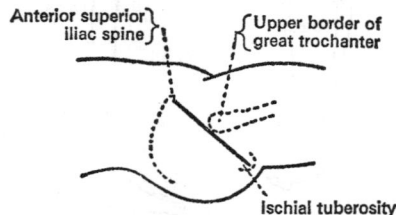

Fig. 563.—Nélaton's line.

TIBIA AND FIBULA: These are readily measured as they are subcutaneous and their extremities can be felt (*Fig. 564*).

BEYERS'S METHOD OF MEASURING THE GIRTH OF THE LIMBS:[1] Beyers is of the opinion that comparative measurements of the circumference of the limbs should follow a standardized routine:

---

[1] A communication to the Johannesburg Junior Clinical and Pathological Club (1930) by the late C. F. Beyers, Surgeon to the Johannesburg General Hospital.

596 A SYNOPSIS OF SURGICAL ANATOMY

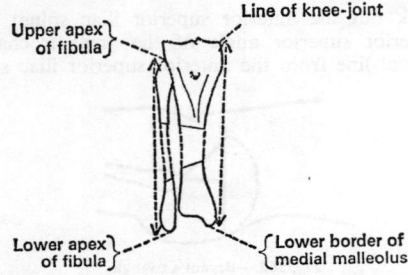

Fig. 564.—Determining the actual lengths of tibia and fibula.

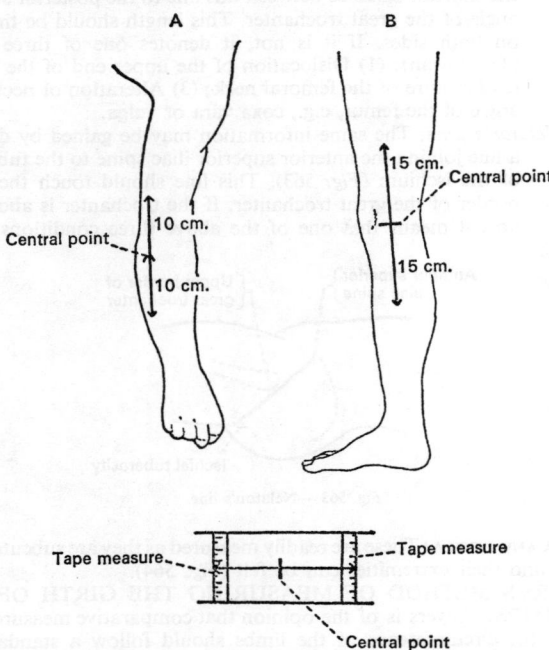

Fig. 565.—Method of measuring the girth of the limbs according to Beyers. **A**, Upper limb. **B**, Lower limb. The lower figure shows how the tape measure is applied in an unvarying manner between the central point and the point where the circumference is to be taken.

Upper limb: The central point is the tip of the olecranon. A point is taken 10 cm. above it and 10 cm. below it. The limb circumference is taken at these two points.

Lower limb: The central point is the joint line (upper border of tibia) on the medial or lateral aspect of the knee. Points are taken 15 cm. above and below the central point and the limb measured.

The tape measure is applied in an unvarying manner with its margin at the level where the measurement is to be made, at right-angles to the long axis of the limb, and between the central point and the point where the record is to be taken (*Fig.* 565).

The method is sound and of great value for teaching. Experienced surgeons agree on the difficulty presented by the anterior superior iliac spine as a point from which to measure, as its accurate localization may be difficult in very stout persons.

Chapter XL

THE ANATOMY GOVERNING THE SURGERY OF THE LYMPHATICS

Anatomical Basis of the Surgical Treatment of Lymphoedema: Lymphoedema results from an interference with lymphatic drainage. This may be:

a. Primary, due to a congenital defect in lymphatic pathways, or

b. Secondary, due to traumatic, inflammatory or neoplastic obstruction of lymphatic flow.

Surgical treatment may consist of mere excision of the lymphoedematous tissue or an attempt to restore lymphatic flow by means of a lympho-venous anastomosis or by reconstruction of lymphatic channels. The latter has been attempted in different ways but the one most frequently used depends on the anatomical fact that the deep fascia forms a barrier to the exchange of lymph between the superficial and deep lymphatic systems.

The lymphoedema seen in the limbs affects only the tissues superficial to the deep fascia and Kondoléon proposed excision of long strips of deep fascia to bring the lymphoedematous superficial tissue into contact with the deep muscles, so enabling the lymph to be removed by the deep lymphatics (*Fig.* 566). Variants of this operation are in use but these operations are only moderately successful.

Lymphatics in Amputations: An important development in the surgery of amputations is the realization of the fact that the lymphatics draining the skin run in the plexus lying on the deep fascia. Therefore the deep

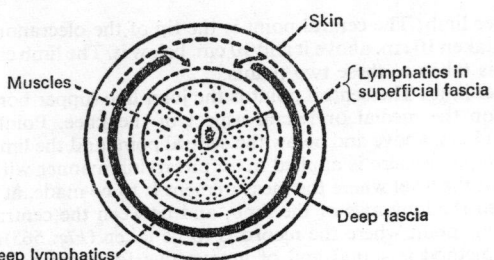

Fig. 566.—Diagram showing anatomical basis of the Kondoléon operation for elephantiasis. At 12 o'clock a segment of deep fascia has been removed to allow the tissues superficial to the deep fascia to be drained by the deep lymphatics as shown by the arrows.

fascia should be dissected up with the skin in amputations and retained in the flaps. This prevents stasis of lymph with swelling of the stump —a matter of prime importance to patient and limb fitter.

Anatomical Principles underlying the Surgery of Colon Cancer: In the preparation of this section extensive use has been made of the article by Morgan and Griffiths,[1] and that by Sonneland, Anson, and Beaton.[2]

Five-year survival statistics for cancer of the colon have greatly improved consequent on wider resections. The aim of the surgeon at operation is twofold: The tumour must be quarantined and not only should the tumour be widely removed, but all the tissues nourished by the artery of supply must also be ablated. Mobilizing the tumour forces cancer cells into the lumen of the bowel and liberates showers of malignant cells into the draining veins. Before the tumour is mobilized the bowel is ligated 30 cm. from it on each side or as far as may be possible. The artery of supply to the area, together with the veins and lymphatics, is divided at its origin from the superior mesenteric artery or the aorta. The tumour is now quarantined and the resection may proceed.

THE EXTENT OF THE RESECTION is governed by several facts. Jamieson and Dobson (1909), in their classic work on the lymph drainage of the colon, showed that cancer cells could skip metastasize, i.e., jump one or more groups of glands draining the cancer area. It must also be appreciated that because the surgeon's impression of the extent of gland involvement is often inaccurate, every case should be treated as though glands were involved. As the proximal groups of glands draining the colon lie in relation to the origins of the colic and inferior mesenteric arteries, their removal implies

---

[1] Morgan, G. N., and Griffiths, J. D., *Surgery Gynec. Obstet.*, 1959, **108**, 641.
[2] Sonneland, J., Anson, B. J., and Beaton, L. E., *Ibid.*, 1959, **106**, 385.

the severance of these vessels where they arise. Extensive lengths of bowel are devitalized and require resection.

THE BLOOD-VESSELS TO THE COLON: These are supplied by the superior and inferior mesenteric arteries. The internal iliac supplies the important middle and inferior haemorrhoidal arteries to the anus and rectum. The usual textbook description of the colic arteries was present in 23·8 per cent of a series of 600 cases reported by Sonneland et al. (1958). There are numerous important variations.

The superior mesenteric artery, which supplies the right and transverse colons, is usually described as giving off three colic arteries: middle, right, and ileocolic (23·8 per cent). In about the same percentage of cases the ileocolic artery is constant but the right colic arises from it (22·7 per cent) or from the middle colic (21·5 per cent).

Less commonly vessels may be duplicated or absent, e.g., the middle colic artery. Morgan and Griffiths (1959) report 2 cases in which the right and middle colic arteries were absent, and the entire colon was supplied by the inferior mesenteric artery which anastomosed via the marginal artery with the ileocolic branch of the superior mesenteric artery.

If for any reason (arteriosclerosis, vascular anomaly, etc.) the collateral circulation to the left colon is deficient, then ligature of the inferior mesenteric artery at its origin may cause ischaemia or gangrene of part of the gut supplied by it. The artery is thus ligated in some cases of cancer of the colon or aneurysmectomy.

The application of a bulldog clamp at the origin of the inferior mesenteric artery at an early stage of operation for cancer of the left colon will demonstrate the adequacy of the superior mesenteric supply.

THE INFERIOR MESENTERIC ARTERY supplies the colon from the splenic flexure to the rectum. It arises from the aorta 3·8 cm. proximal to its bifurcation. It is almost never absent but rarely its origin may be higher—behind the duodenum or pancreas. It soon (3·8 cm.) gives off the large left colic artery which passes up and to the left at an acute angle (not transversely), being crossed by the inferior mesenteric vein, the left ureter being deep to this transit. The vessel bifurcates near the splenic flexure where its branches take an important part in supplementing the marginal artery which is sometimes poor near the flexure. In the 6 per cent of cases in which the left colic artery is absent the marginal arterial arrangements are good. The inferior mesenteric artery supplies several sigmoid arteries to the pelvic colon and ends as the superior haemorrhoidal artery to the rectum.

The sigmoid vessels divide near the bowel and their intercommunications play an important part in supplementing the marginal anastomotic continuity.

THE MARGINAL ARTERY (described by von Haller in 1803 and given its present name by Sudeck, 1907) has been defined by Sonneland et al. as 'the paracolic vessel of anastomosis between colic arteries from which arise the terminal arteries to the colon' (vasa recta). The vessel extends from the ascending colon to the end of the pelvic colon. It is made up by the succession of terminal arterial arcades formed by the arteries to the colon. It lies 2·5–3·8 cm. from the bowel wall.

Singleton[1] has shown that the anastomosis between middle and left colic arteries is absent in 5 per cent of cases, hence the need to maintain the bifurcation of the left colic artery in resections of the left colon.

It is apparent that the integrity of the marginal artery is vital in cases where the inferior mesenteric artery is ligated at its origin and parts of the colon supplied by it are not removed, or when for some reason an arterial trunk must be tied. Even in

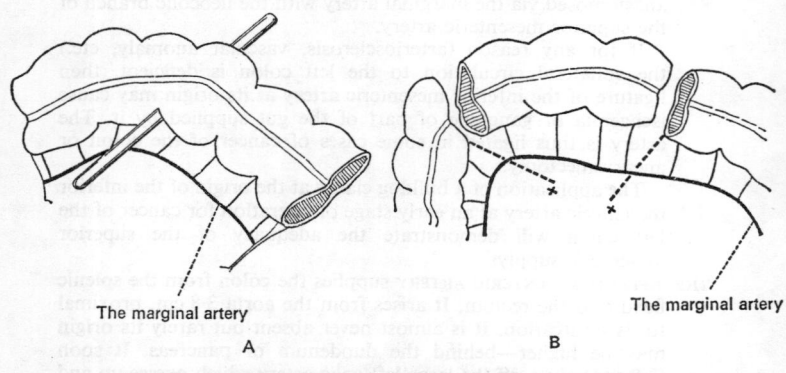

Fig. 567.—Protecting the marginal artery. A, The correct situation of a colostomy rod. B, Method of dividing the mesentery of the colon. (*By courtesy of Morgan and Griffiths.*)

making a loop colostomy, the colostomy rod must be passed through the mesentery immediately medial to the colon so that the marginal artery is not damaged (*Fig.* 567).

The vasa recta are the terminal arteries to the colon. They arise from the marginal artery and penetrate the bowel wall. The

[1] Singleton, Albert O., *Surgery*, 1943, **14**, 328.

SURGERY OF THE LYMPHATICS 601

anastomoses in the bowel are not liberal, therefore end-to-end and not side junctions should be made in colonic anastomoses. In cases where intestinal anastomosis is intended, and one or both of the bowel ends is dependent for its blood-supply on the marginal artery, Morgan and Griffiths advise that the mesentery containing the artery be divided 2·5 cm. distal to the site of division of the colon to maintain the integrity of the vasa recta (*Fig.* 567).

The colonic mucosa has a very rich blood-supply resting on a carpet of blood-vessels. There is an abundant and constant anastomosis between the superior and middle rectal arteries.

The middle and inferior haemorrhoidal arteries are bilateral. They are branches of the internal iliac, the inferior haemorrhoidal coming from its internal pudendal branch.

The middle haemorrhoidal vessels (there may be more than one on each side) are important contributors to the blood-supply of the rectum and pelvic colon. They run in the lateral ligaments of the rectum (rectal stalks), which structures should therefore be preserved in anterior resections of the rectum. These arteries, together with the inferior haemorrhoidals, are responsible for the blood-supply of the terminal colon after ligature of the inferior mesenteric artery at its origin.

PRACTICAL APPLICATIONS:
1. The extent of bowel resection in carcinoma is thus determined by the length of bowel supplied by the arterial trunk to the area involved by the disease, as the veins, lymphatic vessels, and glands draining the part converge on the superior mesenteric or aortic origin of the vessel. It is here the vessel is divided so that the resected bowel and mesentery contains the whole of the

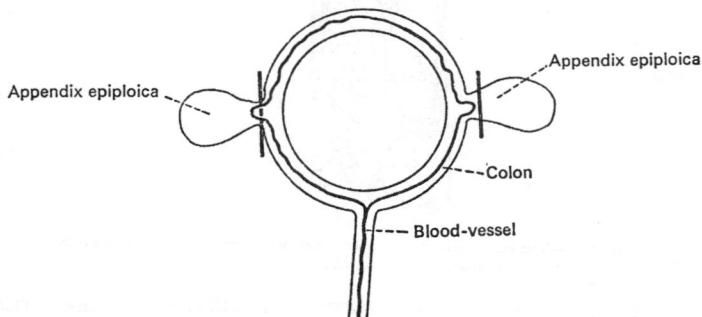

Fig. 568.—Cross-section of colon showing faulty ligation of appendix epiploica on the left. On the right the correct method, which does not damage the blood-supply to the bowel, is shown.

related lymphatic apparatus including the proximal gland group. It has been aptly said that an *honest* resection should be done, i.e., the operator should adhere steadfastly to accepted surgical principles. Whether or not a colostomy can be avoided is a secondary consideration.

2. In view of the great variations in the origin and arrangements of the colic arteries these vessels should be visualized prior to division of arterial trunks. Transillumination is of great assistance.

3. Appendices epiploicae should not be sacrificed as this injures the blood-supply to the bowel. If they must be cut away they should not be shaved off flush with the gut wall, but a few millimetres distal to it, to ensure preservation of the artery passing through the base (*Fig.* 568).

TYPICAL RESECTIONS:

1. CANCER OF CAECUM AND ASCENDING COLON:

    Blood-vessels to the Area for Resection: Ileocolic, right colic, and the right branch of the middle colic. The two branches of the superior mesenteric artery are ligatured and cut at their origin from the parent trunk. The right branch of the middle colic is tied at its origin.

    Resection Necessary (*Fig.* 569): Terminal 15 cm. of the ileum, caecum, and ascending colon, hepatic flexure, to include the proximal third of the transverse colon. Local lymph territory into which this gut drains.

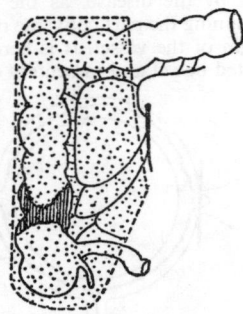

Fig. 569.—The stippled area indicates resection necessary in carcinoma of the caecum or ascending colon. (*By courtesy of Lawrence Abel.*)

2. CANCER OF THE HEPATIC FLEXURE AND RIGHT SIDE OF TRANSVERSE COLON:

    Blood-vessels to the Area for Resection: Ileocolic, right colic, and middle colic.

SURGERY OF THE LYMPHATICS

Resection Necessary: As for cancer of the ascending colon and caecum together with the whole of the transverse colon and splenic flexure. This operation also covers Singleton's observation that in 5 per cent of cases the anastomosis of left and middle colic arteries at the splenic flexure is deficient because of poor development of the left colic artery. Thus when the middle colic is tied at its origin the resection must be made well beyond the splenic flexure where the bowel is viable (*Fig.* 570).

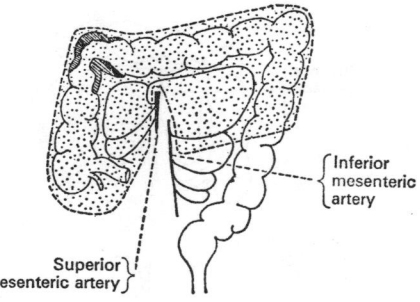

Fig. 570.—Resection for carcinoma of hepatic flexure and right side of transverse colon. (*By courtesy of Lawrence Abel.*)

3. CANCER OF THE TRANSVERSE COLON AND SPLENIC FLEXURE:
Blood-vessels to the Area for Resection: The middle colic artery and the left colic branch of the inferior mesenteric.

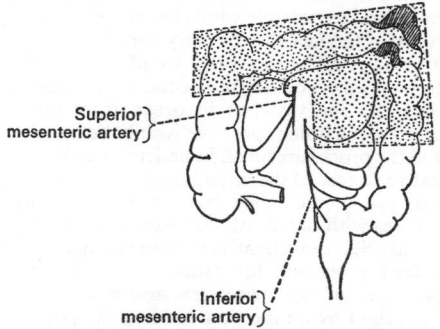

Fig. 571.—Resection necessary for carcinoma of distal transverse colon and splenic flexure. (*By courtesy of Lawrence Abel.*)

Resection Necessary (*Fig.* 571): The bowel is removed from the middle of the ascending colon to the beginning of the pelvic colon. Lymphatic field draining the area.

4. DESCENDING AND PELVIC COLON:

Blood-vessel to the Part: Inferior mesenteric artery.

Resection Necessary: Splenic flexure, descending and pelvic colon with the related lymphatic field. The transverse colon is anastomosed to the rectum (*Fig.* 572).

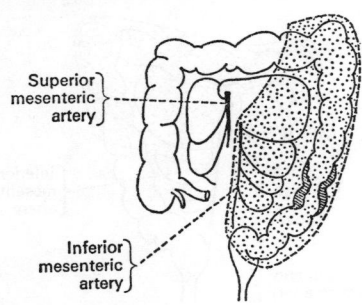

Fig. 572.—Resection necessary for carcinoma of descending and pelvic colon. (*By courtesy of Lawrence Abel.*)

High Ligation of the Inferior Mesenteric Artery: Morgan and Griffiths (1959) point out that the results of resections of the right half of the colon, compared with those on the left, have shown little difference. On the right, however, operation is as radical as possible which has not been the case on the left. In view of the fact that primary lymph drainage of rectum and left colon is along the whole length of the inferior mesenteric artery, and thence to the pre-aortic glands, the logical procedure is to ligate this vessel at its origin from the aorta, and thus secure the maximum possible lymphatic ablation. They recommend the procedure for all fit patients who have an operable and curative cancer of the large bowel below the distal third of the transverse colon. They have performed this procedure in 220 cases with one death but warn against its use in poor-risk patients. Such excellent results imply that this should be the standard procedure for cancer of the left colon.

Technique: The inferior mesenteric artery is exposed, tied and cut at its origin by an incision dividing the peritoneum overlying the terminal aorta. The lymph-glands at the origin of the vessel and in relation to the aorta will be removed as part of the block dissection. The left colic artery is divided proximal to its bifurcation for carcinoma of the pelvic colon or rectum, and the mesentery of the descending colon is divided medial to the marginal artery. This essential vessel may not always be palpable. In such cases the division of the mesentery should be 5 cm. from its colonic attachment. The appearance of the bowel is the best guide to its viability. The colon is then divided at the selected point above, and through the upper part of the rectum below, and an end-to-end anastomosis effected (*Fig.* 573). This procedure ensures the widest lymphatic ablation that can be surgically obtained.

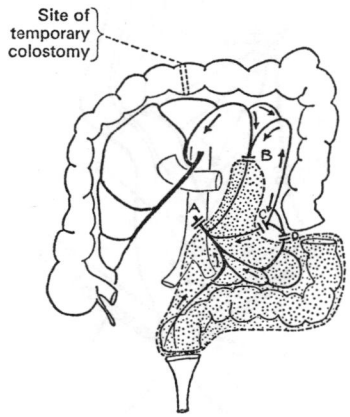

Fig. 573.—High ligation of the inferior mesenteric artery (A) for carcinoma of the sigmoid colon or rectum. B, C, D, indicate the sites of division of branches of this vessel which protect the marginal anastomosis. The arrows show the direction of lymph flow (modified). (*By courtesy of Morgan and Griffiths.*)

5. CANCER OF THE RECTUM: This part of the gut is involved in half of all cases of cancer of the colon.

   Lymphatics of the Rectum: These are: (*a*) Intramural, (*b*) Extramural.

   a. The intramural vessels communicate with a lymph-sinus which lies between the wall of the rectum and the surrounding fat.

   b. The extramural vessels pass:

   i. Across the ischiorectal fossa to the internal iliac glands.
   ii. Across the upper surface of the levator ani to the internal iliac glands.

iii. Posteriorly to glands behind the rectum (sacral glands).
iv. Upwards along the superior haemorrhoidal vessels to the pelvic mesocolon, and so to glands at the bifurcation of the left common iliac artery, and thence to glands along the big vessels up to the glands at the origin of the superior mesenteric.

Extension of Cancer of the Rectum via the Lymphatics: W. E. Miles[1] describes three zones of spread (*Fig.* 574).

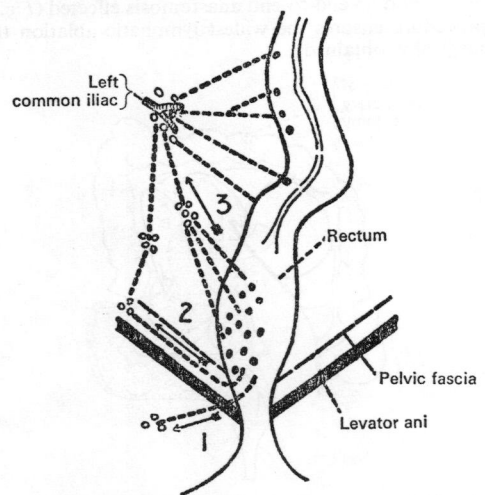

Fig. 574.—The lymphatic drainage of the rectum. The arrows show the three directions in which the efferent lymphatics from the rectum pass: 1, Downward flow through ischiorectal fossa. 2, Lateral flow between levator ani and pelvic fascia. 3, Upward flow in pelvic mesocolon. (*After Miles.*)

a. Downward: Involving perianal skin, ischiorectal fat, and external sphincter ani.

b. Lateral: Involving levatores ani muscles, sacral and internal iliac glands, base of bladder, and seminal vesicles. In women the posterior vaginal wall, cervix, and base of broad ligament are involved also. Miles mentions especially a gland situated on the uterine artery where it crosses the ureter—Poirier's gland. It is often involved in the disease.

[1] Opening Paper, Discussion on Surgical Treatment of Cancer of Rectum, *Br. med. J.,* 1920, Nov., 13.

SURGERY OF THE LYMPHATICS

c. *Upward:* Involves pelvic peritoneum, the whole of the pelvic mesocolon, and glands at the bifurcation of the left common iliac artery.

Resection Necessary: The extent of the operation is necessarily great if the lymph territory under suspicion is removed. *Fig.* 575 shows the scope of the abdominoperineal resection as advocated by Miles. It will be seen that there are removed: the pelvic colon with its mesocolon, the rectum and anus with the surrounding skin, the fat of the ischiorectal fossa, and the levatores ani with their related fasciae. A permanent colostomy is of course necessary.

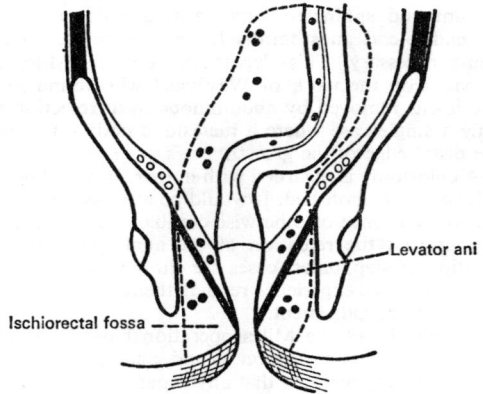

Fig. 575.—Carcinoma of rectum. The extent of operative resection as advised by Miles is indicated by the dotted line. The black dots are lymph-glands.

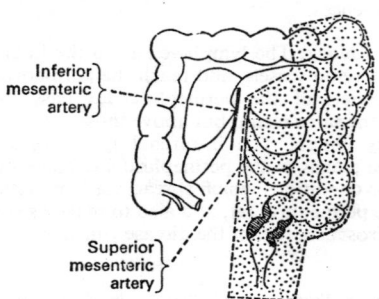

Fig. 576.—Extended resection for carcinoma of rectum.

The tendency is to extend the Miles procedure to include division of the inferior mesenteric artery at its origin from the aorta so that high-lying lymph-glands may be removed. This entails removal of the left colon and rectum from the distal part of the transverse colon. Fat, connective and lymphatic tissues are cleared from the hollow of the sacrum, sacral plexus, etc. Many patients are too frail for such extended procedures. In suitable cases a wider resection may be done as shown in *Fig. 576*.

Anterior Resection of the Rectum: In this operation the bowel is sectioned well clear of the growth below, but the lower rectum and sphincteric apparatus are not interfered with, an end-to-end anastomosis being performed, no colostomy being necessary. This departure from the Miles technique is based on the work of Westheus[1] who found in over 100 specimens removed by abdominoperineal resection there was only a single case where a metastatic node was found below the distal edge of the growth.

A colostomy is regarded with horror. It would be a triumph if it could be abolished. It would be a tragedy if its avoidance led to recurrence of otherwise curable cancer. There are indications that the retention of the anal sphincters may be a reactionary step, unless cases are chosen with the utmost care by those whose experience renders them competent to exercise this nicety of judgement.

The results of the Miles operation have been excellent as the operation is based on sound anatomy and pathology. There is a very real fear that any departure from the principles laid down by Miles, in the desire to spare the patient a colostomy, may be a retrograde step attended with disastrous consequences.

Lymphatics of the Kidney: The lymph-vessels in the kidney pass out, run along with the renal vessels, and reach the para-aortic lymph-glands. The lymph-vessels of the perinephric fat pass independently to the glands of the same chain, but above those which are the recipients of the kidney lymph. The intrarenal lymph-vessels communicate freely with the plexus in the perinephric fat. Therefore in removal of the kidney for conditions which spread via lymphatics, it is essential to remove the perinephric fat, and also to make as sure as possible of removing microscopic foci of the disease which may have reached this fat.

[1] *Pathological Anatomical Foundations of Surgery in Cancer of the Rectum*, 1934. Leipzig.

INJURY TO THE LARGE LYMPH-DUCTS[1]

The surgery of the chest, the diaphragm, and hypertension is conducted near the main lymph-trunks. These structures are sometimes injured and the implications and treatment of the condition are important.

Death due to persistent loss of chyle from the circulation ensues as the result of the loss of fat and protein. Baldridge and Lewis[2] state that it is impossible to maintain adequate serum-protein levels by dietary means when the thoracic duct is incontinent.

Chyle is said to be bacteriostatic as illustrated by the rarity of empyema in chylothorax and the frequency of sterile cultures after repeated thoracocentesis. An important function of the lymphatic system is the continuous formation of lymphocytes. The thoracic duct transmits 5078 million lymphocytes in 24 hours (Yoffey, 1935). The lymphatic system has extraordinary powers of regeneration which play an important part in preventing chronic oedema and elephantiasis. Drinker and Yoffey[3] say, 'it is often thought that ligature of the thoracic duct at the point of venous entrance accomplishes complete obstruction and will result fatally. Nothing can be further from the truth. Ligation of the duct may cause temporary lymph stasis and even chylous collections in the peritoneal, pleural, and pericardial sacs, but ordinarily after a brief period of stasis lymph begins to enter the circulation through collateral lympho-venous connexions. If both the thoracic and the right lymphatic ducts are tied, care being taken that all possible lymphatic branches are secured, lymph may be excluded from the blood-stream for a short time, but ordinarily complete blockage will be a matter of hours only.' It is thus a matter of great difficulty under conditions of normal health to block the entrance of lymph into the venous system. The reasons are anatomical. The embryonic thoracic ducts are bilateral and have numerous cross anastomoses which play an important part following injury or obstruction of the main duct. The usual description of the thoracic duct as being a single channel throughout its course may almost be looked on as an abnormality, so commonly does the duct branch and subdivide.

The Effects of Injury to the Large Lymph-ducts: The thoracic duct may be torn by non-penetrating or penetrating violence. The condition is rare. It may follow hyperextension of the spine or be associated with fractures of the thoracic cage. In closed injury the chylous effusion usually occurs on the right. The reason is thought to be the fixation of the thoracic duct where a fixed and a movable part meet in much the same way as the small intestine tends to rupture at points of fixation. Characteristic symptoms follow. The patient is fairly comfortable for about

---

[1] McGregor, A. Lee, *Br. J. Surg.*, 1953, 40, 569.
[2] Baldridge, R. R., and Lewis, R. V., *Ann. Surg.*, 1948, 128, 1056.
[3] Drinker, C. K., and Yoffey J. M., *Lymphatics, Lymph, and Lymphoid Tissue*, 1941. Cambridge, Mass.

four days, then there is a sudden onset of severe dyspnoea, pallor, cyanosis, and a rapid thready pulse. The condition is immediately relieved on aspiration of the chylous fluid from the thorax only to reappear when it accumulates again. Emaciation occurs rapidly with a progressive decrease in the total protein of the blood. The prognosis is extremely grave. The receptaculum chyli or thoracic duct may be injured during operation. The accident is not serious providing it is recognized and dealt with. All that is needed is ligature and covering with pleura or adjacent tissue.

The Principles governing the Surgery of the Large Lymph-ducts:
1. Lymph is life.
   a. Experimentally it has been found all but impossible to cut off the lymph entry to the vascular system.
   b. Lymph must be conserved or death ensues.
   c. Any flow of chyle should be traced to its origin and appropriate action taken.
   d. In relation to thoracic duct and cisterna chyli stopping the leak is obligatory. In other situations leaks are often insignificant and if not readily closed they may usually be left to look after themselves.
2. The large lymph-ducts are not essential to life.
   a. Injury to cisterna or thoracic duct is only important inasmuch as lymph may be lost to the exterior or into one of the body cavities.
   b. The cisterna chyli may be removed without detriment to the organism.
   c. The thoracic duct may be tied without harmful consequences.
   d. Duct or cisterna may be situated away from commonly accepted positions.
   e. The surgeon should be duct conscious.

Chapter XLI

THE ANATOMY GOVERNING THE SURGERY OF THE SYMPATHETIC[1]

Operations on the autonomic system are now fairly well standardized. It is of interest to note that surgical attack when indicated is almost always upon the sympathetic and seldom upon the parasympathetic. It has become axiomatic that no major surgical procedure on the sympathetic

[1] The study of this chapter will be simplified if its perusal be preceded by reading the anatomy of the sympathetic on p. 170.

should be carried out unless and until its anticipated benefit has been proved by preliminary tests, and of these temporary paralysis of the appropriate ganglia by injection is one of the most important. Such injection may in itself be a valuable means of treatment, as, for example, in cases of femoro-iliac thrombophlebitis.

Vagotomy is the most important operation carried out on the parasympathetic system.

I. REFLEX ACUTE ARTERIAL SPASM RESULTING FROM VASCULAR INSULT

Arterial Embolism or Trauma: When a *clot* lodges in a large artery the vitality of the limb is threatened. The ischaemia is due to two factors: first, the cutting off of the main blood current; and secondly, the spasm of the vessels of the collateral circulation. That such spasm occurs is unquestionable, and it is this additional deprivation which may precipitate gangrene. It should therefore be a matter of urgency to counteract this spasm.

Thrombophlebitis: Of great interest is the knowledge that thrombosis or thrombophlebitis of veins causes reflex vasoconstriction. This may be so great that not only is the blood-supply to the limb diminished, but it may actually be cut off, so that gangrene occurs. The effects of the vasoconstriction are well seen in the 'white leg' of the puerperium or of prolonged hospitalization. The limb is white because of the lessened blood-flow. The swelling is due to three factors: (1) The back pressure in the veins from the blockage; (2) Transudation from the arterioles due to anoxaemia resulting from the lessened arterial stream; (3) Accumulation of tissue fluid due to lymphatic stasis, consequent on diminished arterial pulsation. (Arterial pulsation is an important factor in propelling lymph towards the thorax.) In such cases speedy and sometimes dramatic improvement follows paralysis of the vasoconstrictors to the part by injecting the appropriate ganglia.

II. AUTONOMIC INNERVATION OF THE IRIS

Reference to *Fig.* 577 shows the innervation of the iris.

Parasympathetic fibres arise in the floor of the Sylvian aqueduct with other oculomotor fibres, pass via this nerve to the ciliary ganglion in the orbit, and then by the short ciliary nerves to the constrictor fibres of the iris muscle.

Sympathetic nerves arise from the intermediolateral column at the cervical pupillary centre at the cervicothoracic junction of the spinal cord. They leave the cord by the first thoracic anterior nerve-root, and enter the first white ramus communicans. They pass up the cervical sympathetic chain in the neck to synapse in the superior cervical sympathetic ganglion. The postganglionic fibres ascend in the plexus around the internal carotid artery to the ophthalmic division of the 5th nerve and thence via the nasociliary nerve to the dilator pupillae part of the iris. They carry vasoconstrictor impulses to the retinal vessels. Other fibres supply the choanoid muscle of Müller on the floor of the orbit which protrudes

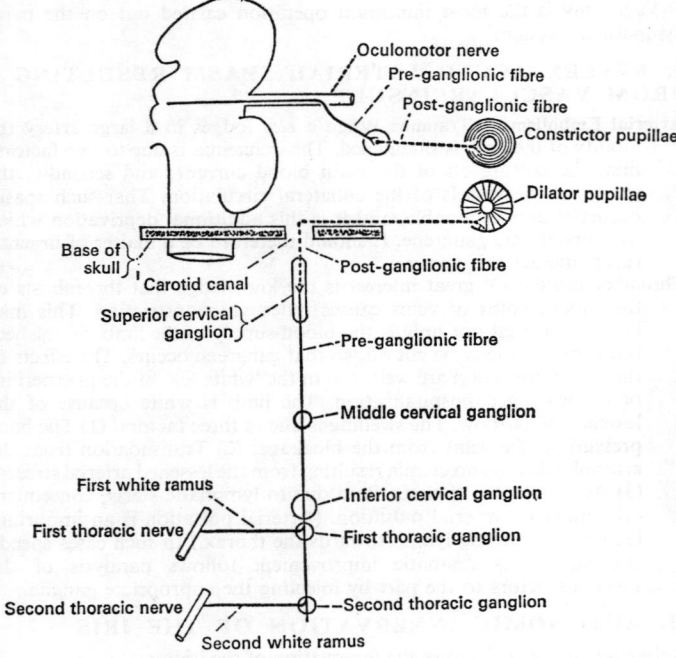

Fig. 577.—The innervation of the iris. The two parts of the muscle are shown as separate circles. Above is the parasympathetic supply to the constrictor pupillae, and below is the sympathetic supply to the dilator pupillae. The ciliary ganglion is shown, but not marked.

the eyeball, and still others supply one-third of the levator palpebrae superioris muscle, thus assisting in the opening of the palpebral fissure.

There are several interesting practical applications of these facts:
1. Injury to the cervical cord may produce pupillary changes.
2. Injury to the lowest trunk of the brachial plexus (C. 8 and T. 1) is usually distal to the intervertebral foramina and does not

result in pupillary changes. Should such changes complicate a lesion of the lowest trunk of the plexus, the pupil on the affected side will be contracted and this implies that the nerve-roots have been avulsed from or so near the cord that operative treatment is impracticable. Unless, therefore, in injuries of this nature, the pupil be examined, useless and unnecessary operation may be undertaken.

3. In cases of permanent facial paralysis the inability of the patient to close the eye is not only unsightly but exposes the cornea to the serious danger of ulceration. By resection of the superior cervical sympathetic ganglion the eye may be almost completely closed, thus obviating the danger of ulceration and improving the patient's appearance. The closure that results from the operation is due to the denervation of that portion of the levator supplied by the cervical sympathetic.

4. Section of the sympathetic in the neck is said by neurological surgeons to cure neuro-paralytic keratitis, following sensory root section of the 5th nerve. It improves the blood-supply by cutting off vasoconstrictor impulses.

5. Horner's syndrome results from paralysis of the cervical sympathetic nerves to the eye. It is evidenced by: (*a*) Constriction of the pupil; (*b*) Narrowing of the palpebral fissure; (*c*) Apparent recession of the eyeball—enophthalmos; (*d*) Frequently a reddening of the conjunctiva due to dilatation of its blood-vessels from paralysis of their vasoconstrictor supply; (*e*) Anhydrosis.

6. The vasoconstrictor nerves to the retinal vessels pass up in the cervical sympathetic. By removal of the cervicothoracic or stellate ganglion these vasoconstrictor fibres are paralysed, and the retinal vessels dilate. In retinitis pigmentosa the vessels to the retina become slowly obliterated with great contracture of the visual fields and night blindness. Removal of the stellate ganglion was at one time practised to improve the blood-supply to the retina and to benefit sight. Adverse reports have led to the abandonment of the procedure.

7. In cases of cerebral compression due to extradural middle meningeal haemorrhage, the presence of a fixed dilated pupil on one side is a valuable indication of the side of the lesion. This fixed dilated pupil is on the *same* side as the lesion and is due to pressure on the oculomotor nerve on the same side by the pushing inwards of a portion of the temporal lobe of the brain by the blood-clot, thus paralysing the parasympathetic nerve-supply to the constrictor pupillae muscle and allowing the dilator pupillae unopposed action.

III. THE CAROTID SINUS PLEXUS

The carotid sinus is a bulge at the bifurcation of the common carotid or at the origin of its internal branch. The sinus is innervated by fibres from the vagus, the glossopharyngeal, and the cervical sympathetic nerves (*Fig.* 578). These nerves form a plexus at the carotid bifurcation. The sinus is the most important peripheral mechanism whence reflex effects are produced which slow the heart-beat and control the blood-pressure.

CLINICAL APPLICATIONS:

1. Attempts at digital control of the carotid artery should never be practised unless urgent need renders such attempts imperative. Pressure on the sinus has caused stoppage of the heart. Pressure

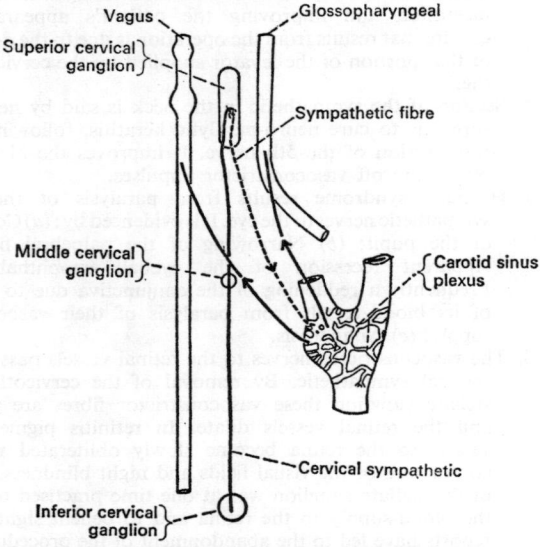

Fig. 578.—The carotid sinus plexus and its nervous connexions.

on the vagus may also be a factor because of the cardiac depressor nerves.

2. The loosening of tight collars in some cases of syncope is reasonable.
3. Cases are sometimes encountered where, as a result of a bout of coughing or other violent expulsive effort, the patient faints. This is occasioned by a reflex slowing of the heart due to increase of pressure in the carotid sinus. The sensitive sinus is usually

unilateral. Should the condition occasion great disability, resection of the sinus plexus is indicated.

IV. THE AUTONOMIC SUPPLY TO THE HEART

The parasympathetic supply is via the vagus, whereas the sympathetic is through the upper three to five (thoracic) white rami communicantes. *All* fibres subserving cardiac pain pass via the sympathetic pathways.

Parasympathetic Supply: Preganglionic motor neurons originate in the dorsal nucleus of the vagus and end in the intrinsic cardiac ganglia. Postganglionic fibres pass from these ganglia along the coronary vessels. Viscero-sensory fibres originate from the intrinsic cardiac ganglia and pass to the ganglion nodosum of the vagus—the depressor nerves, not usually separate in man, but incorporated in the vagus, and responsible for cardiac inhibition (for details *see* p. 152).

Sympathetic Supply: This takes the following origin and course:
1. It arises from the intermediolateral column of the thoracic part of the cord.
2. The fibres leave the cord in the upper three to five thoracic anterior nerve-roots. They pass to the corresponding thoracic white rami communicantes.
3. These preganglionic fibres are destined for the superficial and deep cardiac plexuses.
4. They reach it by two routes:
    a. *The Thoracic Cardiac Nerves:* The first group synapses in the upper three to five ganglia of the sympathetic chain. The postganglionic fibres arise there and pass to the heart via the thoracic cardiac nerves.
    b. *The Cervical Cardiac Nerves:* The second group of preganglionic fibres passes through the thoracic ganglia and synapses in one or other of the three cervical sympathetic ganglia. The postganglionic fibres pass to the heart in the superior, middle, and inferior cervical cardiac nerves (*Fig.* 579). These are the cardiac accelerator nerves. The sensory nerves conveying pain sensations from the aorta, coronary vessels, pericardium, and heart muscle arise in typical end-organs in these structures and pass via the middle and inferior cervical and the thoracic cardiac nerves and thence via the posterior nerve-roots to the spinal cord.[1]

Practical Applications

Cardiac Pain: The pain occasioned by ischaemia of the heart muscle is so common, so terrible, and such a potent cause of death that its treatment has occupied the attention of surgeons since the close of the last century. Owing to the imperfect knowledge of the path taken by the

[1] This account of the nerve-supply of the heart is based on the work of Nonidez and is that given by White and Smithwick in their work, *The Autonomic Nervous System*, 1942, 47. London.

nerves conducting these painful impulses a great variety of operative procedures have been used. Those in use to-day are: (1) Methods of increasing the blood-supply to the heart; (2) Direct attack on the nerves conducting cardiac pain.

The principles underlying these methods are totally different.

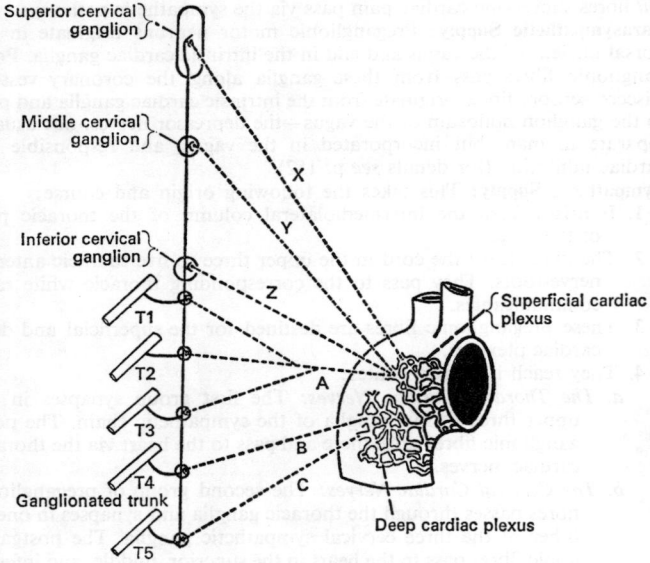

Fig. 579.—The sympathetic supply to the heart. X, Superior, Y, Middle, and Z, Inferior cervical cardiac nerves, respectively; A, B, C, Thoracic cardiac nerves.

ATTACK ON THE PAIN-CONDUCTING NERVES:

1. POSTERIOR RHIZOTOMY: All cardiac pain may be permanently abolished by section of the upper five thoracic posterior nerve-roots on either side (*Fig.* 580). Such a procedure has been carried out many times and permanent results ensue in those who survive. The operation is, however, one of considerable magnitude and the sufferers are poor risks. White has indicated, moreover, that in these people, with their diseased hearts, it is inadvisable that any prolonged operation should be undertaken in the prone position

SURGERY OF THE SYMPATHETIC 617

2. GANGLIONECTOMY: Reference to *Fig.* 579 will show that if the inferior cervical and upper three thoracic sympathetic ganglia are removed, a very large proportion of the sensory supply on one side will be interrupted. This operation can be performed by the anterior route of Gask and Ross or by the posterior approach of Smithwick, and excellent results are reported from it.

Unilateral operation removes the pain on one side only, and it is therefore often necessary that both sides should be done. Sir James Mackenzie warned against operation which would remove the danger signal of pain, but experience has shown that these pain-free cases are warned of impending attacks by mild feelings of oppression, etc.

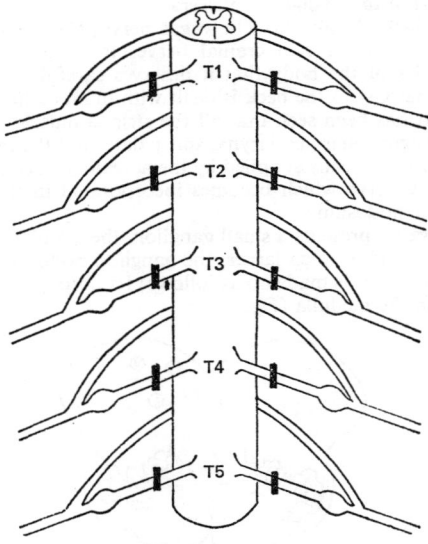

Fig. 580.—A method of removing all pain impulses from the heart by division of the upper five thoracic posterior nerve-roots on both sides.

3. PARAVERTEBRAL ALCOHOL INJECTION: This procedure, introduced by Mandle and Swetlow and developed by White, consists essentially in the destruction of the upper thoracic sympathetic ganglia by alcohol injection. The procedure is a relatively minor one, although it requires expertness and experience for its correct execution. White reports over 50 per cent of cases completely

cured of pain, and less than 10 per cent of failures. The results appear to be permanent. A drawback of the procedure is a troublesome intercostal neuralgia in a small percentage of cases. This is due to irritation of intercostal nerves by the alcohol.

V. THE ABDOMINAL AUTONOMIC SYSTEM

The autonomic system is entirely responsible for the nerve-supply of the viscera and their outgrowths. Only the parietal peritoneum and a small part of the roots of the mesenteries receive a somatic nerve supply. It follows therefore that, except when due to peritonitis, a host of abdominal disorders and diseases produce symptoms which reach the level of consciousness via autonomic sensory nerves.

The Innervation of the Abdominal Viscera

1. Parasympathetic Supply: (*a*) The vagus nerve; (*b*) The nervi erigentes.

VAGUS: This is the Xth cranial nerve. It is so important in the economics of the body that it deserves careful consideration. Its gross anatomy in the neck is dealt with in an earlier section of the work. It has been seen that all the striped muscle in the territory of the vagus, pharynx, larynx, soft palate, and the inhibitory nerve to the heart is really supplied by the accessory portion of the spinal accessory nerve which becomes incorporated in the vagus at the ganglion nodosum.

The vagus presents a small ganglion, the jugular, in the jugular foramen, and a much larger, the ganglion nodosum, just distal to this. The vagus is made up as follows: Its fibres go from or to three nuclei in the medulla (*Fig.* 581):

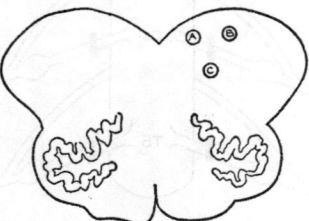

Fig. 581.—The nuclei of the vagus. A, Dorsal or visceral motor nucleus. B, Sensory nucleus or tractus solitarius. C, Nucleus ambiguus—voluntary motor nucleus.

a. The nucleus ambiguus—the voluntary motor nucleus for the supply of the striped muscle referred to above.

b. The dorsal motor nucleus which is responsible for visceral (involuntary) motor innervation (*Fig.* 582).

SURGERY OF THE SYMPATHETIC 619

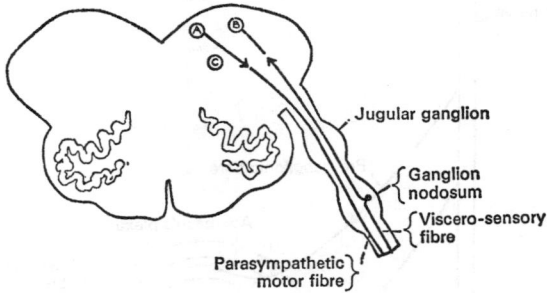

Fig. 582.—To show the parasympathetic efferent and afferent fibres of the vagus.
A, The dorsal motor nucleus. B, Tractus solitarius. C, Nucleus ambiguus.

c. The tractus solitarius—sensory innervation of pharynx and larynx through neurons whose cells lie in the jugular ganglion; sensory impressions from the viscera, the cell-stations being in the ganglion nodosum (*Fig.* 583).
d. The motor or efferent preganglionic fibre commences in the dorsal nucleus of the medulla, runs right through the abdominal plexus, and has its synapse actually in the walls of the viscus it supplies,

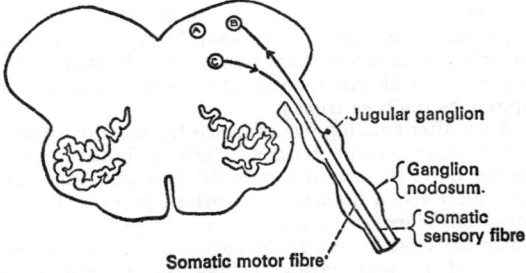

Fig. 583.—To show the somatic afferent and efferent fibres of the vagus.
A, B, C, As in *Fig.* 582.

such as in the plexuses of Auerbach and Meissner in the intestinal wall. There a very short postganglionic fibre begins and ends in the neighbouring muscle. The physiological object of this arrangement is to produce accurately localized effects (*Fig.* 584).

620 A SYNOPSIS OF SURGICAL ANATOMY

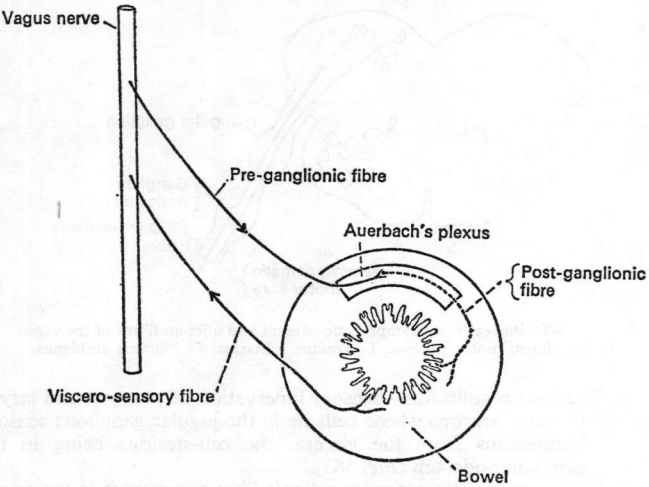

Fig. 584.—Showing the parasympathetic motor and sensory innervation of the gut.

THE ABDOMINAL COURSE OF THE VAGUS:[1] The vagi enter the abdomen through the oesophageal hiatus, the left vagus anterior and the right vagus posterior to the oesophagus. The vagi divide into branches at the cardia of the stomach but this division may occur higher, in which case the vagi at the level of the diaphragm will appear as multiple trunks.

Soon after entering the abdomen the anterior vagus gives off one or more hepatic branches, which run in the lesser omentum to the portal fissure to supply the liver and gall-bladder, and ultimately also a branch to the pyloric antrum. The vagus also gives off branches to the fundus and proceeds in the lesser omentum close to the lesser curvature of the stomach as the nerve of Latarjet, giving off branches to the stomach and ending on the pyloric antrum (Fig. 585).

The posterior vagus runs some distance from the oesophagus and gives off the coeliac branch which accompanies the left gastric artery and goes to the coeliac ganglion to supply the small bowel, proximal colon and pancreas. Branches are given off to the posterior surface of the stomach and the nerve proceeds in a

[1] Burge, H., *Vagotomy*, 1964. London: Edward Arnold.

SURGERY OF THE SYMPATHETIC 621

similar manner to the anterior vagus with branches to the stomach and ending over the pyloric antrum (*Fig.* 586).

A vagotomy can be achieved by section of the main trunks of the vagi (truncal vagotomy) or by sectioning the gastric branches

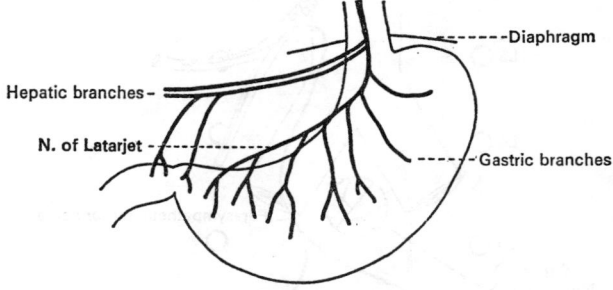

Fig. 585.—The anterior vagus.

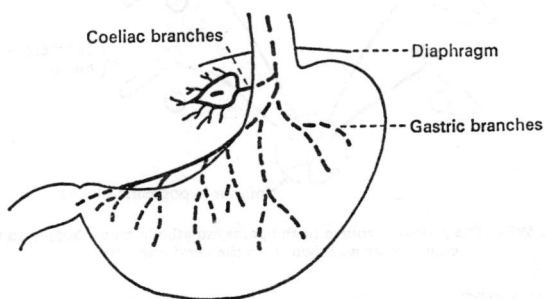

Fig. 586.—The posterior vagus.

and not the hepatic and coeliac branches (selective vagotomy) or by sectioning only the branches leading to the parietal cell area and not the coeliac and hepatic branches nor the nerves of Latarjet (super-selective or parietal cell vagotomy).

FUNCTIONS OF THE VAGUS: The vagus is the parasympathetic supply to the heart and lungs. It is motor to the oesophagus, stomach, gall-bladder, and bowel, and secretory to the stomach and pancreas.

622 A SYNOPSIS OF SURGICAL ANATOMY

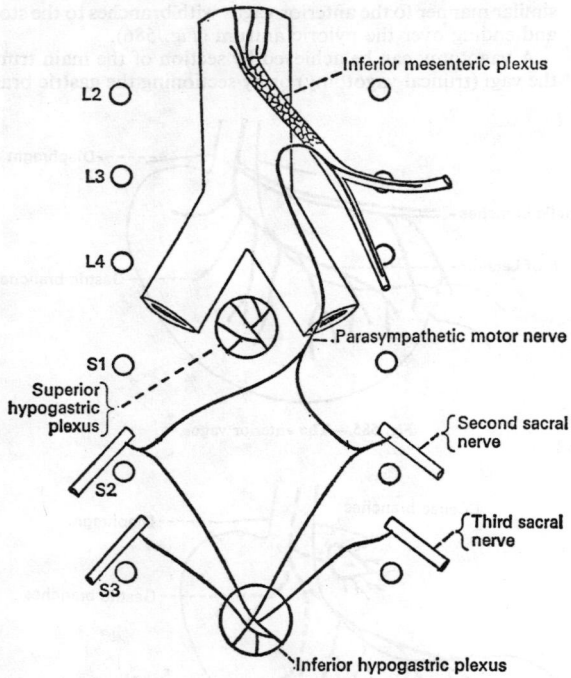

Fig. 587.—The probable course of the parasympathetic motor supply to the left colon. Note its origin from the nervi erigentes.

NERVI ERIGENTES: These constitute the parasympathetic supply to the lower abdominal viscera, such as colon, rectum, bladder, uterus, and sex organs. The nerves come from the 2nd and 3rd or 3rd and 4th sacral anterior roots. The white rami—nervi erigentes— are given off from these roots and run forward along the lateral wall of the pelvis outside the pelvic fascia. At about the middle of the lateral wall of the pelvis the trunks turn medially and pass through the inferior hypogastric plexus at the bladder base to supply the pelvic viscera. Certain of their fibres take an upward course on the left to supply the colon. The course these fibres take is suggested by *Fig. 587*. It will be seen that they pass up from the inferior hypogastric plexus wide of the superior hypogastric plexus, and so to the inferior mesenteric plexus round the artery of that name, and via this vessel to the left colon.

During surgical excision of the rectum the vesical nerves are protected from injury by their position outside the pelvic (Waldeyer's) fascia, but if the operation proceeds in the wrong layer outside this fascia, nerve injury will occur with resultant denervation of the bladder.

2. Sympathetic Supply:

UPPER ABDOMEN:

1. The ultimate origin is from the cells of the intermediolateral column in the lower seven or eight segments of the thoracic part of the cord.
2. The fibres pass out with the thoracic anterior nerve-roots and thence via the corresponding white rami to the lateral chain of sympathetic ganglia usually without interruption. Thence they pass to form the splanchnic nerves.
3. The splanchnic nerves pass to the coeliac and other ganglia around the aorta and its great branches. Many of these fibres have their cell-stations in these plexuses. The postganglionic fibres become associated with the vagal (parasympathetic) fibres and pass with them along the periarterial plexuses to their ultimate distribution. The preganglionic nerves to the adrenal medulla have no synpase on their course but terminate around the chromaffin cells of the medulla. The sympathetic nerves on their way to the bowel, etc., lie at first in the retroperitoneal cellular tissue. Here they may be irritated or injured by collections of fluid, e.g., blood. In fracture of the spine, the upper lumbar vertebrae are frequently broken. Some degree of ileus—intestinal paresis —sometimes complicates these injuries. This is due to irritation of the sympathetic nerve-fibres which are normally inhibitory to the bowel. Irritation causes overaction and thus sympathetic-parasympathetic imbalance results.

   Ogilvie has drawn attention to a type of adynamic ileus which may result from involvement of these nerves by secondary deposits in cases of malignant disease.
4. The sensory fibres of this system arise in end-organs in the viscera and mesenteries and pass via the splanchnic nerves to the lower six thoracic posterior nerve-roots on their way to the cord.
5. *Functions:*
   a. Inhibition of peristalsis and contraction of involuntary sphincters.
   b. Vasoconstriction.
   c. Reflex stimuli.
   d. Nausea.
   e. Carry all visceral pain sensations except such small part as may be conveyed through the nervi erigentes.

PELVIS:
1. The sympathetic supply to the pelvic viscera arises from the area of the thoracolumbar junction of the cord.
2. The fibres pass out via the lower thoracic and the two lumbar white rami to the lumbar and pre-aortic ganglia.
3. The postganglionic neurons arise from sympathetic lateral and pre-aortic ganglia and descend via the so-called aortic plexus. An offshoot, where a ganglion may be situated, passes along the inferior mesenteric artery to innervate the left colon and rectum.
4. Other fibres form the superior hypogastric plexus (Hovelacque) in front of the promontory of the sacrum.
5. From this plexus the two hypogastric nerves pass down in the hollow of the sacrum to the inferior hypogastric plexus behind the bladder base.
6. Sensory fibres take a reverse course through these two plexuses to the posterior roots of the same nerves whence, via the anterior roots, the efferent sympathetic fibres pass.
7. The functions of the sympathetic nerves are: (*a*) Vasoconstrictor; (*b*) Inhibitory to the left colon; (*c*) Motor to the internal sphincter ani (?); (*d*) Transmission of certain types of uterine and colonic pain.

SURGICAL APPLICATIONS IN THE ABDOMEN AND PELVIS

1. Essential Hypertension: Before adequate drug therapy for essential hypertension became available, this condition was sometimes treated by extensive sympathectomy[1] to reduce peripheral resistance (*Fig.* 588). The operation is now no longer necessary because equally satisfactory results can be obtained by drug therapy.

UNILATERAL KIDNEY DISEASE AS A CAUSE OF HYPERTENSION: Regarding the part played by unilateral kidney disease in the causation of hypertension, it is known that experimentally produced hydronephrosis will not in itself cause hypertension. Where nephrectomy produces sustained lowering of the blood-pressure, it is probably due to the removal of a circulatory imbalance which results in the production of a pressor substance which causes the hypertension.

Stenosis of one or both renal arteries is a cause of hypertension especially in young persons. A condition analogous to the Goldblatt kidney exists. The stenosis can be demonstrated by arteriography and blood-pressure may be restored to normal by one of several methods chosen to suit the particular circumstances of the case.

---

[1] White, J. C., and Smithwick, R. H., *The Autonomic Nervous System*, 1942, 12. London.

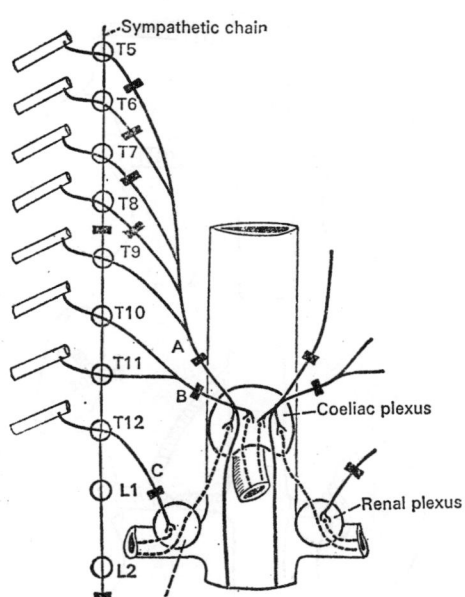

Fig. 588.—Splanchnicectomy of White and Smithwick. The sympathetic chain is removed with the ganglia from T.9 to L.2. The splanchic nerves are dealt with as shown between the black bars. A, Greater splanchnic. B, Lesser splanchnic. C, Least splanchnic.

These are: (*a*) replacing the stenosed vessel by a graft, (*b*) anastomosing the splenic artery to the renal beyond the narrowed area, (*c*) removing the affected kidney if the other is normal (*Fig.* 589).

Platt's law states that in all young hypertensives the hypertension is likely to be secondary. About 75 per cent of all hypertensives under the age of 40 were secondary to some other factor.

2. Bladder and Colon:

NERVE-SUPPLY OF THE BLADDER: Is derived from three sources: (1) The sympathetic (*Figs.* 590, 591); (2) The parasympathetic; (3) The pudendal nerves.

SYMPATHETIC: The sympathetic contribution to the nerve-supply of the bladder is conveyed to it through the presacral nerve of Latarjet. It is essential to realize that this nerve is the 'hypogastric

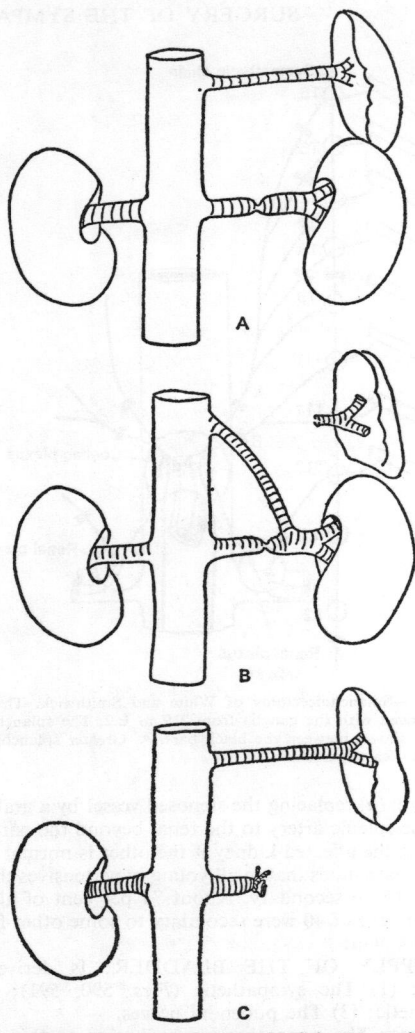

Fig. 589.—Methods of dealing with stenosis of the left renal artery which is causing hypertension. A, The cause of the hypertension; B, Anastomosis of splenic artery to renal distal to the stenosis. C, Nephrectomy when shunt not feasible.

plexus' of anatomy textbooks. The latter term is more accurate, as a plexus exists in 80 per cent of cases and a single nerve in but 20 per cent. As all surgical accounts of the matter speak of the 'presacral nerve', the term will be retained here. The presacral nerve is formed in the midline in front of the body of the 5th lumbar vertebra, between the common iliac arteries, posterior to but not adherent to the peritoneum in an area which is relatively avascular and easy of operative approach. Three roots enter into its formation:

1. The middle root is derived from that part of the sympathetic plexus around the lower part of the aorta known as the intermesenteric plexus. It runs down in front of the aortic bifurcation to join—
2 and 3. Two lateral roots in front of the body of the 5th lumbar vertebra. Each of these roots is formed by the fusion of branches from the 1st and 2nd lumbar sympathetic ganglia.

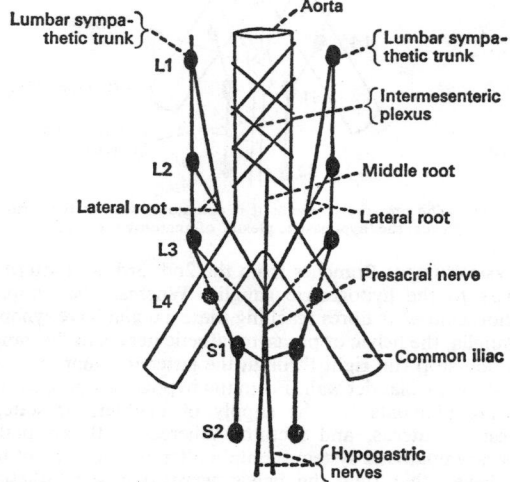

Fig. 590.—The presacral nerve is shown as a single trunk.

The lateral root so formed is familiar to us as the nerve which crosses anterior to the common iliac artery (whereas the sympathetic trunk itself passes into the pelvis posterior to this vessel). The 3rd and 4th lumbar ganglia give small twigs to reinforce the presacral nerve. The mesentery of the small intestine is above the nerve, while the attachment of the pelvic mesocolon is to its left. The presacral nerve runs into the pelvis and soon divides into two branches, the hypogastric nerves, each of which joins a ganglion, the hypogastric ganglion, lying between the lower part of the rectum and the bladder base.

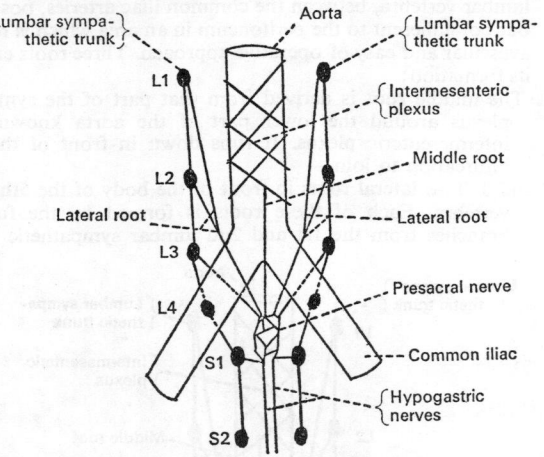

Fig. 591.—The presacral nerve as it is commonly seen in the form of a plexus, the 'hypogastric plexus' of anatomy textbooks.

PARASYMPATHETIC: Branches from the 2nd, 3rd, and 4th sacral roots pass to the hypogastric ganglia. Whereas the sympathetic or thoracolumbar fibres reaching these ganglia have synapses in the ganglia, the pelvic or parasympathetic nerves to the ganglia make a non-stop run right through the latter to synapse round nerve-cells in the bladder wall. From the hypogastric ganglia arise many nerve filaments for the supply of bladder, prostate, seminal vesicles, uterus, and rectum. Whereas both sympathetic and parasympathetic systems contain afferent and efferent fibres, it is believed that only the pelvic nerves (parasympathetic or nervi erigentes) carry afferent impulses dealing with emptying reflexes of bladder and rectum.

PUDENDAL NERVES: Convey motor fibres to the sphincter urethrae membranaceae and sensory to the prostatic urethra.

FUNCTIONS OF THE NERVES: It has till recently been taught that the sympathetic and parasympathetic play antagonistic roles in the rectum and bladder. That this is so in the pelvic colon

SURGERY OF THE SYMPATHETIC

and rectum is accepted, the sympathetic causing relaxation of the bowel wall and contraction of the internal sphincter of the anus. The parasympathetic, on the other hand, produces an opposite effect, being an emptying mechanism, i.e., contraction of the expulsive muscles and sphincter relaxation. In a clear analysis of recent work White and Smithwick[1] conclude that the parasympathetic or nervi erigentes alone mediate impulses for the storage of urine in the bladder and its evacuation. Reflex micturition is inhibited by the pyramidal tracts. Thus cord lesions above the sacral segments or brain lesions may produce abnormal bladder function due to the cutting off of inhibitory impulses. The sympathetic, on the other hand, supplies vasomotor nerves to the bladder and mediates the function of ejaculation, also causing contraction of the bladder neck to an uncertain extent. Pain sensations from the bladder travel exclusively via the sacral autonomic nerves. The sensation of bladder filling probably travels via the sympathetic afferent nerves (*Fig.* 592).

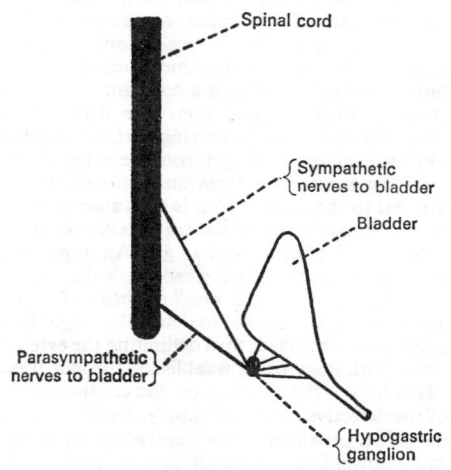

Fig. 592.—Diagrammatic schema of the nerve-supply of the bladder. The sympathetic plays a very subsidiary part in this supply.

NEURECTOMY OF THE PRESACRAL PLEXUS: This operation may be resorted to in: (1) Pain arising from the bladder; (2) Primary dysmenorrhoea.

[1] *The Autonomic Nervous System*, 1942, 92, 380. London.

1. BLADDER PAIN: From the preceding section it is obvious that the operation has little if any application in the treatment of intractable bladder pain. It does improve some cases, not by interrupting afferent pathways, but by relieving spasm of the internal sphincter. In severe cystitis which fails to respond to other forms of treatment, presacral neurectomy may render the sufferer more comfortable in so far as the urine may be retained for longer periods.
2. PRIMARY DYSMENORRHOEA: The causes of pain during the menstrual period are unknown. They have been attributed to the muscular contractions of the uterus. In cases where conservative measures fail, where no organic cause can be found for the pain, and where careful selection generally is exercised, relief of pain follows presacral neurectomy in most cases. It is necessary that the operation be complete and extend as far as the bifurcation of the common iliac arteries on both sides.
3. **Hirschsprung's Disease:** The uncertainty surrounding the cause of this condition has been cleared up by the work of Swenson, Neuhauser, and Pickett[1]. It is now apparent that the ganglion cells of the nerve plexuses in the wall of the colon are congenitally deficient and that the part of the gut so affected receives only a sympathetic supply, the parasympathetic or emptying mechanisms being missing. The affected bowel wall is therefore in a constant state of spasm which is equivalent to a chronic obstruction. The defect begins above the anus, involves the rectum and a varying part of the colon above it; the entire colon and even the entire gut from the outlet of the stomach may be affected. The supposition previously prevalent that the dilated colon, proximal to the obstruction, is the cause of the disease is thus erroneous. This enlargement of the colon is secondary to the obstruction *distal* to it and affects normal gut. An important step forward in elucidating the problem of Hirschsprung's disease was taken when it was found that by running a *small* quantity of barium *slowly* into the anus the radiologist was able to detect the height to which the area of contracted bowel extended, thus delimiting the extent of the disease.

The correct pathology being established, proper treatment became possible. This imples the removal of the contracted bowel which is the area of the defective nerve-cell supply. As this area may involve the dilated bowel just proximal to the contracted segment, about 12 cm. of the dilated bowel is removed for security reasons. The distal level of section is immediately proximal to the anus leaving not more than 2·5 cm. of the anal canal. This ensures continence as the sphincters are not impaired. Furthermore, the lowest inch of anal mucosa is the trigger mechanism which warns the sphincters of advancing bowel content and causes them to come into action. This important area of mucous membrane is preserved (*Fig.* 593).

[1] Swenson, O., Neuhauser, E. B. D. and Pickett, L. K., *Pediatrics*, 1949, 4, 201.

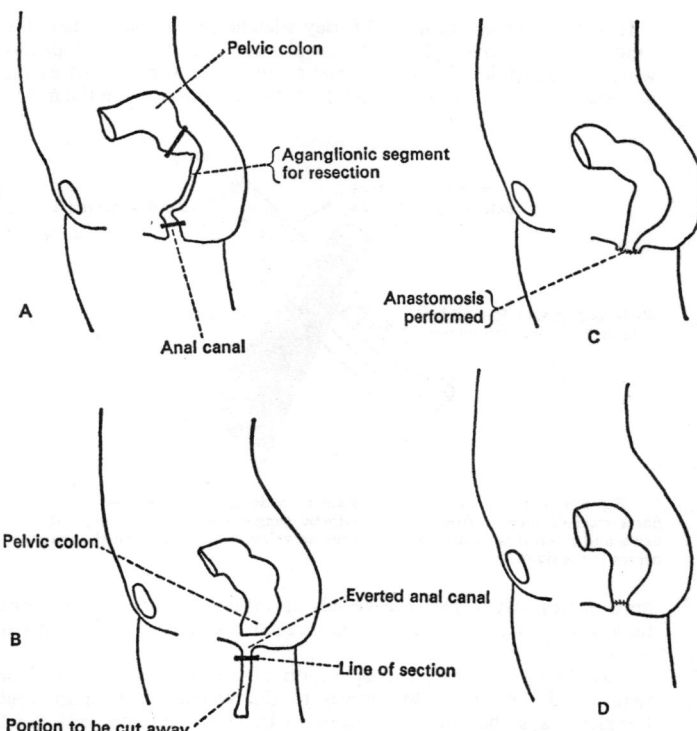

Fig. 593.—The principles of the Swenson operation for megacolon: A, The area lacking in ganglion cells, which is to be resected. The black bars show the proximal and distal lines of section. B, The resection completed proximally. The bowel to be removed has been pulled out through the anus. The black bar shows the distal line of section. C, The anastomosis performed outside the anus. D, The bowel has been allowed to contract, completing the operation.

VI. PERIPHERAL VASCULAR DISEASE

Various measures have been employed to interrupt vasoconstrictor impulses to the limbs.

Periarterial Sympathectomy (Leriche):

   PREMISES: The operation is based on the supposition that the sympathetic fibres to the limb vessels all enter the limb as a plexus around the main artery to that limb.

It is, however, established (Morley Fletcher,[1] Woollard[2]) that the limb vessels receive: (1) A direct plexus from the aortic plexus which accompanies the main vessel to the limb and extends as far as the axilla and the groin (*Fig* 594). (2) Contributions from the mixed

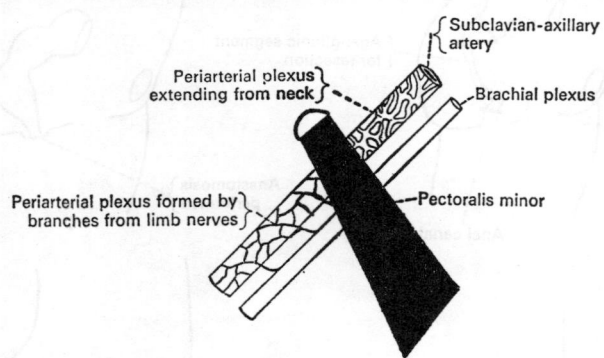

Fig. 594.—The periarterial limb plexus is made up in its proximal part by fibres received directly from the sympathetic ganglionated trunk. Beyond the axilla and groin it is formed by numerous nerve-fibres received from the main nerves to the limbs.

limb nerves, which join the vessels at *different* levels in the limb; these are sympathetic fibres which reach the limb with the mixed nerves to the part.

Such being the case, the operation of sympathectomy does *not* remove all the vasomotor nerves to the vessels of the part, and Langley[3] says that this operation, so far as it removes peripheral vasoconstriction, probably does not do so by severing nerve fibres running with the arteries. J. F. Fulton[4] states that the operation of periarterial sympathectomy is without physiological or anatomical foundation, as no long vasoconstrictor fibres pass distally in the larger limb vessels. Lambert Rogers and Hemingway[5] found that experimental periarterial sympathectomy produces vasodilatation lasting only forty-eight hours. Ogilvie[6] sums up the value of the

[1] *J. Physiol.*, 1897–8 **22**, 259.
[2] *Heart*, 1926, **13**, 319.
[3] Quoted by H. A. Harris, 'Vascular Diseases of the Sympathetic System', *Br. med. J.*, 1927, April 30.
[4] Remarks at the B.M.A. Meeting at Winnipeg in 1930, in the discussion of the surgery of the sympathetic.
[5] *Br. J. Surg.*, 1930, **17**, 473.
[6] *Recent Advances in Surgery*, 1929, 88.

SURGERY OF THE SYMPATHETIC

procedure concisely: 'Praise for the operation appears to be limited to the accounts by individual surgeons of short series of personal cases. Collected series appear to show that the results are on the whole unsatisfactory, and it is clear that, until our knowledge of the course and functions of the sympathetic nerves is more exact, the rationale for sympathectomy stands on very weak ground.'

Sympathetic Denervation of the Limbs: This may be ganglionic or preganglionic. The erstwhile viewpoint that damage to or removal of the synapses in the sympathetic ganglia—so-called postganglionic section—rendered the neuromuscular junctions increasingly sensitive to circulating adrenaline and thus caused relapse of the vasospasm is now known to be not incorrect but unimportant. Thus some surgeons employ ganglionectomy and others preganglionic section in denervating the limbs.

UPPER LIMB: Gask[1] has described an approach from the front. The scalenus anterior is divided, the fascia of the upper aperture of the thorax (Sibson's) torn through, and the apical pleura pushed down.

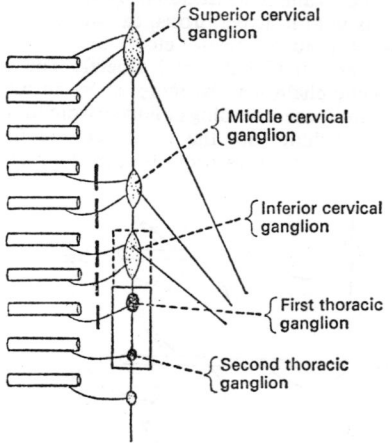

Fig. 595.—Connexions of brachial plexus with sympathetic. The upper limb may be deprived of all its sympathetic nerve-supply by either of two methods: (1) Division of all rami connecting sympathetic with roots of brachial plexus. The rami are shown divided by black bars. (2) Removal of the 1st and 2nd thoracic sympathetic ganglia and their connexions, and sometimes removal of the inferior cervical ganglia also. The area to be removed is shown marked out by an oblong which may be extended to include the inferior cervical ganglion. Both these procedures injure postganglionic fibres.

[1] *Br. J. Surg.*, 1933, **21**, 113.

We have found it a considerable advantage to divide the costo-cervical arterial trunk between ligatures. The sympathetic trunk is exposed to the level of the 3rd thoracic ganglion. The trunk is then pulled down and the 1st, 2nd, and 3rd thoracic and the inferior cervical ganglia are resected. In this way the total sympathetic innervation to the corresponding upper limb is removed. To appreciate the rationale of the operation it must be remembered that the white rami (which go to constitute the sympathetic trunk), arise between the 1st thoracic and 2nd lumbar nerves, so that the fibres constituting the cervical sympathetic all come from the cord below the level of the 1st thoracic nerve, and therefore by removing the 1st, 2nd and 3rd thoracic and inferior cervical ganglia all the sympathetic fibres passing to head, neck, and upper limb are divided (*Fig.* 595).

This operation may be used for the relief of cardiac pain in angina pectoris. To ensure removal of all fibres subserving cardiac pain the stellate plus the upper five thoracic ganglia should be removed. This cannot be achieved by the anterior approach. The operation is used in hyperidrosis, causalgia, traumatic upper limb neuralgia, Raynaud's disease, etc.

AXILLARY APPROACH (Schulze and Goetz): The upper part of the sympathetic chain may be removed by an incision through the second interspace extending obliquely from the outer border of the latissimus behind and the great pectoral in front. The long thoracic nerve requires protection in the mid-axillary line. The

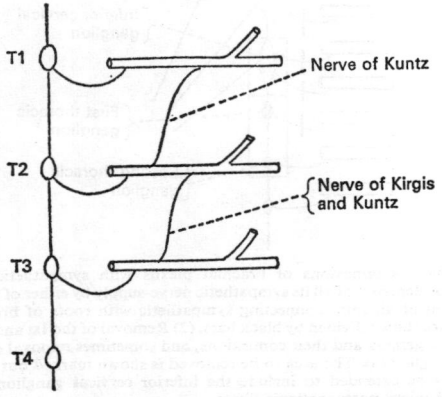

Fig. 596.—The nerves of Kuntz. The grey rami passing from thoracic ganglia to the thoracic nerves are shown.

pleura is opened and the ribs spread. Access to the upper thoracic ganglia is adequate, though the inferior cervical ganglion is less easily dealt with. The scar is well concealed.

Comment:

1. The suggestion has been made that the 8th cervical nerve may supply a preganglionic outflow to the upper limb.

2. The nerve of Kuntz (1927): In about 20 per cent of cases the 2nd thoracic nerve—prior to becoming an intercostal nerve—gives a branch to the first. This is the nerve of Kuntz which is derived from the 2nd thoracic ganglion. It carries sympathetic fibres to the upper limb via the important 1st thoracic nerve contribution to the brachial plexus. Removal of the stellate and 1st thoracic sympathetic ganglia would therefore not impair the sympathetic supply to the upper limb from the nerve of Kuntz (*Fig.* 596). Less commonly the 3rd thoracic ganglion supplies a similar pathway to the upper limb via the 2nd and 1st thoracic nerves (Kirgis and Kuntz, 1942).

Preganglionic Section: There are two routes available to achieve this objective; that of Telford through the posterior triangle of the neck, and that of Smithwick through the back. Both procedures are preganglionic, on the assumption that if the postganglionic fibre is injured symptoms speedily return as the neuromuscular nerve apparatus is rendered over-sensitive to circulating adrenaline. Though this view is hotly contested, it has become correct practice to act as though it were incontestable. In both operations, therefore, the attachments of 2nd, 3rd, and 4th thoracic ganglia are divided, the trunk cut below the 4th ganglion, and the connexions of the 1st ganglion left undamaged. The 1st thoracic ganglion may contain a small sympathetic contribution to the arm. When this is the case, recurrence of symptoms will follow the customary sympathetic denervation, because of the syncytial nature of the architecture of the sympathetic supply to the limb. The 1st thoracic ganglion is fused with the inferior cervical. It is stated that sometimes a waist occurs between the two ganglia, and that amputation through this isthmus or the removal of the lower third of the stellate ganglion (combined with the customary sympathectomy) will completely remove the sympathetic supply to the arm. Horner's syndrome does not occur. This is a postganglionic section (*Fig.* 597).

In the Smithwick denervation, as in the Telford operation, endeavour is made to prevent the ever-present danger of nerve regeneration. Telford swings the freed ganglionated segment upwards and sutures it into the neck muscles.

The Smithwick procedure is a well-conceived anatomical exercise. A vertical incision is made between spines and inner border of scapula. The patient is prone, the incision centred over 3rd rib. Trapezius is divided in the line of the incision. A transverse division would injure

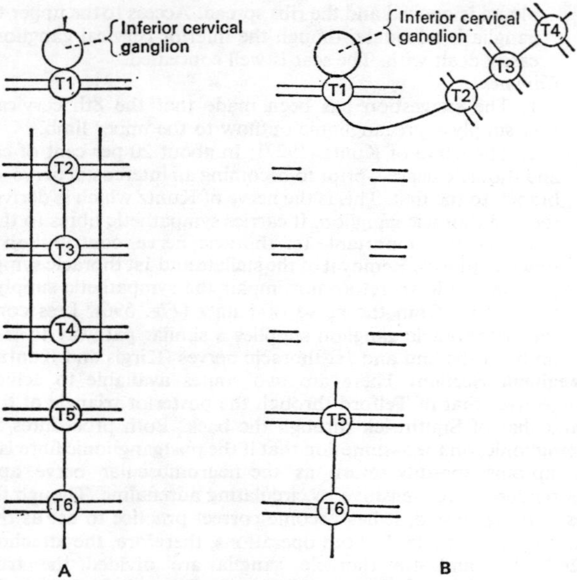

636 A SYNOPSIS OF SURGICAL ANATOMY

Fig. 597.—The general plan of the Smithwick and Telford denervations of the upper limb. A, 2nd, 3rd, and 4th sympathetic ganglia freed from all attachments. B, The mobilized ganglia displaced into muscles of neck or back.

spinal accessory nerve. The rhomboids are split exposing the serratus posterior superior, erector spinae, and posterior chest wall. The costalis tendinous strips are divided and the sacrospinalis mass pulled inwards exposing the third thoracic vertebral transverse process. The intercostal muscles are then cut away from the borders of the 3rd rib between tubercle and angle as also the levator costae insertion to upper border of 3rd rib. The extrapleural connective tissue is thus exposed and it is possible to slip a Doyen raspatory around this rib and free it for 2·5 to 3·8 cm. It is then possible to section the 3rd rib just lateral to the tip of the transverse process and also about 3·8 cm. lateral, thus removing a segment of rib with its periosteum (*Fig.* 598).

The object of removing the periosteum is to expose the pleura, which is then stripped by finger dissection from the sides of the vertebral bodies. The 2nd and 3rd intercostal nerves are now readily exposed at the upper and lower margins of the gap. Each of these is, in turn, grasped with an artery forceps, cut laterally and then freed medially.

SURGERY OF THE SYMPATHETIC

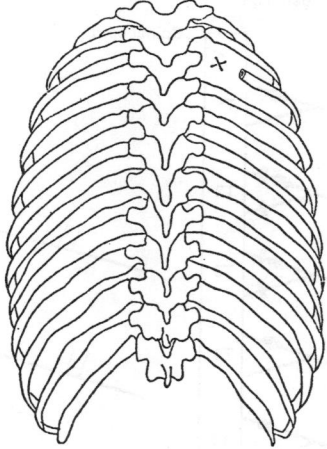

Fig. 598.—The X shows the bone removal in the Smithwick exposure.

The rami, white and grey, connecting each to the related sympathetic ganglion, are cut, and with a special dissector the inner end of the intercostal nerve is teased out of the intervertebral foramen by pushing the dural sleeve away. As soon as the fork of the nerve appears it is carefully snipped with scissors under direct vision. The nerve tissue removed contains the posterior root ganglion on one prong of the fork (*Fig.* 599).

The arachnoid may be cut. A gush of cerebrospinal fluid indicates the event. It is not important. The next step is the picking up of the ganglionated trunk on a hook and the meticulous dissection of 2nd, 3rd, and 4th ganglia. The trunk is secured with a clip below the 4th ganglion, grasped with an artery forceps and cut between this and the clip. By traction on the forceps the rami of the 2nd, 3rd, and 4th ganglia are exposed and divided. These ganglia have now no attachments except to the sympathetic trunk. They are enclosed in a silk bag, the lower end of which is swung upwards and fixed with a stitch at a higher level. The object of the removal of intercostal nerves and their roots is to prevent regeneration of the sympathetic. Should the pleura be punctured it is not important, providing the anaesthetist can keep the lung inflated when asked to and provided the pleural opening is enlarged to a size greater than that of the glottis (2·5 cm.). In this way a tension pneumothorax is prevented. When ready to close the

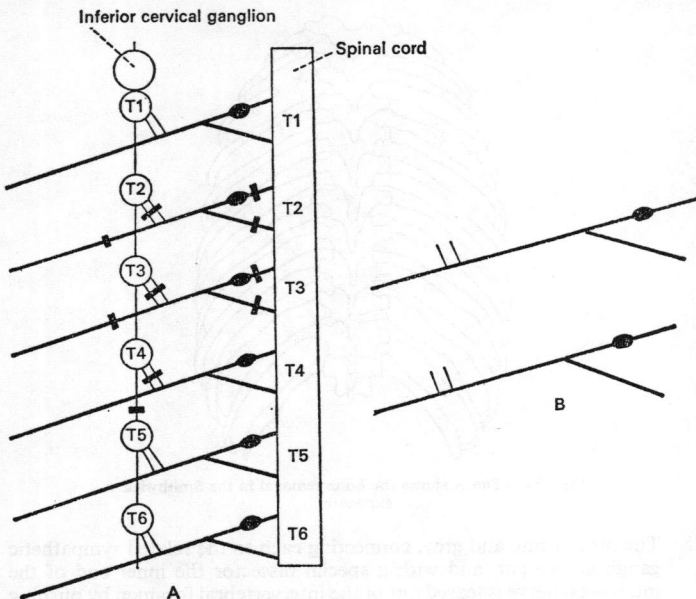

Fig. 599.—A, The black bars delimit the tissue removed in the Smithwick pre-ganglionic upper limb denervation. B, The nerve tissue actually removed.

wound, a catheter is inserted into the opening in the pleura, brought out of the wound, and aspirated by suction, whilst the anaesthetist inflates the lung at the termination of the operation. When the lung is fully expanded the catheter is withdrawn, the opening in the skin closed with a stitch and the wound sealed with collodion. No effort is ever made to suture the pleura. This operation is a brilliant anatomical concept.

LOWER LIMB: Here, as in the upper limb, operations for denervation have become standardized and are for the most part preganglionic in character. The approach is anterior or posterior depending on the age and build of the patient. The lumbar ganglia are removed from the first to the point where the sympathetic disappears under the common iliac vessels (*Fig.* 600).

RECOGNITION OF LUMBAR GANGLIA: The lumbar ganglia are so variable in position and size that Atlas has stated it is not possible even to number the ganglia with anything approaching uniformity. Most

SURGERY OF THE SYMPATHETIC

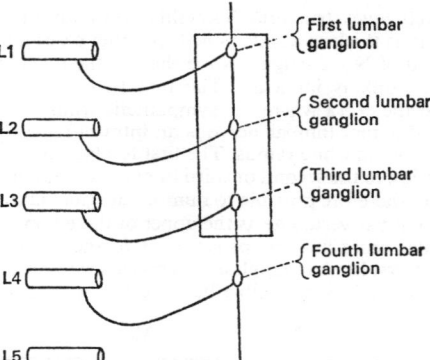

Fig. 600.—The diagram shows the connexions of the sympathetic chain with the lumbar nerves. The sympathetic nerve-supply to the entire lower limb is removed by the operation of lumbar ganglionectomy, i.e., removing the part of the sympathetic shown in the rectangle.

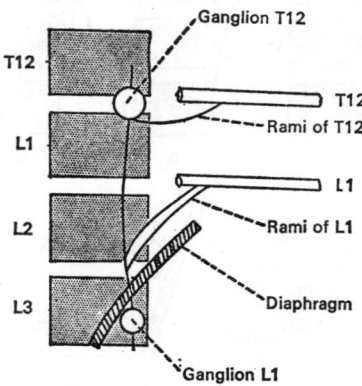

Fig. 601.—Showing that whereas the first lumbar spinal nerve lies in the thorax in relation to the vertebra of the same number, the first lumbar ganglion lies in the abdominal cavity on the third lumbar vertebra. This accounts for the great length of the rami of the first lumbar ganglion.

usually there are four ganglia on each side. The arrangement on one side is not necessarily or most commonly duplicated on the other. Not infrequently the ganglia are aggregated in one or two relatively huge structures. Sometimes the connecting sympathetic trunk is as thick as a slate pencil, in other cases it is as slender as a strand of No. 2 catgut. None the less the practical importance of the trunk is immense. The first two lumbar vertebrae are behind the crura where the sympathetic trunk lies in relation to them. The first lumbar nerve is an intrathoracic structure where it gives off its white ramus. The first lumbar ganglion usually lies in relation to the second or third lumbar vertebra in the abdomen. It is not therefore possible to number the ganglia by their relation to the lumbar vertebrae as the upper of these bones lie behind the muscular crura and the psoas overlaps the others (*Fig.* 601). To find the first lumbar ganglion it is necessary to pick up the lumbar trunk where it is accessible below the crus. It is then traced up

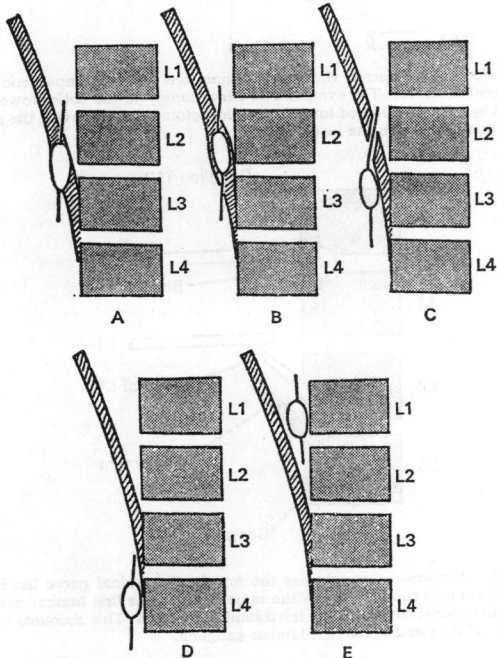

Fig. 602.—The relationships of the first lumbar ganglion to the crus of the diaphragm are shown: A, Partly buried in crus. B, Buried in crus. C, Just below crus. D, Distal to crus. E, Above crus, in thorax.

SURGERY OF THE SYMPATHETIC

into the thorax for at least an inch by teasing away the fibres of the diaphragm with Hartmann's forceps. If no ganglion is found on tracing the thoracolumbar communication into the thorax for 2·5 cm. then the first ganglion in or below the crus is the first lumbar.

The Importance of the First Lumbar Ganglion: It plays an important role in ejaculation and should therefore be preserved during sympathectomy. It is not concerned with vasomotor and sudomotor functions in the foot and lower part of the leg below the knee and resection is thus not necessary in the usual case.

The ganglion is situated in relation to the lower portion of the crus of the diaphragm lying (*a*) on the crus, its upper pole being buried in this structure; (*b*) in the crus; (*c*) immediately below the crus; (*d*) distal to the crus; (*e*) above the crus in the thoracic cavity (*Fig.* 602).

The lumbar chain may be exposed from the back or front.

Posterior Route (*Smithwick*): The patient lies on the opposite side with the loin opened by a pillow beneath it. The upper thigh is flexed to relax the psoas. The incision is a finger breadth

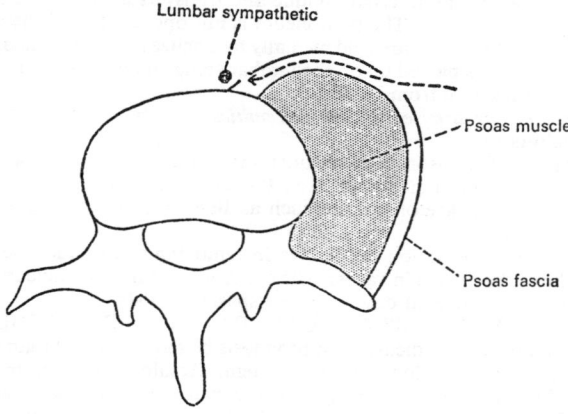

Fig. 603.—Transverse section at the level of the third lumbar vertebra. The arrow shows that in the posterior approach to the lumbar chain the fascia of the psoas is opened twice by the surgeon.

below and parallel to the last rib extending to the iliac crest 3·8 cm. behind the anterior superior spine of the ilium. The posterior border of the external oblique is mobilized, the latissimus cut across, and the aponeurosis of origin of the transversus abdominis exposed. The posterior border of the internal oblique may require division for 2·5 cm. The aponeurosis is cut through in the line of the skin incision, and the division is between subcostal and first lumbar nerves which require careful protection especially in closing the wound. The extra-peritoneal fat is pushed off quadratus and psoas and a roll of 15 cm. gauze packs it forwards. A lighted retractor is inserted. The surgeon defines the fascia over the psoas. This is attached to lumbar vertebrae medially. When the fascia is opened the sympathetic trunk is immediately apparent, its situation being so exact that it may be picked up by a hook even though it is not visible (*Fig.* 603).

The trunk is then followed up and down as explained in the previous section.

Anterior Route: In young, not obese, persons the ganglionectomy may be done on both sides at the same operation. The patient lies supine. The incision extends from just below umbilicus laterally to just below the 10th rib. The flat muscles are dealt with by dividing external oblique in the direction of its fibres and cutting internal oblique and transversus in the line of the skin incision. The peritoneum is not opened. It and the extra-peritoneal fat are held medially by a gauze roll. The sympathetic trunk is picked up on the lumbar spine and dealt with as in the procedure from behind.

Diseases of the arteries of the extremities may be divided into two main groups:
  a. Those of a vasomotor or functional nature in which vasospasm is the important factor, e.g., Raynaud's disease.
  b. Organic disease of arteries such as Buerger's disease and arteriosclerosis.

Sympathetic denervation is effective in removing spasm and sweating. Thus it has value in vasospastic conditions. It has no value in cases of organic arterial disease unless spasm coexists.

PROGNOSIS IN OPERATIONS ON THE SYMPATHETIC: In no field of medicine must prognosis be more guarded than in the realm of operations on this system. Results are often brilliant following surgery but relapse to the *status quo ante* occurs all too often. It is this fact which brought discredit on the surgery of the sympathetic years ago, and although advancing knowledge has improved results, disappointments occur frequently. It is as well to follow certain rules:

1. Indications for operation must be correct.
2. The effects of the proposed operation should be determined by preliminary nerve-block. Occasionally sympathetic denervation has resulted in worsening of the condition of the limb. This has been attributed to various factors, e.g., shunting of blood via

preferential pathways and depleting still further the area of defective supply. Worth-while results may follow denervation even though preliminary nerve-block fails to disclose the existence of vasospasm. The investigator must be on guard should a paradoxical response follow procaine block, i.e., a fall of temperature on the side being tested. This is a contra-indication to denervation.

3. Regeneration can be guarded against by:
   a. Leaving a wide gap in the sympathetic chain.
   b. Covering both ends of the chain by an impermeable barrier, e.g., silk bag or tantalum tube. The value is, however, questionable (*Fig.* 604).

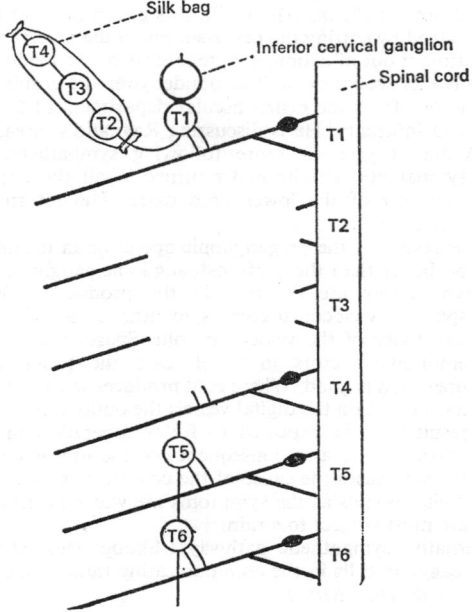

Fig. 604.—Smithwick's device to prevent nerve regeneration.

4. *Intermittent Claudication:* In this condition pain occurs during exercise and is relieved by rest. It is best known as a manifestation of peripheral aorto-iliac obstructive vascular disease. There are

other causes which may produce it. Evans[1] points out that it may be a prominent feature of anaemia, McArdle's[2] disease, the pre-infarctive anterior tibial syndrome, occur as a complication of vasoconstrictive drugs, or be a symptom of a neurological lesion.

Experience has shown that after a lumbar ganglionectomy the limb may improve generally and yet intermittent claudication may continue as the arterioles supplying muscle are too fibrosed to respond to removal of the vasoconstrictor impulses. Patients or near relatives should be warned of this possiblity. Boyd[3] and his co-workers have clarified the matter by dividing claudication into (1) those cases where increase of the blood-supply to the part will relieve the claudication, and (2) cases where such increase will not benefit the patient. In this group of cases relief may be obtained by cutting the nerve-supply to the muscle affected or by putting it out of action, e.g., tenotomy of the tendo Achillis.

5. The reader would do well to ponder over the ensuing remarks of Haxton[4] from the neurovascular department of the Manchester Royal Infirmary. He is discussing Raynaud's disease:

   a. Within a year or more following sympathetic denervation sympathetic activity had returned in all the upper and only very few of the lower limb cases. The return was usually incomplete.

   b. The results of the preganglionic operation in the upper limb are no better than those of postganglionic ganglionectomy.

   c. Two factors are requisite in the production of Raynaud's spasm: Vasoconstrictor sympathetic activity, and local sensitivity of the vessels to cold. Spasm may be induced by emotional factors in which case the prognosis following operation is good. Where cold produces spasm as a result of its local effect on the digital vessels the outlook is poor. The same result may be expected to follow operation in cases where spasm occurs as a consequence of the use of vibrating tools. In these cases the cause of the condition is local injury to the digital vessels as the symptoms are worse in the fingers which are most subject to strain.

6. Alternative sympathetic pathways: Skoog[5] showed the presence of ganglion cells in the communicating rami of the cervical and upper thoracic nerves.

---

[1] Evans, J. G., *Br. med. J.*, 1964, 2, 985.
[2] A disorder characterized by a gross failure of the breakdown in muscle of glycogen to lactic acid—a normal process to supply energy for the contraction of muscle.
[3] Boyd A. M., Ratcliffe, A., Hall. Jepson, R. P., and James, G. W. H., *J. Bone Jt Surg.*, 1949, 31, 325.
[4] Haxton, H. A., *Br. J. Surg.*, 1947, 35, 69.
[5] Skoog, T., *Lancet* 1947, 2, 457.

Alexander, Kuntz, Henderson, and Ehrlich[1] have shown these accessory ganglia in relation to many portions of the sympathetic apparatus, and, of still greater significance, they have demonstrated them in anterior spinal nerve-roots in proximity to the origin of sympathetic rami (*Fig.* 605). Ray and Console[2] showed that the 12th thoracic and first three lumbar dermatomes receive part of their sympathetic nerve-supply through channels

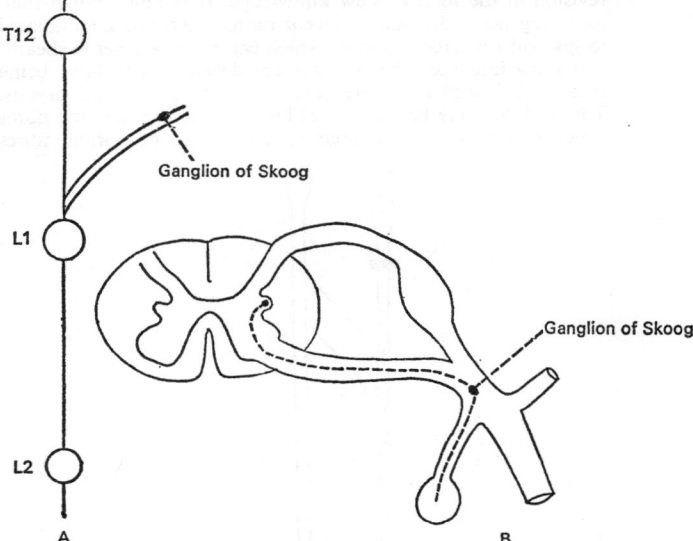

Fig. 605.—A, Skoog's ganglion in the white ramus communicans of the first lumbar nerve. B, Skoog's ganglion in the substance of a spinal nerve.

that do not pass through any part of the paravertebral chain from T.8–L.3. The lower extremity, thus, cannot be completely sympathectomized by any form of attack on the paravertebral chain, as the residual pathways pass via the anterior primary rami of the lumbar nerves. It is apparent that alternative sympathetic pathways do exist in relation to many parts of the paravertebral chain and here probably lies an important cause of relapse following operations on the sympathetic.

[1] Alexander, W. F., Kuntz, A., Henderson, W. P., and Ehrlich, E., *J. int. Coll. Surg.*, 1949, 12, 111.
[2] Ray, B. S., and Console, A. D., *J. Neurosurg.*, 1948, 5, 23.

7. *Collateral Nerve Sprouting:* This concept must be taken into account in considering the causes of return of function following injury to nerve-tissue. Murray's[1] work is summarized here. He states that the nervous system possesses powers greater than those usually understood by the term regeneration.

The accepted physiology that, following the division of a nerve, new fibres grow only from the central end, requires revision in the light of new knowledge. It is now known that, following nerve division, adjacent normal nerves are stimulated to give off tiny side branches which can penetrate nerve-sheaths and grow into the tubes of adjacent degenerating fibres, being thus guided until they may reach and activate effector organs. The stimulus may be a humoral factor from degenerating fibres which can produce a change in the surface of normal fibres

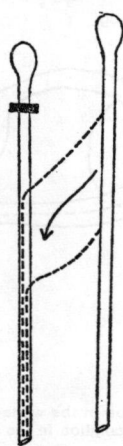

Fig. 606.—Nerve sprouting. A nerve has been divided. Fibres from an adjacent intact nerve are seen growing into the sheath of the injured nerve distal to the line of section. (*After Murray.*)

resulting in nerve sprouting. This process is usually most profuse in relation to delicate nerve terminations. Should it occur more proximally the outgrowing fibrils are less likely to reach effector organs and serve no purpose.

This phenomenon is most prolific in relation to the autonomic system. Murray has shown experimentally that if, during

[1] Murray, J. G., *J. R. Coll. Surg. Edin.*, 1958, 4, 199.

cervical sympathectomy, 10 per cent of nerve-fibres are left intact within one to two months complete re-innervation may occur. This return to function coincides with the disappearance of hypersensivity to adrenaline or noradrenaline (*Fig.* 606). In addition there is rerouting so that unusual functional contacts may occur. The degree of functional recovery is furthermore dependent on the percentage of fibres left intact, so that if only 1 per cent persists, re-innervation will be slower and imperfect.

After cervical sympathectomy sprouting may occur from adjacent nerves, such as the vagus, which may lead to bizarre results. Nerve sprouting is a general phenomenon in the nervous system, the essential factor being the proximity of normal to degenerating fibres.

8. *Physiological Derangements following Sympathectomy:*
   a. Excessive Sweating: Following extensive sympathetic denervation, e.g., lumbodorsal or denervation of two or more limbs, sweating is so extensively paralysed that compensatory sweating occurs in the non-denervated areas. This is troublesome to the patient. It is thus not wise to denervate four limbs. So, too, Raynaud's phenomenon may occur in the hands after operations for hypertension.
   b. In Regard to the Male Sex Organs: Whitelaw and Smithwick,[1] in a paper of great value, deal with some of the secondary effects of sympathectomy. They point out that erection is the result of psychic stimuli together with afferent stimuli from the penis. The latter pass via the internal pudendal nerves to the cord, where a lumbar centre for erection may exist. The efferent pathway is via the nervi erigentes. There ensues dilatation of the arteries to the penis together with engorgement of the corpora cavernosa. The only part the sympathetic plays in the process is inhibition of vasoconstriction of the arteries of the penis.

Mechanism of Ejaculation:
   a. The sympathetic produces contraction of the unstriped muscle of prostate, vesicles, and ductus deferens resulting in seminal fluid entering the prostatic urethra.
   b. The parasympathetic (nervi erigentes) causes contraction of the bulbocavernosus and ischiocavernosus muscles, propelling the ejaculate to the exterior.
   c. The emission takes the path of least resistance, i.e., through the urethra, as the tone of the internal or bladder neck sphincter will not allow it to pass into the bladder. This tone is dependent on parasympathetic impulses (nervi erigentes) together with the reinforcement mediated by the sympathetic via the nerves which pass from the upper lumbar ganglia

[1] Whitelaw, G. P., and Smithwick, R. H., *New Engl. J. Med.*, 1951, 245, 121.

(mainly the first) through the presacral and hypogastric ganglia to the bladder base.

   d. After ejaculation the sympathetic causes vasoconstriction of the penile arteries, thus reducing the blood-supply to the organ, and flaccidity ensues.

Sympathectomy disturbs these mechanisms as follows:

   a. Removal of upper lumbar ganglia, especially the first, reduces the tone of the internal sphincter of the bladder. The ejaculate finds the path of least resistance, which is into the bladder. It is passed with the next urination. This is the cause of dry intercourse.

   b. Following removal of parts of the sympathetic system there is increased tonus of the remaining part of the system. This could increase the vasoconstriction tone of the arteries to the penis impairing the efficiency of erection.

   c. Pooling of blood in denervated areas results in lessening the blood-supply elsewhere which may also impair erection.

   These mechanisms explain why sympathectomy above the diaphragm may impair sexual efficiency. Such disturbances of sex function occur in a relatively small proportion of cases and are frequently temporary in nature. They depend largely on how many lumbar ganglia are removed on both sides.

VII. PARAGANGLIOMA

These are of two types: chromaffin and non-chromaffin depending on whether they are stained by potassium bichromate.

Chromaffin Paraganglioma:

   DEVELOPMENT: The adrenal medulla is formed from the ectoderm of the neural tube. These cells give rise to sympathoblasts which form ganglion cells and phaeochromoblasts which become phaeochromocytes or chromaffin cells. Cells of this type may be diverted from their course and be associated with sympathetic ganglia, usually prevertebral in situation. Kohn[1] applied the term 'paraganglia' to such ectopic collections of chromaffin tissue. A tumour arising from the adrenal medulla is a phaeochromocytoma whereas one arising from ectopic phaeochrome tissue is a chromaffin paraganglioma.

   SITUATIONS OF CHROMAFFIN PARAGANGLIOMAS:

   Theoretically such tumours may occur wherever chromaffin tissue is found. In actuality tumours causing hypertension are found in or near the adrenal gland. Graham[2] collected 198 cases of chromaffin paragangliomas associated with hypertension up to the middle of 1949. The locations were—the right or left adrenal gland, the

[1] Kohn, A., *Ergebn. Anat. EntwGesch.*, 1902, 12, 253.
[2] Graham, J. B., *Surgery Gynec. Obstet.*, 1951, 92, 105.

lumbar paravertebral spaces, in front of the great vessels of the abdomen, the organ of Zuckerkandl (at the origin of the inferior mesenteric artery from the aorta), the left thoracic paravertebral space, and the coeliac ganglion, in that order of frequency (*Fig.* 607). Ten per cent of such tumours are malignant, in 10 per cent more than one is present, and 10 per cent occur elsewhere than in the adrenals.

Pathologists state that the distinction between simple or malignant phaeochromocytomas cannot be made histologically in a proportion of cases. In these it is necessary to wait five years after removal of the tumour to see whether or not recurrence occurs. The only certain sign of malignancy is the existence of local invasiveness or metastases.

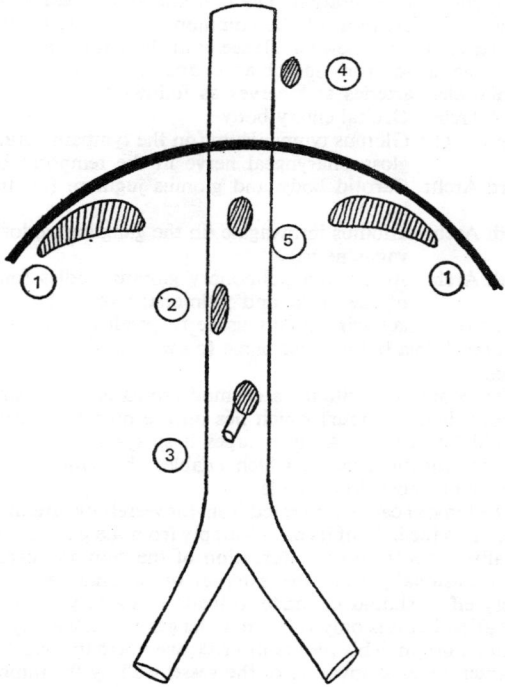

Fig. 607.—Situations where chromaffin tissue may be found. 1, Normal position in adrenal. 2, Lumbar paravertebral space. 3, Organ of Zuckerkandl. 4, Paravertebral space in left thorax. 5, In front of great vessels.

COMMENT: Chromaffin paragangliomas often cause hypertension which may be paroxysmal or sustained. Bartels and Cattell[1] stress the gravity of unsuspected phaeochromocytoma. They report a number of deaths during operations for unrelated conditions consequent on the reactions of the patient who, unknown to the surgeon, harboured such a tumour. The authors state that the occurrence of a hypertensive reaction during the course of an operation should lead to the suspicion of a phaeochromocytoma. This reaction constitutes a response not unlike cardiac arrest which every surgeon should be prepared to meet.

Non-chromaffin Paragangliomas: The non-chromaffin paraganglia are chemoreceptors, responding to alterations in blood gases and pH, with an effect on respiration. The best known of these is the carotid body at the bifurcation of the common carotid artery, but similar structures are found elsewhere. It seems likely that the non-chromaffin paraganglia arise from mesoblastic and neural tissue around the branchial cleft arteries and nerves as follows:[2]

- 1st Arch: Orbital ciliary body
- 2nd Arch: Glomus tympanicum (on the tympanic branch of the glossopharyngeal nerve in the temporal bone)
- 3rd Arch: Carotid body and glomus jugulare (on the jugular bulb)
- 4th Arch: Glomus intravagale (in the ganglion nodosum of the vagus nerve)
- 6th Arch: Aortic and pulmonary glomus bodies (on the arch of the aorta and pulmonary vessels)

Tumours may arise in this tissue to produce a non-chromaffin paraganglioma but a better name to avoid confusion is chemodectoma.

The commonest site for a chemodectoma is in the carotid body (carotid body tumour) which lies on the posterior surface of the carotid bifurcation. As it enlarges it splays out the internal and external carotid arteries which enables the clinical and arteriographic diagnosis to be made.

The tumour can be separated from the vessels by careful dissection. It receives the bulk of its blood-supply from the glomic artery which usually arises from the bifurcation of the common carotid artery but occasionally from the external or internal carotid arteries.[3] Every effort should be made to ligate this artery early during the operation but it is only 1–2 mm. in length and can easily be avulsed from its origin. This results in brisk haemorrhage which is usually misinterpreted as invasion of the vessel wall by the tumour.

---

[1] Bartels, E. C., and Cattell, R. B., *Ann. Surg.*, 1950, **131**, 903.
[2] Szanto, P. B. *Int. Surg.*, 1972, **57**, 236.
[3] Heath, D., and Edwards, C. (1971), 'The Glomic Arteries' *Cardiovasc. Res.*, **5**, 503.

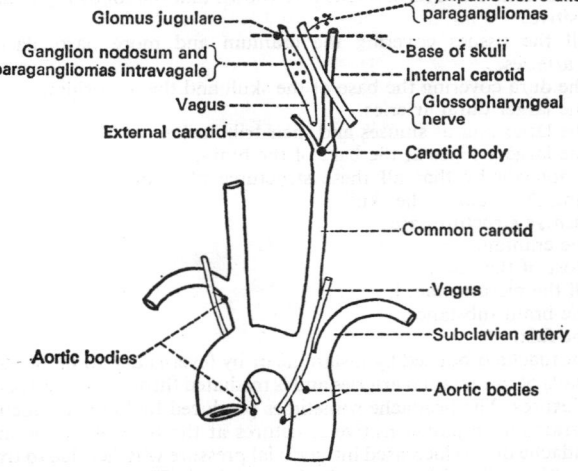

Fig. 608.—The situations in which paragangliomas may be found. (*Re-drawn from Lattes, R., 'Cancer', 1950, 3, 667.*)

Chemodectomas in the other situations (*Fig.* 608) present as a bleeding mass in the ear, a mass at the base of the skull or in the thorax. The tumours are very vascular and can easily be demonstrated by arteriography.

Chapter XLII

THE ANATOMY OF CERTAIN DISEASES

1. HEADACHE

Headache is a common symptom. Only latterly is there some understanding of its underlying causes. Pickering,[1] Symonds,[2] and Wolff and his colleagues have done much in this elucidation. This section is largely a summary of papers by the two former workers.

[1] Pickering, G. W., *J. Am. med. Ass.*, 1948, 137, 423.
[2] Symonds, Sir Charles, *Clin. J.*, Jan.–Feb. 1947, by permission of *Guy's Hosp. Reps.*

Of the cranium and its contents it is known that the following structures are sensitive:
1. All the tissues covering the cranium and more particularly the arteries.
2. The dura covering the base of the skull and the tentorium.
3. The larger dural arteries.
4. The large venous sinuses and their tributaries.
5. The large arteries at the base of the brain.

It is noteworthy that all these structures play an important part in anchoring the brain to the skull.

Insensitive structures are:
1. The cranium.
2. Most of the dura.
3. All the pia-arachnoid.
4. The brain substance.
5. The falx.

The headache produced by histamine or by fever is due to the stretching of the walls of intracranial arteries and is mediated through the perivascular nerve plexuses. The headache sometimes produced by lumbar puncture is due to traction on pain-sensitive structures at the base of the brain. So, too, headache due to increased intracranial pressure whether due to trauma or tumour is explicable on precisely the same basis. Thus a simple explanation is forthcoming for the oft observed clinical fact that following injury to the skull as many headaches are due to low as to high cerebrospinal fluid pressure.

The headache of migraine is due to stretching of the walls of the extra- and intracranial arteries.

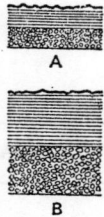

Fig. 609.—Comparison of a section of a cerebral and a peripheral artery. A, Cerebral artery. B, Radial artery.

A raised blood-pressure alone does not cause headache. The headache which occurs so commonly in cases of hypertension is due to variations in the tone of the walls of the cranial arteries.

Pickering makes important observations on the cause of hypertensive encephalopathy. It has been assumed that spasm of cerebral vessels is the precipitating factor. Pickering stresses that from their conformation the vascular structures of the brain are less likely than other vessels to show strong localized vasoconstriction (*Fig.* 609).

The cerebral arteries are peculiar in the thinness of their walls and both anatomical and physiological studies give the picture that these vessels are feebly contractile and would respond weakly or not at all to vasoconstrictor agents.

The encephalopathy of acute hypertension is evidenced by intense headache, vomiting, convulsions and coma and is due to acute oedema of the brain. The latter is more likely to be due to defective than to increased constriction of cerebral arterioles.

In chronic hypertension there sometimes occur attacks of transient paralyses which may be motor or sensory and are often not associated with loss of consciousness. Pickering makes a strong case for regarding such attacks as being organic (e.g., thrombotic) and not of vasospastic origin, and points out their great similarity to the attacks which occur in mitral stenosis and are known to be of embolic origin.

II. INFECTIONS OF THE HAND[1]

The anatomy of the tendon-sheaths of the wrist and hand is dealt with on p. 256.

Fingers: Over the front of the distal phalanx the skin is bound down to the periosteum by dense processes with fatty tissue between. The distal four-fifths of the terminal phalanx receives its blood-supply

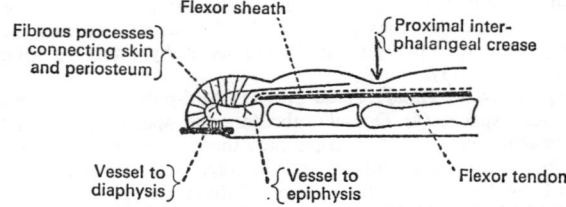

Fig. 610.—A figure to show: (1) The fibrous bands binding skin to periosteum over the last phalanx, and the blood-supply to the shaft of the phalanx traversing these bands. The vessels to the epiphysis do not go through this area. (2) The fact that the flexor sheath is immediately subjacent to the proximal interphalangeal crease, so that a pin-prick in the direction of the arrow may cause tenosynovitis.

from the digital arteries at the sides of the finger. These vessels to the bone reach it by penetrating the dense fibrous processes mentioned. Should infection of this tissue occur (subcutaneous whitlow), there is

---

[1] The perusal of this chapter may be followed by reading the section dealing with the anatomy of palmar incisions on p. 764.

no provision for expansion because of its fibrous nature. The arteries to the bone are compressed by the inflammatory pressure, resulting in necrosis of the part of the bone they supply, i.e., distal four-fifths. The base of the phalanx (the epiphysis in the young) receives its blood-supply by vessels which do *not* traverse this dense tissue—therefore it does not necrose like the rest of the bone (*Fig.* 610).

Interphalangeal Creases: The skin of the creases of the proximal interphalangeal joints of the fingers is closely bound down to the underlying fibrous flexor sheaths. Pricks in these creases therefore may cause thecal whitlow, as the sheath is so intimately related to the skin.

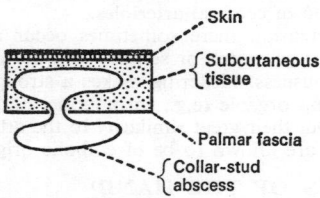

Fig. 611.—Representation of a collar-stud abcess.

Collar-stud Abscess: The relation of skin to palmar fascia is much the same as that of the skin of the scalp to the underlying epicranial (occipitofrontalis) aponeurosis. In each case skin is firmly bound to aponeurosis by dense fibrous tissue which does not admit of distension. Pus under the skin may perforate the palmar aponeurosis, and vice versa, resulting in two pus cavities connected by a stalk—a collar-stud abscess (*Fig.* 611).

Fascial Spaces of the Hand: These are: (1) Mid-palmar; (2) Thenar; (3) Forearm space; (4) Dorsal subcutaneous space; (5) Dorsal subaponeurotic space. The mid-palmar, thenar, and forearm spaces all lie *deep* to the flexor tendons and their synovial sheaths, which therefore form the anterior boundaries of these spaces.

MID-PALMAR SPACE: Lies under the inner half of the hollow of the hand (between the thenar and the hypothenar eminences). Its shape is triangular.

BOUNDARIES (*Figs.* 612–614):

Anterior:

1. Flexor tendons (with their synovial sheaths) of the little, ring, and middle fingers. The tendons of the middle finger are anterior relations of the thenar space also, but are more intimately related to the mid-palmar space.
2. The lumbrical muscles related to the tendons of the ring and little fingers, i.e., 3rd and 4th lumbricals.

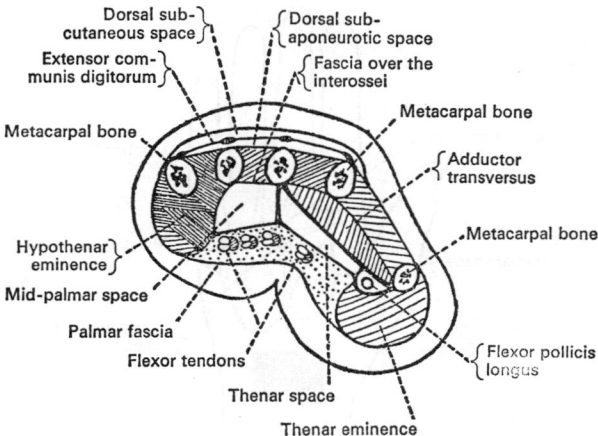

Fig. 612.—Section through the palm to show thenar and mid-palmar spaces. The dorsal subcutaneous and subaponeurotic spaces are also shown.

Posterior: The dense fascia covering the interossei and metacarpal bones.

Radial: The fibrous partition between the thenar and mid-palmar spaces. This partition extends between (1) the fascia on the under-surface of the flexor tendons and (2) the fascia covering the interossei and adductor of the thumb.

Ulnar: The hypothenar muscles.

Proximal: It reaches the level of the distal margin of the transverse carpal ligament. Sometimes this space is continuous with the forearm space by a small tunnel behind the flexor sheaths at the wrist.

Distal: It reaches almost to the level of the distal palmar crease.

The lumbrical muscles have delicate fascial sheaths which are so intimately related to the palmar spaces that infection of the space causes infection of the related lumbrical sheaths. Each lumbrical sheath may therefore almost be looked on as a diverticulum of the space to which it is related. The 3rd and 4th lumbrical sheaths would therefore be diverticula of the mid-palmar space. The 1st lumbrical sheath would therefore be a diverticulum of the thenar space. The 2nd lumbrical sheath may be a diverticulum of either the thenar or the mid-palmar space. Pus in the mid-palmar space is usually drained by slitting the web between the 3rd and 4th or 4th and 5th digits and opening the sheath of the lumbrical in the space.

656 A SYNOPSIS OF SURGICAL ANATOMY

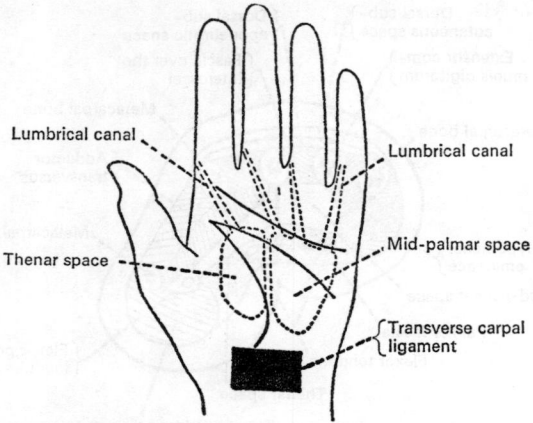

Fig. 613.—The dotted lines indicate the fascial spaces of the palm. The prolongations of the spaces along the lumbrical canals are shown.

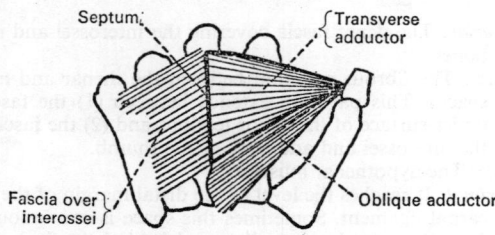

Fig. 614.—The soft tissues of the palm have been removed to show the posterior boundary of the thenar and mid-palmar spaces. On the left is the fascia overlying the interossei which bounds the mid-palmar space. On the right is the transverse part of adductor pollicis which bounds the thenar space. The black line is the septum between the spaces.

THENAR SPACE (*Figs.* 612–614):

POSITION: It lies under the outer half of the hollow of the palm. It is triangular in shape.

BOUNDARIES:

Anterior:
1. Short muscles of the thumb.
2. Flexor tendons of index finger.
3. 1st and 2nd lumbricals.

THE ANATOMY OF CERTAIN DISEASES 657

Posterior: The adductor pollicis, mainly its transverse head.

Radial: The flexor pollicis longus tendon in its synovial sheath which is called the radial bursa.

Ulnar: The septum between the two spaces, mid-palmar and thenar.

Distal: It reaches to the proximal transverse palmar crease. The 1st lumbrical sheath and sometimes the 2nd extend as distal diverticula of the space.

Proximal: It reaches to the distal border of the anterior annular ligament (transverse carpal).

Observe that the digital flexor sheaths of the 2nd, 3rd, and 4th digits begin at the level where the thenar and mid-palmar spaces end. Pus in these tendon-sheaths may therefore burst into and infect the palmar spaces.

FOREARM SPACE: This is merely a fascial interval deep to the flexor tendons in the distal part of the forearm.

BOUNDARIES:

Anterior:
1. The flexor digitorum profundus in its synovial sheath (the ulnar bursa).
2. The flexor pollicis longus in its synovial sheath (the radial bursa).

Posterior: The pronator quadratus and the interosseous membrane.

Distal: It reaches the level of the wrist.

Proximal: It is continuous with the intermuscular spaces of the forearm, and pus may track from the space any distance into the forearm, coming into relationship with the median and ulnar nerves, etc.

Lateral: The space extends to the outer and inner borders of the forearm, and is drained by incisions along these borders.

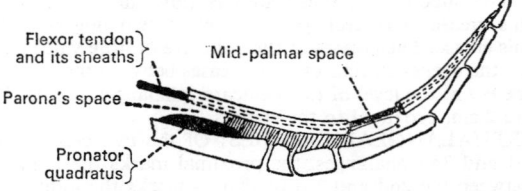

Fig. 615.—Section in the long axis of the hand to show the forearm space—Parona's.

The forearm space becomes infected by extension from the synovial sheaths of the flexors, especially from the common sheath of the flexor digitorum profundus and sublimis, which is called the ulnar bursa. Pus presents *behind* these tendons and not in front of them, because, as is seen in *Fig.* 615, the synovial sheath almost opens into the space behind the tendons, a little connective tissue intervening, whilst in front it is much more firmly attached to the tendons.

DORSAL SPACES (*see Fig.* 612, p. 655): On the dorsum of the hand the areolar tissue is much looser than in the palm, which does not admit of much swelling because of the unyielding nature of the palmar fascia. Therefore in palmar infections the swelling is usually on the dorsum (because of the lymphatic drainage in this direction).

The extensors of the fingers are connected to each other by fibrous tissue, which forms with the extensor tendons an aponeurotic barrier between two spaces—the dorsal subcutaneous and the dorsal subaponeurotic spaces. These spaces are both triangular, with the apex of the triangle at the wrist and the base at the knuckles.

BOUNDARIES:

Proximal: They are continuous with the subcutaneous tissue of the forearm.

Distal: They are continuous with the subcutaneous tissue of the webs of the fingers.

Medial and Lateral: They are continuous with the subcutaneous tissue around the ulnar border of the hand and second metacarpal respectively.

These two spaces are therefore much more extensive and less well circumscribed than the palmar spaces.

Creases of Hand and Fingers: There are two creases just proximal to the thenar and hypothenar eminences:
1. The proximal marks the level of the wrist-joint.
2. The distal marks the level of the proximal border of the transverse carpal ligament.

The superficial palmar arch is three finger-breadths distal to this crease. The deep palmar arch is two finger-breadths below this crease. The creases of the palm are of little value as landmarks for the deeper structures. The creases between the palm and fingers are *not* at the level of the metacarpophalangeal joints. These joints are 2 cm. proximal to the creases.

INTERPHALANGEAL CREASES: Of the two creases between the 1st and 2nd phalanges, the proximal marks the joint. The crease between the 2nd and 3rd phalanges marks the joint.

Dorsum of the Fingers: With the fingers flexed to a fist the prominences at the joints are formed in every case by the *proximal* of the two bones forming that joint.

LEVELS OF THE JOINTS AT THE BACK (*Fig.* 616): With the digits clenched into a fist:
1. The metacarpophalangeal joint is 1·3 cm. distal to the prominence of the knuckle.

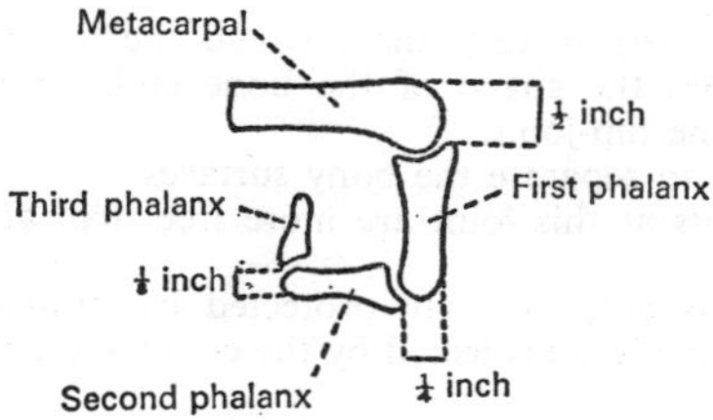

THE ANATOMY OF CERTAIN DISEASES

Fig. 616.—To show that when the fingers are clenched the prominence of the knuckle is always formed by the proximal bone. The distance of the joint from the knuckle is shown.

2. The proximal interphalangeal joint is 0·6 cm. distal to the prominence at the joint.
3. The distal interphalangeal joint is 0·3 cm. distal to the prominence at the joint.

III. COMMON DISLOCATIONS

Clavicle:
   INNER END: This may pass: (1) Forwards and override the sternum, i.e., *anterior dislocation;* (2) Upwards, i.e., *superior dislocation;* (3) Backwards behind the sternum, i.e., *posterior dislocation.*
   OUTER END: The clavicular facet looks down and out, the acromial facet up and in. Dislocation of the clavicle is therefore usually *upwards*. Rarely it may be *downwards* (*Fig.* 617).

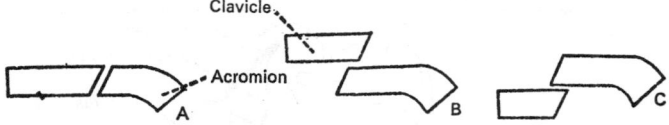

Fig. 617.—A, Normal relationship of bone-ends forming the acromioclavicular joint. B, Common type of dislocation which occurs at this joint. C, A rare type of acromioclavicular dislocation.

Vertebrae: The articular surfaces of the articular processes are perpendicular except in the cervical region, where they are nearly horizontal. Therefore pure dislocation can only be cervical. Elsewhere the articular processes must fracture before dislocation can occur, i.e., fracture-dislocation.

Head of the Humerus: The shoulder-joint has the following characteristics which account for the fact that dislocations at this joint are more frequent than dislocations of all the other bones combined:

660 A SYNOPSIS OF SURGICAL ANATOMY

1. The *glenoid cavity* is very shallow and the articulation gains no strength from the shape of the bone ends forming it, such as obtains in the hip-joint.
2. *Gravity* tends to separate the bony surfaces.
3. The *movements* at this joint are more free than at any other joint in the body.
4. The *capsule* is very strongly protected by muscles in front and behind. Above it is protected by the coraco-acromial arch. Below,

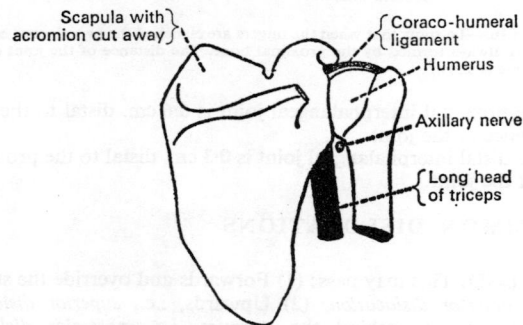

Fig. 618.—Showing certain important structures in the anatomy of the shoulder-joint, notably the coracohumeral ligament and axillary nerve.

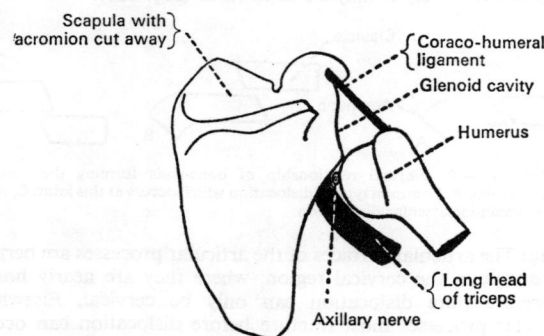

Fig. 619.—To show the danger to the axillary nerve when head of humerus occupies the subglenoid position in dislocation at the shoulder-joint. The intact coracohumeral ligament is shown. Kocher's method of reducing the dislocation is based on the integrity of this band.

however, the capsule is unprotected (*Fig.* 618). This is its weakest part, and the head of the humerus leaves the joint at this place. In all instances, then, the dislocation is first subglenoid.

From the subglenoid position, the head may go up under the coracoid and pectoralis minor—*subcoracoid*.

From the subglenoid position, the head may go up under the coracoid, clavicle, and pectoralis major—*subclavicular*.

From the subglenoid position, the head may go back under the teres muscles—*subspinous*.

From the subglenoid position, the head may continue to pass downwards, coming to lie on the serratus. In these cases, which are rare, the arm is abducted above the head—*luxatio erecta*.

In the subcoracoid and subclavicular dislocations the *coracohumeral ligament remains intact*, and on this fact is based Kocher's method of reduction of dislocations of the shoulder-joint (*Fig.* 619).

NERVE LESIONS COMPLICATING DISLOCATIONS AT THE SHOULDER-JOINT: The brachial plexus is separated from the humeral head by the subscapularis (*Fig.* 620). The axillary (circumflex) nerve which supplies the deltoid lies immediately below the humeral head. It follows that anterior displacements (subcoracoid) of this bone may be associated with grave injury to the nerve-supply of the upper limb. Occasionally such nerve lesions may be associated with an unbearable burning in the palm of the hand, the condition of causalgia. This syndrome is associated with lesions in the territory of two nerves—i.e., median and posterior tibial (internal popliteal). It follows that when causalgia complicates a dislocated shoulder, it is due to injury of those fibres of the median nerve which supply the palm of the hand. Subglenoid displacement of the head of the humerus may injure the axillary nerve and paralyse the deltoid. This injury occurs with remarkable infrequency, considering how exposed the nerve would seem to be in downward displacement of the humeral head (*Fig.* 619).

HABITUAL OR RECURRENT DISLOCATION OF THE SHOULDER-JOINT is a condition where, following a traumatic dislocation, the head of the humerus leaves its socket as the result of quite trivial trauma, e.g., raising the arm to open a door. Many explanations have been offered—e.g., inefficient treatment of the original dislocation, inco-ordination of action of the muscles acting on the joint, etc. Bankart[1] has given an explanation which differs from hitherto accepted views. He states that recurrent dislocation follows that type of dislocation which is caused by violence applied to the back of the humeral head, or which results from a fall on the hand or elbow in such a position that, instead of the head leaving the inferior part of the capsule, it tears the capsule

[1] Bankart, A. S., *Br. med. J.*, 1923, Dec. 15.

from its attachment to the *anterior* lip of the glenoid cavity. The head then lies on the front of the neck of the scapula under the subscapularis. It can be readily understood that, if the capsule does not regain its attachment to the glenoid after the original injury, the head will be liable to slip over the glenoid edge whenever the arm

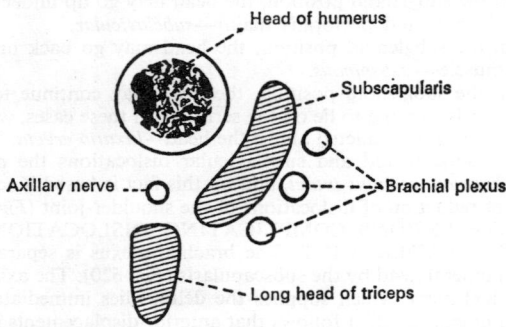

Fig. 620.—To show the relation of the head of the humerus to the brachial plexus and the axillary (circumflex) nerve.

is abducted. This, then, is an exception to the rule that all shoulder dislocations are first subglenoid. It is also apparent that, if Bankart's explanation is correct, the humerus must constantly be in danger of slipping into what may be looked upon as an extension of the joint cavity under the subscapularis. An operation which is calculated to effect a lasting cure is that devised by Bankart, whereby the detached anterior portion of the capsule is fixed to the lip of the glenoid cavity by staples. From our own experience we are in entire concurrence with Bankart's views.

Head of the Radius: Though this bone may be dislocated forwards, outwards, or backwards, in the vast majority of cases the head passes forward, i.e., *anterior dislocation*. The reason is:
1. The circumference of the head is gripped by the orbicular ligament.
2. The capsule is attached to this ligament.
3. To the neck of the bone beyond the orbicular ligament, there is attached, laterally and posteriorly, the radial collateral ligament and the capsule.
4. In front the synovial membrane projects down between the orbicular ligament and neck and is quite unprotected by capsule. This, then, is the weakest part of the joint, and therefore the head of the radius leaves the joint anteriorly (*Fig.* 621).

THE ANATOMY OF CERTAIN DISEASES

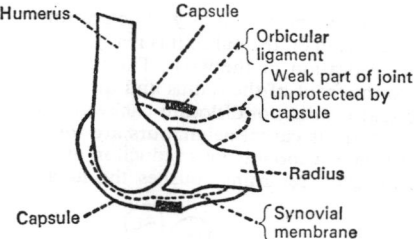

Fig. 621.—Diagram showing the reason why, because of the construction of the radiohumeral joint, the anterior is the commonest type of radial dislocation.

Carpal Bones: The posterior surfaces of the carpal bones are more extensive than the anterior surfaces. They are therefore irregular wedges with the bases behind. The lunate and navicular are exceptions, the anterior surfaces being more extensive than the posterior. When, therefore, dislocations occur, the lunate and navicular tend to be dislocated *forwards*, the other bones when dislocated tend to pass backwards (*Fig.* 622). The lunate, in passing forward, may press on the median nerve, which is normally some distance anterior to it. In dislocation of the lunate, on making a fist the knuckle formed by

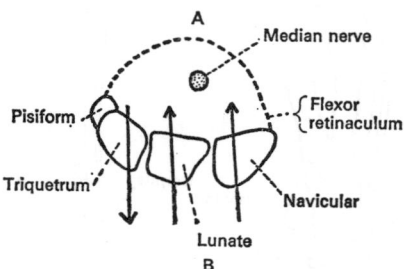

Fig. 622.—Diagram showing first row of carpal bones. The directions in which, owing to their anatomical configuration, they tend to pass if dislocated, are indicated by arrows. Note the relation of the median nerve to the lunate. A, Anterior. B, Posterior.

the head of the third metacarpal may be seen to have receded proximally to a slight extent, so that it is on a level with the adjoining knuckles and does not project distal to them as it normally should. This is known as Murphy's sign.

The commonest injury of the carpus is fracture of the navicular; the second commonest is dislocation of the lunate. The mechanism of the production of this injury is interesting. It is due to great violence, e.g., a fall on the palm. It is really the result of a self-reduced backward dislocation of the wrist. The lunate is much more firmly attached to the front of the radius and ulna than to the other carpal bones, so that it does not dislocate backwards with the wrist, but its connexions with its carpal neighbours are torn. The second stage of the dislocation is a spontaneous reduction of the displacement of the carpus, which, on returning, pushes the lunate forward, the latter

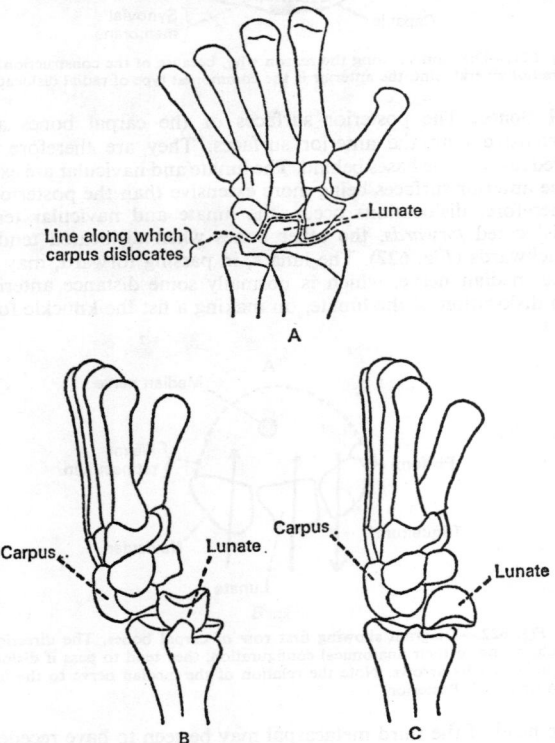

Fig. 623.—The mechanism of dislocation of the lunate (semilunar). A, The dotted line shows the line through which the wrist dislocates backwards. B, The carpus is shown dislocated. C, The dislocated carpus is spontaneously reduced, pushing the lunate forwards and rotating it through 180° (see concave surface). (*After Bankart.*)

rotating round its ligamentous attachment to the radius in such a fashion that its concave distal surface comes to be directed forwards or even upwards (A. S. Blundell Bankart[1]) (*Fig.* 623)

KIENBÖCK'S DISEASE: The ligaments of the lunate (semilunar) offer a remarkable instance of the manner in which the pathology of a region is dominated by the anatomy of the part. It has just been remarked how the anterior ligament of the lunate explains the manner of its dislocation. The posterior ligament of the bone is formed by the deeper fibres of the extensor retinaculum. This ligament is of great importance, carrying, as it sometimes does, the blood-supply of the bone. A fall, or repeated traumatisms incidental to occupation, may injure the blood-supply, producing the changes characteristic of Kienböck's disease—i.e., a progressive degeneration resulting in flattening and increased density as seen in the radiographs.[2]

Metacarpophalangeal Joints: Dislocations, though uncommon, may occur, particularly in the thumb. All the metacarpophalangeal and interphalangeal joints are constructed on the same plan.

The capsule is weak. It is deficient posteriorly, where the extensor expansion fills the gap.

It is protected on each side by collateral ligaments.

It is protected in front by a very strong fibrocartilaginous plate, the palmar ligament. This ligament is very firmly attached to the phalanx and weakly to the metacarpal neck.

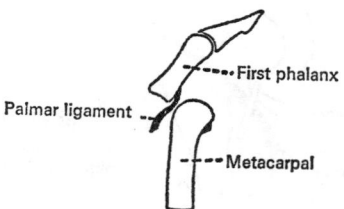

Fig. 624.—Illustrating usual type of metacarpophalangeal dislocation; first phalanx passing back, and palmar ligament remaining attached to phalanx and frequently offering a bar to reduction.

In dislocation at these joints:
1. The base of the first phalanx usually passes backwards because of the nature of the violence.
2. The strong palmar ligament remains attached to the phalanx and passes back with it (*Fig.* 624).

[1] *Manipulative Surgery*, 1932. 115. London.
[2] Mouat, T. B., Wilkie, J., and Harding, H. E., *Br. J. Surg.*, 1923, 19, 577.

666 A SYNOPSIS OF SURGICAL ANATOMY

3. The ligament may and often does act as a bar to reduction.
4. Before reduction can be effected the ligament may have to be divided by a thin-bladed knife pushed in from the back between the bones.

Hip-joint: This joint is as notable for its strength as the shoulder-joint is for its weakness. Therefore it is rarely dislocated. Its strength depends on:

1. The shape of the bones, which interlock like ball and socket.
2. The action of gravity, which holds the bones together.
3. The powerful masses of muscle surrounding the parts.
4. The powerful ligaments.
5. A much smaller range of movements and activity than at the shoulder-joint.

Dislocations are therefore so rare that at some hospitals there is an understanding that if a case of dislocated hip is admitted, the whole surgical staff is notified. These injuries are more common than they used to be owing to the increasing number of motor accidents. A person sitting in the back seat of a car has his hip-joints flexed and also probably adducted. In a collision his knee comes into violent contact with the back of the front seat, and the head of the femur is driven through the lower weak part of the capsule of the hip-joint.

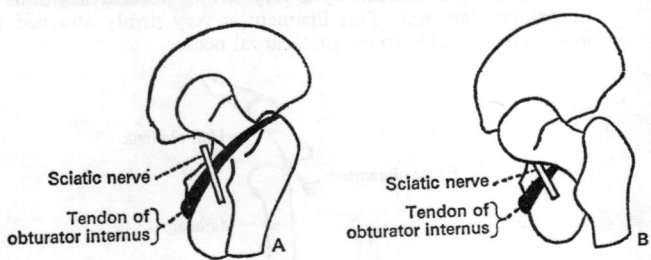

Fig. 625.—Regular posterior dislocations of hip. A, Dislocation 'above the tendon', i.e., on to the dorsum ilii. B, Dislocation 'below the tendon', i.e. into the region of the great sciatic notch. Observe proximity of sciatic nerve to head of femur. It may offer a bar to, or be injured in, reduction.

As in the case of the shoulder-joint, the weakest part of the joint is below, and here the head leaves the capsule. It will then pass forward or backward depending on the line of force.

Passing *forward* it may come to lie on the front of the pubis—*pubic type of dislocation*.

Passing *forward* it may come to lie on the obturator externus—*obturator type of dislocation*.

Passing *back* it may come to lie on the dorsum ilii, above the obturator internus—*high posterior dislocation*.

Passing *back* it may come to lie in the great sciatic notch below the obturator internus—*low posterior dislocation*.

Whether the posterior type becomes high or low depends on the relation of the neck to the obturator internus tendon. If the tendon remains posterior the head will occupy the high position. If the tendon is anterior the head will occupy the low position (*Fig.* 625).

In all these dislocations the iliofemoral or Y-shaped ligament is intact; they are therefore called *regular dislocations*, as the ligament fixes the upper end of the bone and controls its degree of movement. If it is torn, *irregular dislocations* result, and the head may pass up or down or in any direction.

Knee: Displacement of the femur or tibia on each other is prevented by the very powerful cruciate and capsular ligaments. These must be torn before the bones can be displaced. Once they are torn, the bones may move in any direction, as the joint obtains no strength from the configuration of the bone-ends.

Patella: Dislocation of this bone is rare. It may be: (1) Congenital; (2) Traumatic; (3) Recurrent.

1. CONGENITAL: The congenital type is usually one only of a series of developmental abnormalities. It is associated with abnormality of the lower end of the femur, especially the outer condyle. It is as common single as double. The bone is permanently situated on the outer side of the lateral femoral condyle.
2. TRAUMATIC: The traumatic type may be due to direct violence or muscular action, and the bone may pass in any direction.
3. RECURRENT: The recurrent dislocation is the one around which interest is mainly centred. In this condition the bone tends to pass outwards with a greater or lesser degree of frequency, sometimes in fact as frequently as the knee is put through its range of movements. Symptoms may be slight or considerable. Often there is a feeling of weakness and insecurity of the knee.

To understand the aetiology of this condition it is necessary to analyse the extensor mechanism of the knee-joint. The patella is merely a sesamoid bone in the tendon of the quadriceps extensor. Goldthwait[1] has shown that in extension of the knee the quadriceps, in its line of pull, forms an angle with the ligamentum patellae. This is dependent on the fact that, owing to the distance between the acetabula, the femora are oblique, whereas the tibiae are vertical; moreover in women the upper ends of the femora are farther apart than in men, and the angle between the quadriceps extensor and ligamentum patellae is proportionately smaller or

[1] *Boston med. surg. J.*, 1904, Feb.

less obtuse (*Fig.* 626). In extension of the knee it is seen that the patella at first travels over the femoral condyles in a straight line but in the last stages of extension the bone is pulled laterally and rotates out. This is explained on p. 204. There is therefore a natural tendency for the bone to be displaced laterally. This liability is prevented by several factors: one of these is the medial patellar ligament, i.e., the expansion from the fascia lata and vasti which binds the patella and its ligament to the tibial collateral ligament and prevents lateral displacement of the sesamoid. The second factor lies in the shape of the lateral femoral condyle, which is elevated anteriorly to form a prominent buttress which prevents the patella slipping to its outer side. Malkin[1] from a study of the comparative anatomy of the joint, shows that only in man does this bony ridge exist, and he associates it with the erect posture and with the fact that only man walks with extended knees (extension being the position in which displacement of the patella is most likely to occur).

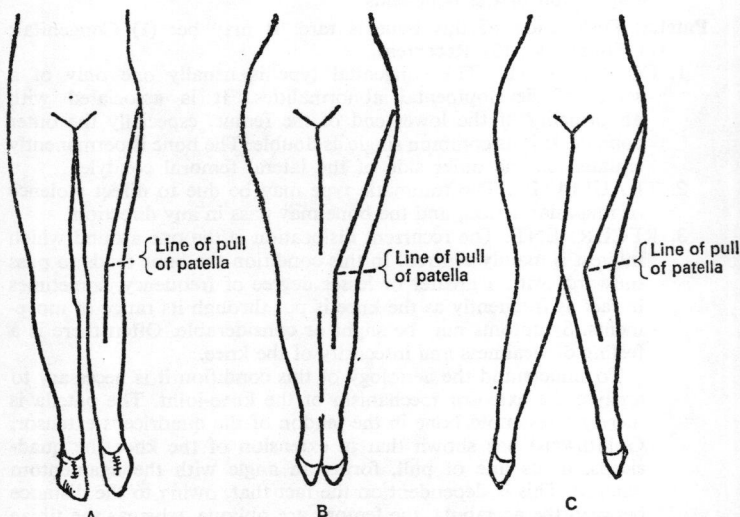

Fig. 626.—To illustrate the genesis of dislocation of the patella. A, Shows that the normal line of pull of the patella forms an angle open outwards. B, Shows this angle to be smaller in women. C, Shows this angle to be much reduced in knock-knee, with a greater liability to dislocation of the patella.

[1] *Br. med. J.*, 1932, July, 91.

It follows, therefore, that the factors which encourage recurrent dislocation of the patella are:

a. Slackness or weakness of the medial patellar ligament or of the vastus medialis, making the line of pull of the quadriceps more angular.
b. Knock-knee, hyperextension of the knee, or a lateral attachment of the patellar tendon.
c. A decrease in the size of the buttress of the lateral condyle which normally prevents displacement.

Treatment will be directed to remedy these defects: e.g., moving the tubercle of the tibia with the patellar ligament to a more medial position; correcting knock-knee; tightening the medial patellar ligament; increasing the prominence of the buttress of the lateral femoral condyle (*Fig.* 627).

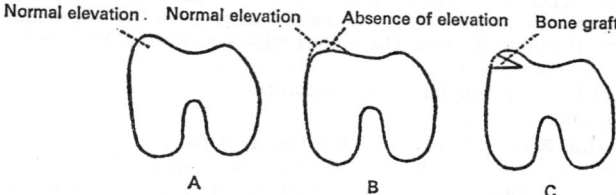

Fig. 627.—To show one cause of recurrent dislocation of the patella—when the normal elevation of the lateral femoral condyle is missing. The femur is seen from below, i.e., the articular surface of the lower end. A, Normal anterior elevation of outer edge of lateral condyle. B, Absence of this elevation. C, The elevation reproduced by raising a portion of the condyle and maintaining the elevation by a bone-graft.

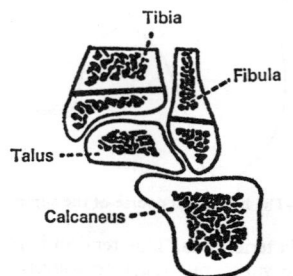

Fig. 628.—Subtaloid dislocation of foot.

Subtaloid: The foot may be dislocated at the joint between the talus and calcaneus, leaving the talus in the tibiofibular mortice (*Fig.* 628).

Ankle: The tibiofibular mortice is shaped to fit the upper articular surface of the talus, which is broader in front than behind; therefore one would expect that in dislocations at the joint the talus would pass more readily forwards than backwards. Despite this fact, posterior dislocation of the ankle, i.e., passage of the whole foot back, is commoner than the anterior because of the nature of the injury, which is usually forcible plantar flexion. If the violence is severe enough, the foot may go in any direction.

IV. LESIONS OF THE SUPRASPINATUS AND SUBDELTOID BURSA

The Supraspinatus

The tendon of the supraspinatus, its injuries and degenerations now comprise an essential and extensive part of the pathology around the shoulder. This knowledge we owe to the investigations over a period of many years by the late E. A. Codman,[1] surgeon to the Massachusetts General Hospital, Boston. The author wishes to express his admiration for this monumental work. In this chapter an attempt is made to represent some of Codman's findings; any inaccuracies are the fault of the writer of this synopsis.

Anatomical Facts: The supraspinatus muscle pursues a horizontal course from the supraspinous fossa, under the acromion process, to its insertion into the *upper* surface of the most anterior of the three muscle impressions on the great tuberosity of the humerus (*Fig.* 629).

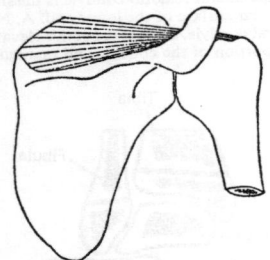

Fig. 629.—The horizontal course of the supraspinatus.

Its distal portion is tendinous. This tendon is fused with the tendons of insertion of the subscapularis, infraspinatus, and teres minor in such a manner that these four tendons are not individual or separate structures except by artificial dissection. They form together a musculotendinous cuff (*Fig.* 630). This cuff is so firmly united with

[1] *The Shoulder*, 1934. Boston, Mass.

THE ANATOMY OF CERTAIN DISEASES 671

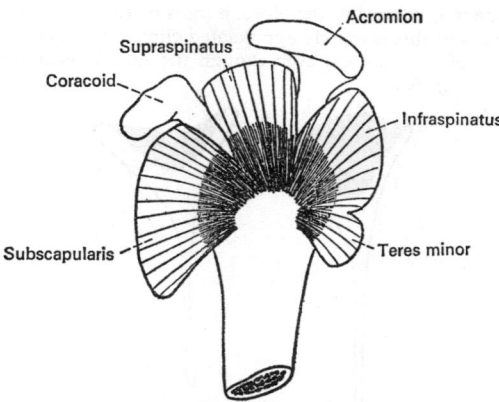

Fig. 630.—The black shading shows the musculotendinous cuff.

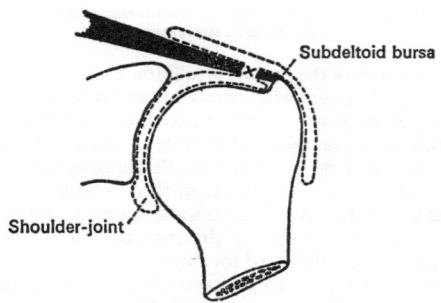

Fig. 631.—Showing that rupture of the supraspinatus tendon converts the shoulder-joint and subdeltoid bursa into a single cavity. X, Rupture of supraspinatus.

the capsule of the shoulder-joint beneath, and the floor of the subdeltoid bursa above, that together they form one structure. It follows that should the cuff be torn, then the shoulder-joint and the subdeltoid bursa become one cavity (*Fig.* 631). It is furthermore apparent that injuries to the musculotendinous cuff may be small or extensive and that in surgical exploration of such injuries the whole cuff and not merely a part of it will be examined.

The supraspinatus is a powerful muscle. It is shaped like the psoas, being covered by a dense fascia which roofs in the supraspinous fossa.

When the muscle wastes, therefore, it loses its roundness and becomes flattened, and this is readily appreciated clinically by flattening above the spine of the scapula, even though the muscle is covered by the trapezius (*Fig.* 632).

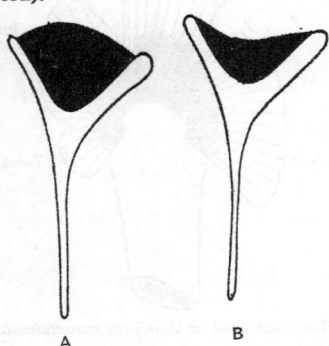

Fig. 632.—A, Shows the normal shape of the supraspinatus. B, The shape of the atrophied supraspinatus.

Function: The function of the muscle is to initiate abduction at the shoulder and to hold the humeral head firmly to the scapula, and that normally is all. It has no rotatory action. In exceptional cases it may take over the function of the deltoid and be able to abduct the arm to a right-angle, but this is a rarity. A moment's consideration will show that the supraspinatus is a very hard-worked muscle. Most movements performed at the shoulder involve some degree of abduction, however small. Think of dressing, eating, driving a car, etc. Think of the typist; her arms are slightly abducted for much of the day. Although a strong muscle has been supplied to perform this work, its tendon is long and relatively thin and, like all tendons, its blood-supply is never profuse. The practial importance of this will be shown later.

Nerve-supply: This is from the upper trunk of the brachial plexus through the suprascapular nerve (C. 5 and 6) which passes through the scapular notch to supply the spinati. Injury to the nerve is rare and results in paralysis of the action of the muscle and internal rotation of the shoulder due to loss of function of the only powerful external rotator—the infraspinatus.

Rupture of the Supraspinatus:
1. This injury always involves the tendon of the muscle.
2. It occurs in males of the working class in 90 per cent of cases. They are more liable to injury.
3. It happens after the age of 40. The average age is 55. The reason given

THE ANATOMY OF CERTAIN DISEASES

for the age incidence is that the tendon is never normal after 40. It has begun to degenerate and has lost elasticity and resilience. The injury is part of the price man pays for the erect posture. Evolution is still advancing. The product is not yet perfect. Because of its structure and the strain on its long tendon, it ages rapidly. Compare the extensor mechanism of the knee-joint: in youth the patellar and quadriceps tendons are so strong that when subjected to violence the bone breaks and the tibial tuberosity may be avulsed; in the years of vigour the sesamoid bone breaks, the tendons are still strong; in old age the quadriceps tendon is degenerate and is likely to snap from the same strain.

4. The violence causing the lesion must be considerable. It is usually a fall, as off a ladder, on that side. There are not usually signs of local bruising or violence, although there may be. It may follow indirect violence, e.g., the rapid elevation of a heavy object with the arm abducted.

5. The lesion should be suspected in *every case of dislocated shoulder*.

6. The mechanism of the injury is twofold:

   a. In most cases it is probably due to violent contraction of the supraspinatus, as in falling, in the natural effort to prevent the head or thorax from being injured, or by taking the impact on the hand. This type of violence causes small rents in the musculotendinous cuff and involves the supraspinatus tendon only (*Fig.* 633, A).

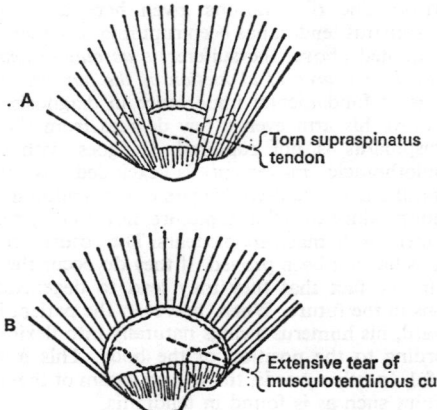

Fig. 633.—Demonstrating (A) a tear confined to the supraspinatus tendon and (B) a more extensive one involving other components of the musculotendinous cuff. The head of the humerus is exposed by the tears.

674 A SYNOPSIS OF SURGICAL ANATOMY

  b. When complicating dislocation of the shoulder-joint the mechanism is quite different. The head of the humerus is so far displaced that the musculotendinous cuff is torn from its attachment to the top of the humerus. Here the gap is considerable and involves several tendons (*Fig.* 633, B).

THE RESULTS OF THE INJURY:

1. There may be a complaint of sudden local pain at the time of the injury but this tends to ease off. Severe pain occurs that night and perhaps following nights. It is referred not so much to the top of the shoulder as to the insertion of the deltoid, where the cutaneous branch of the axillary nerve (C. 5 and 6) is distributed. This interval, before the development of the acute pain, has recently been stressed by Ellis.[1] He quotes Kaufman in regard to the criteria accepted by German Compensation Boards in deciding between trauma as precipitating an injury on the one hand, and trauma which merely activates a pre-existent condition such as fibrositis on the other. In the former case there is a latent interval between the pain caused by the injury and the severe pain which develops some hours later. When, however, a pre-existing condition is reawakened by injury, intense pain occurs and continues. The general value of this statement is considerable. After a few days the pain in rupture of the supraspinatus is not great; the patients are much more comfortable than those with tendinitis.

2. FUNCTION: The observations given here are personal. If the supraspinatus tendon has been ruptured by either of the mechanisms quoted above, the sufferer is *absolutely unable to execute the smallest degree of abduction of the humerus on the scapula.* This is of fundamental importance in diagnosis. If the patient can move his arm even a few degrees from the side then the supraspinatus is not ruptured. (It goes without saying that scapulothoracic movement is excluded by the examiner.) Admitting that microscopic tears of the tendon may occur, these do not produce the clinical picture, nor do they require the same treatment as do macroscopic tears. The occurrence of such minor injuries has not been proved. If they do occur their chief interest lies in the fact that they may lead to degenerative tendinous lesions in the future. When, however, the patient is told to bend forward, his humerus swings naturally into flexion or abduction according to the position of the body. This movement is not painful. In other words, there is no spasm of the muscles around the joint such as is found in tendinitis.

  Moseley's (*see* p. 201) work suggests that the inability to initiate abduction is due to a pain reflex and not to the importance of

[1] John D. Ellis, *The Injured Back and its Treatment*, 56. Springfield, Ill.

supraspinatus function in this action. This does not lessen the diagnostic importance of the loss of this function in acute injury around the shoulder.

EXAMINATION:
1. In chronic cases there is flattening above the spine of the scapula due to the wasting of the supraspinatus.
2. The deltoid may be more prominent on the affected side, due to the fact that the shoulder-joint now communicates with the subdeltoid bursa which may be distended with fluid from the joint, thus pushing out the deltoid (*Fig.* 634).

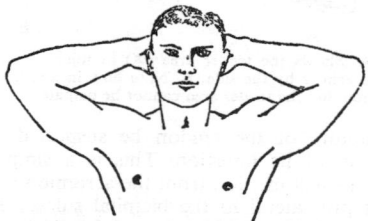

Fig. 634.—The left deltoid appears hypertrophied because it is pushed out by fluid in the subdeltoid bursa which is displaced into the bursa when the supraspinatus tendon is torn and the arm is abducted.

3. There is an accurately localized point of deep tenderness at the insertion of the supraspinatus tendon. This is found as follows (Codman): Standing behind the patient, extend his arm by pulling the elbow back, thus throwing the head of the humerus forward. The forearm, bent to a right-angle, points directly forward. Run the finger along the collar-bone to the acromio-clavicular joint. A line passing from this point straight down the front of the humerus for 7·5 cm. marks out the intertubercular sulcus (bicipital groove). Pressure with the forefinger immediately lateral to the upper end of this line is accurately applied to the insertion of the supraspinatus and is painful when its tendon is damaged. Note that this tenderness is accurately localized. This tender spot vanishes when the arm is abducted as the tuberosity disappears under the acromion (*Fig.* 635).
4. After dislocations examination is less easy. The key to the diagnosis is abduction. If it cannot be executed in its first few degrees, it must be presumed that the supraspinatus is ruptured. Compression of the axillary nerve by the humeral head will also be followed by inability to abduct due to paralysis of the deltoid. In the writer's experience this is one of the rarest accidents in surgery.

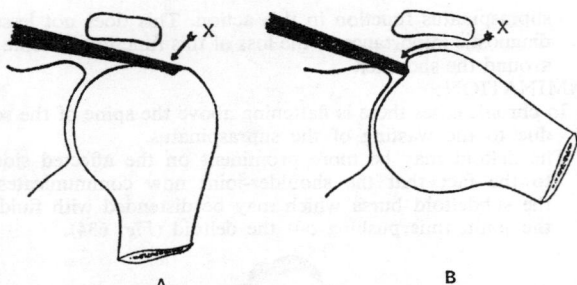

Fig. 635.—A, Shows the tender area (X) in injury of the supraspinatus tendon when the arm is by the side. B, Note how in abduction X disappears under the acromion and the tender area cannot be palpated.

5. Should rupture of the tendon be suspected, Codman advises exploration of its insertion. This is a simple procedure and involves a small incision from the acromion vertically down the humerus just lateral to the bicipital sulcus. The deltoid fibres are separated. The roof of the subdeltoid bursa is opened and the tendon inspected, and necessary action taken. It is to be remembered that:
   a. At operation the patient's affected arm hangs over the side of the table supported by an assistant sitting on a footstool. In this way the upper end of the humerus is thrown forward.
   b. By the assistant rotating the humerus, much of the subdeltoid bursal floor and the tuberosities of the humerus can be brought under the eye of the surgeon.
   c. The tendon ruptures at its insertion to bone. The rupture if it exists is easily seen.
   d. If exploration is delayed retraction occurs.
   e. The floor and the roof of the bursa should always be reconstructed.

The Subdeltoid Bursa

The subdeltoid bursa is the largest bursa in the body. It never communicates with the shoulder-joint (*Fig.* 636). Its floor covers the greater tuberosity of the humerus and the four tendons which pass to the tuberosities; part of it covers the bicipital groove and biceps. Its roof is firmly attached to the under aspect of deltoid, acromion, and coraco-acromial ligament. It extends loosely under deltoid, origin of coracobrachialis and short head of biceps, and coracoid process. It is folded up under the acromion in abduction of the arm to a right angle (*Fig.* 637). Its walls are extremely thin and delicate. Normally they are separated by just a trace of synovial fluid.

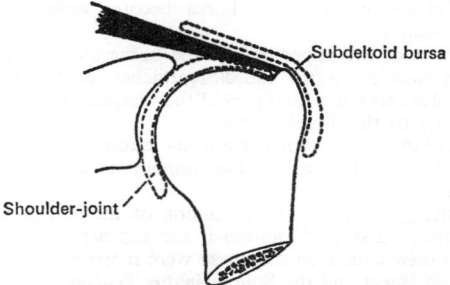

Fig. 636.—To show the relationship of the shoulder-joint and subdeltoid bursa to the supraspinatus tendon.

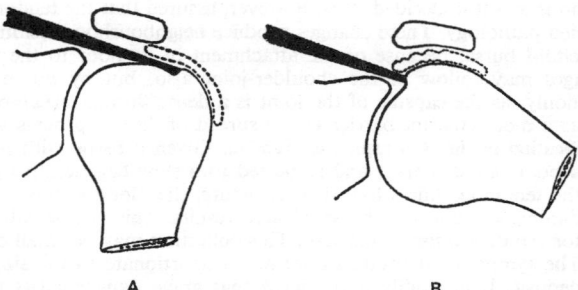

Fig. 637.—To show how the subdeltoid bursa disappears under the acromion in abduction. A, Arm at side. B, Arm abducted.

PRACTICAL FACTS:

1. Tenderness over the bursa, which usually means some pathology of the supraspinatus insertion, disappears when the arm is abducted to 60° or more.
2. There is normally just room for the comfortable movement of the great tuberosity and the bursa under the acromion process. Should there be any factor increasing the thickness of tissue between tuberosity and acromion, abduction will be either impossible or painful as the tuberosity and bursa pass under the acromion, and again painful as they impinge on the acromion in bringing the arm to the side. Clinically, therefore, the sufferer so afflicted will complain of acute pain at a certain angle in abducting or adducting the arm.

3. Should the walls of the bursa become adherent abduction is impossible.
4. Fracture of the upper end of the humerus, extensive contusions and injuries to the muscles attached to the tuberosities, all involve this bursa, and part of the symptomatology and disability is due to this involvement.
5. In thinking of the shoulder and its lesions the practitioner should think of it in terms of two joints, the shoulder-joint and the subdeltoid bursa.
6. All the general causes of bursitis of this cavity taken together could almost be forgotten if the supraspinatus and its lesions and their effects on the bursa were remembered.

The Subdeltoid Bursa and the Supraspinatus Tendon

As a result of its shape, structure, situation, and function, the supraspinatus tendon begins to degenerate early in life—about the age of 40. Whether or not injury produces microscopic tears of the fibres of the tendon is as yet undecided. It is, however, assured that the tendon shows a varied pathology. These changes produce neighbourhood lesions of the subdeltoid bursa, because of the attachment of its floor to the tendon. Changes may follow in the shoulder-joint also, but by no means so commonly, as the capsule of the joint is a dense fibrous structure which acts as a more efficient barrier to the spread of disease processes.

Calcification in the Supraspinatus Tendon: Given a tissue with normally a poor blood-supply, and subjected to a slow degenerative process, the tendinous fibres lose their structure, the blood-supply is further diminished, and an abnormal area results. This is a suitable nidus for the deposition of calcium. This collection may be small or large. The symptoms it produces are not proportionate to the size of the deposit. It is readily appreciated that grave danger exists that the normal 'tight fit' in the passage of the great tuberosity beneath the acromion will be interfered with. Abduction will become painful and may be prevented. The deposit may be in the substance of the tendon and produce no disharmony. It does weaken the tendon. As it grows in size it approaches the floor of the bursa. It then acts as a foreign body—an irritant. It may cause inflammation of the bursal floor. It is not necessary that calcium be present to produce this change. The proximity of the degenerative process may itself do so. It can be understood how pain and difficulty in abduction may ensue on these changes in the bursa. Some such pathology underlies the so-called tendinitis of the supraspinatus. Codman speaks of 'frozen shoulder', an expressive term. It implies spasm, loss of scapulohumeral rhythm.

It produces great pain, worse at night, and gravely impairs movements at the joint. Should the calcified deposit impinge upon the bursal floor and later project into the bursa, the projection is exposed to injury every time it passes beneath the acromion in abduction. Codman

THE ANATOMY OF CERTAIN DISEASES 679

likens it to a volcano. Some day the patient who has been aware of some or perhaps no discomfort in performing abduction is seized with severe acute pain. The volcano has erupted. It has burst and discharged its contents into the bursa—acute bursitis. A radiograph may show the calcium lying in the bursa (*Fig.* 638). It is readily understood that this slow degeneration may extend to other parts of the musculotendinous cuff. Calcification is sometimes seen in other tendons forming the cuff.

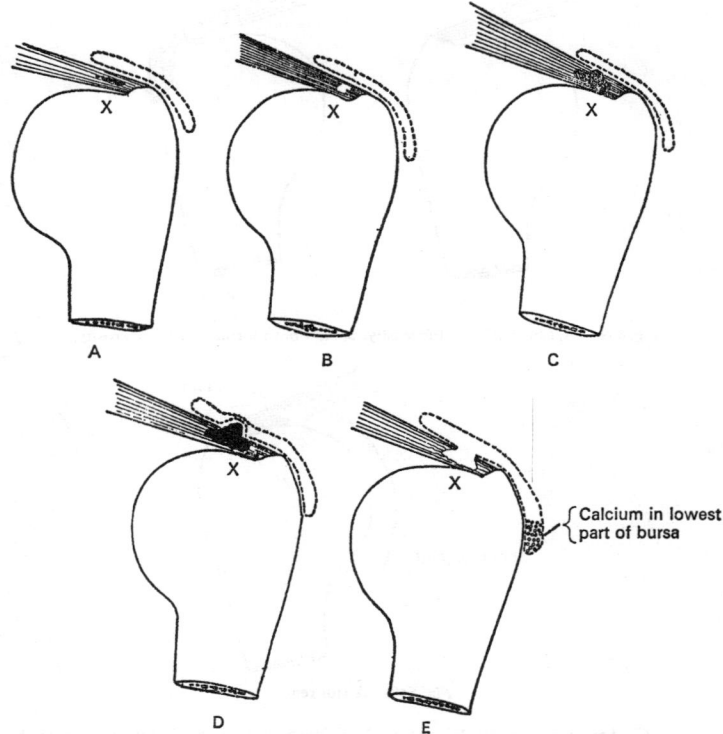

Fig. 638.—To show the sequence of events which may follow a small tear or area of degeneration in the supraspinatus tendon when calcium is deposited in the lesion, X. A, The lesion. B, Calcium deposit. C, Calcium deposit. D, Volcano. E, Eruption—note calcium in bursa.

The avascularity may extend to the insertion of the supraspinatus, into the tuberosity and eburnation of this bone appear, and even irregular bony outgrowth, much as is seen in degenerative arthritis (*Fig.* 639). So the lesion may be extended. The biceps tendon may be slowly worn away by a process of attrition, resulting from such irregularity of the tuberosity which forms its lateral boundary. Ultimately it may rupture.

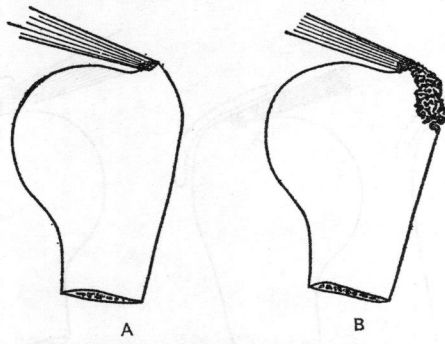

Fig. 639.—A, Eburnation of tuberosity. B, New bone formation on tuberosity.

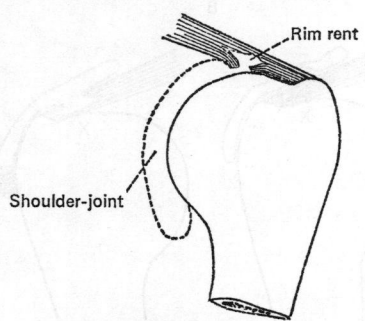

Fig. 640.—A rim rent.

Codman refers to 'rim rents'. Where the musculotendinous cuff meets the tuberosities, there is a very acute angle. He states that some injuries may partially damage the supraspinatus on its inferior aspect at this angle—rim rents (*Fig.* 640). Here now is an injury into the shoulder-joint. A whole genealogical tree may be constructed of how arthritis may date back to a rim rent. Enough has been said to show how important a part is played by the pathology of the supraspinatus tendon in lesions of the subdeltoid bursa.

Abduction of the Shoulder: Abduction is an anti-gravity action. In any painful condition around this joint the arm is held to the side and, if it is very painful, the forearm is held across the body. This is full *internal rotation*. The arm can only be elevated above the head in the position of full *external rotation*. The period of disability of lesions of the supraspinatus and related structures is enormously prolonged by lack of appreciation of this fundamental fact. The original lesion recovers but the patient cannot abduct his arm. The internal rotators and joint capsule have contracted, and until full lateral rotation is secured by stretching these powerful structures (subscapularis, pectoralis major, latissimus dorsi) full abduction is impossible.

Golden rule in the treatment of all shoulder-joint lesions: *Full abduction is only possible if the humerus can be fully rotated outwards.*

The passage of time has strengthened the conviction that this principle is not understood. It cannot be too strongly stressed that after every injury to the shoulder region it should be the doctor's duty to commence external rotation of the humerus early and not to be content until this movement is normal. There is no need to worry about abduction which may be inadvisable soon after the injury. Abduction will be assured if external rotation has been secured.

V. RARE HERNIAE

The abdominal contents occasionally herniate into unusual situations. Rare types of herniae are: (1) Diaphragmatic; (2) Obturator; (3) Pudendal; (4) Sciatic; (5) Lumbar—(a) upper, (b) lower; (6) Ischiorectal.

Diaphragmatic Hernia: This may be: (1) Congenital; or (2) Acquired.

CONGENITAL HERNIA:

DEVELOPMENT OF THE DIAPHRAGM: The diaphragm, pericardium, and heart are formed in the neck and obtain their innervation there (C. 3, 4, 5). They migrate to their ultimate destinations carrying their nerve-supply with them. Five structures go to form the diaphragm and result in the division of the coelom into pleural, pericardial, and peritoneal cavities. These are:

1. The ventral portion of diaphragm is developed from the septum transversum. It is attached to the xiphisternum, forming the central tendon and the central part of the muscle back to the oesophagus.
2. The two dorsal portions form the crura and that part of the diaphragm between the backbone and the oesophagus.
3. The two lateral portions grow in from a ridge on the side wall of the coelom which is connected with the septum transversum. It forms that part of the diaphragm which is attached to the

682 A SYNOPSIS OF SURGICAL ANATOMY

ribs. It constricts the coelom in its growth and ultimately separates pleural from peritoneal cavities. It may fail to reach the dorsal part of the diaphragm especially on the left. Then a canal connects pleural and peritoneal sacs, the pleuroperitoneal hiatus or the foramen of Bochdalek (*Fig.* 641).

Mesodermal tissue forms these various early diaphragmatic structures and later muscle invades this tissue. Congenital diaphragmatic herniae may therefore be sacless if the primitive mesenchyme fails to develop, or the hernial contents may be contained in a hernial sac if muscle does not invade the pleuroperitoneal membrane at a stage when the latter has formed.

Several types of congenital diaphragmatic hernia may be postulated due to errors in the development of the foregoing:

1. *Retrosternal Hernia:* The foramen of Morgagni (1769) is the name given to the space which originally exists between the ventral (xiphisternal) and the lateral (costal) slips of origin. When the diaphragm is fully formed there is a small natural space between these slips. It contains a little areolar tissue and transmits the superior epigastric vessels. This is the space of Larrey. Thus a hernia in this situation may occur on either side

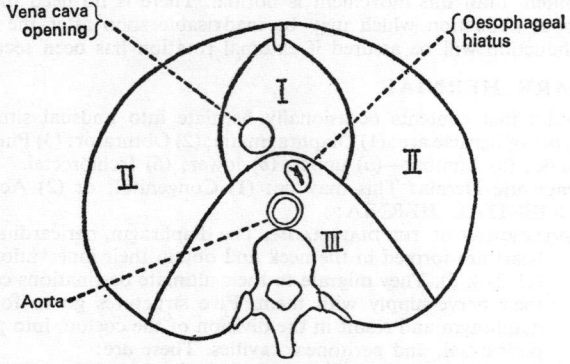

Fig. 641.—The developmental parts of the diaphragm. I, Ventral area. II, Lateral areas. III, Dorsal portion.

It is more common on the right, the reason being that the pericardial attachment is more extensive on the left and offers more protection to the development of a hernia than the liver does on the right. Thus such a hernia usually lies between the pericardium and the right pleura. On occasions the hernia may enter the pericardial cavity due to a related diaphragmatic defect. A sac may or may not exist. Costal cartilages and sternum form the anterior boundary and the diaphragm forms the rest of the circumference of the defect. The situation is usually central and some of these herniae are thought to be acquired, occurring in middle age. Their rarity in children is attributed to the protective barrier of the relatively large liver and the short transverse mesocolon.

2. *Posterolateral Hernia:* Hernia through the pleuroperitoneal hiatus—foramen of Bochdalek (1848). This condition results from failure of fusion of the lateral (costal) with the posterior (crural) components of the diaphragm. It is much commoner on the left. In 9 cases out of 10 there is no hernial sac, there being free communication between pleural and peritoneal cavities. *Fig.* 642, re-drawn from Bingham,[1] shows the site of the defect.

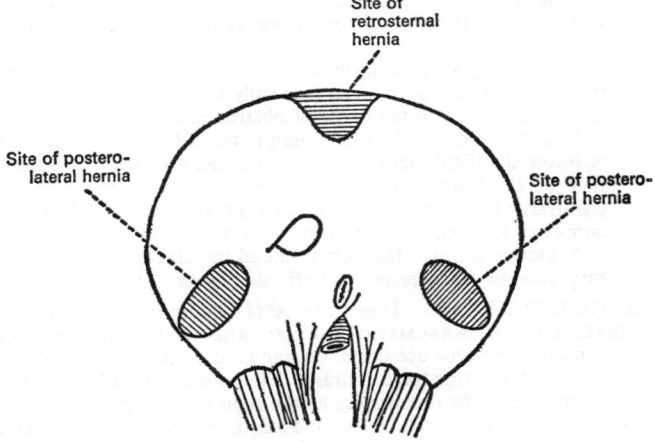

Fig. 642.—Sites of retrosternal and posterolateral herniae. (*Re-drawn from Bingham in the 'British Journal of Surgery'.*)

Bingham points out that 'with notable constancy the defect is situated at the periphery of the diaphragm in the region of its attachments to the 10th and 11th ribs'. This is by far the commonest type of congenital diaphragmatic hernia.

3. *Posterior Hernia—Hernia Diaphragmatica Transversa*: This condition results from failure of development of the posterior

[1] Bingham, J. A. W., *Br. J. Surg.*, 1959, 47, 1.

formative processes of the diaphragm. One or both crura may be absent. The aorta and oesophagus lie in the gap. There is no sac and free communication between the two large serous cavities exists.

4. *Central Hernia—Hernia through the Dome of the Diaphragm:* This rare entity is left-sided. It is thought to result from rupture of the fetal membranous diaphragm. The gap varies in size and may involve the entire left half of the diaphragm.

Comment:

1. Kirkland[1] points out that congenital diaphragmatic hernia may manifest itself clinically in one of two ways. In the infant it is often the cause of death within hours of birth, due to the acute respiratory distress occasioned by abdominal viscera filling the left chest. In older persons symptoms are intermittent and take chronic and bizarre forms.

2. Retrosternal hernia rarely causes symptoms in infants or at any age. Posterolateral hernia may require operation in the first few hours of life.

3. Severe types of congenital herniae are often associated with other maldevelopment, more especially malrotation of the midgut loop, which may be the cause of obstruction.

4. Eventration of the diaphragm is not a true hernia as the gut is below the diaphragm. It is due to absence of muscle in the left half of the diaphragm and may be congenital or result from paralysis of the phrenic nerve. The gut pushes the defective left cupola of the diaphragm well up into the thorax.

5. Hernia through the right dome of the diaphragm is extremely rare because of the protection afforded by the liver.

ACQUIRED HERNIA: These may be (1) Traumatic; (2) Hiatal.

TRAUMATIC DIAPHRAGMATIC HERNIA: This condition may occur following traffic accidents, or war injuries as the result of bullet wounds injuring the diaphragm. The hernia is usually through the left side of the diaphragm, as the right dome is protected by the liver. The scar of a bullet wound may be found over the abdominal wall in a situation which renders it possible that the diaphragm was injured in the passage of the missile. There is usually no sac, and some part of the gut lies in the left side of the chest, usually the stomach. Radiography has been instrumental in the diagnosis of these cases, which were only very rarely detected before radiography was in use.

Acquired diaphragmatic hernia may also follow injury to the muscle such as may be produced by the violent expiratory spasms of whooping cough.

[1] Kirkland, J. A., *Br. J. Surg.*, 1959, 47, 21.

HIATAL HERNIA OF THE DIAPHRAGM: Allison's work[1] has clarified the confusion which existed in regard to the herniae which occur in relation to the oesophageal hiatus. There are two types: (*a*) Congenital; (*b*) Acquired. The congenital type is called 'rolling' by Allison, and the acquired is named 'sliding'.

  a. The Congenital Type: Allison suggests that the genesis of this condition is due to a peritoneal process being left in the posterior mediastinum when the developing stomach invaginates the peritoneum from behind. Thus the cardia is devoid of peritoneum posteriorly and the hernial sac can only be anterior. Providing the cardia retains its normal firm anchorage, the stomach can only enter the sac by its anterior surface rolling upwards until it may be upside-down in the posterior mediastinum. The important features of such a hernia are that it lies

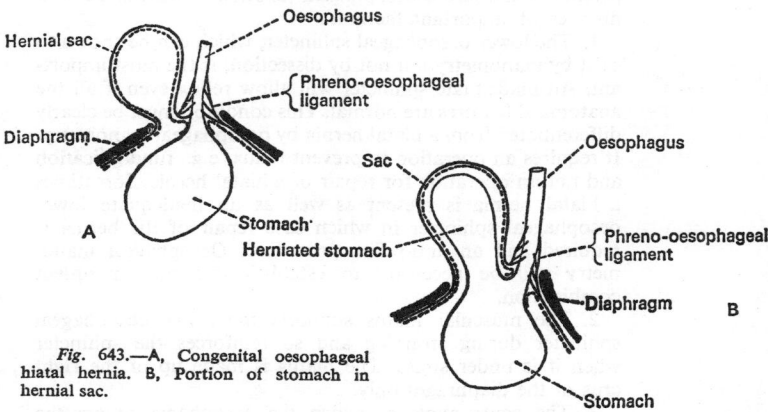

Fig. 643.—A, Congenital oesophageal hiatal hernia. B, Portion of stomach in hernial sac.

in a preformed sac and that the normal relationships of the cardio-oesophageal junction to the diaphragm are undisturbed (*Fig.* 643). This is a rare type of hernia and the only way it can disturb the mechanics of the oesophagus is if it becomes sufficiently bulky to compress this tube against the vertebral column.

  b. The Acquired Type: This is the sliding hernia of Allison. It is far and away the commonest of all internal herniae and its importance in children and adults is immense. To appreciate the factors which cause it and the correct treatment of the

[1] Allison, P. R., *Surgery Gynec. Obstet.*, 1951, 92, 419.

condition, it is necessary to understand the anatomy and physiology of the cardio-oesophageal region.

Maintenance of the Position of the Cardio-oesophageal Junction: The fascia transversalis (endo-abdominal fascia) on the under surface of the diaphragm is reflected on to the lower end of the oesophagus as the phreno-oesophageal membrane which holds the cardio-oesophageal junction in its normal position (*Fig.* 646). This membrane is elastic and allows a fair degree of mobility of the cardia, which is necessary in the process of vomiting. Very vigorous attemps to establish the presence of a hiatal hernia by means of posture and straining may result in such a 'normal' movement of the cardia through the hiatus and must not be misinterpreted as a hiatal hernia.

Factors preventing Gastro-oesophageal Reflux: The competence of the cardio-oesophageal junction is maintained by a number of important factors:

1. The lower oesophageal sphincter, which can be shown to exist by manometry but not by dissection, is the most important. An inadequate sphincter will allow reflux even if all the anatomical features are normal. This condition must be clearly differentiated from a hiatal hernia by oesophageal manometry. It requires an operation to prevent reflux, e.g., fundoplication and not an operation for repair of a hiatal hernia. Sometimes a hiatal hernia is present as well as an inadequate lower oesophageal sphincter in which case repair of the hernia is required and an anti-reflux procedure. Oesophageal manometry will be necessary to establish this not infrequent combination.

2. The muscular hiatus supports the lower oesophageal sphincter during straining and so reinforces the sphincter when it is under stress. The hiatus is made up of the right crus of the diaphragm only.

3. The acute angle at which the oesophagus enters the stomach results in a flap of mucosa which closes off the oesophageal opening when the pressure rises in the fundus of the stomach, and so prevents reflux. This acute angle (of His) is maintained partly by the intrinsic oblique muscle fibres of the stomach and partly by the oesophageal hiatus which acts in much the same way as the puborectalis sling of the rectum (*Fig.* 644).

Mechanism of Sliding Hiatal Hernia: A hernia will result from a weakness of the phreno-oesophageal membrane (e.g., after operations on this area) or an increase in intra-abdominal pressure (e.g., obesity). The cardia will then slide up through the hiatus (*Fig.* 645).

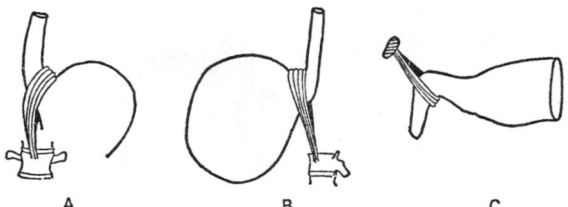

Fig. 644.—A, Crural sling seen from the front. B, Crural sling seen from the side. C, The sling of the puborectalis.

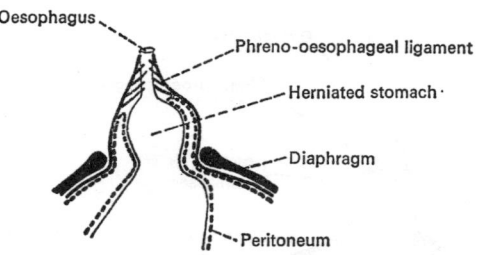

Fig. 645.—Sliding hernia. (*Re-drawn from Allison.*)

Effects of Sliding Hiatal Hernia: The displacement of the cardia into the chest will have the following consequences:

1. Reflux of gastric contents will occur because the inferior oesophageal sphincter will lose the support of the hiatus and will instead be surrounded by the negative pressure in the thorax, the angle of His will be lost (*Fig.* 645) and the pressure in the herniated portion of the stomach will be raised by the compression of the hiatus. Such reflux will result in oesophagitis (with substernal pain) followed in time by chronic ulceration and stricture formation.

2. Compression of the stomach will produce gastric (high epigastric) pain.

3. Stretching of the hiatus will produce somatic pain referred to the lower chest on one or both sides (submammary pain).

4. Displacement of the heart may cause cardiac irregularities and if (rarely) very large, the lung may be compressed to produce dyspnoea.

Repair of the Sliding Hernia: As for all other sliding hernias this requires removal of the sac, reduction of the contents,

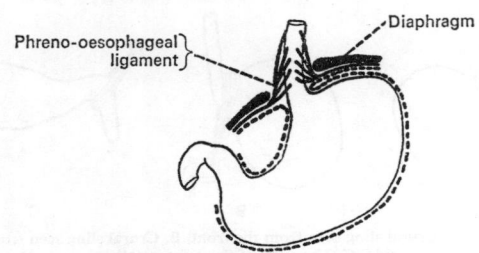

Fig. 646.—The phreno-oesophageal ligament.

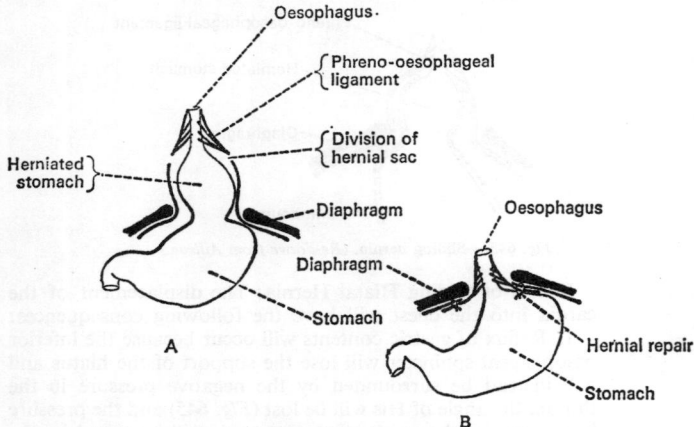

Fig. 647.—A, Repair of sliding hernia. The sac has been cut leaving a fringe attached to oesophagus (phreno-oesophageal ligament). B, The hernia is reduced and the phreno-oesophageal ligament has been sutured to the under aspect of the diaphragm.

closure of the hernial orifice and fixation of the mobile organ. In this case closure of the hiatal orifice cannot be complete and care must be exercised to avoid oesophageal compression (*Fig.* 648). Fixation of the stomach may be achieved by re-attaching the cardia to the hiatal margins (*Fig.* 647), or by fixing the stomach to the under surface of the diaphragm, or on the anterior abdominal wall (Boerema) or on the posterior abdominal wall (Hill). This procedure can be carried out through a thoracic or an abdominal approach.

With the passage of time it has become evident that the abdominal approach has distinct advantages. The chest is not entered, the limbs of the defective crural sling can be clearly defined, the repair is more easily effected, and above all any other intra-abdominal pathology can be detected and dealt with at the same time, e.g., gall-stones.

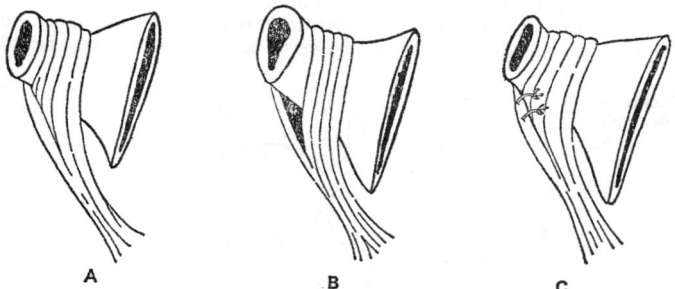

Fig. 648.—A, The normal crural sling. B, The crural sling open below. C, The weakened sling repaired.

Hiatus hernia is associated with peptic ulceration in 20 per cent of cases and with calculous cholecystitis in the same percentage of cases. Hiatus hernia, cholelithiasis, and diverticulosis occur so commonly together that the combination is spoken of as Saint's triad.

Such conditions may be dealt with at the same operation by this approach. The exposure is by a midline incision from xiphisternum to just above the umbilicus. The left triangular ligament of the liver is divided so that its left lobe may be folded to the right. A catheter is passed around the oesophagogastric junction which is retracted to the left. The upper part of the lesser omentum is divided between forceps. The right limb of the sling formed by the right crus is at once apparent and the other limb may be felt and seen. The defect thus defined is readily repaired by interrupted non-absorbable sutures and the surgeon takes such further steps as he deems necessary to anchor the oesophagogastric area.

Care of the Phrenic Nerve: This nerve supplies the diaphragm from its abdominal surface. In addition to its motor function it has a sensory one and supplies the three Ps—pleura, pericardium, and peritoneum.

Perera and Edwards[1] point out that in early life respiration is appreciably assisted by the intercostal muscles but not in adults where the diaphragm is wholly responsible. Although in radical procedures where division of the diaphragm is necessary some injury to the phrenic is unavoidable, it is important to protect it when possible. An example is in the repair of hiatus hernia from above. The condition is common in stout elderly persons where it is of great importance not to impair respiration. The nerve has a complex and variable

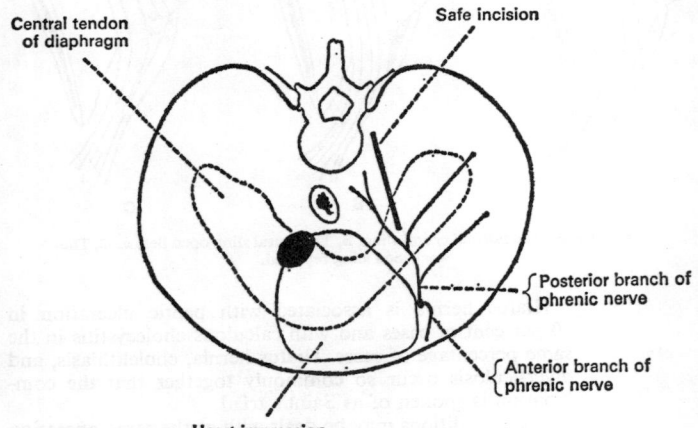

Fig. 649.—A usual type of distribution of the left phrenic nerve. Any extensive division of the diaphragm would damage the nerve. A safe incision for dealing with hiatus hernia from above is shown. (*After Perera and Edwards in the 'Lancet'.*)

intradiaphragmatic distribution. The left phrenic supplies the left half of the diaphragm, the left crus, and the left half of the right crus.

A general plan of its distribution is shown in *Fig.* 649. The nerve divides 0·6 to 2·5 cm. from the superior surface of the diaphragm lateral to the left border of the heart and the pericardial impression on the diaphragm. The small anterior branch supplies the front of the muscle. The long posterior one supplies most of the diaphragm by muscle branches from its lateral aspect. The terminal ones supply the left crus and half of the right crus.

[1] Perera, H., and Edwards, F. R., *Lancet*, 1957, No. 11, 2, 75.

THE ANATOMY OF CERTAIN DISEASES

A safe incision is the left paracrural which runs from the posterior attachment of the diaphragm 2 cm. lateral to the oesophageal hiatus directly forward to the central tendon. It is just lateral to the fibres of the left crus. It gives satisfactory exposure for exploration of the immediate upper abdomen for repair of an hiatus hernia.

If an extensive opening in the diaphragm is required, however, the best incision is a circumferential one which detaches the diaphragm from its attachments to the lateral chest wall, leaving a rim of diaphragm only just large enough to make resuturing possible. In this way good exposure is achieved without the risk of nerve damage.[1]

Spigelian Hernia: Spigelius (1578–1625) was the first to describe the caudate lobe of the liver and the linea semilunaris. Such a hernia escapes through this line. It may protrude through a vascular foramen or a congenital linear slit in the aponeurosis of the transversus where it passes forwards to blend with that of the internal oblique. It may remain interparietal or become more superficial. Such herniae are uncommon, usually small, occur with equal frequency between the sexes and the two sides, may be bilateral, and are sometimes symptomless.

Obturator Hernia: This is a rare type of hernia which occurs as a rule in elderly females who have lost much fat. A process of peritoneum is pushed out of the pelvis through the obturator foramen alongside

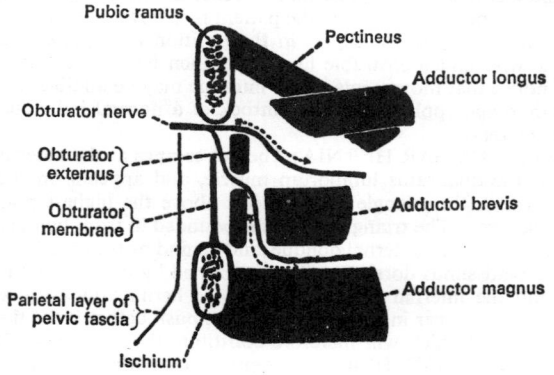

Fig. 650.—Sagittal section of thigh showing course (along the obturator nerve and its branches) which an obturator hernia may follow, as indicated by the arrows.

[1] Scott, R. *Thorax*, 1965, 20, 357.

the obturator vessels and nerve. The hernia may then take one of several courses (*Fig.* 650):

1. It may remain between the obturator externus and the obturator membrane.
2. It may push its way through the obturator externus, which then forms a muscular collar around the neck of the sac.
3. It may pass with the anterior branch of the obturator nerve above the obturator externus muscle.

The hernia is covered by the pectineus and adductor brevis muscles. The obturator artery and nerve are usually lateral to the sac, and the proximity of the nerve renders it liable to be pressed on, and thus pain is caused along the distribution of the nerve which will be felt on the inner side of the thigh and possibly in the knee-joint. Rotation of the abducted thigh inwards causes pain, as this movement tenses the obturator externus muscle.

Pudendal Hernia: This is an extremely rare type of hernia taking place into the labium majus. The hernia escapes between the conjoined ischiopubic ramus and the vagina, and occupies the posterior half of the labium. As herniae here are intensely rare, the swelling will in all probability be mistaken for a Bartholinian cyst.

Sciatic Hernia: This rare hernia presents in the buttock under cover of the gluteus maximus muscle. The gut and peritoneal sac escape from the pelvis at either the upper or lower border of the piriformis. To examine for a suspected abnormality under cover of the gluteus maximus muscle, it is essential to relax the muscle to the full. This can only be done by laying the patient face down with a pillow under his knees so that the hip is in the position of hyper-extension. An otherwise undemonstrable lump may then be detected. It is worthy of notice that movements of the intestine may be audible through the stethoscope applied over the buttock of a normal individual.

Lumbar Hernia:

LOWER LUMBAR HERNIA: The gut escapes at the anterior border of the quadratus lumborum muscle, and appears on the surface through the triangle of Petit, just above the highest point of the iliac crest. The triangle of Petit is bounded in front by the posterior border of the external oblique, and behind by the anterior border of the latissimus dorsi. The floor is formed by the lumbodorsal fascia and the internal oblique. Unless the hernia follows a wound or operation scar in this region, it must push before it the floor of the triangle, which will therefore constitute the coverings of the sac.[1]

UPPER LUMBAR HERNIA: Keith quotes Macready to the effect that a hernia may escape just under the last rib. There exists here a weak area where the aponeurosis of origin of the transversus is covered only by the latissimus dorsi. A hernia here would present

[1] Treves and Keith, *Surgical Applied Anatomy*, 1918, 380. London: Cassell.

just below the 12th rib posteriorly, and have as coverings the latissimus dorsi muscle and the aponeurosis of origin of the transversus abdominis.

Ischiorectal Hernia: This has been dealt with on p. 108.

VI. LOW BACK PAIN[1]

Lumbosacral Region of the Spine: This region is notorious for the frequency of the occurrence there of congenital abnormalities. The following anatomical facts may be noted:
1. The anterior surface of the lumbosacral joint is perpendicularly below the occipital condyles when the body is in the erect posture.
2. The anterior surface of the lumbosacral joint marks the termination of the lumbar convexity (which begins at the 12th thoracic vertebra) and the commencement of the sacral concavity.
3. In the embryo of two months, the sacrum and lumbar region are in the same straight line. The lumbosacral angle begins to form when the child sits up. The lumbosacral angle of the average adult is 120°. The normal range of variation is extensive.
4. The body-weight is borne by the opposing surfaces of the 1st sacral and 5th lumbar vertebrae (the intervertebral fibrocartilage intervening) and by the two articulations between the superior sacral and inferior lumbar articular processes.
5. The lumbosacral articulation is the meeting-place of the movable lumbar spine above with the fixed rigid sacrum below.
6. The two bones entering into the articulation are held together by a host of ligaments: (*a*) Intervertebral fibrocartilage; (*b*) Anterior longitudinal ligament; (*c*) Posterior longitudinal ligament; (*d*) Capsules of the joints between the articular processes; (*e*) Ligamenta flava; (*f*) Interspinous ligaments; (*g*) Supraspinous ligaments; (*h*) Lumbosacral ligaments; (*i*) Iliolumbar ligaments.
7. The anterolateral relation on each side of the lumbosacral joint is the lumbosacral trunk (L. 4 and 5).
8. The 5th lumbar nerve emerges through a bony tunnel which is bounded: (*a*) Anteriorly: by the posterolateral surface of the body of the 5th lumbar vertebra; by the posterior surface of the intervertebral disk; and by the posterior surface of the upper part of the sacrum. (*b*) Posteriorly: by the anterior surface of the articular processes. (*c*) Laterally: by the psoas muscle and iliolumbar ligament.
9. The 4th lumbar nerve crosses in front of the 5th lumbar transverse process to join the 5th lumbar to form the lumbosacral trunk. The nerve (4th lumbar) may be irritated by undue development of this bony mass.

---

[1] Much of the matter in this section is taken from 'Deformities of the Lumbosacral Region of the Spine', by James F. Brailsford, *Br. J. Surg.*, 1929, **16**, 562.

10. The bony canals through which the anterior divisions of the 4th and 5th lumbar nerves emerge are long, and the nerves unprotected by an arachnoid sheath. Each nerve cord is accompanied by a venous plexus which may, if overdeveloped or engorged, irritate the nerve (Forrestier[1]).

Development of the Vertebrae Concerned: A typical vertebra is developed from:

THREE PRIMARY CENTRES: One for the body (10th to 20th week); this centre represents the fusion of what were originally two centres, one for each lateral half of the body. One for each half of the neural or vertebral arch (from seven weeks onwards).

Each of these latter centres forms half of the vertebral arch and the lateral part of the body. Until the age of 4 years this lateral part of the body is separated from the rest of the vertebral body by a plate of cartilage—this junction is the neurocentral synchondrosis.

FIVE SECONDARY CENTRES: These appear at puberty: one for tip of spine (not in cervical region); one at end of each transverse process; one for a plate of bone on the upper surface of the body; one for a plate of bone on the lower surface of the body. They join at 25 years. Mamillary processes of lumbar vertebrae have each a separate centre.

FIFTH LUMBAR VERTEBRA: In addition to the centres for a typical vertebra, the costal element of the transverse process of the 5th lumbar vertebra sometimes appears as a separate bone in children and this is suggestive of a separate ossific centre for the part. Furthermore, the transverse process may remain separate from the vertebral arch and may suggest a fracture when seen on X-rays.

SACRUM: The sacrum has a complicated ossification which has little surgical interest apart from its costal elements. Fusion of bodies takes place from below up between 18 and 25 years.

COSTAL ELEMENTS: These remnants of ribs are represented in every vertebra. The costal element of the 5th lumbar, like that of other vertebrae, is merely the anterior part of its transverse process. The costal elements of the 1st, 2nd, and 3rd sacral vertebrae are very large and form most of the lateral masses. Each has a separate centre of ossification.

Classification of Causes of Low Back Pain: The lumbosacral area of the spine is a frequent source of backache because it is at the junction of the highly mobile lumbar spine with the fixed sacrum and hence is frequently subjected to injury, either a single acute injury or multiple repeated traumata.

---

[1] Quoted by Brailsford.

Anatomical factors are important in the causation of low back pain as the following classification of causes of low back pain indicates:
1. Referred pain from the pelvic or abdominal viscera. This is the reason why a thorough examination of the abdomen and pelvis must be made in all cases of low backache and this examination must include a careful assessment of the main large arteries in the area.
2. Lumbosacral deformities (*see below*).
3. Postural defects, such as leg-length discrepancy, bad posture, paralysis of muscles, pregnancy, pot belly, scoliosis, etc.

All such postural defects should be carefully examined for, but it is important not to confuse postural defects as a cause of backache with those defects which result from a backache.

4. Diseases of the vertebrae, intervertebral discs, ligaments, or muscles.

These diseases might be of traumatic, inflammatory, neoplastic, or degenerative nature.

5. Spinal cord compression.

General Classification of Lumbosacral Deformities: The deformities which may occur in this region may be present without causing any symptoms. The discovery of such deformity cannot therefore be considered the cause of the patient's trouble unless an exhaustive search fails to reveal any other aetiological factor. On the other hand, these deformities may explain symptoms, such as backache, which have long defied explanation. In Brailsford's series of 3,000 cases, deformities were found in 26·4 per cent. These developmental irregularities were due to:

1. DEFECTS IN THE DEVELOPMENT OF THE VERTEBRAL BODY:
   a. Body represented by two hemivertebrae.
   b. Body represented by one hemivertebra.
   c. Two or more vertebrae fused into one.
   d. Vertebra represented by a shapeless mass of bone.
   e. Absence of sacrum and coccyx.
2. DEFECTS IN THE DEVELOPMENT OF THE VERTEBRAL ARCH:
   a. Variation in the direction of the facets of the articular processes.
   b. Defective fusion causing:
      i. Spina bifida.
      ii. Spina bifida occulta.
   c. Anomalies of spinous processes:
      i. Separate ossicle.
      ii. Articulation of adjacent processes.
   d. Anomalies of transverse process of 5th lumbar vertebra:
      i. Traversed by a foramen.

ii. Articulation with the sacrum.
iii. Articulation with the ilium.
iv. Sacralization of 5th lumbar vertebra:
   α. Symmetrical.
   β. Asymmetrical, causing scoliosis (commonest deformity).
   γ. Alterations in segmental formation of nerves arising from lumbar and sacral plexuses.
v. Ossification of iliolumbar ligament.

3. DEFECTS IN THE DEVELOPMENT OF THE SACRUM:
   'Lumbarization' of the 1st sacral vertebra.
4. SPONDYLOLISTHESIS.

Detailed Consideration of Lumbosacral Deformities:

1. DEFECTS OF THE VERTEBRAL BODY:
   a. The body may be represented by two hemivertebrae. The two halves of the vertebra are separated by a vertical hiatus in an X-ray picture. This defect is obviously due to a failure of fusion of the two primary centres for the body.
   b. Only one lateral half of a vertebra exists. A defect of the gravest nature, resulting in a type of scoliosis (laterally bent spine) which is most difficult to deal with, and which usually causes deformity which is incapable of rectification by surgical or other means (*Fig.* 651).
   c. The bodies of several vertebrae may fuse together, the intervening joints being obliterated. The movements of the spine are necessarily restricted. The cause is unknown.
   d. The development of the body is irregular, the vertebra being represented by a shapeless mass of bone in a radiograph.
   e. The sacrum and coccyx are absent.

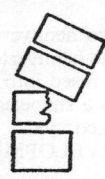

Fig. 651.—Diagrammatic representation of spinal deformity resulting from congenital absence of a hemivertebra.

2. DEFECTS OF THE VERTEBRAL ARCH:
   a. VARIATION IN THE DIRECTION OF THE FACETS OF THE ARTICULAR PROCESSES: The superior articular facets of the 5th lumbar vertebra look backwards and inwards. The inferior ones are about as wide apart as the superior and look in the opposite direction—forwards and outwards. The superior sacral articular

facets look backwards and a little inwards. There is great variability in the direction of the superior sacral facets. One may look backwards, while its fellow looks inwards. Both facets may look directly backwards. When the direction of the facets is asymmetrical, abnormal movements occur at the joint. Abnormalities in the direction of the articular facets may be acquired (e.g., following disuse of one limb) as well as developmental. Putti and others attach importance to these irregularities in the aetiology of backache.

b. DEFECTIVE FUSION OF THE VERTEBRAL ARCHES: The two halves of the vertebral arch should fuse posteriorly in the first year of life. Failure of fusion causes spina bifida (*Fig.* 652).

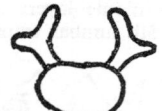

Fig. 652.—Spina bifida.

c. DEFECTIVE DEVELOPMENT OF THE SPINOUS PROCESS: The spinous process is formed by the coalescence of the posterior parts of the laminae in the first year. About puberty a secondary centre appears which fuses with the rest of the spine at 25.

Fusion of the secondary centre with the rest of the process may fail. This results in the posterior part of the spine of the vertebra existing as a separate ossicle.

d. ABNORMALITIES OF THE TRANSVERSE PROCESS OF THE FIFTH LUMBAR VERTEBRA:

i. *Foramen:* Cases have been reported where a foramen (like that in the cervical vertebrae) has traversed the process. It has been noted that all transverse processes represent a fusion of the transverse process proper with a costal element. The foramen is the first stage of an attempt on the part of the costal element to form a separate bone (rib).

ii. *Articulation of the Transverse Process with the Sacrum:* This is the first stage of sacralization and implies merely that the transverse process of the 5th lumbar vertebra makes contact with the upper surface of the ala of the sacrum. It will be noted that when such a lumbosacral transverse articulation exists, the anterior division of the 5th lumbar nerve must emerge through a bony tunnel bounded:

Medially by the lumbosacral joint.
Laterally by the articulation in question.
Below by the ala of the sacrum.

Above by the 5th lumbar process.
Behind by the superior sacral articular process.

It is held by many authorities (Jones and Lovett,[1] etc.) that the 5th lumbar nerve may be pressed on during its course through this tunnel (particularly if the lumbosacral joint is diseased) and be the cause of referred pain (sciatica).

iii. *Articulation of the Transverse Process with the Ilium:* The 5th lumbar transverse processes are directed outwards but also *upwards* to avoid contact with the iliac crest. Such contact does occur in some cases and is a well-known cause of pain in the lower back. A somewhat similar state of affairs may be brought about by ossification of that part of the anterior and middle layers of lumbodorsal fascia which connects the 5th lumbar transverse process to the crest of

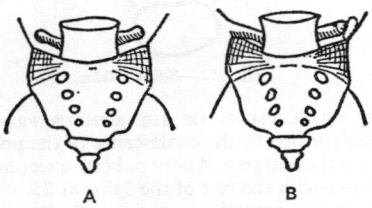

Fig. 653.—A, Normal relation of transverse processes of 5th lumbar vertebra. B, On reader's left—ossification of iliolumbar ligament so that vertebra is fused to the ilium. On right—transverse process articulating with ilium.

the ilium (iliolumbar ligaments) (*Fig.* 653). This produces rigid fixation of the two parts, resulting often in pain in the back. Cases such as those cited in this paragraph have been cured of the backache by operative removal of the cause.

iv. *Sacralization of the Fifth Lumbar Vertebra:* The vertebral formula is not fixed.[2] The lumbar region of man is shorter than that of his nearest (anthropoid) relations. That the process of shortening of the lumbar spine is still continuing is shown by the frequency with which the 5th lumbar vertebra takes on sacral characteristics. Sacralization of the 5th lumbar implies the fusion of its transverse processes with the sacrum. Such fusion may be symmetrical (bilateral) or asymmetrical (unilateral). The effects of these two conditions are vastly different.

---

[1] *Orthopaedic Surgery.* London.
[2] Sir Arthur Keith, *Human Embryology and Morphology*, 1913, 46. London.

THE ANATOMY OF CERTAIN DISEASES 699

α. *Symmetrical sacralization:* This formation is said (Moore)[1] to be architecturally sounder and more able to resist strain than the back with the usual vertebral formula (7, 12, 5, 5, 4).

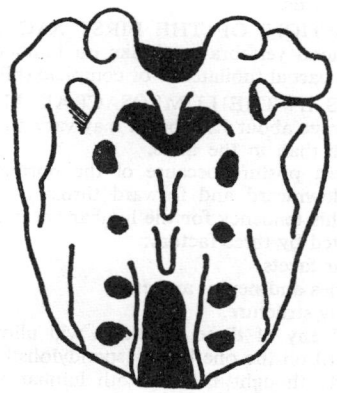

Fig. 654.—Asymmetrical sacralization of 5th lumbar vertebra.

β. *Asymmetrical sacralization* (*Fig.* 654): 'The most frequent deformity associated with a developmental irregularity is the scoliosis due to asymmetrical sacralization of the 5th lumbar transverse process' (Brailsford). Asymmetrical sacralization always leads to scoliosis, which, though not necessarily severe, is yet noticeable, alters muscle balance, and leads to arthritic changes in the joints, pain, etc. The remarks made in connexion with nerve symptoms arising from the existence of a transverse lumbosacral joint apply with even greater force to unilateral sacralization. It has also been shown that the contribution of the 4th lumbar nerve which joins the 5th to form the lumbosacral trunk passes down in front of the 5th lumbar transverse process and may be so tightly stretched over the bone as to give rise to referred pain (V. Putti).[2] In Brailsford's series 8·1 per cent showed sacralization of the 5th lumbar vertebra, 3·4 per cent unilateral, 4·7 per cent bilateral.

[1] Sacralization of the Fifth Lumbar Vertebra', *J. Bone Jt Surg.*, 1925, 7, 271, quoted by Brailsford.
[2] 'New Conceptions in the Pathogenesis of Sciatic Pain', *Lancet*. 1927, July 9, quoted by Brailsford.

γ. *Associated alterations in the lumbosacral plexus:* Just as the brachial plexus may be pre- or postfixed, so may the lumbosacral plexus be 'shunted' one cord segment higher or lower, concomitant with a movement of the sacrum upwards or downwards.

3. 'LUMBARIZATION' OF THE FIRST SACRAL VERTEBRA: The 1st sacral vertebra may take on lumbar characteristics. This may be partial (unilateral) or complete (bilateral).

4. VARIATIONS IN THE LUMBOSACRAL ANGLE: This angle is on an average about 120° but it may vary and is usually greater in the female than in the male.

In the erect posture, because of the normal lumbar lordosis, there is a downward and forward thrust on the lower lumbar vertebrae. This tendency for the lumbar vertebrae to slip forward is counteracted by three factors:

a. The articular facets.
b. Intact pedicles and neural arches.
c. Normal bony structure.

Deficiencies of any of these structures will allow one vertebra to slip forward on the one below (spondylolisthesis).

It was formerly thought that the 5th lumbar vertebra sometimes had two centres of ossification for the vertebral arch and that failure of fusion of these two centres would create a congenital weakness in the pars interarticularis (the part of the arch that lies between the superior and inferior articular processes) allowing the 5th lumbar vertebra to slip forward. This has not been substantiated by extensive examination of still born and neonatal cadavers.[1]

Causes of Spondylolisthesis[2]

Spondylolisthesis can be due to defects in any of the three structures which counteract forward slipping of a lumbar vertebra. Deficiency of the articular facets may be congenital (*congenital spondylolisthesis*)—20 per cent of cases—or degenerative (*degenerative spondylolisthesis*)—25 per cent of cases (*Fig.* 655, A). The latter occurs more often at the level of L. 4 (where the facets are placed obliquely) than at the lumbosacral level (where the facets are in a transverse plane). A defect in the pars interarticularis may be due to an acute fracture (*traumatic spondylolisthesis*), which is very rare, or due to elongation and thinning with later a fracture following on prolonged stress on the 5th lumbar vertebra because of surrounding soft tissue weakness (*spondylolytic spondylolisthesis*)—50 per cent of cases. Rarely a bone disease may weaken the neural arch to allow forward slipping (*pathological spondylolisthesis*) (*Fig.* 655, B).

[1] Rowe. G. G., and Roche, M. B., *J. Bone Jt Surg.*, 1953, 35A, 102.
[2] Newman, P. H., *Ibid.*, 1963, 45B, 39.

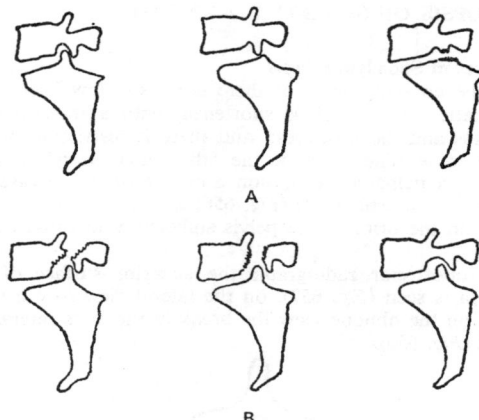

Fig. 655.—Types of spondylolisthesis. A, Normal, congenital, degenerative. B, Traumatic, spondylolytic, pathological.

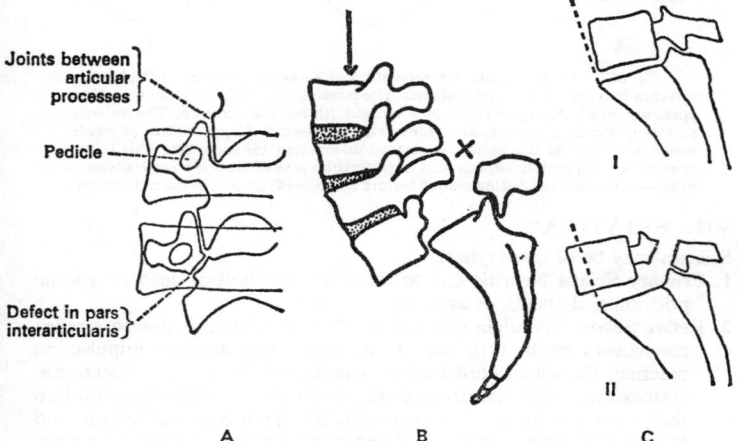

Fig. 656.—Spondylolisthesis with a break in the pars interarticularis. A, On the oblique radiograph the defect in the pars interarticularis gives the appearance of a decapitated 'Scots terrier'. B, On the lateral radiograph there is forward slipping of the 5th lumbar vertebra. The prominent 5th lumbar spine and the gap above it (X) can be appreciated. (The arrow indicates the thrust of the body weight.) C, Normally the body of the 5th lumbar vertebra lies behind a perpendicular line drawn from the front of the sacrum but in spondylolisthesis this line will cut into the body of the 5th lumbar vertebra (*Ullman's Sign*). I, Normal. II, Spondylolisthesis.

Clinical Features of Spondylolisthesis

There may be no symptoms but there is usually low backache, with or without sciatica. The trunk is shortened, with a transverse furrow between the ribs and the iliac crest, and there is restriction of forward flexion of the spine. The spine of the 5th lumbar vertebra is unduly prominent, with a palpable depression above it (in those cases with a defect in the pars interarticularis) (*Fig.* 656) and the 5th lumbar vertebra may encroach on the brim of the pelvis sufficiently to cause obstructed labour.

On an anteroposterior radiograph the superior surface of the 5th lumbar vertebra is seen (*Fig.* 657), on the lateral view forward slipping is evident and on the oblique view the break in the pars interarticularis may be visible (*Fig.* 656).

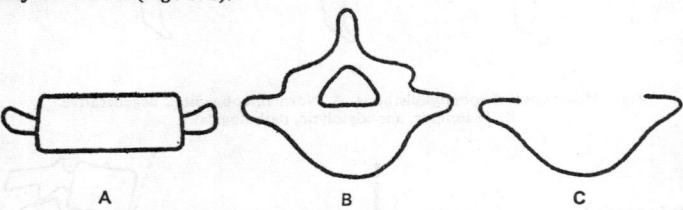

Fig. 657.—Diagrammatic representation of X-ray appearances of 5th lumbar vertebra in a case of spondylolisthesis. The bone is seen from the front (anterior-posterior view). A, Appearance of a normal 5th lumbar vertebra. The *anterior* surface of the body is seen, also transverse processes. B, *Upper* surface of whole vertebra is seen as the bone has rotated downwards through 90°. This is the appearance in spondylolisthesis. C, Characteristic curve of the body and transverse processes which is the distinguishing feature in figure (B) as seen in the radiograph.

VII. SCIATICA[1]

Sciatica may be of three types:

1. **Primary Sciatic Neuritis** due to toxaemia, alcoholism, lead or arsenic poisoning, diabetes, or syphilis.
2. **Reflex Sciatic Neuralgia** where the radiation of pain is due to a reflex mechanism centred in the spinal cord. The afferent impulse on reaching the spinal cord excites synaptically, by way of internuncial connexions, other sensory neurons which project pain sensation into their own territories. This type of sciatic pain does not correspond to a known pattern of nerve distribution and has no objective neurological signs. It may occur from irritation of the structures of the lower back, such as ligaments and muscles, or from disease of the lower abdominal viscera, such as prostate, bladder, uterus, and ovaries.

[1] Steindler, A., *Lectures on the Interpretations of Pain in Orthopedic Practice*, 1959. Springfield, Ill.: Thomas.

THE ANATOMY OF CERTAIN DISEASES

3. **Sciatic Nerve Compression** with referred pain in part or whole of the sciatic distribution. Characteristic features of this type of sciatica are that the pain is referred into a dermatome distribution corresponding to the particular nerve involved and that there are other sensory or motor signs such as anaesthesia, paraesthesia, muscle atrophy, and areflexia. It is this kind of sciatica with which we are concerned here.

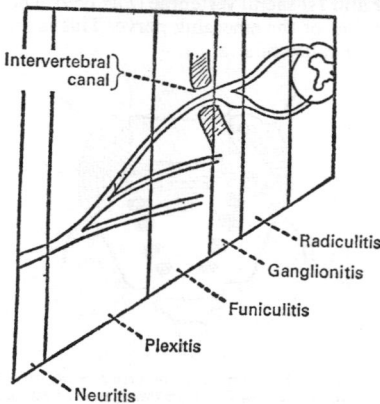

Fig. 658.—Diagram from Putti showing parts of spinal nerve which may be involved in sciatica. (For description *see* text.)

The sciatic nerve is composed of five roots, the 4th and 5th lumbar and the 1st to 3rd sacral roots, and there is a difference in the field of radiation of pain according to the specific root involved (*see Fig.* 156, p. 168).

CAUSES OF SCIATIC NERVE COMPRESSION WITH REFERRED PAIN:

1. Compression by intervertebral disc lesions. (*See* p. 712.)
2. Compression by non-disc lesions within the spinal column.
3. Compression by causes outside the spinal column.

COMPRESSION BY NON-DISC LESIONS WITHIN THE SPINAL COLUMN: This may be caused by pressure on the nerve roots (*radiculitis*) or posterior root ganglion (*ganglionitis*) by intradural or extradural masses.

The commonest anatomical site of compression is to that part of the nerve which traverses the intervertebral canal (*funiculitis*). The term *neurodocitis* is a term used to indicate nerve pain due to irritation of the nerve by the bony foramen or canal through which it passes and funiculitis is thus one form of neurodicitis (*Fig.* 658).

Anatomical Bases of Sciatic Neurodocitis:

1. The fifth lumbar is the principal constituent of the great sciatic nerve (L. 4, 5; S. 1, 2, 3).
2. In sacralization of the 5th lumbar vertebra, its transverse process is wider and deeper than usual, which has the effect of narrowing the intervertebral canal (for the 5th lumbar nerve) between the 5th lumbar and 1st sacral vertebrae (*Fig.* 659). The result is irritation or compression of the emerging nerve. This is an admitted but not very common cause of sciatica.

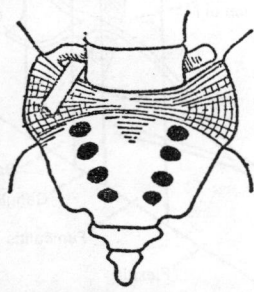

Fig. 659.—Articulation of 5th lumbar transverse process with sacrum on left of figure. Observe the narrow space for emergence of 5th lumbar nerve.

3. Thickening of the ligamentum flavum may compress the 5th lumbar root and symptoms may be relieved by releasing this compression surgically.
4. Putti draws attention to the following facts in the anatomy of the lumbar spine which are relevant to the subject in hand:
   a. INTERVERTEBRAL CANALS: Boundaries:
      Superior: The intervertebral notch.
      Anterior: Posterior part of vertebral body above; intervertebral disc; posterior part of vertebral body below.
      Inferior: Pedicle of vertebra.
      Posterior: The articulation between the inferior articular facets of vertebra above, and superior articular facets of vertebra below. This is a fact to which Putti attaches considerable importance.
   b. THE JOINTS BETWEEN THE ARTICULAR PROCESSES OF THE LUMBAR VERTEBRAE:
      i. The articular facets and therefore the joint cavity are in the saggital plane.
      ii. In the joint between the 5th lumbar and 1st sacral vertebrae the facets are placed in the frontal plane (*Fig.* 660).

THE ANATOMY OF CERTAIN DISEASES

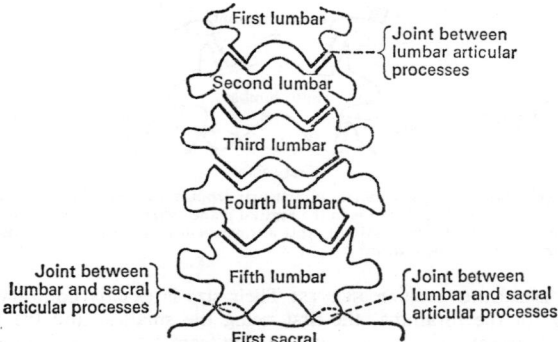

Fig. 660.—Normal arrangement of joints between articular processes of lumbar and 1st sacral vertebrae. The articular facets and joint line are in the sagittal plane, except in the joints between 5th lumbar and 1st sacral articular processes, where the facets and joint line are in the frontal plane. (*After Putti.*)

  iii. Variations from the normal are frequent. Such variations are of great importance when they are of severe degree, and when they are unilateral only.

  iv. The commonest and most important variation is one where one lumbosacral articular joint is in the sagittal plane and the other in the frontal plane. This has been called by Putti 'anomaly of articular tropism' (*Fig.* 661).

c. THE EFFECTS OF SUCH ANOMALIES ON THE INTERVERTEBRAL FORAMEN:

  i. They may alter its shape and reduce its capacity.

  ii. They may induce a localized traumatic arthritis by altering the mechanics of the spine. The swelling and deformity around the joint press on the emerging nerve, producing neurodocitis.

d. INTERVERTEBRAL FORAMINA: These vary in size.

  i. The foramen between the vertebrae L. 5 and S. 1 is always the smallest.

  ii. The foramen between vertebrae L. 4 and L. 5 is the next smallest.

  iii. The foramen between vertebrae L. 3 and L. 4 is the next in size.

  iv. The foramen between vertebrae L. 2 and L. 3 is the second largest.

  v. The foramen between vertebrae L. 1 and L. 2 is the largest.

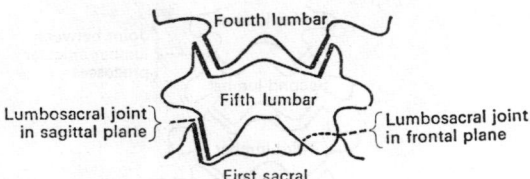

Fig. 661.—Putti's 'anomaly of articular tropism'. Observe that the lumbosacral joint on left of figure is in the sagittal plane, whereas the one on the right is in the frontal plane. Obviously this arrangement is one which lends itself to strain and traumatic arthritis.

e. EMERGING LUMBAR NERVES: Their size is exactly contrary to that of the foramina, the first being the smallest and the fifth the largest, i.e., they increase in size from 1 to 5. In this connexion observe that the 4th and 5th lumbar nerves are, on anatomical grounds, predisposed to neurodocitis more than any of the others. This fact has an important bearing on the pathology of sciatica, as the 4th and 5th lumbar nerves constitute a most important contribution to the sciatic.

The entire acceptance of the views of Sicard and Putti on the pathogenesis of sciatica is rendered difficult by the fact that many authorities consider that the 5th lumbar nerve has no sensory distribution above the knee, and the pain behind the thigh in cases of sciatica is therefore difficult to explain, as this region is said to be supplied by the 2nd sacral nerve. On the other hand, the 5th lumbar root may supply a territory at the back of the thigh, and R. Waterhouse[1] has published a case of herpes in the distribution of the 5th lumbar root where vesicles appeared on the back of the thigh as well as on the outer side of the leg. This is strong evidence that the 5th lumbar assists in the cutaneous supply of the back of the thigh.

f. THE FUNICULUS:[2] This is the part of the nerve which lies in the intervertebral canal. Note:
  i. The 4th and 5th lumbar nerves: the funicular portions of these nerves are longer than in any of the other lumbar nerves.
  ii. The funicular part of the nerve has a dural sheath only, but not an arachnoid sheath like the nerve-root. *The funiculus is therefore not bathed in cerebrospinal fluid.*
  iii. There is a very rich venous plexus around the funiculus. This plexus is much influenced by mechanical conditions outside the funiculus. This part of the nerve having no

---
[1] *Lancet*, 1930, 2, 1015.
[2] Quoted from Bonmot and Forrestier by Putti, *loc. cit.*

THE ANATOMY OF CERTAIN DISEASES

arachnoid sheath and cerebrospinal fluid watershed is exposed to neighbouring mechanical influences, while the venous plexus surrounding the funiculus subjects it to the effects of any congestion or stasis which may occur in the parts around. The nerve-root, being more adequately guarded, is far less subject to such influences.

5. Intervertebral Foramen: Decrease in size of this foramen will compress the funiculus. The 5th lumbar root is specially vulnerable as it is the largest nerve root and the 5th lumbar foramen is the smallest. The intervertebral foramen may be narrowed by intervertebral disc degeneration allowing the vertebral bodies to move more closely to each other, capsular reaction with swelling and oedema following strain on the articular facets, fractures of the vertebrae with callus formation, osteoarthritis of the articular facets with spur formation, and osteophytes on the posterior border of the vertebral bodies (*Fig.* 662).

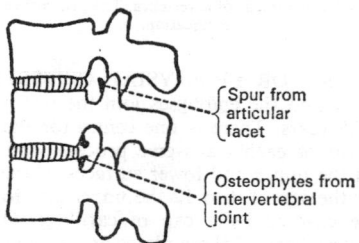

Fig. 662.—Osteoarthritic spurs and osteophytes encroaching on the intervertebral foramen.

COMPRESSION BY CAUSES OUTSIDE THE SPINAL COLUMN: This may cause compression of the lumbosacral plexus (plexitis) or individual nerves arising from the plexus (neuritis), to produce sciatica.

   a. Diseases of the sacro-iliac joint. The lumbosacral trunk (L. 4 and 5) crosses the anterior aspect of the sacro-iliac joint. Disease of this joint may irritate the nerve.

   b. Masses in the pelvis may irritate the plexus or the sciatic nerve.

VIII. LESIONS OF THE INTERVERTEBRAL DISC[1]

To make this section clearer the development of a typical vertebra is described.

---

[1] In the compilation of this section much use has been made of the lucid account given by Walter Mercer, *Orthopaedic Surgery*, 1937, 627. London: Arnold.

Ossification of a Typical Vertebra:

THREE PRIMARY CENTRES: One for the body appears between the tenth and twentieth week. One centre appears on each side at the base of the superior articular process about the same time. From these centres the vertebral arch or ring is ossified (*Fig.* 663).

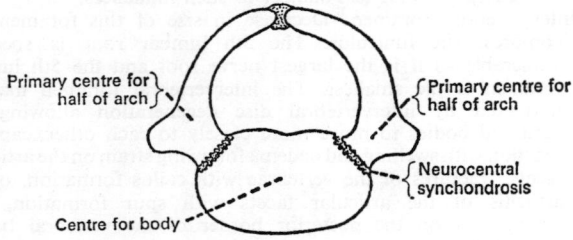

Fig. 663.—Development of a vertebra. The primary centres of ossification.

FIVE SECONDARY OR EPIPHYSIAL CENTRES: These appear about puberty and the epiphyses join the rest of the bone about the age of 25 years. There is one centre for the tip of the spine, one at the tip of each transverse process, and one each in the cartilage on the upper and lower surfaces of the body (*Fig.* 664). Until about the age of 8 to 12 the upper and lower surfaces of a vertebra are covered by a cap of cartilage. Ossification begins then in the periphery of these plates and extends so as to form a ring round a central island of cartilage. By the age of 25 this ring has fused with the vertebra, but the central cartilaginous plate remains throughout life as part of the apparatus of the intervertebral disc (*Fig.* 665).

Until Schmorl in 1928 published the results of his epoch-making investigations, the intervertebral disc appeared to enjoy the same immunity to pathology that characterizes cartilage. To-day the disc ranks high as a cause of pathological spinal conditions. Its pathological lesions are all caused, directly or indirectly, by trauma. It is too inert and avascular a structure to be attacked by toxic, infective, or neoplastic processes. It is insensitive to pain.

Anatomy: Schmorl described the disc as consisting of three varieties of tissue:

1. NUCLEUS PULPOSUS: central in position, firm and elastic, and jelly-like in consistence. It is the remains of the notochord. It is under considerable tension.

THE ANATOMY OF CERTAIN DISEASES

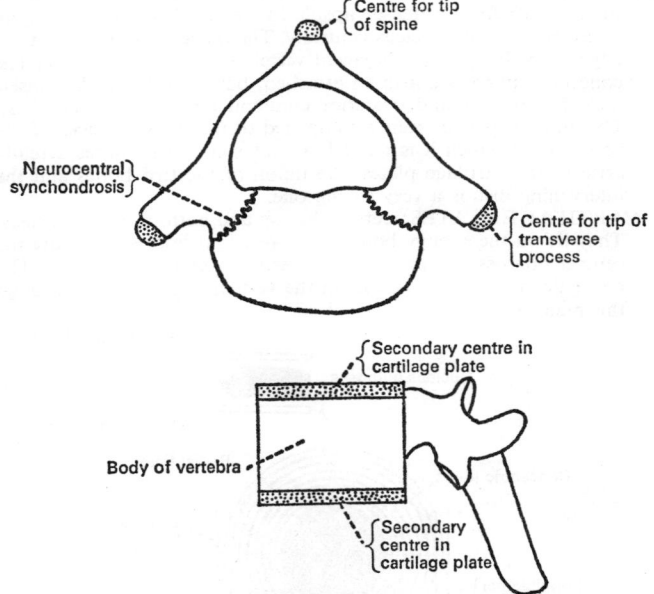

Fig. 664.—Development of a vertebra. The secondary centres of ossification of a vertebra.

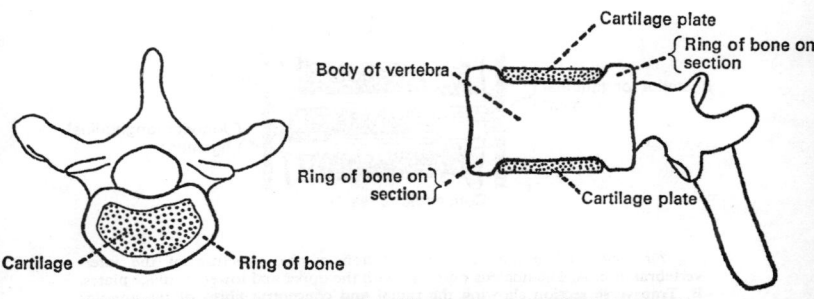

Fig. 665.—Development of a vertebra. The vertebra is completely developed and shows diagrammatically the cartilaginous plates on the upper and lower surfaces of the body.

2. **THE ANNULUS FIBROSUS:** Consists of concentric and radial fibres which form a dense capsule for the nucleus. Both sets gain attachment to the nucleus centrally. The radial fibres turn over the edge of the body of the adjacent vertebra and enter the bone. The concentric fibres are also so attached, but in addition they insert into the anterior and posterior common ligaments of the spine. The annulus is very securely attached to the bony surfaces of the vertebrae to which it is related, and as some of its fibres actually arise in the cartilage plates, the union of the two bones and the intervening disc is a very strong one.
3. **CARTILAGE PLATES:** Set on the top and bottom of the nucleus. They lie on the spongy bone of the vertebral bodies. They are the central non-ossified parts of the vertebral epiphysial plates. The disc gains its nourishment from the vertebra by diffusion through this plate (*Fig.* 666).

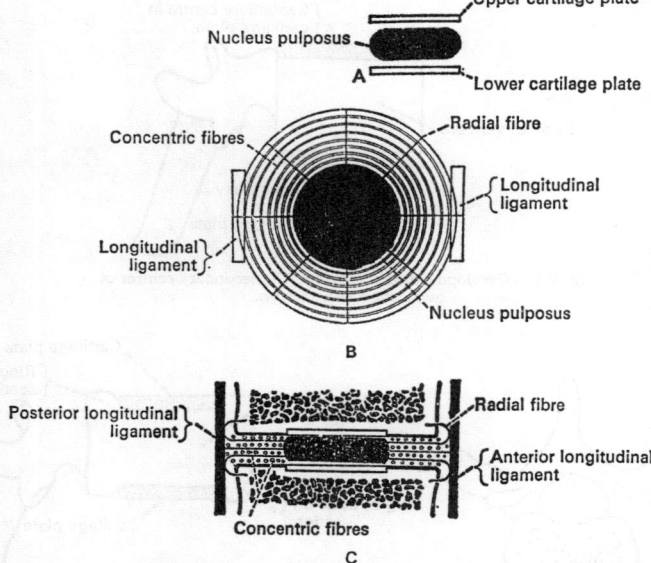

Fig. 666.—Diagrammatic representation of the structure of the intervertebral disc. A, The nucleus pulposus with the upper and lower cartilage plates. B, Transverse section showing the radial and concentric fibres of the annulus fibrosus and their attachment. C, Sagittal section of the disc showing the nucleus and the radial and concentric fibres of the annulus.

THE ANATOMY OF CERTAIN DISEASES

The intervertebral disc has a blood-supply until general development is complete. After that it is nourished by diffusion through the cartilaginous plates from the vessels in the osseous tissue of the vertebrae. O'Connell[1] points out that a cervical intervertebral disc weighs approximately half that of a thoracic one, and a quarter of a lumbar disc. He correlates this with the fact that cervical disc protrusions are smallest, lumbar ones largest, and the thoracic ones intermediate in size.

Function: The discs give shape to the column. They act as a remarkable series of shock absorbers or buffers. Like the tendon of the supraspinatus they are exposed to jars and strains constantly. Even in sleep

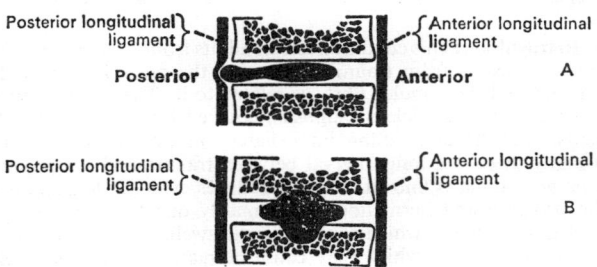

Fig. 667.—A, Shows retropulsion of the nucleus pulposus. B, Nuclear expansion.

they are acted on by every movement of the column. They are under great tension. Each may be likened to a coiled-up spring. Should the confining walls be damaged the spring will bulge at the weak area. It is of interest to consider theoretically the possibilities which may upset normal conditions in these springs.

1. NUCLEAR RETROPULSION: The posterior ligaments may be damaged—the spring forces the weak area back (*Fig.* 667, A).

2. NUCLEAR EXPANSION: The upper or lower cartilage plates lose the support given them by the vertebral cancellous bone. The nucleus bulges into the vertebral body (*Fig.* 667, B).

3. SPONDYLOSIS DEFORMANS: The disc apparatus begins to degenerate because of the effects of multiple minor traumata and age—the spine may take on the aged-gardener shape (*Fig.* 668, A).

4. SENILE KYPHOSIS: Owing to the greater strain on the anterior parts of the discs, they disappear by a slow process of attrition—the anterior parts of the adjacent vertebral bodies come together and fuse (*Fig.* 668, B).

[1] O'Connell, J. E. A., *Br. J. Surg.*, 1955, 43, 225.

712 A SYNOPSIS OF SURGICAL ANATOMY

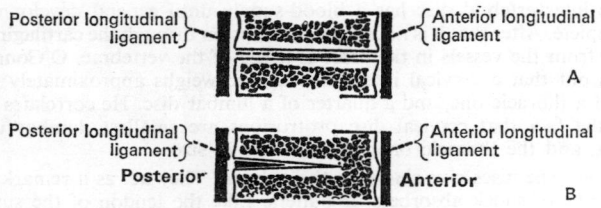

Fig. 668.—A, Showing spondylosis deformans—atrophy of the intervertebral disc. B, Senile kyphosis—note fusion of vertebral bodies anteriorly.

Nuclear Retropulsion: This condition affects adults from 30 to 50, most often males. It results from trauma weakening the posterior longitudinal ligament and the annulus fibrosus related to it. There is a protrusion backwards of the nucleus pulposus, covered by the weakened ligaments. Half the cases follow immediately on a considerable trauma. In many there is a long interval between trauma and symptoms. In some no trauma is known. Naylor[1] adduces evidence to suggest that disc prolapse and herniation are primarily due to biophysical and biochemical factors which cause episodic swelling of the disc by the absorption of fluid which may cause herniation. Later the swelling reduces and may result in some permanent impairment of structure. Trauma is a secondary factor.

The area affected is the lower lumbar. The vast majority affect the disc between the vertebrae L. 5 and S. 1. The disc between L. 4 and L. 5 is the next most vulnerable. It is usually the 5th lumbar nerve which is irritated by prolapse of the 4th disc, and the 1st sacral when the lumbosacral disc is herniated. Prolapse of these two discs comprises 95 per cent of disc lesions producing symptoms. Rarely other areas may be affected.

In compression fractures of the spine there is disc prolapse in three-quarters of the cases. Kümmell's disease of the spine, with consequent kyphosis, is now attributed to damage of the cancellous bone of the vertebral bodies from the prolapse of large fragments of the nucleus pulposus into them.

The symptoms are those of sciatica in most cases. The diagnosis may be any of the general and local causes of this condition and is difficult. There is no easy way to make it. The usual site of the prolapse is lateral in relation to the anterior wall of the vertebral canal. A prolapse here will come into relation with a spinal nerve, usually L. 5 or S. 1. A proportion of cases of disc prolapse (given as one-third by some authorities) may be centrally situated (*Fig.* 669).

[1] Naylor, A., *Ann. R. Coll. Surg.*, 1962, **31**, 91.

1. The signs and symptoms to be expected from this lesion would be pain on raising the pressure in the vertebral canal—e.g., by sneezing. This sign may be absent.
2. Lateral bending of the spine is adopted to ease the pain. It will be towards or away from the lesion depending on whether the protrusion is medial or lateral to the irritated nerve-root[1] (*Fig.* 669, A and B).
3. Sciatica—pain down thigh and leg. Straight leg bending may be, but is not necessarily, painful.
4. The pain may be worse in a particular area—that of the irritated nerve-root. As this is usually L. 5 or S. 1, there is pain at the ankle.

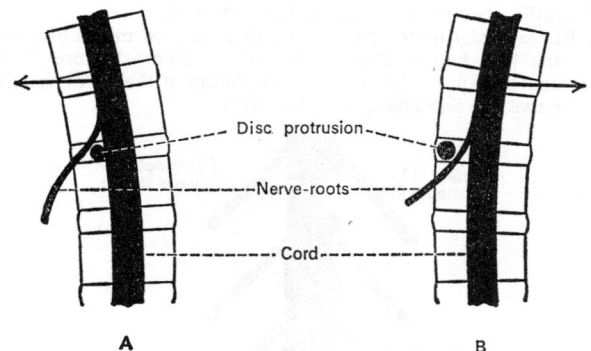

Fig. 669.—The scoliosis will vary, depending on the relationship of the nerve-root to the disc protrusion.

5. There may be numbness in the area of the nerve affected. If this is S. 1 it will be on the outer side of the leg, foot, outer two toes, and sole. The ankle-jerk is lowered. If L. 5 is the nerve pressed on, the area of hypo-aesthesia is more medial over the shin-bone area and extending over the big toe, medial malleolus, and related part of the sole. The ankle-jerk is not depressed. Obviously the distinction between a lesion affecting these two nerves may be most difficult.
6. There is no subarachnoid block as a rule as the prolapse is surprisingly small, perhaps the size of half a pea, and therefore the canal is not much obstructed. There is, however, some stagnation of cerebrospinal fluid, so that its protein content is moderately raised.

---

[1] Mercer, Sir Walter, and Duthie, R. B., *Orthopaedic Surgery*, 1964, 6th ed. London: Arnold.

714 A SYNOPSIS OF SURGICAL ANATOMY

7. There is no constant relationship between the prolapse and a narrow disc space. Often one exists without the other.
8. There may be more than one nuclear prolapse. As herniation backwards of the nucleus pulposus is a recent entity and opinions on many aspects of the matter are divergent and not static, the writer ventures to make a few observations from his own experience:
   a. Like the diagnosis of chronic appendicitis in the abdomen, sciatica should only be attributed to nuclear retropulsion when all other possibilities have been excluded.
   b. There is frequently no pain centrally over the vertebral column in the affected area.
   c. Lipiodol injection is not always necessary. Its use has resulted in irritation of nerve-roots on occasion. There are less irritating radio-opaque media which may be used.
   d. Radiography after lipiodol injection may be misleading even in the best hands. The lesion may be some distance from the constriction of the column. Non-filling of the dural sheath of a nerve is a valuable guide (*Fig.* 670).

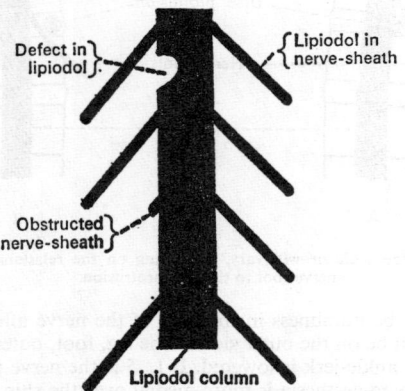

Fig. 670.—Diagrammatic representation of radiograph of lipiodol column in a case where no pathology was found at the site of the defect in the lipiodol column. The nuclear retropulsion was found pressing on the nerve-root on the left, which shows defective filling of its dural sheath with lipiodol.

   e. A nuclear prolapse which is central may produce early symptoms of paraplegia *without any pain at all*.
   f. Where extreme scoliosis exists there is usually some factor present in addition to the prolapse. This is weakness of the ligaments attaching the two vertebrae in the affected area. Some scoliosis

is likely to persist after operation. A well-fitting spinal corset will give rigidity to the weakened area and may effect cure of the symptoms persisting after operation.

9. It is becoming increasingly evident that nuclear retropulsion is the villain of the piece in sciatica. Unless, however, all possible care is used in arriving at a diagnosis, serious mistakes will be made.

10. Operation is by no means always necessary and should not be too strongly pressed on the sufferer, as results are good in only 50 per cent of cases.

MATERNAL OBSTETRICAL PALSY: O'Connell[1] points out that this is a rare condition. The pain in the limb has been ascribed to 'neuritis' due to pressure of the fetal head on some part of the sacral plexus. In his opinion a prolapsed nucleus pulposus is the pathology in many of these cases.

Kyphosis: The remaining disc lesions all have a common result on the spine, especially its thoracic part, tending to increase the normal kyphosis. In youth, true adolescent kyphosis results. In the aged, spondylosis osteoarthritica is the outcome.

Nuclear Expansion or Schmorl's Nodes: Schmorl and his co-workers showed that in 38 per cent of spines there was expansion of the discs into the bodies of the adjacent vertebrae. These workers attributed this to congenital defects in the discs themselves. Lambrinudi considers that strain on the column by forced flexion of the spine in youth is the

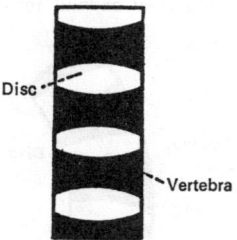

Fig. 671.—Nuclear expansions (Schmorl's nodes) as seen in sagittal section of the spine in adolescent kyphosis or vertebral epiphysitis. Note fish-like vertebrae.

important factor—toe-touching exercises and leapfrog. The thoracic portion of the spine is the part affected. The resulting condition is true adolescent kyphosis, also called Scheuermann's disease or vertebral epiphysitis. It produces anteroposterior curvature of the spine in youth—12 to 17 years. The result is permanent round shoulders. There is multiple expansion of the discs into the vertebral

[1] *Surgery Gynec. Obstet.*, 1944, 79, 374.

bodies, the latter looking like the vertebrae of fish. The effect in youth is to produce proliferation of cartilage and bone which results in spinal deformity (*Fig.* 671).

Disc Changes in the Aged: Depending on the sex and social status, varying changes appear in the spine with advancing years, collectively grouped as senile kyphosis, or spondylosis osteoarthritica by Mercer:

  a. TRUE SENILE KYPHOSIS (*see Fig.* 668, B): The anterior parts of the discs degenerate. Schmorl attributes this to the increased strains which fall on this part of the spine in those who have led lives of heavy labour. There may be bone necrosis of the parts of the vertebral bodies in relation to the degenerated discs. Bone fusion may occur also. The result is a fixed kyphotic spine. The brunt of the process falls on the thoracic spine.

  b. SPONDYLOSIS DEFORMANS (*see Fig.* 668, A): In this condition the whole disc seems prematurely aged and wastes away. As the discs collapse there is a tendency for the spinal ligaments to become lax. The slight movements allowed between adjacent bones result in osteophytic formation at the ligamentous attachments.

  c. SENILE OSTEOPOROSIS OF THE SPINE: This condition is commoner in women. It would seem to affect those whose lives are sheltered from heavy labour. There is an osteoporosis of all the vertebral bodies, which seem to fall together, producing gross deformities. The discs are healthy and unchanged and because of vertebral softening they expand into these bones (*Fig.* 672).

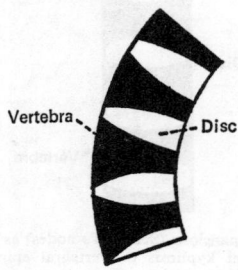

Fig. 672.—Senile osteoporosis, showing kyphosis.

IX. PROLAPSE

The term 'prolapse' implies 'a falling down, partial or complete, of some viscus; in its late stage accompanied by protrusion, so as to be partly external or uncovered'.[1] The term is used to signify the protrusion of a viscus through an anatomical aperture normally present, and also to imply

[1] Lippincott's *New Medical Dictionary*.

THE ANATOMY OF CERTAIN DISEASES

the protrusion of a structure through an aperture not normally existent, e.g., through a wound. Examples of the latter are prolapse of the iris through a corneal wound and prolapse of the testis through a skin wound. We are here concerned solely with prolapse through a pre-existent aperture.

We shall consider: (1) Prolapse of the uterus and vagina; (2) Prolapse of the female urethra; (3) Prolapse of the rectum.

Prolapse of the Uterus and Vagina:

LIGAMENTS OF THE UTERUS: These are the: (1) Broad ligaments; (2) Round ligaments; (3) Uterosacral ligaments; (4) Transverse ligaments of the cervix. The first two are too well known to require further description. They all contain muscle and elastic tissue. The proportion of fibrous tissue, muscle, and elastic tissue varies somewhat with the individual, but more according to age.

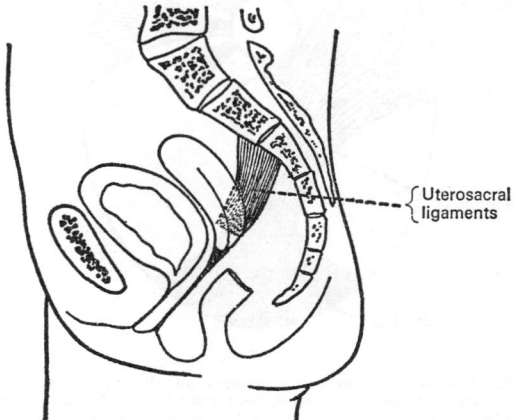

Fig. 673.—To show the uterosacral ligaments.

UTEROSACRAL LIGAMENTS (*Fig.* 673): These structures consist of fibrous and muscle tissue contained in a fold of peritoneum called the recto-uterine, which bounds the pouch of Douglas on each side. They extend backwards from either side of the cervix in the region of the internal os to the sacrum at the level of the 2nd and 3rd sacral vertebrae, embracing the rectum in their course. The ligaments tend to tether the uterus to the sacrum.

TRANSVERSE LIGAMENTS OF THE CERVIX (*Fig.* 674): Also known as the ligaments of Mackenrodt or the retinacula uteri. These bands are really parts of the visceral layer of pelvic fascia. They are strong

718 A SYNOPSIS OF SURGICAL ANATOMY

fibromuscular ligaments radiating fanwise from the cervix at the level of the internal os and cervicovaginal junction out to the side of the pelvis. The centre part is the strongest.

SUPPORTS OF THE UTERUS: Notice particularly that the term is not synonymous with 'the ligaments of the uterus', which play very little part in supporting the organ in its correct position. The actual

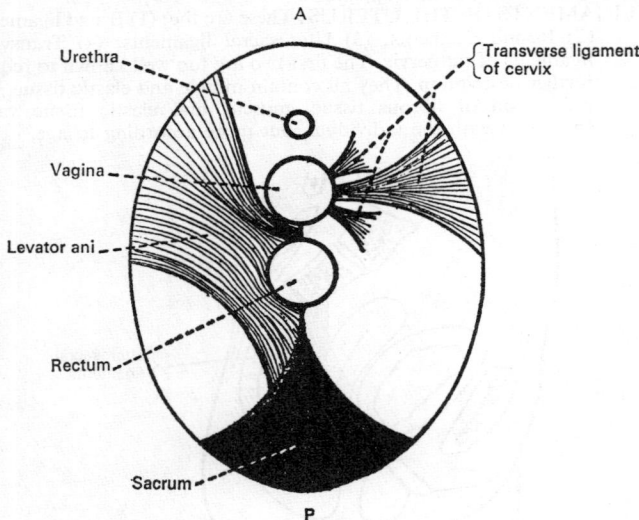

Fig. 674.—A diagrammatic representation of certain important features in the anatomy of the female pelvic floor. On the reader's left the arrangement of the levator ani is shown. On the reader's right the transverse ligament of the cervix is depicted (visceral pelvic fascia). A, Anterior. P, Posterior.

uterine supports are the: (1) Pelvic diaphragm, assisted by the urogenital diaphragm; (2) Fibrous sheaths of the blood-vessels; (3) Fascial bands attached to the cervicovaginal junction, i.e., the uterosacral and transverse ligaments of the cervix.

PELVIC DIAPHRAGM: This is much the most important support of the uterus. It forms a fibromuscular floor to the pelvis. Nature never uses fibrous tissue to withstand constant strain. Muscle tissue is infinitely superior for this purpose. The levator ani, which is the most important constituent of the pelvic floor, is constantly being subjected to strains due to increase of intra-abdominal pressure by such acts as laughing, coughing, straining at stool,

THE ANATOMY OF CERTAIN DISEASES

etc. On the levator, then, mainly falls the task of maintaining the horizontal level of the uterus. The pelvic floor formed by the levator muscle system presents a gap behind traversed by the rectum, and another in front traversed by the vagina and urethra. The anterior gap is protected by the muscles and fascia of the urogenital diaphragm. The muscles of the pelvic floor are unique in as much as they are active continuously, at rest and even during sleep.

FIBROUS SHEATHS OF THE BLOOD-VESSELS: The uterine and vaginal arteries carry with them sheaths derived from the visceral pelvic fascia, and these connective-tissue sheaths form important accessory factors in maintaining the horizontal level of the womb. The transverse cervical ligaments of Mackenrodt are considered by many to be merely condensations of the blood-vessel connective-tissue sheaths. The perineal body does not play an important part in the support of the pelvic contents.

TYPICAL POSITION OF THE UTERUS: As the uterus is a movable organ it is not correct to speak of a normal position, but rather of a typical position with empty bladder and rectum and empty uterus. The body of the uterus should then lie almost horizontal in the standing individual, and a little above the top of the symphysis; the external os being midway between the ends of a line joining the ischial spines. The body and cervix form an angle of 90° to 100° with each other.

The fundus lies nearly 2·5 cm. behind the top of the symphysis and rather above it. It may be said that normally the long axis of the uterus forms a right-angle with the long axis of the vagina.

CAUSES OF CHANGE IN THE POSITION OF THE UTERUS:
1. Pressure from want of space in the pelvis resulting from increase in the size of pelvic or abdominal organs or tissues.
2. Shortening of uterine ligaments.
3. The formation of adhesions.
4. Defects of the normal ligaments, fasciae, and muscles forming the pelvic floor.

VERSION AND FLEXION:

VERSION implies an alteration in the direction of the uterus as a whole, the organ rotating round a coronal axis passing through the external os. It is often associated with inflammatory change.

FLEXION implies an increase or a decrease in the angle between body and cervix.

The direction of the cervix in the pelvis may be normal or altered in these conditions. If the position of the body is altered the cervix naturally lies in front of or behind its typical situation.

Retroversion is apt to bring the uterine axis into line with the vaginal axis and this factor facilitates prolapse.

720 A SYNOPSIS OF SURGICAL ANATOMY

VARIETIES OF PROLAPSE:
1. Prolapse of the posterior vaginal wall. If this is associated with a prolapse of the rectum the condition is a rectocele.
2. Prolapse of the anterior vaginal wall. This usually involves the bladder—cystocele.
3. Prolapse of the uterus.

Two or all of these conditions may be associated.

CAUSATION OF PROLAPSE: Obstetric injury is the main factor in causation. If this results in injury to the pelvic floor from laceration of the perineum and damage to and separation of the levator muscles, the vagina being relatively unsupported below tends to sag downwards and the rectum tends to bulge forwards into the vagina. A rectocele is not necessarily present owing to the loose attachment between rectum and posterior vaginal wall.

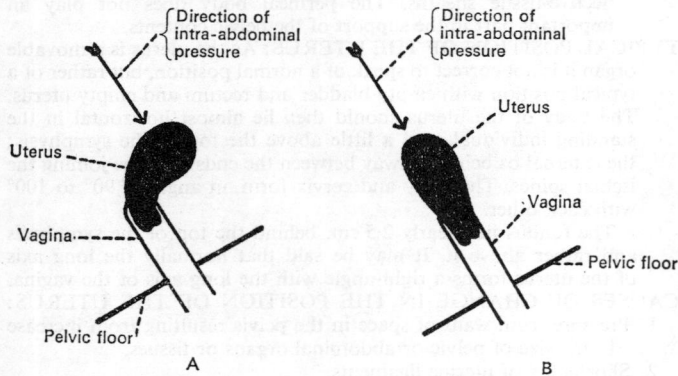

Fig. 675.—Diagrammatic representation of the fact that uterine prolapse is a herniation of the viscus through the pelvic floor via the vagina. In A the normal relationship is shown, the uterus being anteverted, lying parallel with the pelvic floor and at right-angles to the vagina; intra-abdominal pressure is indicated by the arrow. In B the uterus has straightened out and is now lying in the axis of the vagina and at right angles to the pelvic floor; the direction of intra-abdominal pressure is such that it tends to push the uterus into the vagina.

Damage and separation of the levator and fasciae in front of the uterus and around the base of the bladder will remove the normal support in that region, and this lack of support is more pronounced if perineal damage also exists. This is the genesis of prolapse of the anterior vaginal wall.

For the uterus to descend it is almost a *sine qua non* that it should first become retroverted so far as to bring the axes of uterus and vagina into line (*Fig.* 675). The uterus will then be able to descend along the vaginal canal, gradually inverting the vagina from above downwards, as its weight, constantly thrown on the fibrous ligaments, weakens them till they are no longer able to support it alone. Further, the damaged pelvic floor, perineum, levator ani, and fasciae no longer close the pelvic outlet in the normal manner. Should vaginal prolapse precede uterine prolapse, as is often the case, the drag of the vagina on the uterus will also tend to bring down this organ. The extruded body of the uterus is covered by the vagina.

Prolapse of the Female Urethra: This condition is due to loss of tone in the sphincteric musculature permitting the mucosa to glide on the underlying tissues and ultimately prolapse or herniate through the meatus (Bryden Glendining). It is found in emaciated children and as a result of parturition in women. Tumours growing from the mucous membrane may project to the exterior and pull the mucosa after them.

Prolapse of the Rectum: Normally the act of defaecation is accompanied by a tendency to eversion of the anal mucosa. When this becomes excessive the term 'prolapse' is used.

SUPPORTS OF THE RECTUM: The end gut is held in position by:
1. The attachments of the levatores ani between the internal and external sphincters.
2. The visceral layer of the pelvic fascia.
3. The recto-urethralis muscles of Roux, which attach it to the urogenital diaphragm and perineal body.
4. The *rectal stalk* (Prof. J. W. Smith). On each side of the back of the rectum 2·5 cm. above the levator, is a dense fibrous cord running from the third piece of the sacrum to the rectal wall. It contains the nervi erigentes (S. 2, 3) and the middle haemorrhoidal arteries, and is an important structure in holding up the rectum. The surgeon cannot draw down the rectum in the operation of perineal excision till this 'stalk' is divided.
5. The fatty tissue of the pelvis and ischiorectal fossae.

FACTORS CAUSING PROLAPSE OF THE RECTUM:
1. Tumours growing from the mucous membrane (adenoma or polyps) which are forced down by peristalsis, become gripped by the sphincters, and pull the mucosa after them.
2. Excessive contraction of the bowel wall causing relaxation of the submucosa, thus loosening the attachment of the mucous membrane—e.g., diarrhoea.
3. Loss of perirectal and perianal fatty tissue, causing relaxation of the supporting tissue, e.g., following emaciating illness, such as enteritis in children.

4. Increased intra-abdominal pressure tending to force the rectum down, e.g., whooping-cough, straining from constipation, piles, urethral stricture.

DEGREES OF PROLAPSE:
1. Incomplete or anal prolapse, where the mucosa only is extruded.
2. Complete or rectal prolapse, where all the bowel coats are prolapsed. In this condition the peritoneum may be pulled out of the

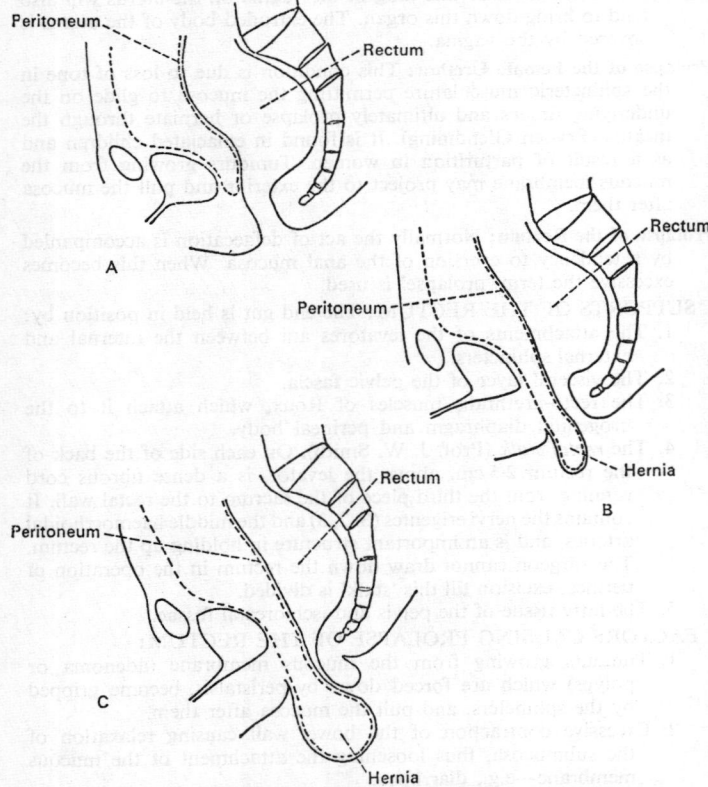

Fig. 676.—A, Normal relationships of pelvic peritoneum to pelvic floor. B, Anterior rectal wall prolapsing between levatores ani and taking pelvic peritoneum with it. C, Extensive rectal prolapse with peritoneum pulled down. Note the prolapse is mostly at the expense of the anterior rectal wall.

anus by the rectum so that a cul-de-sac of peritoneum is actually prolapsed beyond the anus, a point to be carefully remembered in the surgical treatment of the condition.

3. *Massive rectal prolapse:* The late Roscoe Graham of Toronto[1] drew attention to the huge prolapse which may follow obstetrical injury or may develop in infancy or later consequent on long continued diarrhoea. This occurs at the expense mainly of the anterior rectal wall and is really a herniation to the exterior of the peritoneum of the pouch of Douglas, passing down between the separated edges of the levator ani muscles (*Fig.* 676).

DIAGNOSIS: The only condition with which a prolapse may be confused is that where a piece of intussuscepted gut protrudes at the anus. This is easily distinguished by the fact that there is a space between the protruded gut and the anal margin, into which a probe may be inserted. This cannot be done in prolapse, as the mucous membrane of the prolapse becomes continuous with the skin of the anal margin.

X. COLD ABSCESSES OF THE SPINE

In tuberculosis of the bones of the vertebral column there frequently accumulates debris which forms a collection of fluid known as a 'cold abscess' because it is devoid of the acute symptoms such as heat, redness, pain, etc., which attend the development of ordinary abscesses. As a result of the disease of one or more of the bodies of the vertebrae, such bodies can no longer support the weight transmitted through them, and consequently they collapse. The debris in their interior is squeezed out by this collapse and travels along paths which are determined by the anatomy of the surroundings, and which can often be predicted by knowledge of this anatomy. The anatomical fact that the vertebral column is made up of a series of separate bones, all of which transmit weight, combined with the pathological fact that one or more of these bones is weakened by disease and crushed by this weight, accounts for the great frequency with which cold abscesses appear in tuberculosis of the spine.

Position and Course of Cold Abscesses of the Spine in Different Regions:

IN ANY REGION: A cold abscess may appear: (1) Just in front of the bodies of the vertebrae—a prevertebral abscess; (2) Within the vertebral canal, and compressing the spinal cord. Though the latter may occur it is very exceptional.

IN THE CERVICAL REGION: A cold abscess may appear:
1. RETROPHARYNGEAL: This is a cervical prevertebral abscess. Note that:
    a. It may bulge into the mouth or pharynx.
    b. It is central in position and *behind* the prevertebral fascia,

[1] Graham, R. R., *Ann. Surg.*, 1942, 115, 1007.

differing from the acute retropharyngeal abscess, which is to one side of the midline and *in front of* the prevertebral fascia (*Fig.* 677).

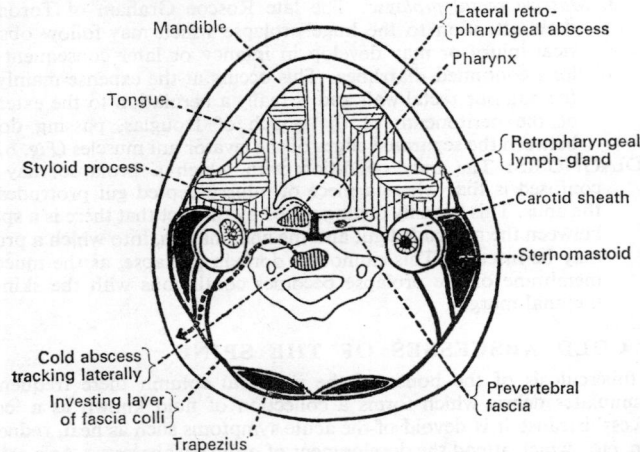

Fig. 677.—Horizontal section through skull at a level below tongue showing situation of pus in acute retropharyngeal abscess, and the route taken by a cold abscess arising in the vertebra. Observe that the retropharyngeal abscess bulges the lateral wall of the pharynx, and that the cold abscess presents at the posterior border of the sternomastoid.

2. AT THE POSTERIOR BORDER OF THE STERNOMASTOID: The abscess tracks laterally behind the prevertebral fascia and appears on the surface at the posterior border of the sternomastoid.
3. IN THE MEDIASTINUM: The abscess tracks down behind the prevertebral fascia and is guided by it into the posterior mediastinum of the thorax.
4. AT THE BACK OF THE NECK: The abscess tracks back along the posterior divisions of the spinal nerves and appears on one side of the midline on the back of the neck.
5. IN THE AXILLA: The pus tracks back under the prevertebral fascia and enters the open mouth of the axillary sheath and thus gains the axilla or arm.

IN THE THORACIC REGION: A collection of fluid here may take the following courses:
1. Remain prevertebral in the posterior mediastinum.
2. Tracking down from here it finds at the lower end of the posterior mediastinum three openings which it may enter—gaps behind the:

THE ANATOMY OF CERTAIN DISEASES 725

(*a*) Lateral lumbocostal arch; (*b*) Medial lumbocostal arch; (*c*) Median arcuate ligament (*Fig.* 678).

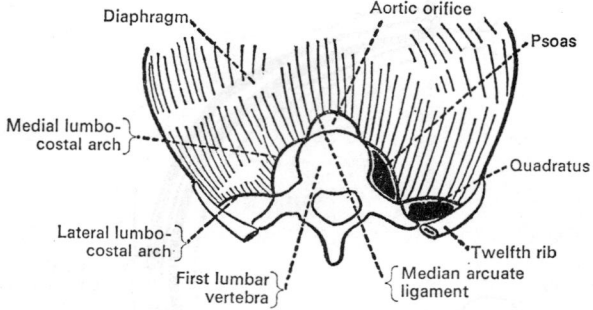

Fig. 678.—Diaphragm seen from above showing lumbocostal arches. On the left the psoas and quadratus are removed. These arches often serve to direct the flow of tuberculous pus.

- *a.* Passing behind the lateral lumbocostal arch it extends down between the anterior layer of the lumbodorsal fascia and the quadratus lumborum, and may remain here on the quadratus behind the kidney, or may extend forwards along one of the three nerves which lie behind the kidney, i.e., the 12th thoracic, the ilio-inguinal, or iliohypogastric. In the latter case it may extend on to the lower anterior abdominal wall along these nerves.
- *b.* The medial lumbocostal arch is the open upper end of the psoas sheath. Having entered this 'stocking' it extends downwards, being unimpeded in its course as far as the insertion of the psoas into the lesser trochanter. It is therefore seen in the thigh as a swelling pushing forwards the femoral artery which here lies on the psoas.
- *c.* The median arcuate ligament crosses over the aorta. The fluid having traversed the arch may extend down along the vessel into the abdomen and may remain in relation to this great trunk or extend along any of its branches.
3. The contents of the cold abscess may extend along the course of one of the thoracic nerves (*Fig.* 679). If it follows this course it may:
    - *a.* Extend half-way round the thorax along the course of an intercostal nerve and present: (i) In the thorax at the anterior end of an intercostal space (not in the midline); or (ii) In the

726 A SYNOPSIS OF SURGICAL ANATOMY

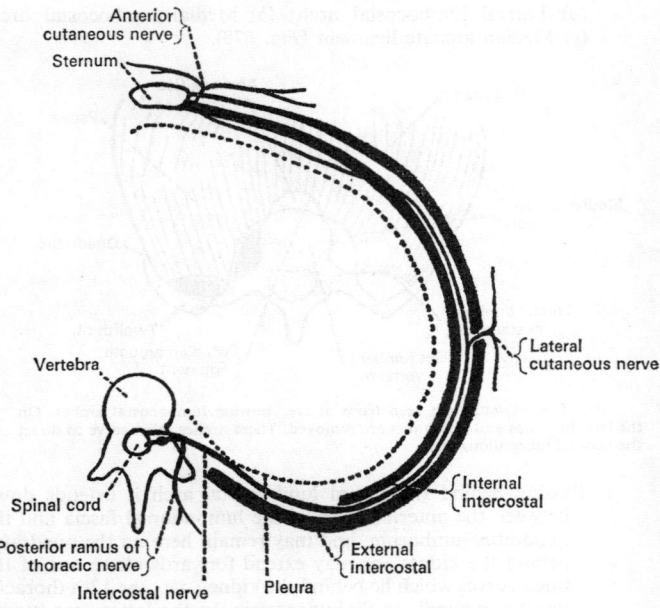

Fig. 679.—Course of an intercostal nerve.

abdominal wall in the rectus sheath. Having reached the rectus sheath, the fluid may extend along the sheath behind the rectus for a considerable distance.

b. Extend along the lateral cutaneous branch of the intercostal nerve and present in the mid-axillary line where the lateral cutaneous nerves become subcutaneous.

c. Extend into the back along the posterior division of a thoracic nerve and present either 2·5 cm. or 7·5 cm. from the line of the spines of the vertebrae, depending on whether it follows the medial or lateral branch of the posterior division.

IN THE LUMBAR REGION: The collection may:
 1. Extend along the aorta and then along any of its branches, so that, for example, the abscess may present in the ischiorectal fossa along the internal pudendal artery, or in the buttock along the superior gluteal artery.
 2. Extend into the sheath of the psoas or quadratus lumborum.

3. Follow the course of one of the lumbar nerves, so that it may appear in the thigh along the femoral or obturator nerve, or in the back.
4. Extend between the flat muscles of the abdominal wall and present in the triangle of Petit, i.e., the lumbodorsal triangle.

XI. SUBPHRENIC ABSCESS

In relation to the periphery of the liver, six spaces may be defined. They are of great surgical importance because pus may collect in them, forming abscesses. Such abscesses are termed 'subphrenic' because they are all related to the diaphragm. The ligaments of the liver take a large part in delimiting these spaces. Of these six spaces, three are on the right and three are on the left. They are named: (*a*) Right anterior intraperitoneal compartment; (*b*) Right posterior intraperitoneal compartment; (*c*) Right extraperitoneal compartment; (*d*) Left anterior intraperitoneal compartment; (*e*) Left posterior intraperitoneal compartment; (*f*) Left extraperitoneal compartment (*Fig.* 680).

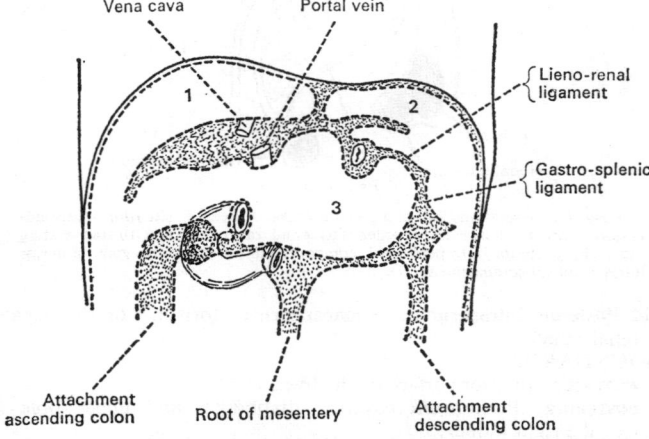

Fig. 680.—Anatomy of the subphrenic spaces, the viscera having been removed. 1, Right anterior intraperitoneal compartment. 2, Left anterior intraperitoneal compartment. 3, Lesser sac. (*After Strode, by courtesy of the Editor of 'Surgery'.*)

Right Anterior Intraperitoneal Compartment:
BOUNDARIES:
ANTERIOR: Diaphragm and anterior abdominal wall.
POSTERIOR: Liver (anterior surface).

SUPERIOR: Coronary ligament (anterior layer).
LEFT: Right side of the falciform ligament.
RIGHT: The fossa communicates with the right posterior intraperitoneal compartment by the potential space between the diaphragm and the right lateral surface of the liver.
BELOW: The fossa is open.

Observe that the right anterior intraperitoneal compartment is continuous with the right posterior intraperitoneal compartment round the anterior sharp margin of the liver. In cases where an abscess forms in one of these compartments, it is usually prevented from extending round this sharp margin by the formation of adhesions between the transverse colon and great omentum to the anterior border of the liver, which serve to limit the abscess to one compartment (*Fig.* 681).

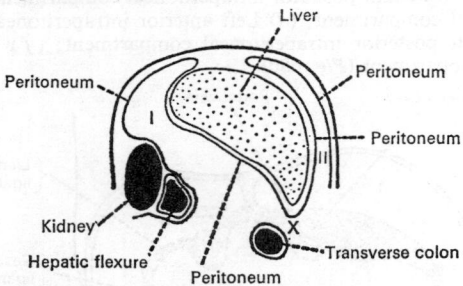

Fig. 681.—Anatomy of subphrenic abscess. X denotes situation where adhesions form between anterior border of liver and transverse colon, thus separating the right posterior intraperitoneal compartment (I) from the right anterior intraperitoneal compartment (II).

Right Posterior Intraperitoneal Compartment: Morison's or the hepatorenal pouch.
BOUNDARIES:
ANTERIOR: Inferior surface of the liver.
POSTERIOR: Peritoneum covering diaphragm and upper pole of the right kidney.
ABOVE: Coronary ligament (posterior layer).
BELOW: The pouch is open into the general peritoneal cavity.

Left Anterior Intraperitoneal Compartment:
BOUNDARIES:
ANTERIOR: Abdominal wall.
POSTERIOR: Liver.
ABOVE: Left triangular ligament.
RIGHT: Falciform ligament.

THE ANATOMY OF CERTAIN DISEASES 729

    LEFT: The fossa is open. The spleen is some distance away.
    BELOW: The fossa is open.
The left and right anterior compartments are separated from each other, therefore, by the falciform ligament.

Left Posterior Intraperitoneal Compartment: This is the lesser sac of the peritoneum and is open into the main peritoneal cavity through the foramen epiploicum (Winslow). This foramen is 3 cm. in size and is situated opposite the 12th thoracic vertebra.
    BOUNDARIES OF THE FORAMEN OF WINSLOW:
        ANTERIOR: Right free border of the lesser omentum containing the bile-duct, the vertical part of the hepatic artery, and the portal vein.
            The *duct* is *dexter*.
        POSTERIOR: Vena cava and the right adrenal gland.
        SUPERIOR: Caudate process of the liver.
        INFERIOR: Horizontal part of the hepatic artery and below that the first part of the duodenum.

Right Extraperitoneal Compartment: The area between the bare area of the liver and the diaphragm.
    BOUNDARIES:
        ANTERIOR: Superior layer of the coronary ligament.
        POSTERIOR: Inferior layer of the coronary ligament.
        LEFT: Vena cava inferior.
        RIGHT: Fusion of the two layers of the coronary ligament to form the right triangular ligament which terminates the fossa.
        ABOVE: Diaphragm, which is in actual contact with the lower boundary.
        BELOW: Posterior surface of the liver.
    This area is entirely shut in, and if it be distended by fluid, the liver tends to be pushed down and the diaphragm up.

Left Extraperitoneal Compartment: This space is merely the connective tissue around the upper pole of the left kidney. It is seldom infected and is the least important of the six spaces.

XII. OSTEOARTHRITIS

The term 'osteoarthritis' is used in a strict sense, excluding the arthritis of tuberculosis and syphilis. The anatomical conformation of joints accounts for the changes which occur in the articulations in osteoarthritis.[1]

Development of Joints: In the mesoblast occupying the limb bud there appears a paraxial condensation which is the *anlage* or forerunner of the bones of the limb. At the site of the future joints there is a breaking down of this paraxial condensation. The mesenchyme abutting on the ends of the future bones becomes converted into articular cartilage,

---

[1] The author wishes to record his indebtedness for the facts set forth in this section to the work of A. G. Timbrell Fisher, *Chronic Non-tuberculous Arthritis*, 1929, London.

whereas that at the periphery forms the joint capsule, accessory ligaments, and synovial membrane. The fact that the articular cartilage and synovial membrane arise from similar undifferentiated tissue cells explains the readiness with which, under pathological conditions, cartilage or bone may on the one hand form in synovial membrane, or on the other hand articular cartilage may undergo metaplasia into fibrocartilage or connective tissue.

Synovial Membrane and Fluid: Fisher compares the synovial membrane of a diarthrodial joint to a sleeve, clothing the inner surface of the capsule, with two surfaces and two circumferences. Macroscopically the latter terminate at the margins of the articular cartilage, but microscopically *the synovial membrane is seen to cover the periphery of the articular cartilage:* this is a fact of prime importance in the anatomy of the joint.

THE LAW OF THE SYNOVIAL MEMBRANE: This membrane clothes all intra-articular structures which are not covered by articular cartilage. It follows that intra-articular tendons or ligaments are invariably clothed by the membrane.

STRUCTURE OF SYNOVIAL MEMBRANE: This consists of two layers:

EXTERNAL: Lax connective tissue blending insensibly with the joint capsule.

INTERNAL: A shiny layer resembling pleura or peritoneum and covered by flattened cells, which do not, however, form a homogeneous layer but are absent in some places and reduplicated in others.

SYNOVIAL VILLI: These are projections into the joint which give a shaggy appearance to parts of the synovial membrane. A villus is a slender synovial process with a core of delicate connective tissue containing blood-vessels, nerves, and often fat. The distribution of the villi is instructive, being confined largely to the neighbourhood of the articular margins, so that their secretion is readily available for the lubrication of the articular surfaces. The villus is not covered by an endothelial layer, but by connective-tissue cells known as synovial cells. The mucin gains the articular cavity in three ways.:

1. The surface cells rupture, discharging their contents into the joint.
2. The deeper cells discharge their secretion into the connective tissue of the villus, whence it is expressed into the joint cavity by the movements of the joint.
3. Some of the synovial cells are detached, and they discharge their contents while free in the joint cavity. The cell bodies form the debris normally present in synovial fluid.

The secreting synovial cells are especially plentiful in the synovial membrane covering the fat pads which are found in various joints, e.g., knee, hip, shoulder.

The synovial membrane may be divided into a villous portion, near the articular margin, and a more remote non-villous area. This latter area, in contradistinction to the former, is covered by a single layer of flattened endothelial-like cells between the adjacent members of which stomata can be seen.

LYMPHATICS OF SYNOVIAL MEMBRANE: These vessels form a fine network just beneath the endothelium, and a second free network in the outer layer of the synovial membrane, where they come into intimate relationship with the capillaries of the joint. The lymphatics end in neighbouring glands.

NERVES OF SYNOVIAL MEMBRANE: There is a delicate subendothelial plexus of nerves, amongst which end-bulbs may be seen, differing, however, from the pacinian corpuscles found in the tendons and ligaments around the capsule.

BLOOD-SUPPLY OF JOINTS: Vessels are always numerous, and inosculate freely in the capsule and outer layer of the synovial membrane. At the place where this membrane passes from the capsule to the bone—the synovial reflection—they are especially plentiful, forming an anastomosis called the 'circulus vasculosus'.

LOOSE BODIES IN JOINTS: The fate of a loose body in the joint is governed by the synovial membrane. The following are the facts:
1. A metallic foreign body remains unaffected, being quite free in the joint.
2. Non-metallic foreign bodies become surrounded by a glistening connective-tissue sheath and become secondarily attached to the synovial membrane.
3. Bony or cartilaginous loose bodies derived from the articular surface actually increase in size in the joint cavity. The increase in size takes place through the intermediation of the synovial membrane to which the body becomes attached; should the body remain or become free in the cavity, it may grow by means of the nourishment it receives from the synovial fluid which bathes it.

Articular Cartilage: Articular cartilage is hyaline cartilage. There are important differences between the central and peripheral parts of the cartilage which line the articular end of a bone.
1. CENTRAL PORTION OF ARTICULAR CARTILAGE: Here three strata may be distinguished:
    a. A superficial stratum which consists of flattened cells arranged in groups of two to four which lie parallel to the surface in the cartilaginous matrix. There is no covering membrane or perichondrium. The cells of this layer are normally all vigorous and healthy.
    b. The intermediate layer of cells is irregular in disposition.

732 A SYNOPSIS OF SURGICAL ANATOMY

   c. The deepest cells are arranged vertically and abut on the underlying bone.
2. PERIPHERAL PORTION OF THE ARTICULAR CARTILAGE: This part of the cartilage is covered by a delicate extension of the synovial membrane forming a perichondrium. The cartilage here becomes fibrillated, gradually merging into fibrous tissue. The thin synovial extension over this part of the cartilage contains capillary vessels. The important fact emerges that the periphery of the joint cartilage comes into intimate relationship with blood-vessels, whereas the central cartilage does not.

NUTRITION OF ARTICULAR CARTILAGE (*Fig.* 682): Fisher's conclusions are:

1. That part of the cartilage lying nearest the bone which it clothes is nourished by delicate vessels from the blood-vessels of the bone.
2. The central (superficial) part of the articular cartilage is nourished by the synovial fluid only.

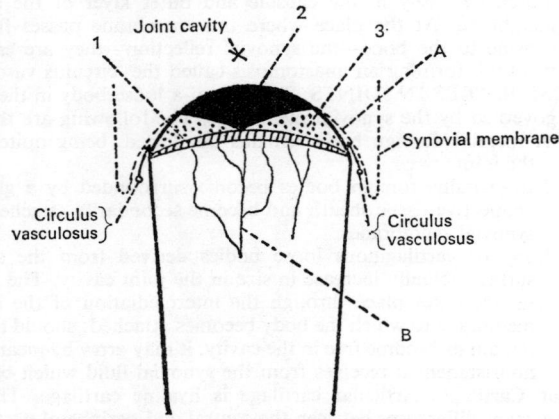

Fig. 682.—The nutrition of articular cartilage. A diagram constructed to show the facts brought out by Timbrell Fisher. 1, Part of cartilage lying nearest the bone and supplied by the blood-vessels (B). 2, Central portion of cartilage dependent on the synovial fluid for its nutrition. 3, Peripheral portion of cartilage supplied by blood-vessels from the circulus vasculosus which run in the extension from the synovial membrane (A) which forms a perichondrium for this part of the cartilage.

3. The periphery of the articular cartilage is nourished by the fine vessels which ramify in the membrane overlying it, which vessels are derived from the circulus vasculosus.

4. The fundamental fact is that the periphery of articular cartilage has a vastly better system of nourishment than has the central portion.
5. Incisions in articular cartilage take a long time to heal, and are repaired by the cartilage cells of the part changing to connective or fibrous tissue cells, *no new cells being formed.*
6. Lateral incisions heal much more readily than central ones.

Chapter XLIII

THE ANATOMY OF SURGICAL PROCEDURES

I. THE ANATOMY OF PUNCTURES

It is of daily importance in medical practice to withdraw fluid from a joint or cavity of the body for purposes of examination, diagnosis, or drainage. For this purpose a needle puncture is made. The anatomy of the part governs the site of insertion of the needle. It is of importance to realize that in the vast majority of cases the cavity to be punctured is in a state of distension by the contained fluid.

The procedure is resorted to in the following situations: (1) Joints; (2) Central nervous system—ventricles of brain, cisterna magna, spinal subarachnoid space; (3) Pleural cavity; (4) Pericardium; (5) Peritoneal cavity; (6) Liver; (7) Spleen; (8) Urinary bladder; (9) Maxillary antrum; (10) Pouch of Douglas; (11) Tunica vaginalis testis.

1. Joints:

SHOULDER-JOINT (*Fig.* 683):
  a. A needle is entered just lateral to the tip of the coracoid process and pushed in a direction backwards, upwards, and outwards.
  b. A needle is entered just lateral to the angle formed by the junction of the acromion with the spine of the scapula. This, like the coracoid, is a bony point always distinguishable. The needle is pushed in an inward and upward direction.

ELBOW-JOINT: The part of the joint which is nearest the surface lies posteriorly, between the head of the radius and the capitulum (lateral condyle) of the humerus. The head of the radius can always be distinguished and the needle is entered just proximal to the head, in a direction directly forwards (anteriorly), the joint being flexed to a right angle and the forearm semi-pronated (*Fig.* 684). When the elbow-joint is distended with pus the capsule bulges to either side of the triceps and may be easily and efficiently drained in this situation.

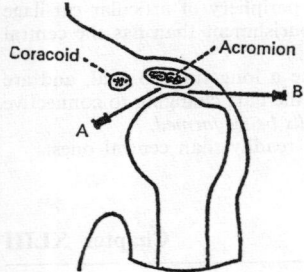

Fig. 683.—Anterior (A) and lateral (B) routes for puncture of shoulder-joint.

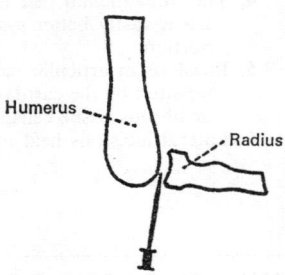

Fig. 684.—Puncture of elbow-joint.

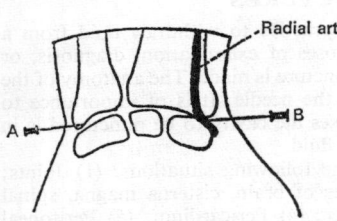

Fig. 685.—Puncture of wrist-joint. A Below ulnar styloid. B, Below radial styloid.

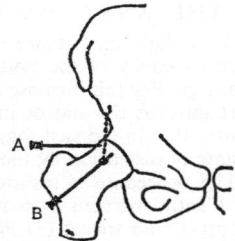

Fig. 686.—Puncture of hip-joint. A, Lateral route. B, Anterior route.

WRIST-JOINT: The needle is inserted immediately below either the radial or the ulnar styloid process and pushed in at right angles to the process (*Fig.* 685). It is better to insert the needle below the ulnar styloid, as the radial artery passes just distal to the radial styloid.

HIP-JOINT (*Fig.* 686):

a. The needle is entered at a point 5 cm. below the anterior inferior iliac spine and pushed upwards, backwards, and medially.

b. The needle is entered from the side just above the upper border of the great trochanter and pushed inwards and slightly upwards, in a line almost parallel with the femoral neck.

KNEE-JOINT:

a. The needle is pushed into the suprapatellar bursa. This extends three finger-breadths above the level of the patella and almost always communicates with the joint. The needle is pushed into it through the quadriceps muscle which overlies the bursa (*Fig.* 687).

b. The needle is entered on either side of the ligamentum patellae immediately below the patella, and pushed directly backwards (*Fig.* 688).

ANKLE-JOINT: The needle is inserted just below the tip of either malleolus and pushed in an upward direction so that it enters the joint between the malleolus and the corresponding articular surface of the talus (*Fig.* 689).

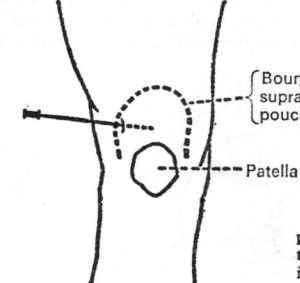

Fig. 687.—Puncture of suprapatellar pouch. The needle is entered through the vastus lateralis, in an inward and backward direction.

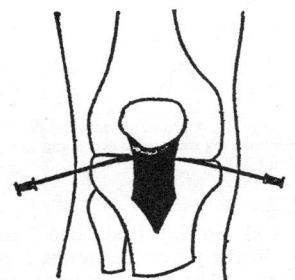

Fig. 688.—Puncture of knee-joint.

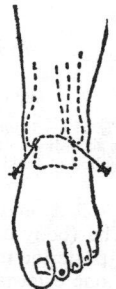

Fig. 689.—Puncture of ankle-joint.

2. Central Nervous System:

PUNCTURE OF THE VENTRICLES OF THE BRAIN:

LATERAL VENTRICLE: In the child below the age of two years the anterior fontanelle is still open and a needle is pushed through its lateral angle and passed in a direction downwards and outwards until fluid is found. After the age of two years a small circle of bone must be removed with a trephine at the site where the needle is to be entered.

  a. The needle is entered at a point 3 cm. behind the external auditory meatus and the same distance above Reid's base line (a line drawn back from the lower margin of the orbit through the centre of the auditory meatus). The needle is directed towards the tip of the opposite auricle. The ventricle is 5 cm. from the surface[1] (*Fig.* 690, A).

  b. A line is drawn vertically up for 5 cm. from the external auditory meatus. A point is taken 2 cm. behind the upper end of this line. The needle entered here for 5 cm. strikes the body of the lateral ventricle at its junction with the descending and posterior horns[2] (*Fig.* 690, B).

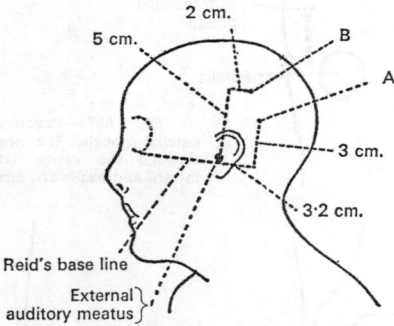

Fig. 690.—Tapping the lateral ventricle of the brain. A, Point for entering the needle according to Keen's method. B, Point for entering the needle according to the method of Jenkins. (*See* text for explanation.)

This may be put in another way:

  c. The (body or) vestibule of the lateral ventricle is situated 3 cm. posterior to a line drawn perpendicularly over the vertex from one external auditory meatus to the other, and at a horizontal level along this line 5 to 7·5 cm above the meatus.

  d. A method in general use to-day is as follows: The needle is entered at a point 1·8 cm. above the superior nuchal line of the occipital bone, and 2·5 cm. from the midline, and pushed horizontally forwards and slightly outwards. It strikes either the posterior horn or body of the lateral ventricle at a distance of 4 to 5 cm. from the surface.

[1] Keen, quoted by Stiles, 'Surgical Anatomy', in Cunningham's *Anatomy*, 1906, 1227.
[2] Jenkins, quoted by Treves and Keith, *Surgical Applied Anatomy*, 1918, 48.

THE ANATOMY OF SURGICAL PROCEDURES

CISTERNAL PUNCTURE: The patient is sitting or lying on one side with the head flexed forwards. The needle is entered in the midline just above the first palpable cervical spinous process—that of the axis or second vertebra (*Fig.* 691). It is directed forwards and upwards, parallel to an imaginary line joining the external auditory meatus with the nasion. The point of the needle strikes the occipito-atlantoid ligament in the adult at a depth of 4 to 5 cm. from the surface and is felt to pierce the ligament and enter the cistern. The posterior surface of the medulla is fully 2·5 cm. anterior to the posterior atlanto-occipital ligament.

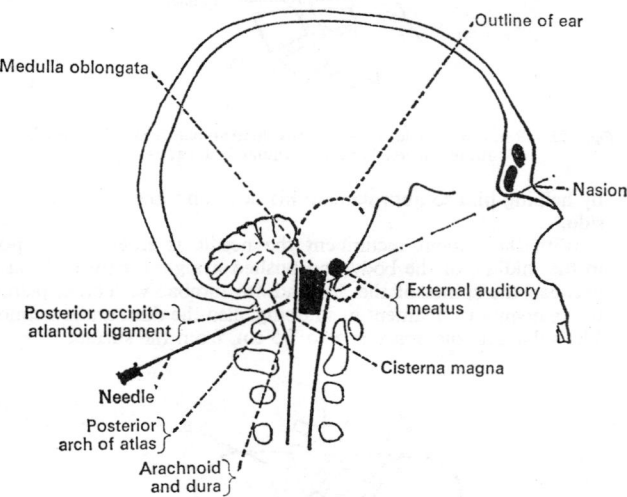

Fig. 691.—Cisternal puncture.

LUMBAR PUNCTURE: In this procedure the spinal subarachnoid space is tapped below the level of the spinal cord, so as to avoid injuring this important structure. The cord ends at the level of the 2nd lumbar vertebra. The subarachnoid space ends at the level of the 2nd sacral vertebra. The needle is entered anywhere between these two points (*Fig.* 692). The usual spot chosen is between the 3rd and 4th lumbar vertebrae. The spine of the latter vertebra corresponds to the level of the line connecting the highest points of the iliac crests (*Fig.* 693). The column must be acutely flexed to obtain separation of the spinous processes and arches of the vertebrae. This is ensured by getting the patient to bend forward if sitting, or

738 A SYNOPSIS OF SURGICAL ANATOMY

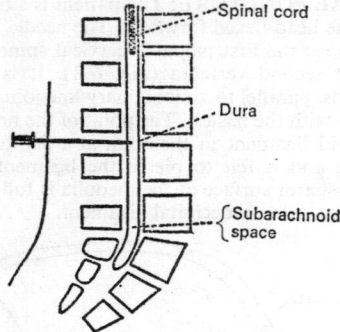

Fig. 692.—Route of needle in performing lumbar puncture. The cord is out of danger. The cauda equina is not shown.

by helping him to approximate his head and knees if lying on his side.

With the patient recumbent the needle is entered at a point in the midline of the body and pushed straight forwards. It passes between the spines of the 3rd and 4th lumbar vertebrae, piercing the interspinous ligament in so doing, also the dura and arachnoid. The subarachnoid space is 5 to 7·5 cm. from the surface.

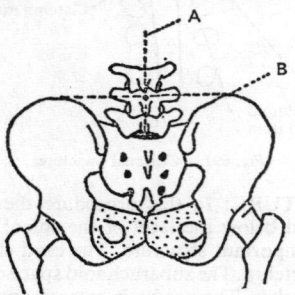

Fig. 693.—Determining classic site for lumbar puncture in the region of intersection of mid-vertical line (A) with line joining the highest points of iliac crests (B).

3. **Pleural Cavity:** A needle is pushed into the pleural cavity through an intercostal space. The site usually chosen is in the anterior, mid-, or posterior axillary line in the 5th, 6th, or 7th space. These sites are

THE ANATOMY OF SURGICAL PROCEDURES 739

selected because the thorax is here less covered by muscle than elsewhere. The site of puncture depends on the situation of the fluid which requires tapping. In inserting the needle, it is necessary to remember that the pleura in the mid-axillary line reaches as far down as the 10th rib.

4. **Pericardium:** This sac is only punctured when distended with fluid, and a point is chosen lateral to the apex of the heart so that it shall be unscathed. The usual site is the 5th or 6th space in the mammary line. The mammary line is 10 cm. from the midline. The apex of the (normal-sized) heart is 9 cm. from the midline.

5. **Peritoneal Cavity:** This cavity is punctured to evacuate fluid or to insert some inert gas. The customary site chosen is a point 2·5 cm. below and 2·5 cm. to the left of the umbilicus. The needle can be felt to pierce first the anterior sheaths of the rectus, then the posterior sheath and peritoneum as it enters the cavity. The bowel in this situation is the small intestine. This gut is freely movable, and if it be encountered is displaced by the needle without injury.

6. **Liver:** It is necessary to puncture the liver to obtain a core of tissue for histological study or to locate abscesses. The procedure is only practised on the right side. The needle is inserted in the mid-axillary line. It may be entered in the 10th, 9th, or 8th space. Above this it will injure the lung. In any of these three spaces the needle traverses the intercostal muscles, then the parietal pleura covering the chest wall, then the pleural recess below the lung (costophrenic sinus), next the

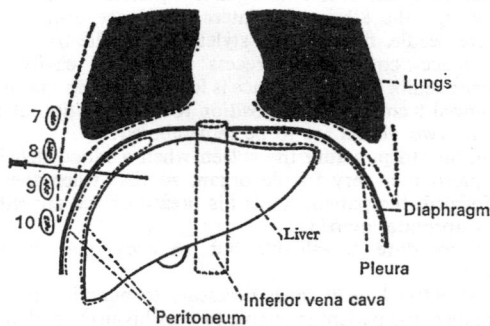

Fig. 694.—Showing that in exploring the liver by the right lateral route the needle traverses both pleural and peritoneal cavities.

pleura covering the diaphragm, and then the diaphragm. Then it pierces the peritoneum over the under-surface of the diaphragm, then passes through the peritoneal recess between the liver and the diaphragm, then the peritoneum on the liver, and lastly the liver (*Fig.* 694). The needle should never traverse the tissues for a greater distance than 8·2 cm. for fear of damaging the inferior vena cava. Fatal haemorrhage has resulted from neglect of this precaution.

7. **Splenic Venography:** This organ may be punctured when it is enlarged. It then lies in contact with the anterior abdominal wall, and a needle pushed into it passes through the abdominal muscles, the parietal peritoneum, and the peritoneum covering the spleen, there being merely a potential peritoneal space between these two peritoneal layers (*Fig.* 695). The procedure is valuable in cases of portal hypertension to visualize the portal and splenic veins.

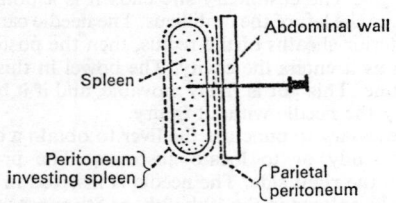

Fig. 695.—Showing how puncture of the spleen necessarily means traversing the peritoneal cavity with the needle.

When the spleen is not enlarged it is punctured in the mid-axillary line through the 8th or 9th intercostal space using a fine lumbar puncture needle, fitted with a stylet. The needle traverses the intercostal space, costophrenic recess of pleural cavity, diaphragm, and peritoneum. Slight resistance is felt on entering spleen. The needle is advanced 8 cm. and is in position for the injection of the contrast medium. Two points are to be remembered:

  a. It is unsafe to puncture the spleen when a blood deficiency exists.
  b. The spleen is a very friable organ, so that when the puncture is performed, the patient holds his breath or the anaesthetist maintains absolute apnoea.

  The procedure is valuable but an occasional death has been reported.

8. **Urinary Bladder:** It is at times necessary to puncture the bladder—if, for instance, the patient is unable to pass his urine and an instrument cannot be inserted from below. In the adult the bladder is, when empty, entirely a pelvic organ (*Fig.* 696). When it fills it rises and becomes partly an abdominal organ. Puncture is made possible by the fact that the surface which comes into contact with the anterior abdominal wall (inferolateral surface) is devoid of peritoneum, as the bladder in rising pushes the peritoneum before it. The needle pierces: skin,

linea alba, fascia transversalis, space of Retzius containing extraperitoneal fat, bladder.

9. **Maxillary Sinus:** The natural orifice of this sinus is in the middle meatus of the nose, considerably above the level of the floor of the sinus. In disease, therefore, the contents of the cavity are apt to

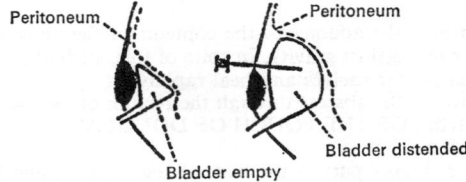

Fig. 696.—Demonstrating how the distended bladder lifts up the peritoneum, enabling a trocar to be inserted through its anterior surface without entering the peritoneal cavity.

stagnate. The cavity may be explored or drained by puncturing that part of its inner wall which forms the outer wall of the inferior meatus of the nose (*Fig.* 697). The needle is introduced through the nostril, and passed in an outward and backward direction. It pierces the bone under cover of the inferior nasal concha (inferior turbinate), and enters the sinus at a level considerably lower than that of the natural orifice of the cavity.

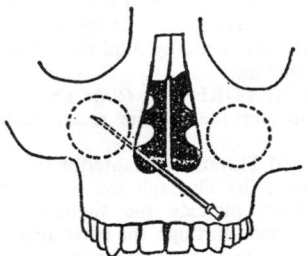

Fig. 697.—Draining maxillary sinus through its inner wall via inferior meatus of nose.

10. **Pouch of Douglas:** This peritoneal recess, also called 'rectovesical' in the male, and 'recto-uterine' in the female, is the lowest part of the peritoneal cavity. For that reason, fluid in the peritoneal cavity, whether it be blood or pus, tends to enter this pouch by gravity. Modern surgery encourages this by putting all patients in a suitable

position after abdominal operations. The peritoneum of the pelvis has more power of resistance than the peritoneum elsewhere in the abdomen; also fluid in this situation is localized and can do comparatively little harm. Because of the tendency of fluids to collect here, abscesses in the pouch of Douglas may occur. They are called *pelvic abscesses*. When they form they must be evacuated. This may be done:

a. By opening the abdomen—the contents of the abscess have then to escape against gravity. In spite of this, such abscesses usually do empty themselves and heal rapidly.

b. By opening the abscess through the rectum or vagina.

BOUNDARIES OF THE POUCH OF DOUGLAS:

IN THE MALE:

Anterior: Upper part of the base of the bladder, and here lie the upper parts of the seminal vesicles and the ducti deferentes. Superior surface of the bladder.

Posterior: Anterior wall of the rectum.

Floor: Reflection of peritoneum from the bladder to the rectum.

IN THE FEMALE:

Anterior: Posterior surface of the uppermost part of the posterior vaginal wall, i.e., that part of the vagina which forms the posterior wall of the posterior fornix of the vagina. Uterus.

Posterior: Anterior wall of the rectum.

Floor: Reflection of the peritoneum from the rectum to the vagina and uterus.

In both sexes the floor of the fossa is 7·5 cm. from the anus. It may therefore just be reached by the tip of a finger inserted into the rectum. When distended by fluid the collection is easily felt per rectum or vaginam.

ROUTES FOR PUNCTURE (*Fig.* 698): The pouch may be entered:

a. In the male through the anterior rectal wall, about 7·5 cm. from the anus.

b. In the female: (i) Through the anterior rectal wall, about 7·5 cm. from the anus; (ii) Through the posterior vaginal wall at its uppermost part, piercing the vaginal wall and immediately entering the pouch through the peritoneum of its anterior wall.

In both *a* and *b* (i) the needle traverses the rectal wall and then immediately enters the pouch by perforating the peritoneum of its floor.

Drainage of such collections through rectum or vagina is frequently used. It will be observed that abscesses opened in this way drain by gravity as the opening is situated at the lowest level of the peritoneal cavity; also the weight of the viscera and gut pressing downwards tend to cause the collapse of the walls of the abscess cavity, which is obliterated.

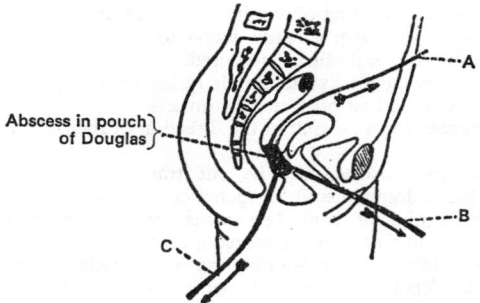

Fig. 698.—Showing routes whereby an abscess in the pouch of Douglas may be evacuated. Tube A, drainage through anterior abdominal wall. Tube B, Drainage through vagina. Tube C, Drainage through rectum.

Although drainage of a pelvic abscess in this way is easy and satisfactory it must be kept in mind that if a loop of bowel is lying in or below the abscess it may be damaged and result in a fistula or it may prolapse. Drainage through the rectum or vagina must therefore only be carried out if the operator, having displaced the bowel upwards, is certain that the abscess is in fact in the most inferior part of the pouch of Douglas.

11. **Tunica Vaginalis Testis:** There is normally a small amount of fluid in the tunica vaginalis testis. This may become greatly increased—the condition known as *hydrocele*. The testis lies free in the cavity formed by the tunica vaginalis, excepting posteriorly, where it is attached to the epididymis. A collection of fluid in the tunica may be withdrawn through a needle which may be entered at any part over the swelling, excepting posteriorly, where the epididymis, vessels, and vas are situated. The needle pierces the coverings of the testis, which are: (*a*) Skin; (*b*) Dartos muscle; (*c*) External spermatic fascia; (*d*) Cremaster fascia; (*e*) Internal spermatic fascia or infundibuliform fascia; (*f*) Parietal layer of tunica vaginalis testis. Inversion of the testis is described on p. 413.

II. THE ANATOMY OF ABDOMINAL INCISIONS

Incisions through the abdominal wall are based on anatomical principles. The intra-abdominal pressure is considerable, and the surgeon aims at leaving the abdominal wall as strong as possible after operation, otherwise there exists a very real fear that portions of the abdominal contents may leave the abdominal cavity through the weak area which is caused by a badly placed incision, resulting in a condition known as scar, incisional, or ventral hernia.

744 A SYNOPSIS OF SURGICAL ANATOMY

The principles governing abdominal incisions are:

1. The incision must give ready access to the part to be investigated, and should admit of extension if required.

2. The incision must traverse muscle rather than fascia, as the scar left in the peritoneum is best protected by muscle.

3. The muscles must be split in the direction of their fibres, rather than cut across.

4. The rectus muscles may be cut transversely without seriously weakening the abdominal wall, as such a cut passes between two adjacent nerves without injuring them. The rectus has a segmental nerve-supply, so that there is no risk of a transverse incision cutting off the distal part of the muscle from its nerve-supply, as would obtain if a muscle were divided which depended on a single nerve (e.g., one of the limb muscles) (*Fig.* 699).

5. The incision must divide no nerves.

6. The openings made by the cut through the different layers of the abdominal wall must, as far as possible, not be superimposed. This will be explained below.

7. Drainage-tubes should be inserted through separate small incisions, as their presence in the main wound may seriously prejudice the strength of the ultimate scar. For the same reason a colostomy should be made through a separate incision and not through the main wound.

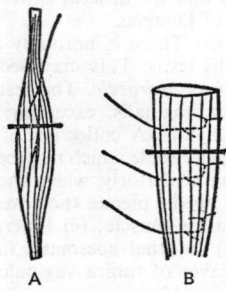

Fig. 699.—Demonstrating that division of a muscle (A) with a single nerve-supply causes paralysis distal to the section, whereas division of a muscle (B) such as the rectus, with a segmental supply, produces no paralysis, as the nerves are uninjured.

Classification: Abdominal incisions may be classified as follows:
1. INCISIONS THROUGH THE ANTERIOR ABDOMINAL WALL:
   a. DIVIDING NO MUSCLES: (i) Median; (ii) Paramedian; (iii) Pararectal; (iv) Through linea semilunaris.

THE ANATOMY OF SURGICAL PROCEDURES 745

   b. DIVIDING MUSCLES: Transrectal: (i) Superior or subcostal; (ii) Middle or umbilical; (iii) Inferior or suprapubic.
   c. SPLITTING MUSCLES: (i) Paramedian or Mayo-Robson; (ii) Lateral: (α) McBurney, (β) Lanz; (iii) Inferior: (α) Hernia incision, (β) Ureteric incision.
2. INCISIONS THROUGH THE POSTERIOR ABDOMINAL WALL:
   a. KIDNEY INCISIONS: (i) Oblique; (ii) Vertical.
   b. URETERIC INCISIONS: Horizontal.
   c. COMBINATION OF VERTICAL AND HORIZONTAL (Royle).

1. INCISIONS THROUGH THE ANTERIOR ABDOMINAL WALL

Incisions Dividing no Muscles:

MEDIAN INCISIONS: These traverse the abdominal wall in a vertical direction above or below the umbilicus. They have been and are very extensively used. The incision divides: (1) Skin; (2) Linea alba; (3) Fascia transversalis; (4) Extraperitoneal fat; (5) Peritoneum (*Fig.* 700).

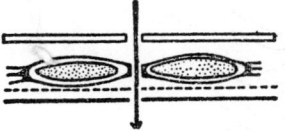

Fig. 700.—Median incision.

The supra-umbilical incision gives access to the stomach and duodenum. The infra-umbilical incision gives access to the intestines, appendix, bladder (distended), and pelvic organs. In exposing the bladder the incision may stop short of the peritoneum so that the bladder is dealt with through its anterior surface which is devoid of peritoneum in the region of the space of Retzius (prevesical).

Midline upper abdominal incisions are sound. Midline lower abdominal incisions are unsound. The linea alba above the umbilicus is a dense strong structure 1·3 cm. wide formed by the interlacing fibres of the rectus sheaths. It is relatively avascular. It holds sutures well. It gives excellent approach to the more centrally situated upper abdominal organs. It is the incision of choice where speed is essential, e.g., perforated peptic ulcer. The gall-bladder and bile-ducts can be dealt with through this approach if necessary although better access can be had to these structures through more laterally placed incisions. The stomach, duodenum, pancreas, and left lobe of liver are directly related to the incision. It may be extended upward by removing the xiphisternum and

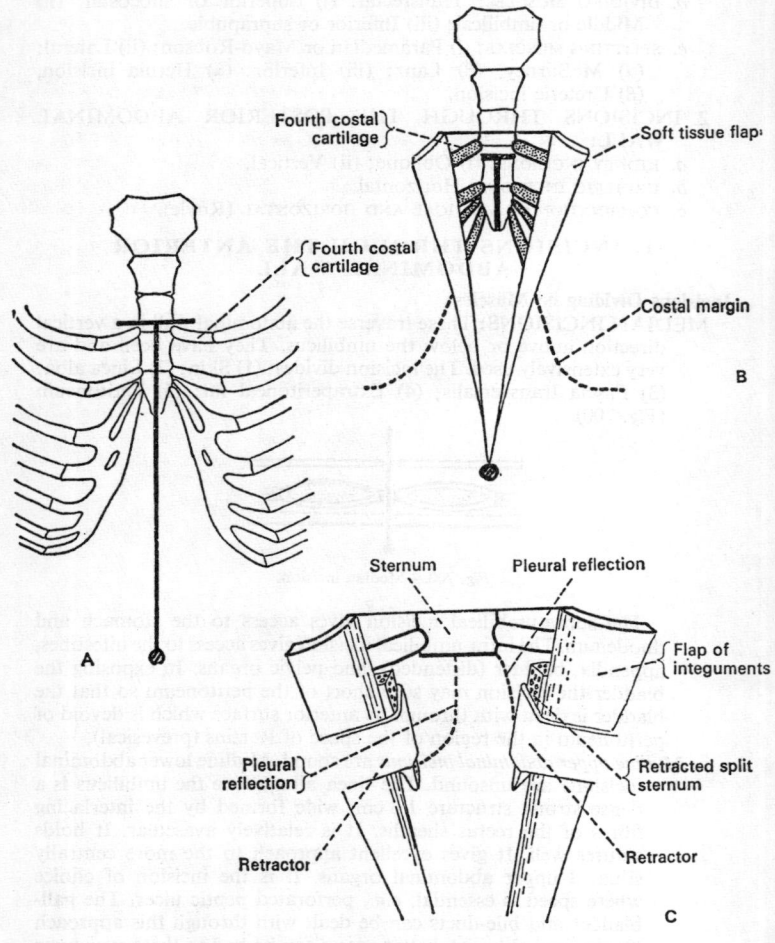

Fig. 701.—A, The skin incision. B, Soft tissues retracted to show lines of sternal section. C, The sternum has been divided and split and the portions held open by a rib spreader.

the writer has, in following the suggestion of Wangensteen, found this route a very suitable one for total gastrectomy by extending the incision up to the fourth costal cartilage where a small transverse incision is made. With a Lebsche knife the sternum is split in the midline up to the fourth interspace. The tissues here are separated from the sternum to its outer borders where the chisel is re-inserted first on one side and then on the other and the bone divided in a medial direction to meet the vertical incision (*Fig.* 701). A small rib spreader holds the sternal halves apart. The anterior fibres of the diaphragm may be cut if necessary. Opening the pericardium is unimportant. Should the pleura be opened, the tear is enlarged so that it is an inch long to prevent tension pneumothorax developing. No attempt is made to suture the rent. The lung can be kept inflated through the operation and the wound closed with a catheter in the pleural cavity which is withdrawn as the final stage of the operation after the skin is sutured and blood and air have been aspirated. The sternal sections are readily approximated with one or two wire sutures passed around them. The abdominal surgeon works with greater facility with the patient supine. For difficult high gastrectomies or total ones where partial oesophagectomy is unnecessary the midline exposure is excellent and can be made and closed in a fraction of the time taken by thoracotomy.

The midline lower abdominal incision is frequently followed by an incisional hernia particularly at the lower end just above the pubis. A major reason for this is that at the time of closure of the incision the surgeon sutures the external oblique fascia (Gallaudet's fascia)[1] instead of the linea alba. The external oblique fascia lies on the outside of the external oblique aponeurosis. It is adherent to the external oblique aponeurosis, is given off over the cord as the external spermatic fascia at the external ring and extends over the pubis into the perineum. It is not as strong as the linea alba and unless the linea alba is sutured a hernia will develop immediately above the pubis and with time will descend over the pubis.

PARAMEDIAN INCISION: This is made vertical, parallel to the midline, and about 2·5 cm. away from it to one or other side. It is a very popular and well-planned incision. The resulting scar is strong. It may be made of any length, and even if extended from costal margin to pubis, the scar does not greatly weaken the abdominal wall. The incision traverses: (1) Skin; (2) Anterior rectus sheath; (3) Rectus; (4) Posterior rectus sheath; (5) Fascia transversalis; (6) Extraperitoneal fat; (7) Peritoneum (*Fig.* 702).

---

[1] Condon, R. E. (1964), *Hernia* (Ed. Nyhus, L. M., and Harkins, H. N.), Philadelphia: Lippincott.

748 A SYNOPSIS OF SURGICAL ANATOMY

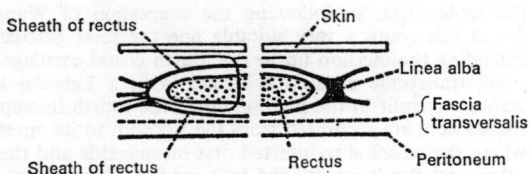

Fig. 702.—Structures divided by the paramedian muscle-splitting incision.

DEALING WITH THE RECTUS:
1. The muscle may be divided in the line of the incision. As has been shown in a previous section, the nerves to the rectus enter it from the side or back about its middle. Should the incision through the rectus be made too far laterally, the nerves will be divided and the muscle paralysed (*Fig.* 703). If the muscle

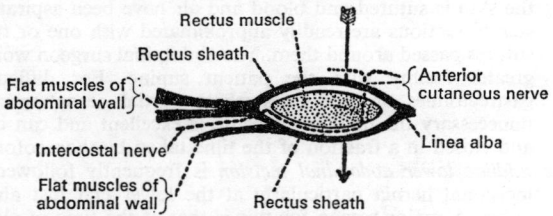

Fig. 703.—Schematic representation of the fact that opening the abdomen by vertical division of the rectus abdominis too far laterally will paralyse this muscle by cutting off its nerve-supply. The arrow represents an incision which endangers the nerve-supply.

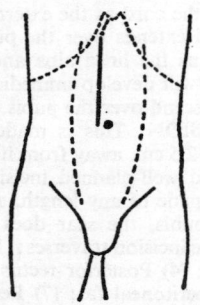

Fig. 704.—Mayo-Robson incision; a paramedian incision, the upper end of which may be extended, if necessary, to the xiphisternum.

is divided in the line of incision, the part medial to the cut is deprived of its nerves and disappears by atrophy. This incision presents the advantage that it can be rapidly carried out, e.g., in emergencies; it also lends itself to strong reconstruction. The rectus-displacing exposure is more difficult to carry out than the rectus-splitting one. It requires meticulous care in dissecting the rectus sheath from the tendinous inscriptions so that the muscle is not damaged. It may be mentioned here that any vertical incision to give efficient access to the gall-bladder *must reach the costal margin*.

2. The muscle may be displaced outwards intact without any further interference with it. When the wound is closed the muscle returns to its bed, and forms the most efficient protection possible to the line of the incision, which it directly covers (*Fig.* 705). This is a sound incision extensively used on the right or left of the midline. When used to deal with the terminal part

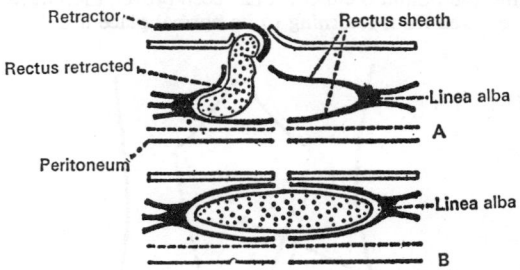

Fig. 705.—A, Structures encountered in approaching peritoneal cavity by paramedian route with retraction of rectus. B, Shows how incision line in the aponeuroses is protected by rectus muscle on closing the wound.

of the pelvic colon or for excision of the rectum, the incision extends low down so that the rectus may be mobilized down to its insertion to the pubis.

EXPLORATORY INCISION: In cases where it is suspected that an intra-abdominal lesion exists, but its situation cannot be determined, an incision is made which gives sufficient access for exploratory purposes to every part of the abdominal cavity. The best incision for this purpose is a paramedian incision of whatever length may be necessary to one side of the umbilicus.

PARARECTAL INCISION: This is an incision medial to the outer border of the rectus. It is most often used for approach to the appendix and is also called 'Battle's incision'. The incision crosses the line joining the umbilicus to the right anterior superior iliac

750 A SYNOPSIS OF SURGICAL ANATOMY

spine at a right-angle at the junction of its inner and middle thirds. One-third of the incision is above the line, two-thirds below it (*Fig.* 706). The incision divides: (1) Skin; (2) Anterior rectus sheath in the line of the skin cut; (3) The rectus is pulled inwards; (4) The posterior rectus sheath—in the line of the skin cut; (5) Fascia transversalis, extraperitoneal fat, and peritoneum in the line of the skin cut.

The opening in the posterior sheath is made with care so that the nerves which are running between the sheath and muscle are not cut. The inferior epigastric vessels are sometimes found coursing upwards much farther laterally than usual, and may readily be injured in dealing with the posterior sheath or by too forcible retraction of the rectus. The incision may be prolonged up or down, or both, to give access to the pelvis and ascending colon. Its value depends on the fact that the rectus is not cut, and that this muscle protects the incisions in the peritoneum and fasciae after the wound is closed. It has been proved that the rectus may be prevented from returning to its normal place if a drainage-tube is

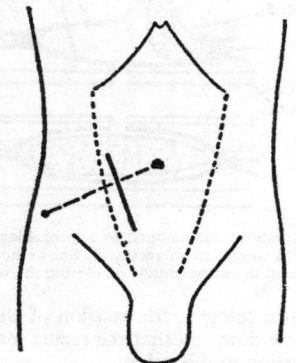

Fig. 706.—Line of pararectal (Battle's) incision.

put into the wound. In this case all the benefit of the manœuvre of displacing the rectus is lost, as the muscle is prevented from returning to its normal place by the drainage-tube (*Fig.* 707). The resulting scar is therefore unprotected by muscle. Note that this incision gives access to the pelvis as well as to the iliac fossa.

There is no recorded instance of inguinal hernia having followed the use of this incision (cf. p. 757—'Inguinal Hernia following the McBurney Incision').

THE ANATOMY OF SURGICAL PROCEDURES 751

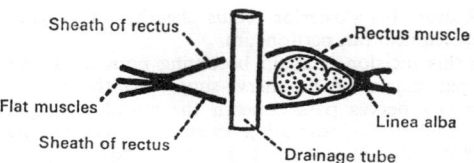

Fig. 707.—Showing that the pararectal incision loses all its advantages if a drainage-tube traverses the incision, as the rectus is prevented from covering the scar in the fasciae.

INCISION THROUGH THE LINEA SEMILUNARIS: This line is at the outer border of the rectus. It is formed by the aponeuroses of the oblique muscles after the muscles have given place to fascia. It is a bad incision. The incision passes entirely through fascia, and crosses at right-angles the line of the nerves going to the rectus, so that some of them must inevitably be injured (*Fig.* 708).

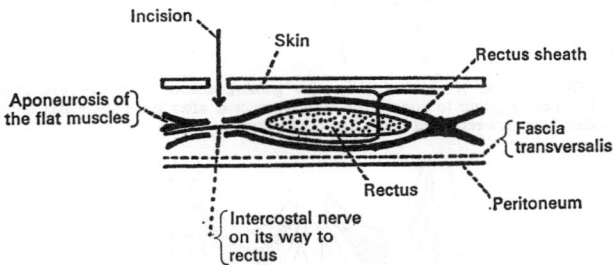

Fig. 708.—Demonstrating that an incision in the linea semilunaris is anatomically unsound, as the nerves to the rectus are cut.

Incisions Dividing Muscles:

SUPERIOR TRANSRECTAL: This is Kocher's incision for approach to the liver, gall-bladder, and bile-ducts. The incision commences at the tip of the xiphoid process and passes down and to the right, parallel to the costal margin and two finger-breadths below it. The rectus is cut across in the line of the incision (*Fig.* 709). Deep to it are seen one or two of its nerves which are passing downwards and inwards. They are preserved by being drawn carefully aside. (This advice, though excellent in theory, usually fails in practice, as the nerves are so easily snapped by the manipulations necessary to the operation.) On the left the incision may be used to approach the spleen. The incision divides: (1) Skin; (2) Anterior rectus sheath;

(3) Rectus; (4) Posterior rectus sheath; (5) Fascia transversalis, extraperitoneal fat, peritoneum.

As this incision is again becoming popular, it may be well to give particulars of the nerve-supply to the upper rectus. The intercostal nerves pass beneath the costal cartilages to gain the abdominal wall, insinuating themselves between the digitations of the diaphragm and the transversus abdominis. Coyte[1] showed

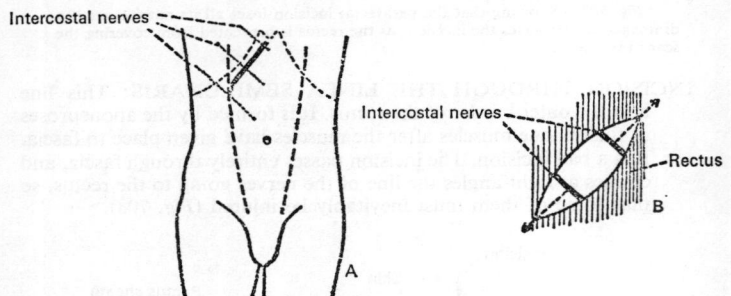

Fig. 709.—A, Kocher's incision for gaining access to biliary passages. B. The nerves going to supply the rectus, exposed after the muscle has been divided. They are retracted in the line of the arrows.

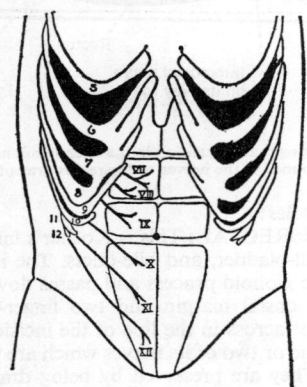

Fig. 710.—To show that the 7th, 8th, and 9th intercostal nerves enter the rectus sheath in relation to the 9th costal cartilage.

[1] *Lancet*, 1922, November.

that these nerves, having reached the abdominal wall, loop upwards in a manner reminiscent of the costal cartilages. Moreover, *half the nerve-supply of the rectus enters it in relation to the 9th costal cartilage:* the 7th intercostal nerve just above its tip, the 8th and 9th beneath it. The remaining intercostal nerves enter beneath their corresponding cartilages (*Fig.* 710).

MIDDLE TRANSRECTAL:
1. Where a supra-umbilical median incision gives insufficient access, it may be combined with a second incision carried laterally at right-angles to the first. The incision then becomes a right-angled one. The vertical limb divides the structures in the midline, the horizontal limb divides the rectus and its sheaths. On the right the incision gives excellent access to the right hypochondrium, bile-duct system, and right kidney region (*Fig.* 711). On the left it may be used for removal of the spleen.
2. When still more room is required, e.g., in the removal of large kidney tumours from the front, the lower limb of this incision may be carried from the umbilicus to the tip of the tenth costal cartilage. In addition to dividing the rectus this splits the lateral flat muscles largely in the direction of their fibres and divides no nerves (*Fig.* 712). A large triangular flap is raised with its apex at the umbilicus and its base at the costal margin. In cases where not quite so much room is required the lateral limb only of this incision may be used.

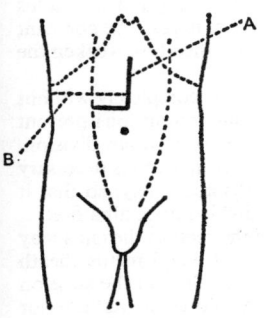 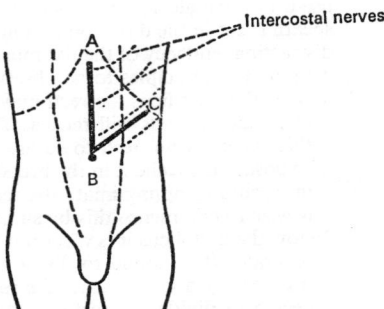

Fig. 711.—A, Method of enlarging a supra-umbilical incision by a right-angle extension through the rectus. B, The dotted line shows Rutherford Morison's incision for difficult operations on the bile-ducts.

Fig. 712.—Angular incision used for gaining access to a very large spleen or kidney. AB, Median supra-umbilical incision. BC, Incision joining the umbilicus to the tip of the tenth costal cartilage. C, Observe that no nerves are injured in the incision.

3. For difficult operations on the gall-bladder and bile-ducts, Rutherford Morison[1] advised and practised a transverse incision extending from 2·5 cm. below the tip of the 12th rib to the upper part of the middle third of a line joining the xiphoid process to the umbilicus (*Fig.* 711, B).

INFERIOR TRANSRECTAL: An incision used when free exposure of the pelvis is required. The skin cut is made transversely across the lower abdomen, just above the pubis and inguinal ligaments, stopping short of the anterior superior iliac spine on each side. The cut falls in the natural skin crease which exists here. The rectus sheath is divided in the line of the skin incision. There is then a choice of procedures. The recti may be divided transversely, or merely separated from each other in the midline without division, and the peritoneum is then opened transversely or vertically, depending on the method of access through the muscles.

Incisions Dividing the Flat Muscles: An incision, or part of it, extending from outer border of sacrospinalis to umbilicus and midway between rib margin and iliac crest gives good exposure of laterally situated tumours, such as those of kidney or peripheral colon. The flat muscles are cut across, no nerves are divided. If necessary the rectus sheath may be opened, its components divided, and the muscles retracted in or the muscle may be cut across.

The Present Status of Muscle-cutting Incisions: It is correct to say that transverse or muscle-cutting incisions are becoming more generally used. Physiologically this is sound. No nerves are cut and the rectus sheath is cut in the direction of and not across its fibres. The constant distracting tendency of the flat muscles does not therefore weaken the wound. The principles to be observed are:

1. Above the umbilicus the recti may be cut across completely without fear that the ends will retract. The tendinous inscriptions prevent this. There is no need to suture sheath to muscle before division. Exposure is excellent in the broad sthenic person. Care is necessary in closure to approximate the rectus sheaths accurately, so that it is wise to commence this by suturing the divided linea alba first.

2. Below the umbilicus it is wiser not to divide the recti as the ends may separate. It is sound to divide the flat muscles and rectus sheath transversely and to retract the rectus inwards. Should the surgeon decide to divide the rectus it should be anchored to its anterior sheath by sutures above and below the line of proposed section.

3. Approach to the stomach, liver, pancreas, spleen, etc., may be obtained by a curvilinear incision dividing skin and both recti. It has a gentle upward convexity reaching to within an inch of the costal margin and extends from the outer border of one rectus to

---

[1] *Surgical Contributions*, 1916, 2, 398. Bristol.

the outer border of the other (Welch[1]). This gives high access where approach to the inferior surface of the diaphragm is sought, e.g., total gastrectomy. The transverse incision dividing both recti has the advantage that it may be continued across the costal margin into the chest, giving excellent access to the oesophagus for oesophago-gastrectomy.

Muscle-splitting Incisions:

McBURNEY'S GRIDIRON INCISION (1894): This is the classic incision for approach to the appendix and right iliac fossa. It is associated with the names of McBurney and Roux. It is in common use on the left side for bringing the pelvic colon outside the abdomen in the operation of left inguinal colostomy. The incision

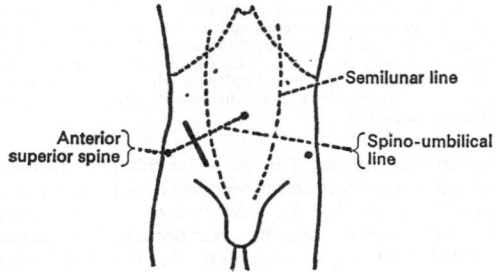

Fig. 713.—McBurney's incision.

is made at right angles to the spino-umbilical line, crossing this at the junction of its outer and middle thirds (*Fig.* 713). One-third of the incision is above the line, two-thirds are below it. It is therefore very oblique in direction. Having divided the skin, the external oblique muscle is split in the direction of its fibres, and next the internal oblique and transversus are also split in the direction of their fibres, i.e., transversely. The peritoneum is divided in the direction of the original skin incision, i.e., down and in. The advantage of the incision is that it leaves an unimpaired abdominal wall when the wound is closed. The incision would therefore be ideal but for the disadvantages alluded to below. This method of opening the abdomen embodies the principle mentioned above, that the openings through the various layers of the abdominal wall should not, if possible, be superimposed. Its greatest disadvantage is that it gives but a limited exposure and it is difficult to get at the

Welch, G. E., *Surgery of the Stomach and Duodenum*, 38. Chicago: The Year Book Publishers Inc.

756 A SYNOPSIS OF SURGICAL ANATOMY

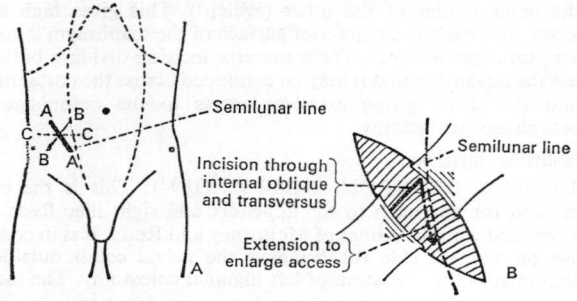

Fig. 714.—A, Showing how in McBurney's incision the structures of the abdominal wall are divided or merely split in different directions. AA, Line in which skin, external oblique, and peritoneum are divided. BB, Line in which internal oblique is split. CC, Line in which transversus is split. B, Showing a method of increasing access when employing McBurney's incision, viz., by extending the cut through the parietes downwards along outer border of the rectus in the semilunar line.

pelvis through the cut. If it has to be enlarged, all the advantages of the incision are lost and it becomes a bad one, as enlargement is obtained by extending the inner end of the opening through the deep muscles, down along the outer border of the rectus (*Fig.* 714). Now this latter cut goes through the fascia of the linea semilunaris where there is no muscle, and this is therefore a weak area of the resultant scar. It is therefore advised that the incision be used only when the diagnosis is beyond question and where access will be sufficient without extension of the wound. Also if some other condition exists in addition to the appendix lesion, it may not only be impossible to deal with it through the cut, but even impossible to explore it. For these reasons, Sir Harold Stiles, in using this incision in cases where the removal of the appendix entailed a difficult operation (e.g., acute appendicitis in poor risk cases), advised and practised that the muscle-splitting principle be abandoned and the flat muscles be divided in the line of the skin incision. When this cut is carried down to the inguinal ligament, it will divide the inferior epigastric vessels at its lower end. At its upper end it divides the ascending branch of the deep circumflex iliac artery. This gives wider exposure, and the length of the incision may be increased upwards or downwards. As the muscles have to be extensively divided in the latter procedure, the incision through the flat muscles is not widely used.

Another plan for improving the 'access' is to extend the original incision (through the internal oblique and transversus) in an inward direction across both layers of the rectus sheath. The rectus is pulled in or divided. This is a sounder plan than incising the linea semilunaris, but is not advisable in septic cases for fear of infecting the whole rectus sheath. As these are precisely the cases where it is most necessary, the method is not of wide applicability.

INGUINAL HERNIA FOLLOWING THE MCBURNEY INCISION: Inguinal hernia unquestionably follows the muscle-splitting incision in a percentage of cases; some authors put this as high as 30 per cent, though we think this figure is high. A consideration of the anatomy of the incision explains this complication. The ilio-inguinal and ilio-hypogastric nerves play a very important part in supplying those portions of the internal oblique and transversus abdominis muscles which constitute the falx inguinalis or conjoint tendon. This muscle mass is the most important constituent of the inguinal canal, being responsible for the 'shutter action' whereby the muscle descends, protecting the posterior wall of the canal, during coughing or straining. Atrophy of this muscle follows injury to its nerve-supply, and the risk of inguinal hernia occurring is considerable. The ilio-hypogastric and ilio-inguinal nerves lie between internal oblique and transversus precisely at the site of the McBurney incision, and may be damaged by cutting, retraction, or strangulation in scar tissue in septic cases. The division of the ilio-inguinal nerve practised as a routine by many surgeons in hernia operations is devoid of harmful effects, as the nerve is purely sensory by the time it reaches the inguinal canal (*Fig.* 715).

ARTIFICIAL ANUS: The right-sided muscle-splitting incision is in general use for the performance of right inguinal colostomy, or caecostomy, i.e., bringing out the caecum on to the surface of the abdominal wall. An artificial anus is made in the right iliac fossa as a temporary measure. When such an outlet is permanently required the colon is brought out through a left-sided McBurney incision. In either situation it is of great advantage that it should pass through several muscle layers, as they control the effluent from the opening and act to some extent as a sphincter opening. On the left side, where the contents of the colon are solid, the new anus may in time act only once or twice a day, the opening being efficiently controlled at other times by the flat muscles.

LANZ INCISION: This incision for approach to the appendix is a modification of McBurney's. The incision begins at the right anterior superior spine and extends to the left in the interspinous fold. The flat muscles are split in the direction of their fibres.

It may here be pointed out (in case the student be confused by the number of incisions used to approach the appendix) that there is need for approaching the appendix via varying incisions,

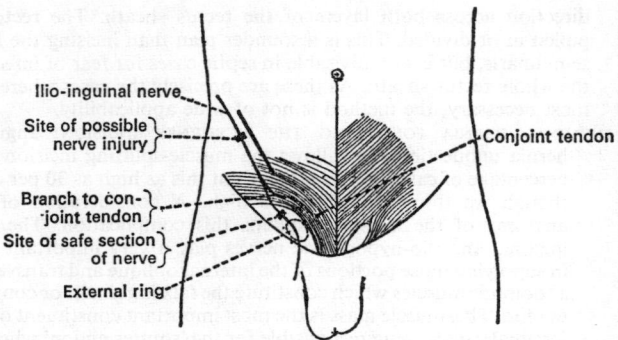

Fig. 715.—Showing the genesis of inguinal hernia consequent on the McBurney incision. The black bar indicates the incision. Observe the proximity of the ilio-inguinal nerve to the wound; also that injury to the nerve here paralyses its branch to the conjoint tendon (falx inguinalis), whereas injury at the external ring leaves the nerve-supply to the tendon unimpaired.

for not only may the organ occupy different positions, but the difficulties which may be encountered at the operation for its removal depend on whether it is removed during an attack of acute appendicitis or during a quiescent period ('interval operation'). What is usually the simplest of abdominal operations, when the appendix is not inflamed, is frequently difficult when an acute process is going on. McBurney's access, then, may be suitable in cases where the diagnosis is beyond question, but may be inadequate when the appendix is in an unusual situation, e.g., under the liver, or when the diagnosis is uncertain. Furthermore, there is the danger already referred to that this incision may be followed by inguinal hernia owing to the nerve-supply of the muscles bounding the inguinal canal (ilio-hypogastric and ilio-inguinal) being damaged.

INFERIOR MUSCLE-SPLITTING INCISIONS:

MEDIAL: An incision one finger-breadth above the inner half of the inguinal ligament is the classic incision for dealing with an inguinal hernia (*Fig.* 716, A). It is also the classic skin incision for dealing with the testicle, cord, or tunica vaginalis (hydrocele). When used for the cure of hernia, the incision divides the skin and two layers of superficial fascia (Camper and Scarpa). It exposes the external oblique aponeurosis, the external abdominal ring, and the cord at the inner end of the inguinal ligament. The external oblique aponeurosis is split in the line of its fibres and the cord is exposed lying in the inguinal canal.

THE ANATOMY OF SURGICAL PROCEDURES

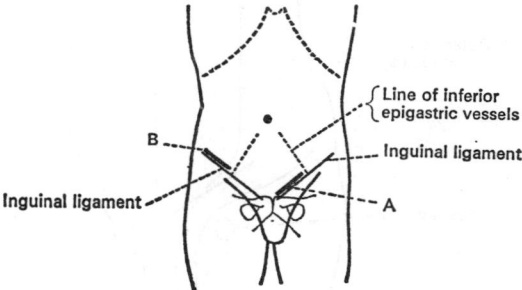

Fig. 716.—A, Incision for inguinal hernia. B, Incision for gaining access to lower end of ureter or iliac vessels.

Lotheissen Operation (1898): The same incision is widely used in the Lotheissen operation for the cure of femoral hernia. The steps of the operation are the same as those for inguinal hernia up to the exposure of the cord in the canal. The cord or round ligament is then drawn aside and the fascia transversalis is exposed, forming the posterior wall of the outer half of the canal. This fascia is divided, exposing the femoral canal lying behind the inguinal ligament. The sac of the femoral hernia is found in this canal.

McEvedy Operation:[1] This is a valuable advance in the surgery of femoral hernia. It is carried out through the same incision. The upper skin flap is elevated and the anterior rectus sheath exposed. In this situation the aponeuroses of the flat muscles of the abdomen are all anterior to the rectus. This sheath is incised 1·25 cm. medial to the lower fourth of the linea semilunaris, and the rectus retracted inwards, which exposes the fascia transversalis. When this is incised the inferior epigastric vessels are seen and the neck of the femoral hernial sac. The inferior flap of the skin incision may be retracted down to expose the hernia itself should this be necessary. If the hernia is irreducible the lacunar ligament (Gimbernat) may be divided under direct vision and an abnormal obturator artery secured if required. Should it be necessary the peritoneal cavity can be widely opened and the suture of the inguinal ligament to Cooper's ligament is readily effected. A further considerable advantage of this approach is the fact that the inguinal canal is not disturbed (*Fig.* 717).

[1] McEvedy, P. G., *Ann. R. Coll. Surg.*, 1950, 7, 484.

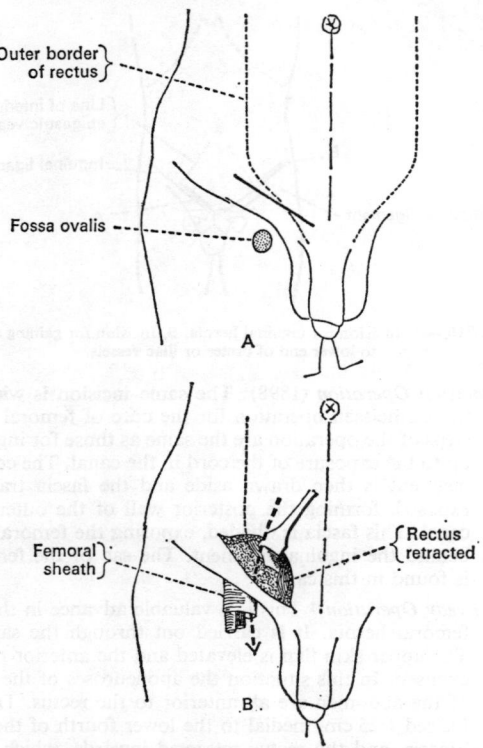

Fig. 717.—Anatomy of the McEvedy operation. A, The incision. B, The exposure. The arrow shows the path of a femoral hernia through the femoral canal.

When Henry introduced his suprapubic extraperitoneal approach to both femoral rings, he pointed out that repair of the femoral canal from above does not weaken the floor of the inguinal canal. Liability to the subsequent development of inguinal hernia is therefore not caused by this approach. The McEvedy type of incision may also be used for the repair of inguinal hernia and is especially useful in recurrent ones.

LATERAL: An incision 2·5 cm. above the outer half of the inguinal ligament is the classic approach to the lower part of the ureter and external iliac artery (*Fig.* 716, B). The incision splits the flat muscles in the direction of their fibres. It is not usually carried medial to the middle of the inguinal ligament because of the presence of the inferior epigastric vessels, though this may be done if more room is needed, the vessels being tied. Having separated the muscles, the fascia transversalis is divided in the line of the incision and the peritoneum is pushed inwards and is not divided. The ureter is found lying in the extraperitoneal fat, crossing the common iliac artery. It will be observed that this incision gives good exposure to the iliac vessels, both internal and external. It admits of liberal extension backwards.

Sherren's Suggestion: Through this incision a finger can be pushed up behind the peritoneum towards the region of the kidney fossa. In abscesses around the kidney, such as may follow tears of this organ from accidents, it is necessary to drain the abscess. Sherren suggested that the abscess may be drained through this incision. Both gravity and respiration assist in its speedy evacuation.

The Ease with which the Peritoneum Strips: The peritoneum can be stripped off the anterior or posterior abdominal wall with ease. This fact is taken advantage of in the planning of some abdominal incisions, e.g., in the incision for exposure of the ureter above the outer half of the inguinal ligament. Sir John Thomson-Walker advises a midline suprapubic incision for exposure of the terminal ureter and the bladder. The peritoneum is not opened, but is stripped off the anterior abdominal wall and from the side wall of the pelvis.

2. INCISIONS THROUGH THE POSTERIOR ABDOMINAL WALL

These are used in the exposure of the kidney, ureter, and adrenal gland.

Kidney Incisions:

OBLIQUE INCISION: The oblique incision is the favourite. It extends from the kidney angle in a direction obliquely downwards and outwards towards the anterior superior spine (*Fig.* 718, B). The kidney angle is the angle formed by the outer border of the sacrospinalis muscle at its junction with the 12th rib. The incision is planned to run in the direction of the fibres of the external oblique muscle. It divides: (1) Skin and superficial fascia; (2) Latissimus dorsi and serratus posterior inferior; (3) External oblique is split in the direction of its fibres; (4) Internal oblique and transversus are divided in the line of the skin incision; (5) Fascia transversalis; (6) Extraperitoneal and perirenal fat; (7) The lateral cutaneous branch of the 12th thoracic nerve is cut and there results an area of anaesthesia the size of the palm of the hand over the gluteal region. The incision may divide also the ilio-inguinal and ilio-hypogastric nerves. The outer border of the quadratus is exposed at the upper part of the cut. Care must be exercised towards the lower part of the cut that the peritoneum is not injured, as it lies exposed when the fascia transversalis is divided.

The incision gives good exposure to the kidney and also to the upper half of the ureter. Its great advantage is that it may be extended forwards above and parallel to the outer half of the inguinal ligament to expose the lower half of the ureter and the base of the bladder. The incision and its continuation allow exposure of the whole length of the kidney and ureter.

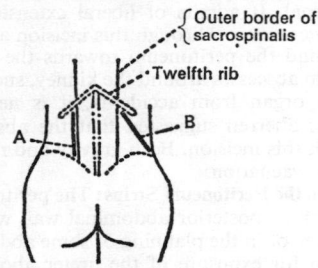

Fig. 718.—Posterior approaches to kidney; A, By vertical incision. B, By oblique incision.

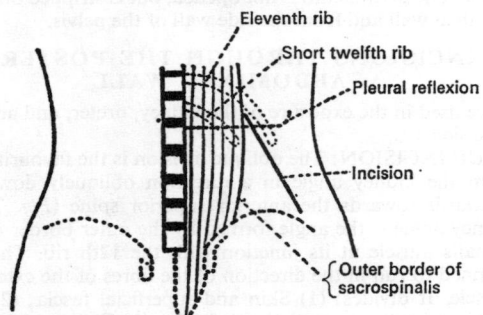

Fig. 719.—To show danger of opening pleura by oblique kidney incision when the 12th rib does not project beyond outer border of sacrospinalis.

DANGER AT THE KIDNEY ANGLE: The pleura crosses the inner half of the 12th rib. If the 12th rib is very short, as it not uncommonly is, then the kidney angle is formed by the sacrospinalis and the 11th rib and the pleura crosses this angle (*Fig.* 719). The ribs are not usually enumerated from above downwards to find out if the lowest rib felt is or is not the 12th. In the event, then, of the 12th rib not being palpable, the incision commences between the 11th rib and the outer border of the sacrospinalis and the pleura may be opened. This may cause infection of the pleural cavity if there is inflammatory kidney disease. Such an accident has resulted in many fatalities.

VERTICAL INCISION: This extends perpendicularly along the outer border of the sacrospinalis from the 12th rib to the iliac crest (*Fig.* 718, A). The incision divides: (1) Skin and fascia; (2) Latissimus dorsi and serratus posterior inferior; (3) The three layers of lumbodorsal fascia; (4) The fascia transversalis and

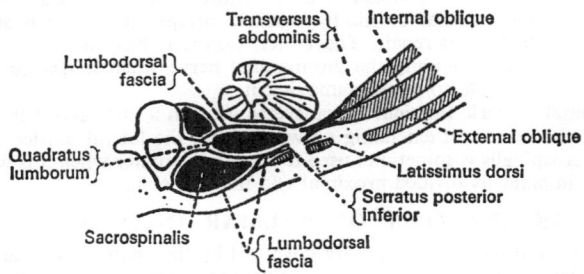

Fig. 720.—Anatomical structures encountered in exposing kidney by vertical incision along outer border of sacrospinalis. The kidney capsules are not shown.

extraperitoneal fat (*Fig.* 720). The incision is planned to interfere as little as possible with the muscles. It has the disadvantage that it does not give exposure of the ureter, and cannot easily be extended to effect such exposure.

PAINFUL SCARS: White[1] draws attention to the occasional painful scar following a surgical incision. Paraesthesiae may develop of such intensity that they lead to disability or drug addiction. He makes the following observations:

1. The condition is due to injury of a sensory or mixed peripheral nerve. The sympathetic is not involved as blocking of the related ganglia has no effect on the pain. It is therefore not a causalgia. Sympathectomy is useless.
2. The condition may resist all forms of treatment.
3. Pain is transmitted by (*a*) the rapidly conducting myelinated delta and (*b*) the slowly conducting C fibres. The first type are less resistant to trauma, and when damaged, residual

[1] White, J. C., *Ann. Surg.*, 1958, 148, 422.

sensation may have a peculiarly disagreeable character. This is the best explanation offered of the disturbance (Landau and Bishop[1]).
4. Incisions close to the midline are not affected as there are no nerves there of any size to be damaged.
5. Certain areas are much more likely to be affected, i.e., those that injure the superficial radial, intercostal, saphenous, or the inguinal nerves (in herniorrhaphy).
6. It follows that every care must be taken to protect nerves related to an incision, even though the nerve may not be seen. In thoracotomy the blades of the retractor must be separated from the intercostal structures by swabs. The intercostal nerve must not be included in the sutures closing the muscles. The ilio-inguinal or ilio-hypogastric nerves should be protected in hernial repair. The writer, however, has had no cause to regret dividing the ilio-inguinal nerve when it has not been possible to avoid damaging it.

Horizontal Ureteric Incision: A transverse incision a little above the level of the iliac crest extending outwards from the lateral border of the sacrospinalis is sometimes used to expose the ureter when it is wished to implant its divided proximal end into the skin.

III. THE ANATOMY OF PALMAR INCISIONS

Incisions in hand or fingers are governed by the anatomy of the part. This is dealt with on p. 653, and may with advantage be read before perusing this section. It is necessary to state here that in the treatment of infections of the hand a general anaesthetic is used and the part is rendered bloodless by a constricting bandage. The tendon-sheaths of the wrist and hand are described on p. 256.

Principles: Incisions on the flexor aspect of limbs or digits should be avoided. They are subject to longitudinal stresses and the scars may become redundant or keloid. Incisions on the fingers should be midlateral on the appropriate side. Thus they will be behind the ends of the interphalangeal creases and the digital vessels and nerves (Bunnel). A flap may be formed by a right-angled extension of this incision to the other side just beyond the distal flexion crease. In the palm incisions are made in the flexion creases. They are subjected to no stresses and heal with little scar.

Terminal Phalanx:

PALMAR SURFACE: Infections of the pulp space comprise over 20 per cent of hand infections and are very much commoner than infections of the tendon-sheaths or palmar spaces. An infected pulp space may be drained by the excision of a small ellipse of skin over the area of maximum tenderness. The well-known lateral,

[1] Landau, W., and Bishop, G. H., *Archs Neurol. Psychiat.*, 69, 490. Quoted by White.

THE ANATOMY OF SURGICAL PROCEDURES

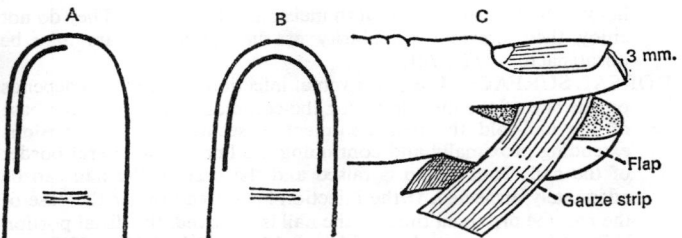

Fig. 721.—Incisions for opening whitlows on the volar aspect of the terminal phalanx. A, Half horseshoe. B, Horseshoe. C, Shows the flap raised.

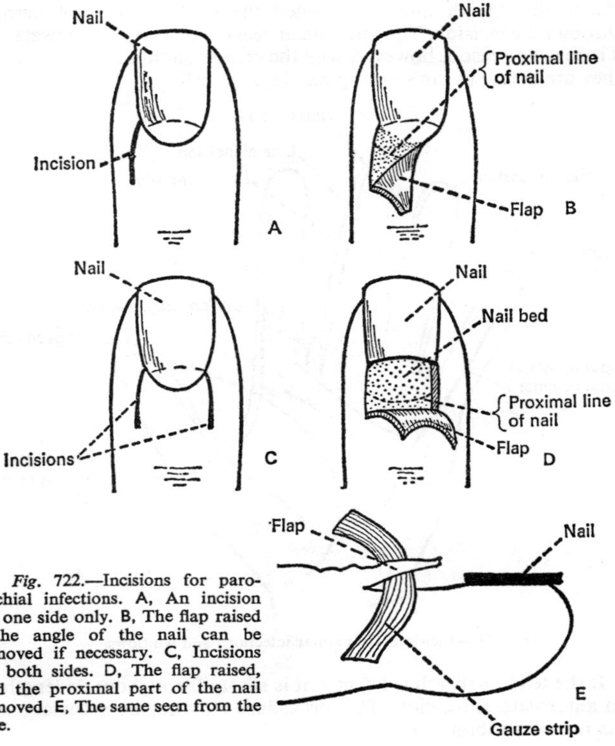

Fig. 722.—Incisions for paronychial infections. A, An incision on one side only. B, The flap raised—the angle of the nail can be removed if necessary. C, Incisions on both sides. D, The flap raised, and the proximal part of the nail removed. E, The same seen from the side.

hockey-stick or alligator mouth incisions may be used. They do not enjoy their previous popularity as the resultant scars may be unsatisfactory (*Fig.* 721).

DORSAL SURFACE: For paronychial infections the incision depends on the site of the infection. For the common infection at the base of the nail-fold the best treatment is secured by two incisions extending proximally and continuing the line of the lateral border of the nail. Thus a flap is raised and the base of the nail can be adequately inspected. If the infection has spread under the base of the nail the proximal third of the nail is removed, the distal portion being left to protect the highly sensitive nail bed (*Fig.* 722).

First and Second Phalanges: Incisions are midlateral just behind the vessels and nerves. The resultant scar is not subject to pressure and if the tendon-sheath must be opened the tendon does not herniate through the incision. The interphalangeal creases are not transgressed. There is no reason, however, why the creases should not be divided if they are acting as constricting bands (*Fig.* 723).

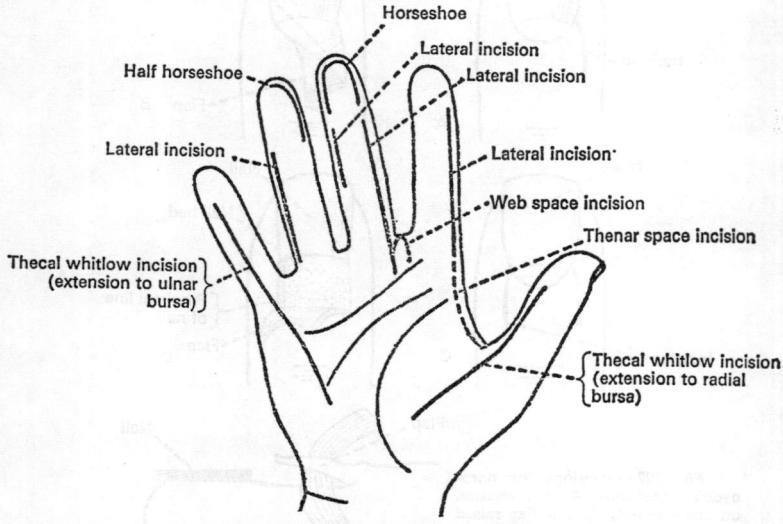

Fig. 723.—Incisions for palmar infections and whitlows.

If the tendon-sheath is infected it is slit up throughout its length by an anterolateral incision. This procedure may not be necessary with the use of antibiotic drugs.

Radial and Ulnar Bursae:

THECAL WHITLOW OF THUMB: This is opened by an anteromedial incision. When the infection extends into the proximal part of the tendon-sheath, the radial bursa, the above incision is continued up along the line of the tendon on the inner border of the thenar eminence. The incision must stop 3 cm. distal to the lower wrist crease to avoid the branch of the median nerve which crosses the tendon-sheath to supply the thenar muscles (*Fig.* 724).

ULNAR BURSA: When a thecal whitlow of the little finger extends proximally to involve the ulnar bursa it is opened as shown in *Fig.* 725. The incision is anteromedial on the finger, and extends proximally as far as the transverse carpal ligament on the ulnar side of the flexor tendons to the fifth digit. The deep branch of the ulnar nerve is not in danger.

Palmar Spaces:

THENAR SPACE: This is readily opened by an incision in the line of the web between thumb and index finger. The incision is deepened to expose the space anterior to the adductor pollicis (*Fig.* 726). If the site of maximum tenderness is in the palm, the incision is made through the skin crease which marks out the thenar eminence.

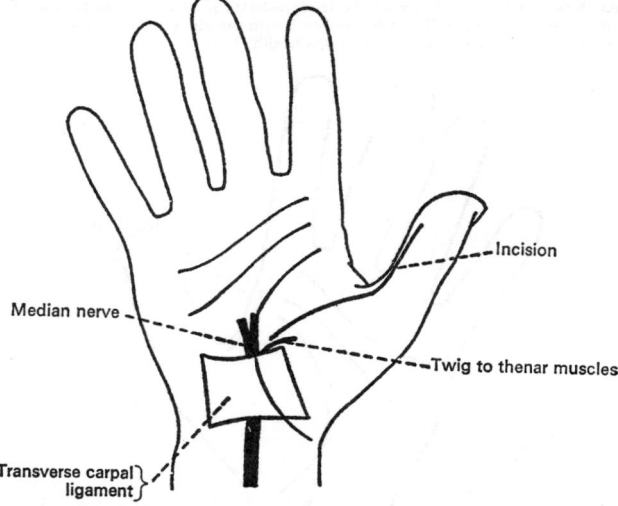

Fig. 724.—Incision for opening a thecal whitlow of the thumb with involvement of the radial bursa. Observe that the incision stops short of the median nerve branch to the thenar muscles.

768 A SYNOPSIS OF SURGICAL ANATOMY

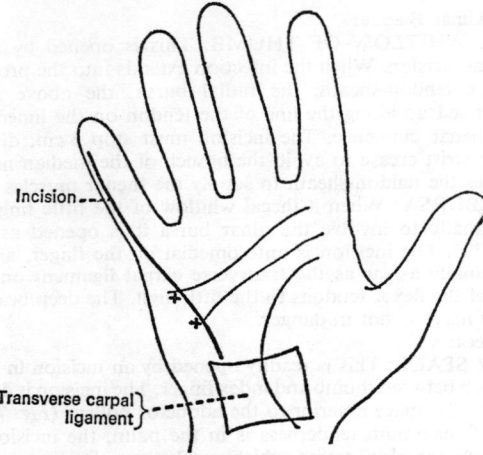

Fig. 725.—Incision for thecal whitlow of the little finger involving the ulnar bursa. Between the crosses the tendon-sheath may sometimes be absent, so that continuity of the digital flexor-sheath with the ulnar bursa does not exist. Care is then necessary to avoid infecting a healthy bursa.

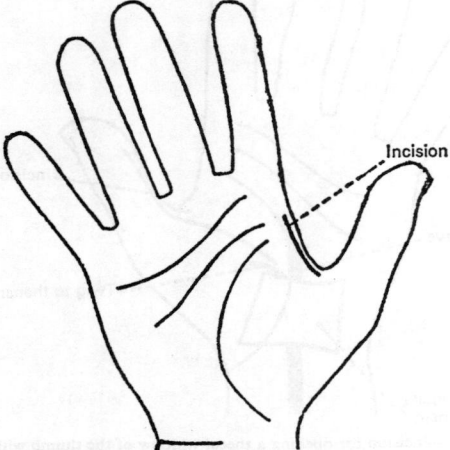

Fig. 726.—Incision for opening the thenar space.

THE ANATOMY OF SURGICAL PROCEDURES 769

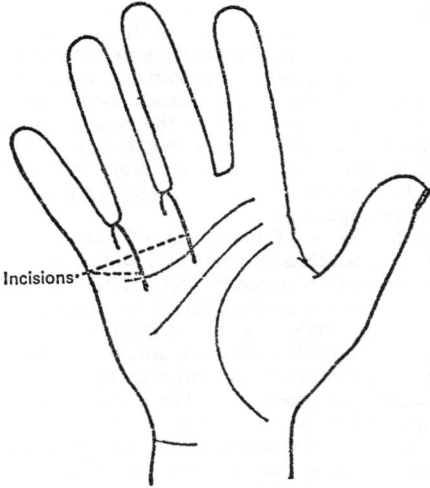

Fig. 727.—Incisions for opening the mid-palmar space.

MID-PALMAR SPACE: This is best dealt with by splitting the web between the middle and ring fingers and exposing the lumbrical muscle. As we have seen, the sheath of this muscle is a diverticulum of the mid-palmar space, and by pushing a pair of forceps up along the muscle the space may be drained. The web between the ring and little fingers may be opened if the physical signs point to that as the most favourable site to institute drainage (*Fig.* 727). If the point of maximum tenderness so indicates, a generous incision is made in an appropriate palmar crease and skin and palmar fascia incised.

IV. THE ANATOMY GOVERNING AMPUTATIONS
General Principles

There are certain facts which guide the surgeon in choosing the site for amputations. The first of these is, of course, the extent and nature of the disease or trauma. Secondly, he is guided by certain anatomical principles. Lastly, and of very great importance, is the view of the artificial-limb maker; he it is who has to make the most suitable substitute for the lost limb, and his task may be assisted or rendered difficult or impossible by the nature of the stump. The wise surgeon will bear these facts in mind in planning amputations.

The efficient functioning of artificial limbs, therefore, requires that stumps be of a certain length and shape. In the leg a long stump is always inferior to a 14 cm. one, so that frequently more of the leg is removed than is demanded by the lesion *per se;* contrariwise, a very short stump (*see below*) may make the fitting of a prosthesis very difficult or impossible. So it is better in some cases to sacrifice the joint above rather than that the patient should be handicapped by too short a stump.

Should the joint immediately above the projected stump be the site of arthritis it may be advisable to sacrifice the joint, e.g., do an *above-* rather than a below-knee amputation.

Weight-bearing: May be: (1) End bearing; (2) Lateral bearing—(*a*) tibial, (*b*) ischial; with which is combined (3) Diffuse bearing.

Until comparatively recently there existed a complete lack of technical knowledge of artificial limbs, and the surgeon was obsessed by the desire to obtain *end-bearing* stumps, i.e., where the weight is transmitted through the end of the stump. The experience gained in recent wars has resulted in an entire change in our conceptions as to what constitutes a good stump. This is evidenced by the fact that all artificial-limb makers and most surgeons have given up direct or end-bearing stumps, and plan amputations so as to obtain weight-bearing at the accessible bony points of the joint above the amputation—*lateral bearing;* for example, an artificial limb correctly fitted to the subject of a lower-leg amputation takes about 85 per cent of the weight at the tuberosity of the tibia. It follows, therefore, that the classic dictum that the stump should be covered with skin capable of weight-bearing no longer applies, with the single exception of the Syme amputation, the disadvantages of which are stated below. In the through-thigh amputations weight is borne by the ischial tuberosity and not by the end of the stump. The reason why end bearing is disappointing is that the skin at the end of the stump cannot bear the pressure of the body-weight without suffering from trophic disturbances and pressure sores. End-bearing stumps cannot as a rule function efficiently.

A well-fitted prosthesis for the lower limb takes weight all round that part of the limb above the amputation site which is embraced by the bucket. This is called *diffuse bearing*, and is due to the friction between the skin and the prosthesis. Only a small part of the weight can be taken in this way, otherwise a tendency would exist for the skin to be pulled upwards.

Requirements of a Good Stump:
1. It must be covered by healthy skin which is not adherent to the stump.
2. There must be no muscles or tendons in the flaps. Muscle may, however, be included in elderly people with atherosclerosis as more blood is carried to the stump.
3. The tissues covering the bone-end must not be capable of active movement. They must not form a bulky mass.

4. The scar must be painless, non-adherent, and in such a position that it is not subjected to pressure in the prosthesis.

Fashioning of the Stump (*Fig.* 728):

FLAPS: These consist of skin and fascia only. They are planned so as to fit accurately without tension and without being flabby. Right-angled corners are avoided. The old rule that the flaps should be together equal in length to $1\frac{1}{2}$ times the diameter of the limb at the level of bone section allows for too much skin. The lengths of the flaps will depend therefore on the mobility of the skin at the site of section, and flaps will be trimmed, if necessary, after they are cut.

Perkins[1] stresses the importance of the deep fascia in the movement of the stump in the socket. Piston action occurs, not between socket and skin, but between skin and the deep tissues. If the skin is adherent to deeper tissues, piston action is transmitted to them as also to the end bulbs which form on the divided nerves, and this causes pain and disability. He advises that the deep fascia be sutured separately because of its importance in amputations.

LEG AND THIGH: In a leg or thigh amputation the golden rule to follow is to make long anterior, short posterior flaps. This allows of a scar tucked away at the back of the stump. A single anterior flap may sometimes be necessary. It may suffer from circulatory disturbance at its distal margin.

MUSCLES: These are trimmed off in such a fashion as to give a cone-shaped appearance to the stump. Distally they are severed about

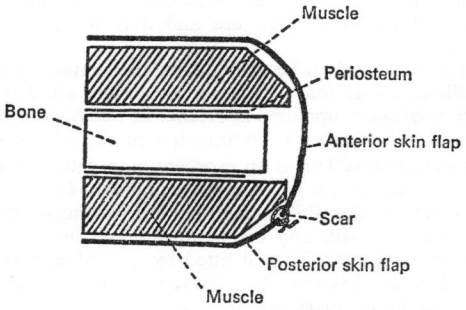

Fig. 728.—Method of fashioning an amputation stump. *See* text.

1·25 cm. below the bone-end (*Fig.* 728). Muscles are not sewn over the end of the stump. Following amputations in the fingers it is not advisable to suture flexors to extensors over the end of the bone.

[1] *Br. J. Surg.*, 1944, 31, 377.

This leads to stiffness and does not improve function; moreover, each of the phalanges has its own flexor and extensor. Muscles in the end of the stump cause a bulky, mobile, and possibly tender mass of fibrous tissue which makes efficient fitting of the prosthesis very troublesome.

NERVES: These are no longer pulled out and crushed. They are not pulled on but sought between muscles, divided with a sharp knife, and generally treated as gently as possible. It is never advisable to ligature a nerve to control bleeding from the arteria comes nervi.

BONE: The periosteum is cut round the end of the bone 1·25 cm. above the section so that the distal 1·25 cm. of the bone is bare of periosteum. This is to prevent the formation of bony spurs; other surgeons, however, cut the periosteum at the level of bone division. The bone is cut so as to avoid projections which may damage the skin of the stump—e.g., the sharp anterior margin of the tibia is bevelled off.

It must not be forgotten that flexors are stronger than extensors. The common practice of putting a pillow under the knee in below-knee stumps, and under the thigh in above-knee stumps, may give the flexors so great an advantage as to result in a flexed stump—a very troublesome complication.

Lower Limb Amputations

Toes:

1. Amputations through the first interphalangeal joint of the outer four toes or through the first phalanx are not advised, as the remaining stump is of little use and may form a troublesome projection.
2. When three toes need to be amputated, the remaining two are at such a disadvantage that it is better to sacrifice all. The great toe, however, is of such supreme importance in weight-bearing that it is probably wise to retain it even though it be the only toe remaining.

At Tarsometatarsal Joints: This is an excellent amputation providing the scar is dorsal and muscle balance is maintained—i.e., by preserving the attachments of the tibilias anterior and peroneus longus to the first cuneiform and stitching the peronei brevis and tertius to the cuboid. Such a foot can be well fitted by an ordinary boot with a piece of cork in the fore part. It is therefore of little more expense to the owner than an ordinary boot.

Pirogoff's Amputation: Of historical value only.

Just above the Ankle-joint (Syme's): This is the classic example of an end-bearing stump. It has enjoyed a great popularity. From the point of view of permanent efficiency, however, it is not a good amputation. The opinion of authorities best fitted to judge is as follows: A perfect Syme's amputation—e.g., where the skin forms a firm non-mobile pad, the scar is anterior, there are no end bulbs in the pad, and the nutrition is good—has a life of 6 to 10 years. At the end of that time the stump is giving so much trouble that a re-amputation with a 14 cm. tibial stump is necessary, and the patient welcomes the change.

The Syme's amputation is well thought of by Gillis[1] and others of great experience. It can be done if the tissues around the heel are sound. The end of the stump is formed by the skin of the heel which is used to weight-bearing. The patient wears an elephant boot. He can get up at night without artificial aid. The operation is a difficult one.

Supramalleolar amputation (Silbert[2]) is a valuable procedure in cases where owing to the serious general condition of the patient a more radical procedure cannot be undertaken. A guillotine amputation is made just above the malleoli. It inflicts minimal trauma and may be primary or final, depending on the condition of the patient (*Fig.* 729).

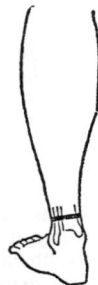

Fig. 729.—Supramalleolar amputation.

At the Site of Election in the Leg:

'OLD' SITE OF ELECTION: This was an amputation through the upper third of the leg. In the old days the patient wore a wooden leg after recovery, and his limb was in a kneeling position in the bucket of the splint, so that he walked about on the tubercle of the tibia with the leg flexed to a right-angle at the knee, the end of the stump projecting behind. This type of splint is now obsolete, and the stump is so planned as to be embraced by the bucket of an artificial leg (*Fig.* 730).

'NEW' SITE OF ELECTION: This is at a point 14 cm. from the joint line (knee). This length of leg gives a useful lever with which to control the new limb. A much shorter stump may still be useful in the leg. There is a limit, however, to this shortness. The shortest leg

---

[1] Gillis, L.. *Amputations*, 1954, 86. London: Heinemann.
[2] Silbert, S., and Haimovici, H., *J. Am. med. Ass.*, 1954, **155**, 1554.

stump which can be efficiently fitted with a prosthesis is 6 cm. of tibia, or alternatively it must be possible to hook two fingers round the stump (when flexed to a right-angle) on the *inner* side, as the medial hamstrings extend farther distally than the biceps on the outer side. If the stump is too short to permit of this it is better to amputate above the knee. Whereas the preservation of the knee-joint is of the utmost value to the patient, it is worthless if an artificial limb, efficiently activated by a tibial lever, cannot be fitted distal to the joint, or if the bucket of the prosthesis is pushed off the stump every time the knee is bent.

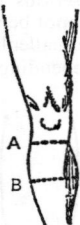

Fig. 730.—Showing old (A) and new (B) 'site of election' for amputation below the knee.

STUMP OF THE FIBULA: It has been stated that in amputations which leave a very short stump it is better to remove the fibula stump because the head of the fibula will not bear pressure, because the biceps abducts it, and because its removal may enable sufficient slack of skin to be obtained to section the tibia at a lower level than would otherwise have been possible. Authoritative opinion is, however, opposed to this procedure for several reasons: firstly, its removal leaves a scar which may cause trouble later; secondly, because the tibial tuberosity takes 85 per cent of the weight-bearing; and lastly to avoid 'pistoning' of the stump in the bucket. Artificial-limb makers tell us that one of the most troublesome complications of stumps is when they are so cone-shaped that they move up and down in the bucket—'pistoning'. The fibular projection is just sufficient to prevent the stump from being completely cone-shaped, and its presence, with a well-adapted prosthesis, prevents this up-and-down movement. The fibular head may, of course, need removal if diseased.

At Knee: Amputation through the knee, Gritti-Stokes, and amputations through the broad end of the femur, are obsolete. There are important reasons for this: if the amputation is through the knee, an artificial joint in the prosthesis has to be below the normal joint level. The large femoral condyles bear pressure badly. The prosthesis is bulky and ugly. Disarticulation through the knee may be advisable in the elderly or in growing persons. The end of the stump is covered by skin which is used to weight-bearing in kneeling and the blood-supply is good. Growth continues longer at the lower end of the femur and it is an advantage to retain the epiphysis.

Through the Shaft of the Femur: The site of election is one which gives a 25 cm. femoral stump. The femur is measured for purposes of amputation from the top of the great trochanter. The site may also be estimated as a hand-breadth above the patella or 10 cm. above the joint line. The amputation is done on general principles, with this important addition, that the adductors must be fixed to the periosteum. If this is not done they retract upwards and form a bulky mass on the inner aspect of the thigh which cannot be kept in the bucket of the prosthesis. It becomes chafed and irritated, and painful adventitious bursae form in it.

When it is necessary to remove more femur it should be borne in mind that the shorter the thigh stump the more inefficient does it become as a lever to activate an artificial limb. Therefore not every length of thigh stump is useful. The irreducible limit for a useful stump is a bone section 6·5 cm. below the perineum or 11·5 cm to 12·5 cm. distal to the tip of the great trochanter. If this length of thigh stump is unobtainable, then the patient cannot wear a 'thigh leg', but must be fitted with a tilting table—that is to say, the bone section must be made through the great trochanter.

At Hip-joint: This should be modified, if possible, to retain the head, neck, and part of the great trochanter of the femur in the stump—transtrochanteric amputation—as it leaves a stump which is more comfortable to the patient. Such amputees are fitted with a limb on the top of which is a platform called a tilting table. If the hip-joint is disarticulated (as may be necessary, e.g., in sarcoma of the femur), then the outer surface of the hip bone is so smooth that the patient has a constant sensation of slipping in his splint. If the upper end of the femur is left, then the stump has a square end on which the patient sits much more securely. In these amputations most of the muscles are cut away from the os innominatum, and the flap is a single *posterior* one with the scar lying below and parallel to the inguinal ligament.

Amputation in the Presence of Ischaemic Gangrene

The better understanding of the problems of peripheral vascular disease and the use of antibiotics has made it possible to operate more distally in many cases of gangrene, diabetic or otherwise, where above-knee amputations were formerly advised. In cases of gangrene of two or more toes the *transmetatarsal amputation* (McKittrick,[1]) is sometimes

[1] McKittrick, L. S., McKittrick, J. B., and Risley, T. S., *Ann. Surg.*, 1949, 130, 826.

advisable. Whether the flaps are closed without drainage or left open depends on the condition of the toes and whether the gangrene is static or not. The procedure is not advised where severe pain radiates up the limb from the necrotic area. The metatarsus is cut through and in suitable cases previously prepared flaps are sutured. Silbert[1] states that the advantages of transmetatarsal amputation cannot be over-emphasized, pointing out that it is the only major amputation which enables an amputee to walk without a prosthesis or crutches (*Fig.* 731).

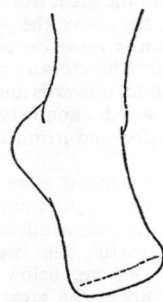

Fig. 731.—Transmetatarsal amputation.

Upper Limb Amputations

Fingers: The work of Couch,[2] of Toronto, has entirely changed existing concepts on this important matter. Hitherto, as Couch says, the whole matter has been covered by a blanket rule, 'save all you can'. The surgeon has thought in terms of anatomy instead of in terms of physiology. Function is more important than form. What is the value of a portion of a digit which is useless or in any way subject to repeated injury? Couch's main conclusions are as follows:

INDEX FINGER:
  1. The loss of part or all of the distal phalanx of the index finger is no handicap to the patient. No compensation is paid for such loss, as the earning capacity of the patient is not impaired.
  2. Should injury force amputation proximal to the distal interphalangeal joint, not only should the entire finger be sacrificed but the distal part of the metacarpal should also be removed. The reasons are that the patient never learns to use the short index stump. It is just a nuisance. Moreover the angular projection caused by the head of the metacarpal, in a metacarpophalangeal

[1] Silbert, S., and Haimovici, H.. *J. Am. med. Ass.*, 1954, 155, 1554.
[2] Couch, J. H., *Surgery of the Hand*, 1939, 59 et seq. Toronto: University of Toronto Press.

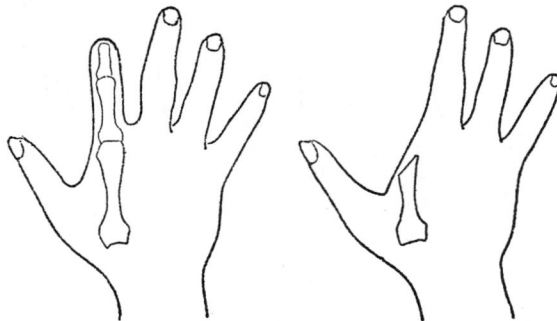

Fig. 732.—Showing two commendable amputations of the index finger.

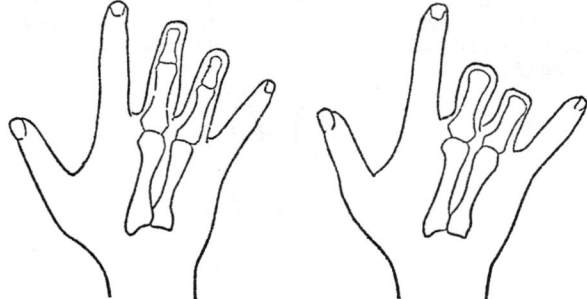

Fig. 733.—Commendable amputations of the middle and ring fingers. They would also be sound in principle if amputation was confined to but one of the digits.

amputation, gets in the way. The patient never learns the proper clearance to protect it. Furthermore, the metacarpal head tends to be dislocated backwards. There are then only two advisable amputations in relation to the index (*Fig.* 732).

The rules set forth above do not apply in the presence of contra-indication such as infection, where it is inadvisable to cut through bone.

MIDDLE AND RING FINGERS: Here conditions are different. Amputations at all levels are good as far proximally as the first interphalangeal joint. The stump lends strength to the hand and prevents the adjacent fingers from falling together (*Fig.* 733).

778 A SYNOPSIS OF SURGICAL ANATOMY

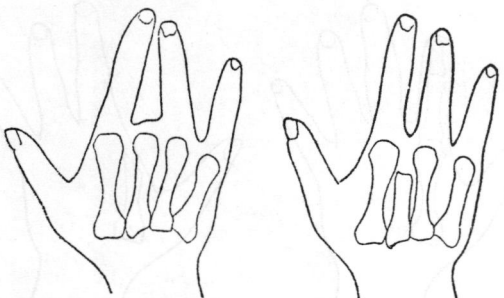

Fig. 734.—The left-hand figure shows a poor amputation. The defect is rectified in the right-hand figure.

Amputation through the metacarpophalangeal joint is not good. The adjacent fingers fall together and the metacarpal head tends to be displaced dorsally. This is prevented by removing the metacarpal head (*Fig.* 734).

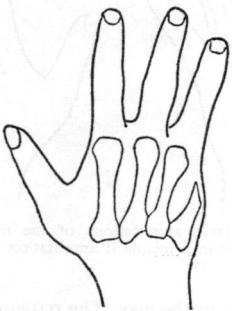

Fig. 735.—Sound amputation of the little finger.

LITTLE FINGER: Amputation may be carried out at any level where good flaps are available. Metacarpophalangeal amputation is bad. It leaves an unsightly projection which is readily injured. Removal of the metacarpal head is advisable (*Fig.* 735).

In amputations through fingers the tendons should not be sutured over the bone-end. For the effective functioning of groups of tendons acting together, such as those of the long flexors of the fingers, it is essential that the free gliding of all the tendons of a group should be maintained. Failing this, movements of the unaffected fingers may be sufficiently impaired to warrant the surgical release of tendons which have been sutured across the bone end.

THUMB: The value of this member is almost as much as the rest of the fingers put together. As much as possible should always be preserved.

Hand: Conservation of tissue must be the key-note of the surgery of the hand.

Through Forearm: There is some difference of opinion in regard to preserving the lower third of the forearm. This portion is apt to become blue and cold and to give trouble from nutritional disturbance. Muirhead Little sums up the matter aptly by saying that the advantages of a long forearm stump with its attendant possibilities of nutritional disturbances must be weighed against the disadvantages of a sacrifice in length with nutritional security. The optimum length of radius and ulna should be 18 cm. measured from the olecranon prominence. Short forearm stumps may also be of value, but the shortest length compatible with the efficient activation of a prosthesis is a stump with 7·5 cm. of ulna. Any shorter stump cannot be effectively used, as the muscles bunch up on contraction and the stump jumps out of the bucket. Pronation and supination should be retained in forearm amputations whenever possible. Ability to rotate adds considerably to the value of a forearm stump. Rotation is lost if the bone-ends become joined by fibrous or bony ankylosis.

Through Arm: The optimum length of an arm stump measured from the tip of the acromion is 20 cm. The shortest length of humerus which can be fitted with a useful prosthesis is a 13 cm. stump, measured from the tip of the acromion. Put in other words, if 2·5 cm. of humerus can be retained measuring from the lower border of the anterior axillary fold, an efficient limb can be fitted.

If it is not possible to keep quite sufficient humerus to activate a prosthesis, a further 1·8 cm. may be gained by dividing the tendon of the major pectoral (and possibly latissimus dorsi) where it is attached to the intertubercular sulcus.

Disarticulation at the Upper Limb-joints: As in the lower limb, disarticulations are not advisable as artificial limbs are difficult to fit and long stumps are prone to trophic troubles.

Maximal and Minimal Length for Amputation Stumps

	MEASUREMENT FROM	MAXIMUM	MINIMUM
Leg	Knee-joint	14 cm.	8 cm.
Thigh	Top of trochanter	25 cm.	15 cm.
Forearm	Tip of olecranon	18 cm.	10 cm.
Arm	Acromion	20 cm.	13 cm.

It will be noted that the site of election advised in the leg is shorter than that heretofore accepted.

V. THE ANATOMY OF INJECTIONS INTO NERVES

Objects: Injections are made into nerve-trunks for two purposes:
1. An anaesthetic solution is injected to procure a temporary anaesthesia of the area supplied by the nerve, so that an operative procedure may be carried out.
2. Strong alcohol, 90 per cent, is injected into the nerve-trunk with the deliberate purpose of destroying it. This produces anaesthesia in the area of distribution of a sensory nerve. The nerve regenerates and sensation returns in six or more months. The procedure is resorted to in cases of intractable neuralgia. The 5th nerve is the one usually affected and the condition is called 'trigeminal neuralgia'. One or more of the divisions of the nerve may be affected. Injections to destroy the nerve are therefore made: (*a*) Into the affected division; (*b*) Into the semilunar (Gasserian) ganglion—in this case all divisions are rendered anaesthetic as the entire ganglion is destroyed.

Second Division of the 5th Nerve:

METHOD:
1. The nerve is injected where it emerges from the foramen rotundum into the pterygopalatine fossa.
2. Two points are marked out (*Fig.* 736):

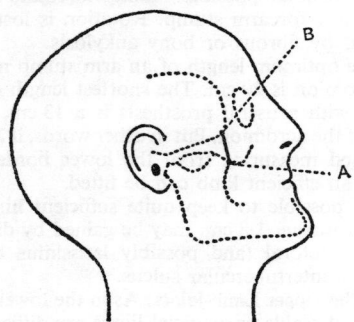

Fig. 736.—Injection of 2nd division of the 5th nerve. (For description *see* text.)

  a. The coronoid process of the mandible is felt for and a mark (A) made in the angle between its anterior border and the lower border of the zygomatic arch.
  b. A mark (B) is made in the angle between the upper border of the zygoma and its frontal process.
3. Join A and B by a straight line. The needle is entered at A and passed upwards and inwards at an angle of 45° with the horizontal.

The needle is kept in the direction of the line AB. The needle passes behind the maxilla, enters the pterygopalatine fossa, and strikes the bone forming the margin of the foramen rotundum at a depth of 5 to 7·5 cm. from the surface. The injection is made here.

Third Division of the 5th Nerve: The foramen ovale through which the nerve emerges lies 5 cm. from the surface.

METHOD (*Fig.* 737)

1. Mark out the lower border of the zygomatic arch—line AA'.
2. Join the incisura notch of the ear to the lower border of the ala nasi—line BB'. This line corresponds in level to the lower border of the notch between the head and coronoid process of the mandible.
3. Take a point 2·5 cm. in front of the external auditory meatus on line AA', and draw a line downwards in front of the ear at right angles to line AA', crossing the line BB' at D. This is line CC'.
4. A needle entered at D, passing slightly upwards, reaches the foramen ovale and therefore the mandibular nerve at a depth of 5 cm. from the surface. (Varies from 4 to 6·7 cm. in depth from the surface.)

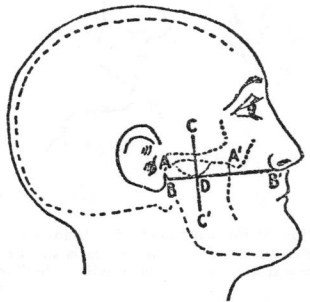

Fig. 737.—Harris's method of injecting 3rd division of 5th nerve.
(For description *see* text.)

Semilunar Ganglion: The same landmarks are taken as for injection of the third division. When the needle strikes the margin of the foramen ovale, it is pushed through for 0·6 cm. It has then entered the ganglion.

THE METHOD OF HÄRTEL: The needle is entered at a point on the face 3 cm. lateral to the angle of the mouth (*Fig.* 738). Two lines have been made on the face: one joining the point of insertion of the needle to the pupil, the patient looking directly forward; the second joins the point of entry to the articular tubercle. The needle is advanced towards the centre of the zygomatic arch in the plane joining the point of entry of the needle to the pupil, the patient being viewed from the front. The needle strikes the infratemporal bony plane at a depth of 6 cm. It is gently withdrawn slightly, and then pushed up in a more posterior direction until when viewed from the front the needle is in the plane of the first of the lines indicated (i.e., to the pupil), and when viewed from the side the needle is in the plane of the second line (that to the articular eminence). The needle then enters the foramen ovale, and if advanced 1·2 cm. farther enters the semilunar or Gasserian ganglion.

Infra-orbital Nerve: The nerve is reached by entering a needle 0·6 cm. above and 0·6 cm. lateral to the angle of the ala of the nose. The

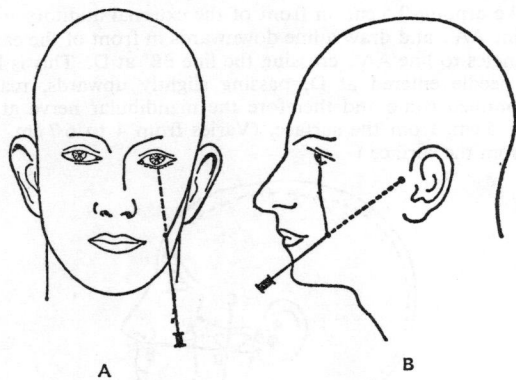

Fig. 738.—Injection of the semilunar (Gasserian) ganglion by the method of Härtel. A, Viewed from the front the needle is in line with the forwardly directed pupil. B, Seen from the side the needle is in line with the articular tubercle. (*See* text.)

needle is pushed back and slightly up. The point of the needle is felt to slip into the infra-orbital foramen and therefore into the nerve. A finger is kept on the lower border of the orbit to prevent the needle entering the orbit in the event of the foramen being missed.

Supra-orbital Nerve: This is the only part of the ophthalmic division of the 5th nerve which ever requires injection. The supra-orbital notch may be felt at the junction of the inner and middle thirds of the upper border of the orbit. When the nerve traverses a foramen instead of a notch, it passes up at a point in the upper orbital margin 2·5 cm. from the midline. The nerve may be injected here where it lies just under the skin.

THE ANATOMY OF SURGICAL PROCEDURES 783

Posterior Inferior Alveolar Nerve: This nerve is sensory to all the teeth of the lower jaw. It is therefore often anaesthetized by dentists in working on the lower teeth. The nerve is struck just above its entrance into the mandibular foramen by entering a needle 0·6 to 1·2 cm. above the crown of the last molar tooth and just medial to the ramus of the mandible and passing it backwards and slightly outwards.

The *lingual nerve* (sensory to mouth and tongue) may be anaesthetized at the same place as the alveolar nerve. Thus an injection at this site renders the lower teeth, floor of the mouth, and anterior two-thirds of the tongue sufficiently insensitive for the performance of small operations.

Mental Nerve: This nerve emerges through the foramen of the same name which is situated at the level of the second premolar tooth midway between the upper and lower borders of the body of the mandible. A needle entering the skin here and passed directly inwards strikes the nerve.

Sacral Nerves: The sacral nerves supplying the pelvic viscera—bladder, prostate, uterus, etc.—may be anaesthetized by entering a needle through the gap over the lower part of the back of the sacrum—

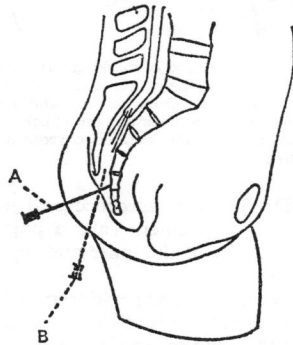

Fig. 739.—Epidural injection. A, Direction in which needle is first inserted. B, Ultimate direction of needle.

hiatus sacralis—which is easily felt, pushing the needle into the sacral part of the vertebral canal, and injecting an anaesthetizing solution around the sacral nerves in the canal (*Fig.* 739). The lower sacral roots are alone anaesthetized, as they are shut off from the nerves above by the dural sac.

784 A SYNOPSIS OF SURGICAL ANATOMY

Great Sciatic Nerve:

FIRST METHOD: The upper part of the nerve is mapped out as follows (*Fig.* 740):

POINT A: A point midway between the ischial tuberosity and the small trochanter.

POINT B: A point on the upper border of the great sciatic notch is marked out by taking a point 10 cm. lateral to the upper part of the natal cleft and 10 cm. above the ischial tuberosity.

Points A and B are joined; the nerve commences on this line about 3·7 cm. below point B, and may be injected on the line AB anywhere below this level at a depth of about 7·5 cm. from the surface.

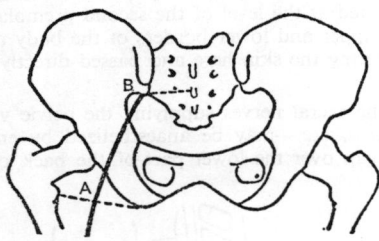

Fig. 740.—Demonstrating method of marking out great sciatic nerve when it is desired to inject it. A is midpoint between ischial tuberosity and small trochanter of femur. B is 10 cm. from midline and 10 cm. above ischial tuberosity. A line joining A and B maps out the upper part of the nerve. The portion of the nerve seen in the sciatic notch is covered by the piriformis and lies therefore in the pelvis.

SECOND METHOD: Join the sacrococcygeal joint to the posterior border of the great trochanter. Take a point a finger's breadth external to the junction of the inner and middle thirds and enter the needle here vertically.

THIRD METHOD: Exit of sciatic nerve from pelvis is at the junction of the middle and lower thirds of the line connecting the posterior superior spine of the ilium to the tip of the great trochanter.

Pudendal Nerve: This nerve is sensory to the perineum and vagina, and motor to the levator ani, anal, and perineal muscles. The vaginal mucous membrane, above the level of the hymen, is insensitive to pin-prick in 90 per cent of cases. The pudendal nerve is one of the two terminal branches of the sacral plexus, arising from the anterior primary rami of S. 2, 3, 4. It leaves the pelvis through the great sciatic foramen, but soon re-enters it through the lesser one, in company with the internal pudendal vessels, crossing the sacrospinous ligament medial to the ischial spine. This neurovascular bundle enters the pudendal canal (Alcock's) where the nerve immediately divides into the inferior haemorrhoidal, the dorsal nerve of penis or clitoris, and the

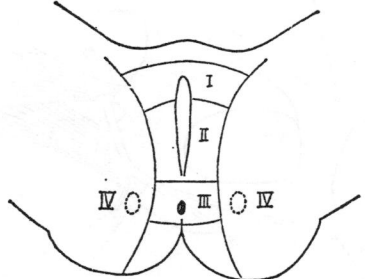

Fig. 741.—The nerve-supply of the perineum. I, Dorsal nerve of clitoris. II, Perineal nerve. III, Superior haemorrhoidal nerve. IV, Perineal branch of posterior cutaneous nerve of the thigh. (*By courtesy of Huntingford and the Editor of the 'Journal of Obstetrics and Gynaecology of the British Empire'.*)

perineal division. Frequently the inferior haemorrhoidal nerve takes an independent origin and course, piercing the sacrospinous ligament and crossing the ischiorectal fossa on its way to the anal region. Perineal anaesthesia may be produced by the percutaneous or transvaginal route. The method has its greatest value in obstetric practice and in operations on the external female genitalia (*Fig.* 741).

PUDENDAL NERVE BLOCK:[1] The object of the procedure is to infiltrate the pudendal nerve where it crosses the ischial spine before it enters Alcock's canal. By so doing the inferior haemorrhoidal nerve, which sometimes arises before the pudendal nerve enters the canal, does not escape the blockade. The patient is prepared for operation and lies in the lithotomy position. A 15 cm. flexible spinal type needle is used. The surgeon inserts the right forefinger on the tip of the ischial spine per vaginam. His other hand directs the needle, with syringe attached, to the tip of the right forefinger. When the needle is at the tip of the spine it is advanced 0·6 cm., now lying over the sacrospinous ligament. The tip of the finger now deflects the flexible needle sharply, enabling it to pierce the vaginal wall. The needle is slowly advanced and can be felt to penetrate the sacrospinous ligament, where the injection is made. The procedure is then carried out on the opposite side (*Fig.* 742).

---

[1] According to the account of Huntingford, P. J., *J. Obstet. Gynaec. Br. Emp.*, 1959 96, 26.

786 A SYNOPSIS OF SURGICAL ANATOMY

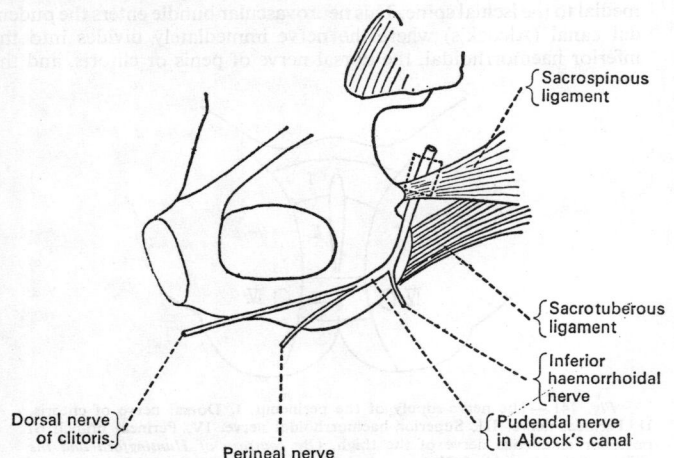

Fig. 742.—The anatomy of pudendal nerve block. The dotted square is the site of injection. (*By courtesy of Huntingford and the Editor of the 'Journal of Obstetrics and Gynaecology of the British Empire'.*)

Areas I, II, and III in *Fig.* 741 are anaesthetized by pudendal nerve block. Vaginal sensation is also lost, and the levator ani, perineal, and anal muscles are relaxed. The ilio-inguinal and the genital branch of the genitofemoral nerve take no part in the supply of the female external genitalia.

Chapter XLIV

THE ANATOMY OF SURGICAL APPROACH

I. SURGICAL APPROACH TO THE BRAIN

Routes: As the vast majority of operations on the brain are undertaken through a normal skull, the problems of approach are purely anatomical. The operative routes have become standardized. Six routes of approach were used by Cushing. These are the: (1) Lateral osteoplastic flap; (2) Frontal osteoplastic flap; (3) Transfrontal

THE ANATOMY OF SURGICAL APPROACH

osteoplastic flap; (4) Occipital osteoplastic flap; (5) Suboccipital exploration; (6) Trans-sphenoidal operation.[1]

Craniectomy: Implies the removal of a portion of the skull, leaving a permanent gap.

A permanent bony defect over an area unprotected by muscle may be attended with serious consequences, such as herniation of the brain. In cases, therefore, where it is desired to give the brain room for expansion by craniectomy the operation is so planned that the defect is covered by muscle. As the temporal muscle is the most conveniently situated for this purpose, the decompression, as such an operation is called, is usually made subjacent to it—subtemporal decompression.

Osteoplastic Craniotomy: Implies the raising of a portion of the skull, which is replaced when the operation on the brain is completed, leaving therefore no bony gap in the brain case.

LATERAL OSTEOPLASTIC FLAP (*Fig.* 743): This exposure, used much the most commonly, gives access to the: (1) Greater part of the convexity of a cerebral hemisphere; (2) Adjacent subcortical regions; (3) Outer aspects of the temporal lobe; (4) Falx cerebri; (5) Medial aspect of the hemisphere.

INCISION: This forms three-fourths or four-fifths of a circle. It commences just above and behind the ear, and, having outlined the flap to be raised, terminates above the middle of the zygomatic arch. The circle can be made to demarcate however much skin

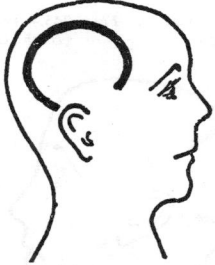

Fig. 743.—Incision for lateral osteoplastic craniotomy by the lateral osteoplastic flap. (*Hugh Cairns, after Cushing.*)

it is desired to raise. The temporal artery enters the base of this flap and ensures a liberal blood-supply. The entire blood-supply to the flap may be controlled by pushing an instrument, such as

[1] Hugh Cairns, *A Study of Intracranial Surgery*, Special Report Series No. 125, Medical Research Council, 1929, 58. London.

an intestinal occlusion clamp, across the base of the flap under the skin and gripping the base of the flap in the clamp.

FRONTAL OSTEOPLASTIC FLAP (*Fig.* 744): This incision is much the same as the last, but exposes more of the frontal lobe.

TRANSFRONTAL OSTEOPLASTIC FLAP (*Fig.* 745): This exposure gives access to the: (1) Frontal lobe; (2) Olfactory groove; (3) Optic chiasma; (4) Optic nerve; (5) Pituitary gland; (6) Region above the pituitary (suprasellar region).

INCISION: This is rectangular. It commences at the front part of the temporal fossa just above the zygomatic bone and passes along the line of the eyebrow to the glabella, then vertically upwards for 13 cm., then outwards to finish just above the ear. The temporal artery is in the base of the flap.

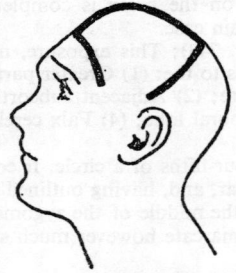
Fig. 744.—Frontal osteoplastic flap. (*Hugh Cairns, after Cushing.*)

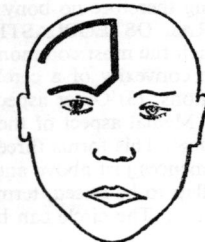
Fig. 745.—Transfrontal osteoplastic flap (*Hugh Cairns, after Cushing.*)

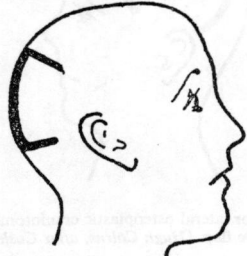
Fig. 746.—Occipital osteoplastic flap. (*Hugh Cairns, after Cushing.*)

OCCIPITAL OSTEOPLASTIC FLAP (*Fig.* 746): The approach exposes the lateral part of the hemisphere, i.e., the parietal and occipital lobes.

THE ANATOMY OF SURGICAL APPROACH 789

INCISION: Consists of a posterior limb corresponding to the superior nuchal line, an anterior limb extending from above the ear to the midline, and a connecting limb in the sagittal plane. The flap contains the posterior branch of the temporal artery.

COMMENT: Observe that each of the foregoing flaps consist of: (1) A large scalp-flap; (2) A slightly smaller bone-flap; (3) A muscle-flap on which the bone-flap hinges, which muscle conveys blood-vessels to the bone; (4) The temporal artery in the base of the flap. In any of these flaps, particularly the first, if the part of the bone covered by muscle is permanently removed, an ideal decompression ensues.

Suboccipital Exploration: This approach gives access to: (1) Cerebellum; (2) Cerebellopontine angle; (3) Fourth ventricle; (4) Medulla; (5) Other parts of the posterior cranial fossa; (6) The upper part of the spinal cord.

INCISION: The 'cross-bow' cut of Cushing (*Fig.* 747). The horizontal limb connects the bases of the mastoid processes, passing 2·5 cm. above the superior nuchal line. The vertical limb passes from the centre of this incision, exactly in the midline, to the 6th cervical

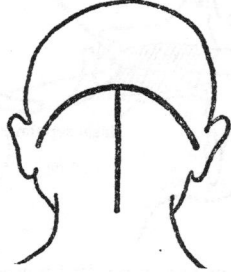

Fig. 747.—Cross-bow incision for bilateral cerebellar exposure or suboccipital exploration or decompression. (*Hugh Cairns, after Cushing.*)

spine. The suboccipital muscles are cleared from the occipital bones and the cerebellum is displayed by removing the exposed parts of these bones. The posterior margin of the foramen magnum is exposed, and if necessary the posterior arch of the atlas. This is not an osteoplastic craniotomy but a craniectomy, as the bone is permanently removed.

COMMENT: So completely does the tentorium cerebelli divide the posterior from the other fossae of the skull that a decompression above the tentorium is useless for a lesion below it, and vice versa. Therefore for a tumour of the posterior fossa the decompression must be such as has just been described.

790 A SYNOPSIS OF SURGICAL ANATOMY

Trans-sphenoidal Operation: Pituitary tumours may be removed by the transfrontal operation or by the trans-sphenoidal route. As the tumour does not admit of complete removal, the part left goes on growing and soon causes symptoms again unless this can be prevented. This is best achieved by removing the *floor* of the sella turcica so that the remains of the tumour tend to be extruded by intracranial pressure into the sphenoidal sinus. The floor of the pituitary fossa can only be removed by the trans-sphenoidal route. This is also the route favoured for the insertion of pellets of radio-active substances into the pituitary.

TECHNIQUE (*Fig.* 748): A small incision is made in the mucous membrane between the upper lip and gum. The anterior edge of the nasal septum is exposed. The mucoperiosteum is separated from each side of the septum nasi and the whole of the latter removed.

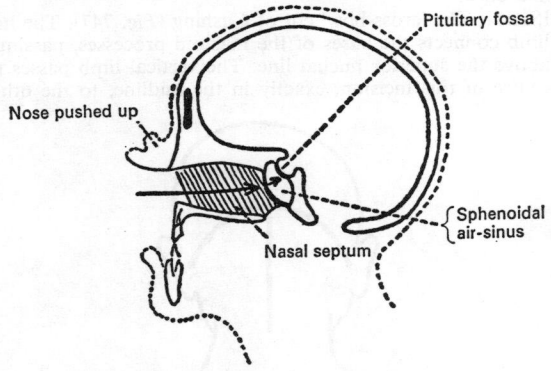

Fig. 748.—Nasal route to pituitary gland is indicated by arrows.
(*Hugh Cairns, after Cushing.*)

The anterior wall of the sphenoidal sinus is cut away, exposing the bulging floor of the sella turcica, which is removed. This exposes the *dura* beneath the pituitary, excision of which lays bare the tumour. The cavity of the nose is not entered, so that the approach is not through a septic cavity.

The transfrontal approach is in general use for the surgery of pituitary tumours.

II. TRANSTHORACIC APPROACHES

Approach to the Superior Mediastinum: This may be required for tumours of different kinds. The area is adequately exposed by an incision splitting the manubrium and body of sternum as far as the 4th costal

THE ANATOMY OF SURGICAL APPROACH

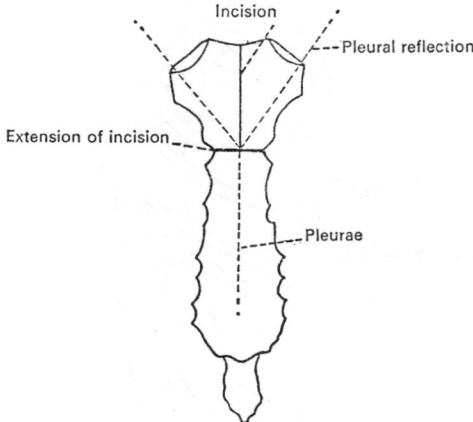

Fig. 749.—Showing the line for splitting the manubrium and the lateral extension sometimes necessary.

cartilage and extending it laterally by incisions at right-angles. The thymus is removed through such an incision (*Fig.* 749).

Lateral Transthoracic Approach: The greatest value of transthoracic procedures is exemplified by this route; here chest wall is covered by the big padding muscles such as latissimus, serratus anterior, great pectoral, trapezius, and external oblique. Wide access is obtained by removal of any rib from 5th to 9th. Brock considers that the removal of healthy ribs is unnecessary. Comparable access is obtained by intercostal division. Incision must be generous and extend the whole length of the rib. The scapula is readily lifted upwards once the latissimus is divided. The iliocostalis is mobilized posteriorly by dividing the tendons attaching to the rib to be removed and retracting the muscle back. Thus rapid subperiosteal removal from costal cartilage to tip of transverse process may be carried out. Additional room may be gained by dividing ribs above and below just lateral to the costotransverse region. Smithwick, in transthoracic sympathectomy, removes 6th rib and 2·5 cm. of 5th rib at its anterior end, and 2·5 cm. of 7th rib at its posterior end. The entire pleural cavity is widely exposed and the ganglia from the stellate to the 12th thoracic plus all the splanchnic nerves can readily be removed (*Fig.* 750). Thus all types of lung, oesophageal, and aortic surgery may be carried out through lateral thoracic exposure.

792 A SYNOPSIS OF SURGICAL ANATOMY

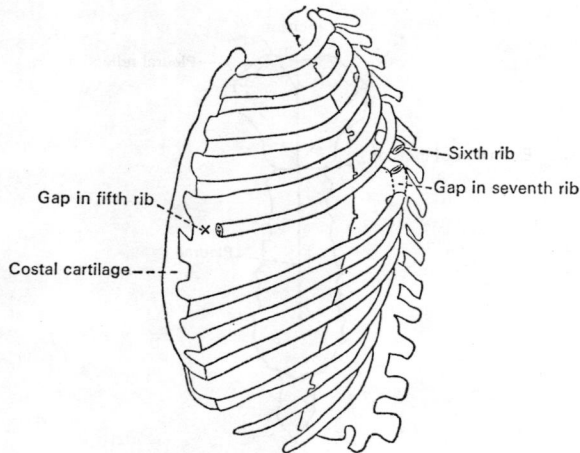

Fig. 750.—The bone removed in the transthoracic sympathectomy of Smithwick.

Transthoracic Route to the Upper Abdomen: Surgery has taken a noteworthy step forward by the development of the transthoracic transdiaphragmatic approach. It is one of the remarkable advantages of this route that it is well tolerated even by the old and enfeebled persons in whom it is so often indicated. It is correct to say that conditions hitherto considered inoperable have entered the range of practical surgery since the introduction of this approach, e.g., cancer of the lower oesophagus. Furthermore, procedures attended with great technical difficulty and hazard may be more easily dealt with by the new route, e.g., total gastrectomy. Transthoracic diaphragmatic procedures require great surgical skill and experience in their performance, but there is usually more room to work in by this route and the difficulty, so great by the abdominal route, of carrying out an anastomosis just under the diaphragm, is obviated. High oesophagogastric anastomosis in relation to the aortic arch is, of course, a procedure which may be attended with great difficulty. The route is indicated in conditions such as diaphragmatic hernia, lesions of the upper reaches of the stomach such as carcinoma and leiomyoma, ulcer, diverticulum, etc. So too, lesions of oesophagus, e.g., carcinoma, stricture, diverticulum, etc., splenectomy, in difficult cases, are best dealt with thus.

In all surgery where the pleural cavity is widely open the lung collapses. As positive pressure is essential, it is of the first importance to ensure that the collapsed lung is inflated each half-hour to prevent postoperative complications, such as atelectasis.

INCISION: The patient lies on the sound side. The incision depends on the case. Routinely one of the lower ribs is removed, e.g., 8th or 9th. If oesophagogastric anastomosis is contemplated then the 8th rib is resected by an overlying incision and if the anastomosis is to be high, the incision will curve up between scapula and vertebral column to admit of section of 7th, 6th, and 5th ribs lateral to costo-transverse articulations. It is unwise to resect the 7th rib as it is then difficult to obtain easy access to the upper abdomen. Thus if the operation is mainly abdominal it will be found more advisable to take out the 9th rib.

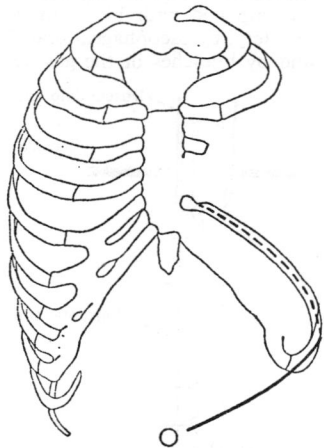

Fig. 751.—Showing the laparotomy incision (thick black line) and its extension for rib removal (dotted line).

About one-third of cases of cancer of oesophagus or upper stomach are found at operation to be inoperable and it is wise to avoid a wide thoracotomy if inoperability is determinable by simpler means. This is not always possible, but in cases of carcinoma of gastric fundus or lower oesophagus it is good practice to commence the operation by an oblique incision from costal margin towards umbilicus, retract rectus medially and divide the peritoneum and lateral flat muscles in the line of the fibres of external oblique, insert the hand and palpate for liver or other secondaries or operability of a subdiaphragmatic neoplasm. If inoperability exists, the patient has been little disturbed. Should it be decided to proceed, the incision is extended back along the chosen rib, which can then be removed (*Fig.* 751). The diaphragm is opened from costal margin to oesophageal hiatus. In many cases rib resection is sufficient as it is advisable to maintain the integrity of costal margin when possible, e.g., splenectomy. Furthermore, by incising the diaphragm widely the upper abdomen can be adequately explored and a procedure such as gastro-enterostomy may be combined with supradiaphragmatic vagotomy. The incision from outer border of rectus to spine with division of costal margin and removal of a rib is a standard approach for total gastrectomy.

Oesophagogastric Anastomosis: The accomplishment of this procedure entails the observation of certain anatomical knowledge.

1. *The oesophagus* is supplied with blood in its upper part by the inferior thyroid artery, by oesophageal branches of the aorta in its main extent, and by branches of the gastric arteries and inferior

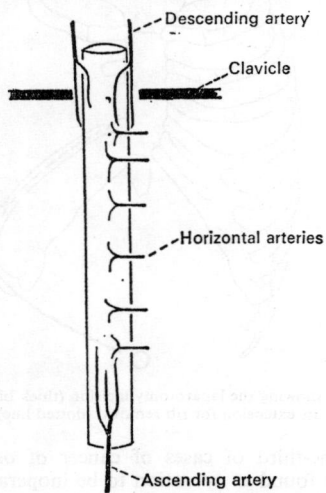

Fig. 752.—Schematic representation of the blood-supply of the oesophagus.

phrenic below. It is to be remembered, therefore, that rough handling or wide mobilization of the oesophagus may imperil its blood-supply, especially over its main extent where the aortic branches are distributed in a segmental manner (*Fig.* 752). There are not more than two or three aortic oesophageal arteries. They are slender, tenuous vessels.

2. In resecting the oesophagus it may be mobilized in its whole extent having regard to its relations. In its midzone the right pleural sac is in contact with it and may readily be torn especially in cases of cicatricial stenosis. This is not a serious matter unless infection

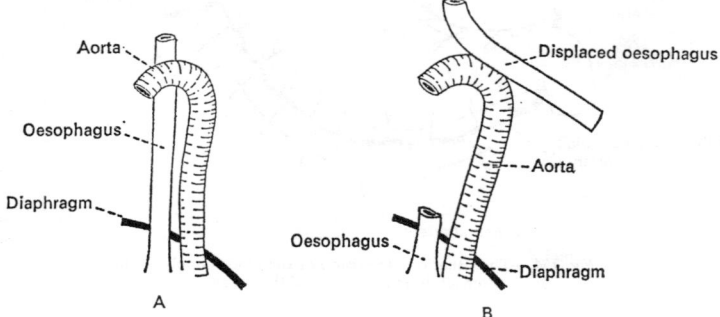

Fig. 753.—A, The normal relationship. B, The divided oesophagus has been displaced lateral to the aortic arch.

exists and providing the anaesthetist can cope with possible temporary collapse of both lungs. The thoracic duct crosses behind the oseophagus from the 7th to the 5th vertebrae and then continues up along its left border. It enjoys a remarkable immunity to injury. Should it be torn, as indicated by an escape of milky fluid, its ends should be tied. The lymph finds alternative routes to the venous system and the accident is usually not attended with any dire consequence if it be recognized and dealt with as outlined. The oesophagus may be dissected free behind the aortic arch by finger dissection. The pleura is incised above the arch just posterior to the left subclavian artery where the oesophagus may be freed and, if disconnected from stomach, threaded through under the arch and pulled out above it (*Fig.* 753).

3. *The stomach* has a lesser curve which is short and relatively immobile because of fixation by the left gastric artery and its branches. When this vessel is cut there is considerable mobility of this curvature. If the stomach is now freed from its omental and ligamentous ties and diaphragmatic attachments it can be brought to the upper aperture of the thorax. The blood-supply is adequately maintained if the two arteries entering from its right are preserved—the large right gastro-epiploic and the small right gastric. It is necessary,

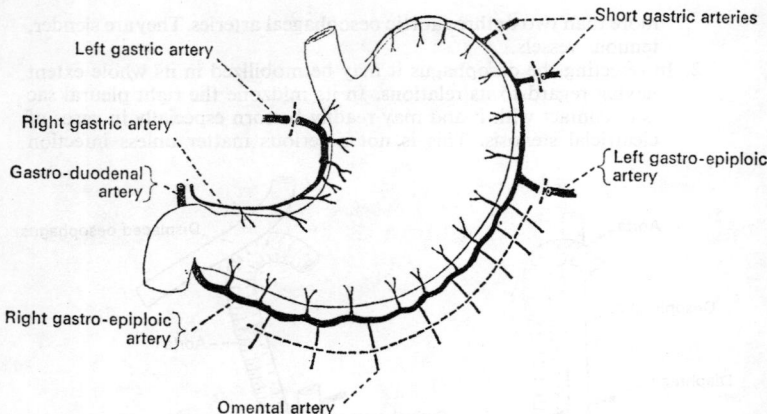

Fig. 754.—The situation of division of the blood-supply to the stomach in mobilization of the organ.

however, to preserve carefully the vascular arcades to ensure a free passage for the collateral circulation (*Fig.* 754).

In such a manner then it becomes feasible to bring the stomach up to any desired level in the left pleural cavity and oesophagogastric anastomosis may be carried out below or above the aortic arch. Sweet brought the stomach through the upper aperture of the thorax and joined it to the cervical oesophagus. The intrathoracic stomach is well tolerated. It tends to take on a tubular shape in this situation.

4. It happens on occasions that most or all of the stomach is removed. In such cases the jejunum is anastomosed to the oesophagus. It is usually possible to bring a loop of jejunum through the transverse mesocolon and join it to the oesophagus. If the loop will not reach high enough two courses are possible:
   a. Divide the main arteries to the loop, protecting the arcades which will carry the collateral (Sweet).
   b. Divide the jejunum and perform an anastomosis in Y (Roux) (*Fig.* 755).

Owing to the anatomical fact that the oesophagus has no serous covering, the new suture line is a cause of concern. It may be rendered more secure by using one of two procedures. If enough stomach is available, this organ may be pulled up and sutured to the oesophagus in such a way that the new suture line is buried; or the brilliant device of Roscoe Graham may be used of suturing the one limb of the small gut loop to the other over the anastomosis (*Fig.* 756).

THE ANATOMY OF SURGICAL APPROACH 797

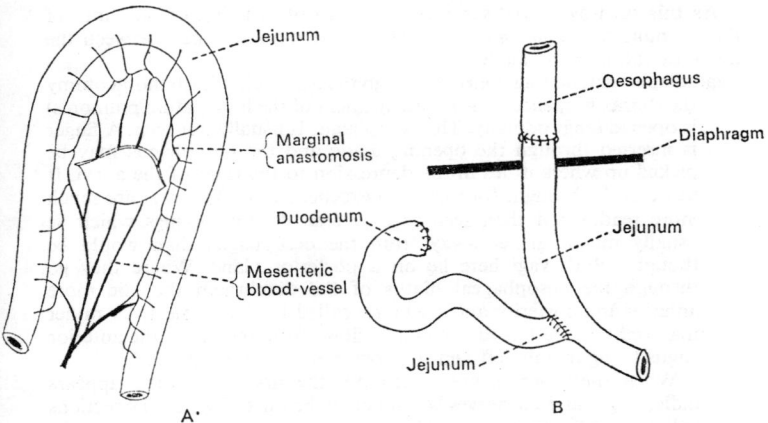

Fig. 755.—A, Lengthening the small gut loop by dividing its arteries, the marginal anastomosis being preserved. B, Anastomosis in Y.

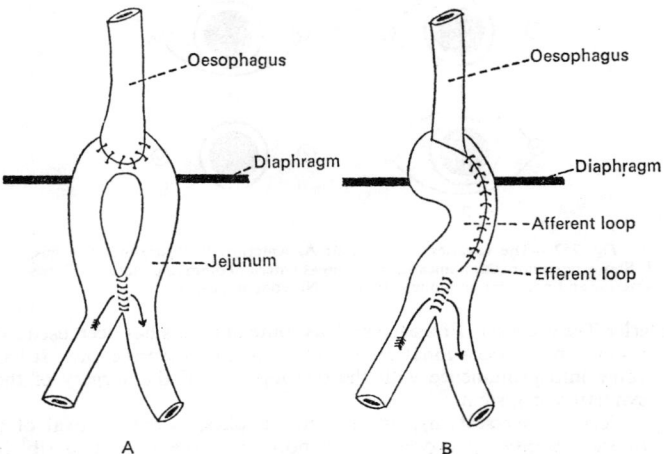

Fig. 756.—A, Oesophagojejunal anastomosis. The entero-anastomosis shown is unnecessary. B, The Roscoe Graham manœuvre. The entero-anastomosis is obligatory.

798 A SYNOPSIS OF SURGICAL ANATOMY

As this turn-over necessarily produces an obstruction of one limb of the jejunum it is a *sine qua non* that an entero-anastomosis between the limbs of the loop be made.

Supradiaphragmatic Vagotomy: Through the usual left 9th rib thoracotomy the thorax is opened. The broad ligament of the lung (latum pulmonis) is opened longitudinally. The oesophagus is usually not seen. A finger is inserted through the opening made and the oesophagus may be picked up where it lies in the depression to the right of the aorta. It can then be brought forward into excellent view. The vagi are much more readily felt than seen as they feel like taut strings which lie usually much farther away from the oesophagus than would be thought. Both vagi here lie on a posterior plane. Where they go through the oesophageal hiatus of the diaphragm they lie more anterior and posterior and are better called by these adjectives rather than right and left as each contains fibres from the other, the anterior vagus being mainly left and the posterior mainly right trunks.

When these nerves are pulled on, the first bifurcation appears indicating that if the nerves be cut below their first division the sections will be subdiaphragmatic. The anatomical arrangements over the lower oesophagus are very variable. They fall into the following groups (*Fig.* 757):

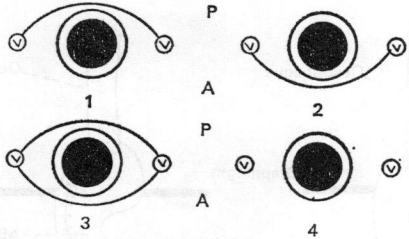

Fig. 757.—The vagaries of the vagi: A, Anterior. P, Posterior. V, vagus. 1, Shows posterior communications. 2, Shows anterior communications. 3, Shows anterior and posterior communications. 4, No communications.

Posterior Transthoracic Procedures: This route of access has been used for a long time in occasional cases such as costotransversectomy. It has come into prominence with the development of the surgery of the sympathetic system.

Costotransversectomy, as the name implies, is the removal of a thoracic transverse process and a portion of the associated rib. It finds its usefulness in the drainage of prevertebral abscess, due to causes such as tuberculosis or mediastinitis. The incision is transverse and divides the outer components of the erector spinae after trapezius

THE ANATOMY OF SURGICAL APPROACH

and perhaps latissimus dorsi have been split in the direction of their fibres. The erector receives a segmental nerve-supply and is not therefore deprived of its nerve-supply if divided transversely. The transversus spinalis has a similar nerve-supply and may be dealt with in the same way. Transverse process of vertebra and inner end of rib are thus exposed and may be removed. The posterior mediastinum and vertebral body are thus brought into the operative field. Operations on the sympathetic system to the limbs are dealt with in Chapter XLV, p. 633.

DENERVATION OF THE HEART: The accelerator nerve impulses to the heart[1] travel from the cord to the heart via the thoracic cardiac nerves passing through the 2nd to 5th thoracic ganglia on the way via the white rami communicantes of the corresponding intercostal nerves. Fibres carrying impulses of cardiac pain pass through the upper 3rd to 5th thoracic ganglia and some of the fibres run express through the upper thoracic ganglia to reach the inferior and middle cervical ones. From there the impulses travel via the middle and inferior cervical cardiac nerves from the heart.

It follows that removal of the 2nd to 5th thoracic ganglia on both sides will prevent any accelerator impulses reaching the heart and that removal of the inferior cervical and upper 3rd to 5th thoracic sympathetic ganglia on both sides will prevent any fibres conducting cardiac pain from reaching the sensorium (*Fig.* 758).

Smithwick et al.[2] make the following observations regarding the cardiac accelerator nerves:

a. Sympathetic cardiac denervation has no adverse effect on the coronary circulation.

b. All sympathetic cardiac nerves can be interrupted and still leave the heart an adequate accelerator response through reduction in vagal tone and the chemical mediation of adrenaline.

c. All accelerator fibres arise below the stellate ganglion—none travel via the cervical cardiac branches and few if any come from ganglion T. 1.

d. The outflow from ganglion T. 2 is most important.

e. The outflow from the right is slightly greater than from the left.

f. Unilateral denervation is probably of no therapeutic value in the control of a rapid heart rate.

g. Resection of the cardio-accelerator fibres in man is helpful in hypertensives with unusual degrees of tachycardia, and in patients with exertional or emotional tachycardia.

The nerve-supply of the heart is interfered with surgically in two conditions: for ischaemic pain (angina) and for tachycardia

---

[1] Cannon, W. B., and associates, *Am. J. Physiol.*, 1926, 66, 326.
[2] Smithwick, R. H., Chapman, E. M., Kinsey, D., and Whitelaw, G. P., *Surgery*, 1949, 26, 727.

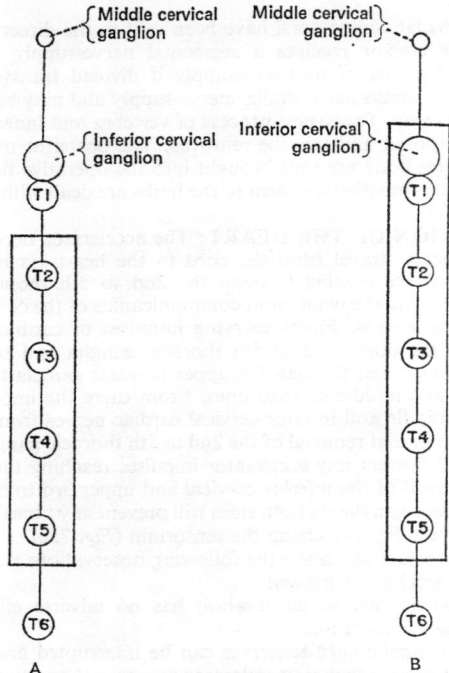

*Fig. 758.—A, The neurectomy necessary to cure tachycardia.
B, The neurectomy necessary to remove cardiac pain.*

such as is sometimes associated with hypertension either before or after operation. In either case relief of symptoms is secured by attack on the upper thoracic sympathetic ganglia as through these structures pass the fibres conducting cardiac pain and also the cardiac accelerator fibres. The operation is sometimes indicated in people with gravely damaged hearts who are unable to tolerate much surgical insult. There are two routes available—anterior and posterior—just as for upper limb denervation. It is wise that prior to deciding on the approach the patient be tested to see whether he can tolerate the prone position for two hours, as this position puts an increased strain on the heart. Should the heart not stand up to this strain the anterior route should be used.

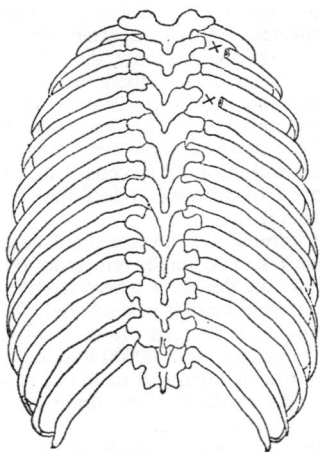

Fig. 759.—The marks X show bone removal in performing cardiac denervation by the Smithwick approach.

The posterior operation is essentially the same as that for upper limb denervation excepting that 3·7 cm. each of the 2nd and 4th ribs are removed. The intercostal nerves are not interfered with (*Fig.* 759).

The operation is performed first on the side where most pain is felt. At a later date it can be done on the other side if pain there is severe.

The relief from or reduction of pain consequent on the ganglionectomy is not the only benefit to the victim of angina. The removal of the sympathetic motor innervation results in increased myocardial performance with abolition of or delay in the appearance of ischaemic changes in the electrocardiogram during exercise (Birkett et al.[1])

ADRENALECTOMY: There are several noteworthy features in the surgical anatomy of the glands. They may or may not have a fascial investment separate from that of the kidney and it is not advisable to open the fascia covering the kidney when separate (Cattell). This organ is better retracted and protected if the renal fascia is left intact. In one in each 250 cases the kidney and adrenal rest in a common compartment and are attached to each other (*see* p. 94) and care is then necessary to find the connective-tissue

[1] Birkett, D. A., Apthorp, G. H., Chamberlain, D. A., Hayward, G. W., and Tuckwell, E. G., *Br. med. J.*, 1965, **2**, 187.

cleavage line between the organs, through which separation should be effected. As there is often advanced renal pathology in cases requiring adrenalectomy, the kidney should be protected from bruising, etc., during operation.

The adrenal has a characteristic canary yellow colour. This should be recognized as it has happened on the left side that portions of the pancreas have been removed by mistake. The adrenal gland will not hold forceps. Parts of its investing fascia can be gripped by forceps to facilitate removal of the gland without tearing it.

The three adrenal arteries are small, and give off numerous tenuous branches. The single vein is as thick as a lead pencil and very short on the right where it enters the vena cava. It deserves great respect and is best secured after the gland has been mobilized. Should it be torn the accident is best dealt with by suturing the vena cava with 00000 braided silk.

Cade[1] has drawn attention to abnormalities of the adrenal veins. These may be double and drain into unusual situations, e.g., the inferior phrenic vein.

The approach to the adrenals by a transverse abdominal incision above the umbilicus is finding increasing favour. It presents the advantage that both adrenals can be explored or removed as a one-stage procedure, and exploration of the abdomen can be carried out. Another point is that the adrenal vein can be secured before removal of the gland is begun—a factor of importance in dealing with phaeochromocytoma where handling of the gland before securing the vein is fraught with danger.

ABNORMALITIES: One adrenal may be congenitally missing. It is important to determine this in cases where it is not planned to carry out total adrenalectomy. This purpose may be achieved by opening the peritoneum and palpating the opposite side. Sometimes a second incision is necessary. Accessory adrenal tissue— see p. 432.

Congenital Atresia of Oesophagus: The posterior transthoracic approach is advised by Ladd and Swenson[2] in certain cases of congenital oesophageal atresia and tracheobronchial fistula. The operation must necessarily be performed as soon as the diagnosis is established, i.e., a day or two after birth. The infant lies on the left side, a folded towel under the chest. The incision begins at 2nd right rib, runs down between vertebral spine and inner border of scapula to the level of the 6th rib and then tails off laterally for 2·5 cm. Trapezius and rhomboids are divided. Two cm. each of 2nd to 6th ribs are resected.

[1] Cade, Sir Stanford, *Ann. R. Coll. Surg.*, 1954, 15, 71.
[2] Ladd, William E., and Swenson, Orvar, *Ann. Surg.*, 1947, 125, 23.

The intercostal structures are tied and cut and the pleura carefully pushed away from the inner ends of ribs and vertebral column, exposing the sympathetic chain and azygos vein. The latter structure is surprisingly large and is divided or retracted in. The vagus nerve is then seen lying on trachea and oesophagus.

III. SURGICAL APPROACH TO THE JOINTS

Operative surgery is largely the application of anatomical knowledge. In no branch of surgery does anatomy play a greater part than in the approach to the joints. It is a principle of the construction of the body that big vessels and nerves lie on the flexor aspects of joints, being afforded better protection thus. The surgical corollary follows that joints are never 'approached' from their flexor surfaces. The surgical approach to a joint is therefore from its extensor aspect or to one side, usually lateral. We owe to Theodore Kocher, anatomical and surgical master, many of the best joint incisions. The debt of surgery is no less to Langenbeck.

We shall consider the surgical approach to the: (1) Shoulder-joint; (2) Elbow-joint; (3) Wrist-joint; (4) Hip-joint; (5) Knee-joint; (6) Ankle-joint.

1. Shoulder-joint: There are three lines of approach to the articulation: (*a*) Anterior incision; (*b*) Posterior incision; (*c*) Superior incision.

ANTERIOR APPROACH: The method of Ollier. This is the most generally used of the three. It gives access to the upper part of the humeral shaft and subdeltoid bursa, as well as to the joint.

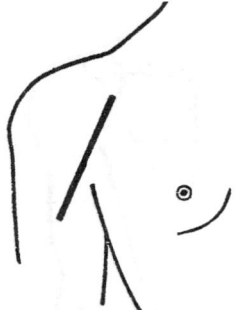

Fig. 760.—Anterior approach to shoulder-joint.

INCISION: Made in the sulcus separating the deltoid from the great pectoral (*Fig.* 760)—in other words, in the line of the upper part of the cephalic vein. It begins at the coracoid process and extends for 10 – 14 cm. down the arm.

STRUCTURES ENCOUNTERED: The cephalic vein is exposed and retracted inwards with the pectoralis major. The deltoid is retracted outwards. Several structures are exposed in the depths of the incision. From above down these are: (*a*) Tip of the coracoid giving origin to the coracobrachialis; (*b*) Tuberosities of the humerus on rotating the limb in and out; (*c*) Surgical neck of the humerus, mostly covered by—(*d*) Tendon of the great pectoral; (*e*) Bicipital or intertubercular sulcus containing the long tendon of the biceps. N.B.—The long head of the biceps is *covered* by the pectoral tendon.

Note that the muscles attached to the tuberosities (subscapularis to lesser, and supraspinatus, infraspinatus, and teres minor to the greater) conceal the joint capsule. The latter is exposed by detaching the muscles from the tuberosities or by detaching the tuberosities themselves. The joint can then be opened. Note that the vessels and nerves of the axilla are not seen.

POSTERIOR APPROACH: We owe this to Kocher. It is used when the glenoid cavity is involved by the disease or if the latter is very diffuse.

INCISION: A curved one commencing over the acromioclavicular joint, extending back along the inner border of the acromion, then curving over the junction of the acromion with the spine of the scapula, towards the posterior axillary fold, ending 5 cm. above it (*Fig.* 761).

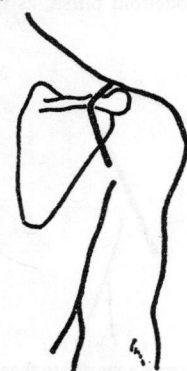

Fig. 761.—Posterior approach to shoulder-joint.

STRUCTURES ENCOUNTERED: The upper part of the cut enters the acromioclavicular joint, by dividing the superior ligament of the joint. The trapezius is then encountered and divided from its

THE ANATOMY OF SURGICAL APPROACH 805

acromial attachment. Below the scapular spine the deltoid is found and is detached from the spine. The supra- and infraspinatus are now exposed and freed from the acromion, which is chiselled through at its junction with the spine and can then be thrown laterally with the deltoid, exposing the upper, outer, and posterior aspects of the joint, covered by spinati and teres minor. These muscles are detached from their insertions, giving free access to the capsule.

Observe that no important vessels or nerves are exposed, though the suprascapular nerve may be seen passing from supra- to infraspinatus through the great scapular notch.

SUPERIOR APPROACH: Is used only in those cases where the action of the deltoid (abduction of the arm to a right-angle) is lost or will not be subsequently required. It is used almost solely where the surgeon wishes to secure bony union (ankylosis) of the humerus with the scapula—arthrodesis. The operation is most often necessitated by poliomyelitis.

INCISION: Extends right across the top of the shoulder (*Fig.* 762).

STRUCTURES ENCOUNTERED: The deltoid muscle is seen, divided, and turned down, exposing the head of the humerus and great tuberosity with the muscles attached. By separating these the capsule is widely exposed. The axillary nerve and anterior and posterior circumflex humeral vessels are seen.

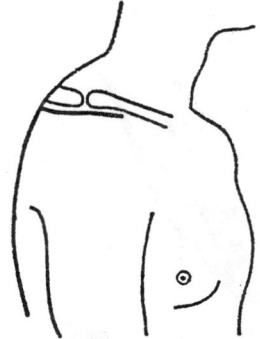

Fig. 762.—Superior approach to shoulder-joint.

2. **Elbow-joint:** Two methods are in general use: (*a*) Kocher's method—used for wide exposure of the joint, e.g., to excise the whole articulation; (*b*) Langenbeck's method—used for a lesser degree of exposure, e.g., to remove a piece of loose bone from the joint.

KOCHER'S METHOD:

INCISION: Commences 5 cm. above the joint line over the lateral epicondylar ridge and extends vertically down to the head of the radius between the brachioradialis and radial extensors laterally and the triceps medially (*Fig.* 763). It then trends inwards, passing along the outer border of the anconeus between that muscle and the extensor carpi ulnaris, tailing off on to the inner aspect of the forearm. The muscles around the back and sides of the joint are separated from the bones, exposing the whole posterior aspect of the capsule and the bone-ends. No structures are exposed other than those mentioned, if we except the supinator and the interosseous recurrent artery, which may lie between the anconeus and the extensor carpi ulnaris, though it is usually under the anconeus. The planning of the incision was a surgical inspiration. It passes between those muscles supplied by the radial nerve before it pierces the lateral intermuscular septum, which is medial to it, while the muscles lateral to the incision are supplied by the nerve after it has pierced the septum.

LANGENBECK'S METHOD:

INCISION: A vertical centrally placed one at the back of the elbow (*Fig.* 764). Its centre is at the tip of the olecranon. It divides the triceps in the direction of its fibres above and the anconeus below.

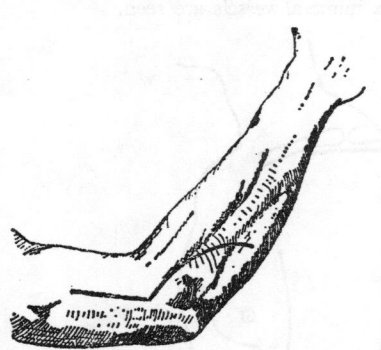

Fig. 763.—Posterolateral aspect of right arm and forearm showing Kocher's method of approach to elbow-joint.

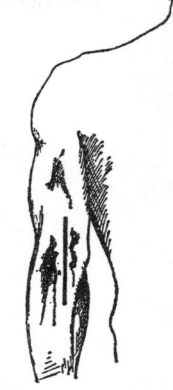

Fig. 764.—Langenbeck's approach to elbow-joint.

The joint is exposed by separating the muscles from the bones. The incision may injure the nerve to the anconeus, which runs in the line of the cut in the substance of the triceps. The incision

is a good one, very generally used for the more minor operations on the joint.
3. **Wrist-Joint:** From the anatomical relations round the joint, incisions can be neither anterior (because of flexor sheaths and large vessels and nerves) nor on the radial border (because of the radial vessels). The approach is therefore: (*a*) Dorsal; or (*b*) Medial.

DORSAL APPROACH: The Bockel-Langenbeck method.

INCISION: Passes in the long axis of the limb just radial to the extensor indicis proprius (*Fig.* 765). The dorsal carpal ligament is encountered beneath the skin. To the outer side of the cut is the extensor pollicis longus and beneath that are the radial extensors. The tendons are retracted and the joint capsule, on which is the dorsal carpal arch, is exposed. The volar interosseous artery and dorsal interosseous nerve lie in the groove for the extensor indicis, between it and the bone.

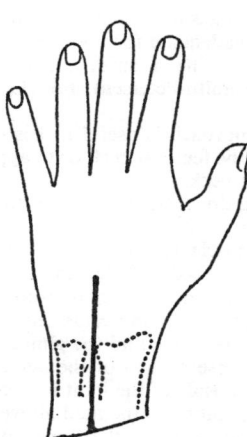
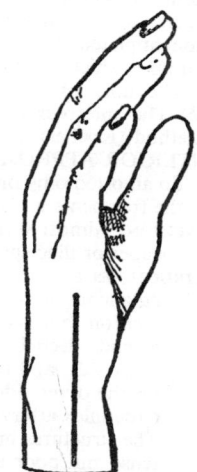

Fig. 765.—Dorsal approach to wrist-joint.

Fig. 766.—Medial approach to wrist-joint.

MEDIAL APPROACH: The method of Sir Patrick Heron-Watson.

INCISION: A vertical one on the ulnar border of the hand and forearm with its centre at the wrist-joint (*Fig.* 766). It begins 5 cm. above the ulnar styloid and extends to the middle of the fifth metacarpal bone.

STRUCTURES ENCOUNTERED: The dorsal branch of the ulnar nerve is met at the proximal end of the incision. It is important and is preserved. The incision passes between the extensor and flexor carpi ulnaris. The former is divided at its insertion into the base of the fifth metacarpal, and it is then possible to clear the whole of the dorsal aspect of the carpus by raising the extensor tendons. The same process is carried out on the front of the carpus, though in so doing it is necessary to sever the pisiform and hook of hamate from the carpus. The whole carpus may now be removed if necessary and also the bases of the bones with which it articulates. No important vessel or nerve is seen in the operation.

4. Hip-joint: This joint is anatomically the most stable of all the limb joints. It lies a long way from the surface, and the acetabulum and head of the femur make a very close articulation. It is therefore the most difficult of access of all the limb joints and its approach in an adult subject is always a formidable undertaking. The methods of access are planned according to the magnitude of the procedure contemplated, a certain type of incision being adequate for one purpose which would be wholly inadequate for another.

The lines of approach are: (*a*) The anterior method (Huter); (*b*) The antero-external method (Smith-Petersen); (*c*) The posterior method (Kocher).

ANTERIOR APPROACH: This approach is useful if it is desired to do an osteotomy or division of the femoral neck or to approximate the fragments in fracture of the neck.

INCISION: Almost vertical, passing down the thigh from the anterior superior iliac spine (*Fig.* 767).

STRUCTURES ENCOUNTERED: The fascia lata is exposed. The lateral cutaneous nerve is to the inner side of the upper end of the incision, but is cut a little below as it passes outwards. The cut extends deep between the sartorius and rectus femoris on the inner side, and the tensor fasciae latae and the gluteus minimus on the outer side. The transverse branch of the lateral femoral circumflex artery is cut. The capsule of the joint is then exposed. The structures in front of the joint (enumerated above) are very tense and poor exposure is obtained, so that no very extensive procedure can be attempted by this route.

ANTERO-EXTERNAL APPROACH (*Fig.* 767): The addition of an external limb to the vertical incision gives vastly better access than the anterior approach. This method is especially useful for operations in case of congenital dislocation of the femoral head, e.g., making a ledge above the acetabulum to prevent the head slipping out.

INCISION: Precisely as in the anterior method, with the addition of a 7·5 cm. extension backwards from the upper end along the crest of the ilium.

THE ANATOMY OF SURGICAL APPROACH

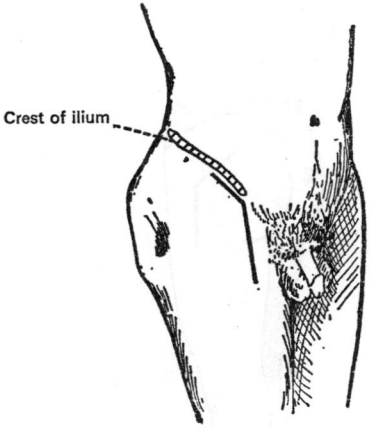

Fig. 767.—The lower limb of the incision is the anterior line of approach to the hip-joint. The addition of the lateral extension at the upper end of the incision transforms it into the antero-external (Smith-Petersen) approach.

STRUCTURES ENCOUNTERED: The same as in the vertical part of the cut. The external limb of the incision goes through tensor fasciae latae down to the bone, and this muscle and the anterior parts of the two lesser glutei are stripped off the outer aspect of the dorsum ilii, carrying with them the superior gluteal nerve. Thus the superior surface of the joint and femoral neck are exposed in addition to the front of the joint.

POSTERIOR APPROACH: This approach is much the best and most popular for extensive operative procedures on the joint, e.g., excision.

INCISION: This is an angled one (*Fig.* 768). The angle is at the tip (anterior or posterior) of the great trochanter. The lower limb of the incision extends vertically down the limb axis for 7·5 cm. The upper limb extends towards the posterior superior iliac spine in the direction of the fibres of the gluteus maximus.

STRUCTURES ENCOUNTERED: The tendinous insertion of the gluteus maximus is divided where it meets the fascia lata, and here are found branches of the lateral circumflex artery. The gluteus itself is divided in the direction of its fibres, many branches of the gluteal arteries being cut in the process. Kocher[1] states that when the gluteus maximus is poorly developed it need not be divided but its upper

---

[1] *Text-book of Operative Surgery*, 1911, 304. London.

810 A SYNOPSIS OF SURGICAL ANATOMY

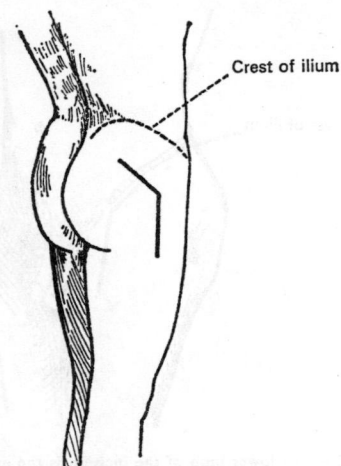

Fig. 768.—Kocher's method of approach to hip-joint.

border exposed and pulled downwards. Having dealt with the great gluteus and with a layer of fat beneath it, there appears the interval between the two minor glutei above and the piriformis below. The two former muscles are detached from their trochanteric attachment, or alternatively the trochanter with its muscles is chiselled off and retracted up and back. The obturators and piriformis are pulled down. Thus the entire posterior, lateral, and even anterior aspects of the capsule and neck of the femur are displayed. No large vessel or nerve is seen throughout. The operation is thus far merely an anatomical exercise.

5. **Knee-joint:** The type of incision varies greatly according to the procedure to be carried out.

CLASSIFICATION OF METHODS OF APPROACH TO THE JOINT:

1. FOR EXCISION OF THE BONE-ENDS FORMING THE JOINT:
    a. Lateral J incision—Kocher's incision.
    b. Horizontal incision—Volkmann's incision.
2. FOR EXTENSIVE INTRA-ARTICULAR MANIPULATIONS AND SOME OPERATIONS ON THE MENISCI:
    a. Patella-splitting method—Sir Robert Jones's incision.
    b. Patella-displacing method—Timbrell Fisher's incision.
3. FOR NON-EXTENSIVE INTRA-ARTICULAR PROCEDURES:
    a. For Dealing with the Menisci in Uncomplicated Cases: An

incision in the interval between the anterior border of the tibial collateral ligament and the inner border of the patella and patellar ligament.

b. *For Dealing with Loose Bodies in the Joint:* (i) In the anterior part of the joint—parapatellar incision; (ii) In the posterior part of the joint—lateral incision.

EXCISION OF BONE-ENDS:

KOCHER'S LATERAL J INCISION: This method gives exposure of the entire joint, having the great advantage of retaining intact the quadriceps extensor mechanism. The incision begins over the vastus lateralis 10 cm. above the upper border of the patella, passing vertically down 1·8 cm. lateral to that bone, then curving in to end at the anterior border of the tibia just below the tubercle (*Fig.* 769). The cut is deepened through skin and muscle, splitting the vastus lateralis and its tendinous expansion and thus exposing the interior of the joint. The tibial tubercle is detached, carrying with it the patellar ligament, and the quadriceps tendon, the patella, and its ligament are turned medially. The whole interior of the joint is exposed.

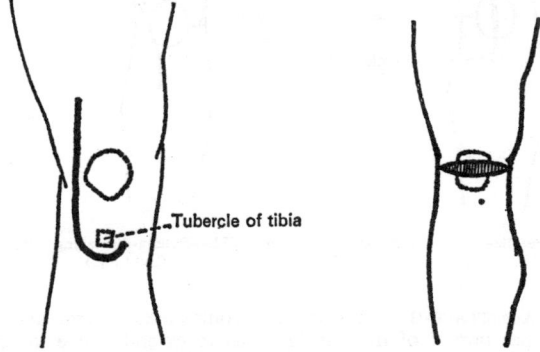

Fig. 769.—Kocher's lateral approach to knee-joint. (Right leg.)

Fig. 770.—Horizontal elliptical incisions for excision of knee-joint. The integuments defined by the ellipse are removed. (Right leg.)

HORIZONTAL INCISION: This is a transverse incision crossing the patella, or it may consist of two curved incisions, meeting at the sides, the ellipse of skin so outlined being removed if it is anticipated that the integuments will be redundant after the operation (*Fig.* 770). The patellar ligament is divided, and the lateral ligaments and the joint so exposed, or the patella may be removed with the skin ellipse.

FOR EXTENSIVE INTRA-ARTICULAR MANIPULATIONS:

PATELLA-SPLITTING INCISION: This is a vertical or slightly curved incision extending from a point 7·5 cm. above the patella to the tibial tubercle (*Fig.* 771). It inclines outwards in its upper part, following the direction of the main fibres of the quadriceps tendon. The quadriceps tendon, patella, and its ligament are divided longitudinally. The outer half of the patella should be bigger than the inner half, as the two halves are to be dislocated, and the outer half is easier to displace than the inner. The infrapatellar pad of fat is next encountered and divided to the inner side of the plica patellaris synovialis.

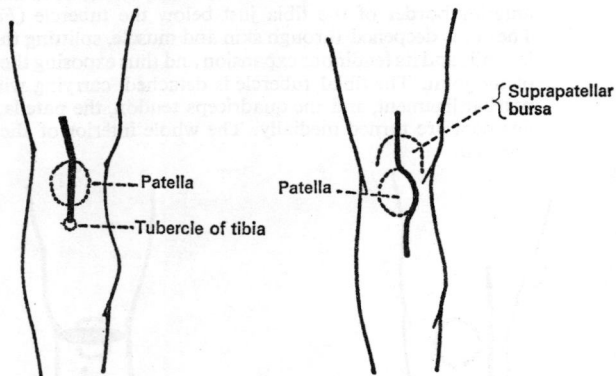

Fig. 771.—Patella-splitting incision. (Right leg.)

Fig. 772.—Patella-displacing incision. (Right leg.)

PATELLA-DISPLACING INCISION: This commences 10 cm. above the upper border of the patella so as to extend above the suprapatellar pouch, curves along the inner border of the patella, and ends medial to the tibial tubercle (*Fig.* 772). This cut is semilunar in shape. The capsule is divided 0·6 cm. from the inner border of the patella. The incision through the capsule is extended down medial to the patellar ligament and into the quadriceps tendon above, and the patella and its ligaments are displaced out, exposing the whole joint.

The incision is planned to damage the quadriceps and its extensions as little as possible and to avoid an incision through the cartilage of the patella, as it has been seen (p. 733) that such traumata are slow to heal.

THE ANATOMY OF SURGICAL APPROACH

APPROACH TO THE MENISCI: All incisions to approach the medial meniscus (which is the injured one in the vast majority of cases) are made in the space bounded above and below by the inner condyles of the femur and tibia, laterally by the inner border of the patella and its ligaments, and medially by the anterior border of the tibial collateral ligament.

INCISION: This may be: (1) Transverse, between the bone-ends; (2) Oblique, sloping upwards and forwards; (3) Curved with

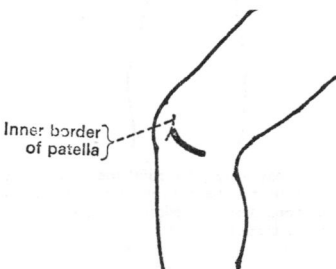

Fig. 773.—Incision recommended by Sir Robert Jones for gaining access to the medial meniscus.

the convexity forwards (*Fig.* 773); (4) Curved with the convexity backwards (*Fig.* 774); (5) Vertical.

When skin and fascia are divided, the capsule is exposed, and under it the synovial membrane, which is separated from the capsule by a fair amount of fat.

An incision 7·5 cm. long, or less, is sufficient for dealing with injuries to the menisci.[1] Any method of approach to these structures which entails injury to the collateral ligament is unsound,[2] as the integrity of this ligament is essential to the stability of the joint.

Similarly planned incisions to the above, but lateral to the patella, are used for dealing with the lateral meniscus. Where both may be injured, the medial should be explored first, as it is possible to examine the lateral meniscus from the medial incision, but not vice versa.[3] Fairbanks[4] states that the split-patella operation is better avoided when both menisci are to be examined. It is better to make two incisions, the one medial and the other lateral to the patella.

---

[1] Jones and Lovett, *Orthopaedic Surgery*, 1923, 84. London.
[2] A. G. Timbrell Fisher, *Internal Derangements of the Knee-joint*, 1924, 60. London.
[3] P. Jenner Verrall, Carson's *Modern Operative Surgery*, 99.
[4] *Br. med. J.* 1930, 1, 582.

814 A SYNOPSIS OF SURGICAL ANATOMY

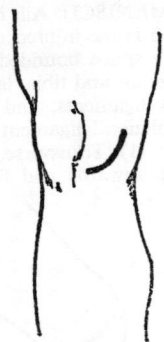

Fig. 774.—Incision for exposure of medial meniscus as recommended by Timbrell Fisher. This incision has the advantage of avoiding the infra-patellar branch of the long saphenous nerve, division of which may be followed by a painful neuroma. (*Naughton Dunn.*)

APPROACH TO THE BACK OF THE JOINT: This may be needed for loose or foreign bodies which remain at the back of the joint, or for drainage of the joint.

INCISION: A longitudinal one on the inner or outer side as the case may be. On the outer side the capsule is exposed in front of the biceps tendon, while on the inner side the incision goes down between the semimembranosus and semitendinosus. In each case the capsule is opened behind the corresponding collateral ligament.

6. **Ankle-joint:** The ankle-joint may be opened through: (*a*) The lateral J incision of Kocher; (*b*) The anterior incision of McCrae-Aitken. The former gives much more extensive exposure and is used for excising the bone-ends forming the joint.

LATERAL J INCISION OF KOCHER:

INCISION: Begins 10 cm. above the lateral malleolus midway between the fibula and tendo Achillis and curves round 2·5 cm. below the lateral malleolus, ending at the outer border of the peroneus tertius, thus avoiding the superficial peroneal nerve (*Fig.* 775).

STRUCTURES ENCOUNTERED: The peronei and their sheaths are exposed below. The sheath is slit up and the tendons are pulled out of the way or they are divided. The capsule is exposed in front of the fibula, and the three bands of the lateral ligament (anterior and posterior talofibular and calcaneofibular ligaments) are divided. The tendons on the front of the tibia are pulled inwards, and the front of the capsule is opened. In a similar way the back of the

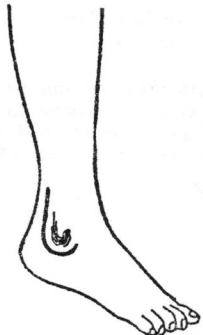

Fig. 775.—Kocher's lateral J-shaped incision for excision of ankle-joint.

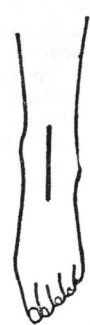

Fig. 776.—Anterior approach to ankle-joint.

tibia is exposed by retracting the tendons and dividing the capsule, and the foot can then be dislocated in on the leg and the entire joint surface rendered accessible, without an artery or nerve being seen.

McCRAE-AITKEN METHOD: For less extensive procedures in the ankle-joint.

INCISION: A vertical one 10 cm. long on the front of the joint (*Fig.* 776). The tendons and their sheaths are hooked aside and the anterior part of the capsule is exposed.

IV. SURGICAL APPROACH TO THE LONG BONES

Humerus: The shaft of this bone is much more difficult to expose than that of the femur. The reasons are:
1. The axillary and brachial neurovascular bundle is related to the inner part of the shaft above, and the front of the shaft below.
2. The musculocutaneous nerve crosses the front of the shaft very obliquely from medial to lateral.
3. The radial (musculospiral) nerve crosses the back of the shaft from medial to lateral.

EXPOSURE OF THE HUMERAL SHAFT:
UPPER THIRD: The incision is the same as that for the anterior exposure of the shoulder-joint, i.e., between contiguous borders of deltoid and pectoralis major, along the upper part of the cephalic vein.
LOWER TWO-THIRDS: An incision is made in the line of the medial or lateral intermuscular septum. If the incision is a lateral one, the radial nerve is in the same line as the cut. If it is medial, the incision is between the median and ulnar nerves.

WHOLE SHAFT: The incision devised by Arnold K. Henry[1] is ideal and anatomically sound. It permits of the exposure of the humeral shaft in whole or part.

To expose the whole shaft the skin incision follows the *cephalic vein* from the tip of the coracoid process to the level of the bend of the elbow, and continues in the midline of the flexor aspect of the forearm in its upper third (*Fig.* 777).

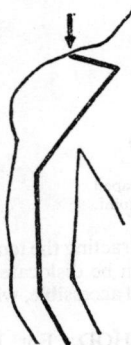

Fig. 777.—Henry's incision for exposure of whole length of humeral shaft. The black line represents the cut through skin and deep fascia. The arrow marks the acromio-clavicular joint. If it is desired to expose the shoulder-joint an incision is carried outwards (from the upper end of the main incision) along the anterior border of the clavicle, and the deltoid is detached from this bone and thrown laterally as a muscle-flap.

(The incision will of course be shorter if it is required to expose less of the shaft). The incision is deepened between the deltoid and pectoralis major above, and then along the outer edge of the biceps. The outer one-fourth of the brachialis muscle projects lateral to the biceps. This part of the brachialis is separated from the rest of this muscle by deepening the incision to the bone (*Fig.* 778). This part of the incision slopes inwards, reaching the bone in the midline. The outer part of the brachialis is in reality a migrated part of the triceps and is supplied by the radial nerve. Thus the nerve-supply of the brachialis is not impaired by this exposure.[2] The outer part of the brachialis forms a protection for the radial nerve when the muscles are stripped from the shaft. Note that the incision through the brachialis stops 3·7 cm. above the epicondyle so as not to enter the elbow-joint.

[1] *Br. J. Surg.*, 1924, **12**, 84.
[2] This is not Henry's explanation.

THE ANATOMY OF SURGICAL APPROACH

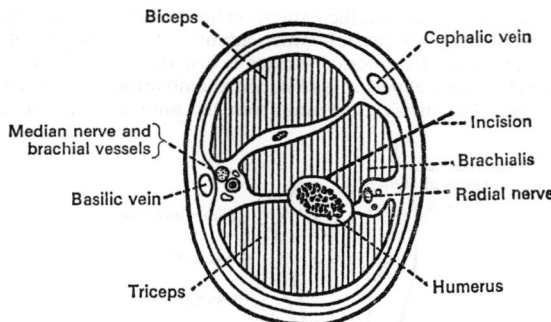

Fig. 778.—To show the manner in which Henry's incision for exposure of the humeral shaft avoids the radial nerve by splitting the brachialis.

Radius: This bone may be exposed in its whole length by an incision along the anterior border of the brachioradialis. This landmark is the frontier line between the structures on the inner side (flexors) supplied by the median nerve, and those on the outer side (extensors) supplied by the radial.[1] The incision in its lower two-thirds is also that for ligature of the radial artery. This artery and the superficial branch of the radial nerve lie in the line of the cut and are actually exposed by it, being retracted inwards. In the lower half of the forearm the nerve is retracted out and the artery in, as here the nerve is passing backwards and outwards. The supinator is exposed above and its fibres are detached and retracted out, care being taken of the dorsal interosseous nerve which is in the muscle at the level of the neck of the radius. The pronator quadratus below is detached and retracted in.

Ulna: The dorsal border is subcutaneous throughout its length. The bone may be exposed by an incision in this line, the extensor carpi ulnaris being lateral and the flexor carpi ulnaris medial.

Femur: The shaft may safely be exposed by an incision from the trochanter major to the outer condyle. This incision divides the iliotibial band and is deepened to the bone along the posterior border of the vastus lateralis, i.e., in the line of the lateral intermuscular septum. The incision cuts the transverse branch of the lateral femoral circumflex artery above and the superior lateral geniculate artery below. This incision passes through the vastus lateralis, in which lie the terminations of the perforating arteries and the descending branch of the lateral circumflex. The area of the cut is therefore vascular and the

---

[1] Kocher, *Text-book of Operative Surgery*, 1911, 312. London.

818 A SYNOPSIS OF SURGICAL ANATOMY

bone difficult to expose with the patient on his back. For these reasons Henry[1] has planned an incision which admits of the exposure of the femoral shaft along its anterior surface below the level of the small trochanter. Excellent exposure is obtained and no important structures are damaged. The incision extends from the anterior superior iliac

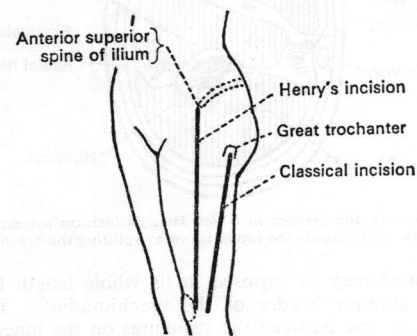

Fig. 779.—Showing classic incision for exposure of femoral shaft, and that suggested by Henry.

spine to the outer border of the patella (*Fig.* 779). The deep fascia being divided, the vastus lateralis is separated from the rectus femoris. Under these muscles lies the vastus intermedius. The nerve to the vastus lateralis and the descending branch of the lateral circumflex artery form a neurovascular bundle crossing the upper part of the vastus intermedius. They are retracted up and the muscle is divided down to the bone. The suprapatellar pouch extends three fingerbreadths above the upper patellar border. The cut is not extended so far down. If necessary the pouch may be separated from the femur without injury and this part of the shaft exposed, though efforts to free the pouch from the overlying quadriceps tendon will result in injury to the bursa and an opening into the knee-joint. Because of the existence of this extension from the knee-joint there can be no question that in cases of infection the lateral incision is safer, at least as far as the lower third of the bone is concerned.

Tibia: Like the ulna, the tibia may be exposed in its whole length along its subcutaneous anterior border or anteromedial surface.

Fibula: In exposure of this bone, it is necessary to remember that the common peroneal nerve winds round its neck, and that the superficial peroneal is related to the upper two-thirds of the lateral aspect of the shaft, lying between the peronei.

[1] *Br. J. Surg.*, 1924. 12, 84.

UPPER AND MIDDLE THIRDS: The incision is along the postero-lateral border in the line of the posterior intermuscular septum, exposing the peroneus longus in front and the soleus behind in the upper third, and the flexor longus hallucis behind in the middle third of the bone. At the upper part of the incision care is taken of the common peroneal nerve.

LOWER THIRD: The incision extends along the anterolateral border between the peroneus tertius in front and peroneus brevis behind.

WHOLE SHAFT: This may be exposed by an incision behind the peroneal muscles (Kocher).

INDEX

Abdomen, dermoids of, 427
— intercostal nerves supplying, 167
— lymph-glands of, (*Figs.* 331–333) 333
— sympathetic plexuses in, (*Fig.* 164) 176
— transthoracic approach to upper, (*Fig.* 751) 792
— upper, sympathetic supply to, 623
Abdominal aorta, aneurysms of, exposure and resection of, (*Fig.* 536) 561
— approach to sliding hernia, 689
— autonomic system, (*Figs.* 581–593) 618–631
— — — surgical applications of (*Figs.* 588–593) 624–631
— cavity of child, (*Figs.* 127, 128) 135
— course of vagus, (*Figs.* 585, 586) 620
— dislocation of testis, (*Fig.* 404) 415
— incision(s), anatomy of, (*Figs.* 699–717) 743–761
— — classification of, 744
— — dividing muscles, 745, (*Figs.* 702–704) 747, (*Figs.* 709–712) 751
— — — flat muscles, 754
— — — no muscles, (*Figs.* 700–706) 744
— — exploratory, 749
— — median, (*Figs.* 700, 701) 745
— — midline lower, 747
— — — upper, (*Fig.* 701) 745
— — paramedian, (*Figs.* 702–705) 747
— — principles governing, (*Fig.* 699) 744
— — splitting muscles, 745, (*Figs.* 713–717) 755
— — transverse, in adrenalectomy, 802
— inflammation in child, danger of, 135
— (internal) inguinal ring, 97, 406
— muscles, paralysis of, limp of, 578
— organs, palpation of, in testing for abnormalities, 590
— respiration in child, 133
— ring, subcutaneous (external), 219
— viscera, innervation of, (*Figs.* 581–587) 618
— — lower, parasympathetic supply to, (*Fig.* 587) 622
— — pain from, referred to low back, 695
— wall, anterior, extravasation of fluid in, 221
— — — incisions through, (*Figs.* 700–717) 461, 744
— — — superficial fascia of, (*Figs.* 203–205) 218

Abdominal wall, cold abscess at, 725, 726
— — posterior, incisions through, 745, (*Figs.* 718–720) 761
Abdominoperineal resection of rectum ligature of hypogastric arteries in, 554
Abducens nerve (6th), loss due to division of, 451
Abduction at shoulder, (*Figs.* 188, 189) 201
— of shoulder, 681
Abductor minimi digiti quinti, 286
— pollicis brevis, (*Fig.* 168) 182
— — longus, 258, 287
— — — origin of, 274
— — — stenosis of, 259
Aberrant breast tissue, cancer of, 374
— renal arteries, 534
— right ovarian vein compressing ureter, 536
Abridged left inferior vena cava, (*Fig.* 523 C, D) 543
Abscess(es), anorectal, (*Figs.* 110–113) 120
— cold (*see* Cold Abscesses)
— ischiorectal, (*Fig.* 114) 122
— pelvic, 742
— pelvirectal, (*Fig.* 115) 123
— subphrenic, (*Figs.* 680, 681) 727
Accessory bile-duct, (*Figs.* 70, 382 B) 81, 388
— — in lever, (*Fig.* 75 D) 85
— bones, (*Figs.* 212–222) 229–240
— — of foot, (*Figs.* 212–219) 229n, 230
— — hands, (*Fig.* 220) 236
— — true, 230, 236
— breast tissue, 372, 373, 374
— endometrial tissue, 432
— hepatic arteries, right or left, 526, 558
— — and cystic arteries, (*Fig.* 72 E) 83
— kidneys, 400
— ligaments of ankle-joint, (*Figs.* 283, 284) 281
— — foot, (*Figs.* 292–294) 290
— organs, (*Figs.* 417, 418) 428
— — multiple, 432
— pancreatic duct, (*Fig.* 488) 494
— — tissue, (*Figs.* 417, 418) 428
— peritoneal bands, (*Figs.* 62–68) 73–78
— ribs, (*Figs.* 209–211) 224
— saphenous vein, 308
— spleens, 432
— thyroid(s), 367
— — arteries, 19

821

822 INDEX

Accessory thyroid tissue, 428
Accoucheur's position of hand in hemiplegia, 463
Acetabulum, 254
— fusion of parts of, (*Fig.* 234) 249
Achalasia of kidney, 499
— oesophagus, 492
Achillodynia, 260
Achondroplasia, 582
— level of umbilicus in, 52
Acromioclavicular joint, dislocations of, (*Fig.* 617) 659
Acromion, failure of union in, 248
— process limiting abduction of humerus, (*Fig.* 188) 201
Adamantinomata, 353
Adduction deformity due to coxa vara, 477
Adductor(s) canal, occlusion of femoral artery in, 555
— hallucis, maintenance of transverse arch of foot by, 295
— magnus tendon injuring popliteal artery, 565
— pollicis, (*Figs.* 169, 170) 183
— — space anterior to, incision giving access to, (*Fig.* 726) 767
— — testing integrity of, (*Fig.* 170) 183
— of thigh, treatment of, in amputation through thigh, 775
Adenoid(s), (*Fig.* 324) 325, 326
— relation of spinal accessory nerve to glands draining, (*Fig.* 144) 154
— tissue, (*Fig.* 324) 325
Adenomyoma of rectovaginal septum, 432
Adherent tonsil, 28
Adhesions, blood to tendon graft from, 546
— causing duodenal diverticula, (*Fig.* 430 B) 445
— limiting spread of subphrenic abscess, (*Fig.* 681) 728
Adolescent kyphosis, (*Fig.* 671) 715
Adrenal fascial capsule, (*Fig.* 84) 94
— glands, (*Figs.* 85, 86) 95
— — abnormal, 94, 801, 802
— — autonomic supply of, 172
— — blood-supply of, 95
— — chromaffin paraganglioma in, (*Fig.* 607) 648
— — development of, 95
— — relations of, (*Fig.* 86) 95, 96
— — — to kidneys, (*Fig.* 78) 90, (*Figs.* 85, 86) 94, 95
— — surgical anatomy of, 801
— medulla, preganglionic fibres to, 172
— — sympathetic supply of, 623
— — tumour arising from, 648
— tissue, accessory, 432

Adrenal veins, abnormal, 802
Adrenalectomy, 801
Adrenergic receptors of oesophagus, 492
Adventitia of aortic, blood-supply to, (*Fig.* 538) 562
Adventitious bursae, 265
Adynamic ileus, 623
Afferent side of autonomic system, (*Fig.* 165) 178
Aganglionic lower colon causing Hirschsprung's disease, (*Fig.* 593) 630
Aged, intervertebral disc changes in, (*Fig.* 672) 716
Air-sinuses, development of, in child, (*Figs.* 122, 125) 131, 132
Albarran, subcervical glands of, 102
Alcock's canal, (*Figs.* 95–98, 742) 107, 108, 785
— — relations of, 348
Alcohol injection of fifth nerve, sensory loss due to, (*Fig.*) 450
— — into nerve-trunk, (*Figs.* 736, 737) 780
— — paravertebral, 617
Alderman's nerve (*see also* Auricular Nerve), 139
Alimentary canal, development of, 197
— — diverticula of, (*Figs.* 426–430) 440
— — nerves of, autonomic, 171
— tract, duplications of, 442
Allison, sliding hernia of, (*Figs.* 644–649) 685
Alveolar nerve, posterior inferior, 783
Amastia, complete and unilateral, 372
Amphiarthrosis, (*Figs.* 236, 238) 251
Ampulla of Vater (*see* Vater, Ampulla of), (*Figs.* 69, 74) 78
Amputation(s), anatomy governing, (*Figs.* 728–735) 769–786
— at hip-joint, 775
— knee, 774
— lower limb, (*Figs.* 729–731) 772
— lymphatics in, 597
— in presence of ischaemic gangrene, (*Fig.* 731) 775
— principles governing choice of site for, 769
— stump(s), cone-shaped, 774
— — forearm, 779
— — length of, 770, 773, 779
— — method of fashioning, (*Fig.* 728) 771
— — requirements of good, 770
— — weight-bearing, 770
— upper limb, (*Figs.* 732–735) 776
Anaemia causing intermittent claudication, 644
Anaesthesia due to combined lesion of hand and arm, 457

INDEX 823

Anaesthesia of upper limb in whole brachial plexus palsy, 458
Anaesthetic, injection of, into nerve-trunk, 780
Anal canal, anatomical, (*Fig.* 105) 116
— — development of, 109
— — incision of, 119, 120
— — muscles of, (*Fig.* 105) 115
— — surgical, (*Fig.* 105) 116
— columns, (*Fig.* 99) 110, 111
— dimple or pit, (*Figs.* 385 C, 388) 393, 396
— fascia, 106, 110, 224
— fissure, 119
— fistula (*see* Fistula in Ano)
— intermuscular space, abscess in (*Figs,* 111–113) 121
— intramuscular glands, 111, (*Fig.* 110) 120, 121
— — — aberrant, (*Fig.* 114) 122
— membrane, 109
— papillae, 111
— plate, 421, 422
— prolapse, 722
— region, (*Figs,* 99–115) 109–123
— sinuses, 111
— sphincter(s), (*Figs.* 105–109) 113–120, 491
— — nature of, (*Fig.* 108) 117
— — palpation of, 584
— stenosis, 394
— valves, (*Fig.* 99) 110
Anastomosis round semispinalis capitis, (*Fig.* 181) 193
Anatomical angles, (*Figs.* 463–479) 475–487
Aneurysm of common hepatic artery, (*Fig.* 511) 525
— subclavian, 226, 564
— within liver, ligation of hepatic artery in, 560
Angina pectoris, ganglionectomy to relieve cardiac pain in, 634
— sufferer, relief to, from ganglionectomy, 801
Angle of Louis as landmark to deeper structures, 41
Ankle, adventitious bursa at, 265
— binding bands at, 284, (*Figs.* 290, 291) 288
— compression of tibial nerve at, 471
— flare, 307
— fracture at, restoration of horizontal joint lines, (*Fig.* 475) 484, 485
— optimum position for ankylosis of, (*Fig.* 486) 489
— perforating veins (*Fig.* 310) 307, 310, 316
— tendon-sheaths of, (*Figs.* 251–253) 259
— ulcers, pathology of, 313

Ankle-joint, amputation just above, (*Fig.* 729) 772
— dislocation of, 670
— ligaments around, (*Figs.* 281–284) 281
— puncture of, (*Fig.* 689) 735
— spread of disease between fibula and, 270
— surgical approach to, (*Figs.* 775, 776) 814
Ankylosis, optimum positions of joints for, (*Figs.* 480–486) 487
Anlages of developing pancreas, (*Fig.* 417) 431
Annular pancreas, (*Figs.* 417 D, 418) 428
Annulus fibrosus, (*Fig.* 666) 710
Anococcygeal body, 198
Anomaly of articular tropism, (*Fig.* 661) 705
Anorectal abscess resulting in fistula in ano, (*Figs.* 111–113) 120
— junction, 106, (*Fig.* 103) 114
— ring, (*Fig.* 104) 115, 116
— — palpation of, (*Fig.* 108) 117
Anoxaemia from lessened arterial stream in 'white leg', 611
Ansa hypoglossi, 155, (*Fig.* 149) 160
— subclavia, 157
Antecubital fossa, relations of, 348
Anterior arterial tract, (*Figs.* 491, 492, 494, 495) 502, 503, 506
— clinoid processes, (*Figs.* 8, 13) 12
— communicating artery, (*Fig.* 11) 15
— facial vein, (*Figs.* 299, 300) 298, (*Figs.* 303, 304) 301
— fontanelle, (*Figs.* 120–121) 129
— inversion of testis, (*Fig.* 403 C) 414
— lobe of pituitary, (*Fig.* 7) 11
— longitudinal ligament of spine, (*Fig.* 118) 125
— temporal diploic vein, 296
— tibial compartment, (*Fig.* 533) 556
— — syndrome, 556, 644
— triangle, 207, 209
— vein of leg, (*Fig.* 311) 307
Anterolateral vein, (*Fig.* 311) 307
Anus, artificial, 757
— congenital deformities of rectum and (*Figs.* 384–388) 392–397
— covered, (*Fig.* 385) 392, 397
— deformities of, (*Figs.* 385, 387, 388) 394
— development of, 392, (*Fig.* 387) 395
— ectopic, or failure of migration of, 392, (*Figs.* 387, 388) 395
— imperfect, (*Figs.* 385, 387, 388) 394
— imperforate, 392
— line dividing rectum from, 394
— migration of, (*Fig.* 387) 395
— muscle control of, (*Figs.* 102–104) 113

INDEX

Anus, relationship of internal and external, at lower end of, (*Fig.* 108) 119
Aorta, abdominal, gradual occlusion of, 553
— — occlusion of, 553
— — — collateral circulation in, 554
— anastomosis of, to pulmonary artery, 509
— ascending, development of, 515
— blood-supply to, (*Fig.* 538) 561
— coarctation of, (*Figs.* 507, 508) 520
— cold abscess tracking along, 725, 726
— descending, development of, (*Fig.* 599) 511
— excision and reconstruction of, in coarctation, (*Fig.* 507 C) 522
— hepatic artery arising in, 525
— oesophageal branches of, (*Fig.* 752) 794
— overriding of, in Fallot's tetralogy, 508
— position of inferior vena cava in relation to, 543
— relationship of, with oesophagus, (*Fig.* 753) 795
— saddle emboli of, 505
— site of traumatic rupture of, 565
— transection of, (*Fig.* 539) 564
Aortic aneurysm(s), dissecting, (*Figs.* 538, 539) 561
— — exposure and excision of, (*Figs.* 536–539) 561, 564
— — resection of, and neurological damage, 506
— arch, cervical, 516
— — complex of embryo, (*Fig.* 498) 510, 511
— — development of, (*Figs.* 498–499) 510, (*Fig.* 502) 515
— — 'double', (*Figs.* 504, 505) 518
— — landmark to, 41
— — position of, in relation to sternum, 41
— — right, (*Fig.* 503) 516
— — — with left ligamentum arteriosum, (*Fig.* 505) 518
— — system, anomalies of, (*Fig.* 501) 511, 512, (*Figs.* 503–505) 516
— bifurcation, occlusion of, sudden, 553
— glomus bodies, (*Fig.* 608) 650
— lymph-glands, (*Fig.* 333) 334
— occlusion, and blood-supply to cord, (*Figs.* 493–495) 504, 505, 506
— opening in diaphragm, (*Fig.* 184) 197
— orifice of diaphragm, relations of, 347
— plexus, 176, 177, 624, 632
— sac, (*Fig.* 498) 510, 515
— stenosis, ventricular pressure in, 509
— surgery, approach to, 791
— — neurological complications of, 499, 500, (*Figs.* 493–495) 503

Aortic vascular ring, embryonic, (*Figs.* 498–500) 511, 512, (*Fig.* 504 A) 517
— — — persistence of, (*Fig.* 504) 518
Aorto-iliac atherosclerosis, 564
— exposure, (*Fig.* 540) 564
— obstructive vascular disease causing intermittent claudication, 643
Apical lymphatics of tongue, 330
Aponeurosis of epicranius, (*See* Galea Aponeurotica)
— origin of sacrospinalis, (*Fig.* 178) 190
— transversus abdominus, 97, 98
Aponeurotic layer of scalp, 1, 2
Appendages of rete testis, (*Fig.* 405) 417
Appendicitis, incisions for, (*Fig.* 706) 749, (*Figs.* 713–715) 755, 757
— infection of gall-bladder from, 87
— inflamed Meckel's diverticulum simulating, 390
— obstructed flow of urine simulating pain of, 405
— tests, for 591
Appendicular artery, 60, 62
Appendix(ces), (*Figs.* 46, 47) 59
— abscess, interstitial, causing diverticulum, 445
— diverticula of, 445
— epididymis, (*Fig.* 405) 417
— epiploica, blood-supply of, (*Fig.* 439) 443
— — preservation of arteries at base of, (*Fig.* 568) 602
— incisions giving access to, (*Fig.* 706) 749, (*Figs.* 713–715) 755, 757
— kinking of, by genitomesenteric fold, 74
— lymphoid tissue of, 59
— mesenteries of, 60
— positions of, (*Fig.* 47) 59
Aqueductus cerebri, blockage at, (*Fig.* 6) 10
Arachnoid mater, (*Fig.* 4) 7
Arachnoidal granulations, 7
— processes, 7
— villi, 7
Arches of foot, (*Figs.* 295–297) 292–296, (*Figs.* 472–474) 482
— — support of, (*Figs.* 295–297) 293
Arcuate ligament, median, coeliac artery compression by, 447
— — — cold abscess tracking through, (*Fig.* 678) 725
Argyll Robertson pupil, 145
Arm(s) (*see also* Upper Limb)
— abduction movements of, impossible with ruptured supraspinatus, 674, 675
— — painful, 677, 678
— amputation through, 779

INDEX 825

Arm(s) injury, Volkmann's ischaemic contracture following, 324
— nerve-supply of, cutaneous, 166
— route of blood to, in occlusion of innominate artery, 557
— in sling position, restricting shoulder mobility, 571
— veins of, (*Figs.* 306, 307) 303, 304
Arnold's nerve (*see* Auricular Nerve)
Arteria radicularis magna, (*Fig.* 491) 501, 502, (*Fig.* 495) 506
Arterial branches of distribution, (*Fig.* 528) 548
— collateral circulation, (*Fig.* 528) 548
— diseases of extremities, 642
— embolism causing spasm in collateral circulation, 611
— enlargement in coarctation of aorta, 522
— entrapments, (*Fig.* 432) 447
— occlusion, gradual, in atherosclerosis, 553
— — sudden, results of, 553
— pulsation causing movement of lymph, 611
— spasm, reflex acute, due to vascular insult, 611
— supply of kidneys, (*Figs.* 514–516) 531
— trauma causing spasm in collateral circulation, 611
— trunk, longitudinal branches of, (*Fig.* 528) 548
Arteries to ileum and jejunum, arrangements of, (*Fig.* 44) 57
— of thyroid gland, (*Figs.* 16, 17) 17
— muscles, tunica media to, 561
Arteriomesenteric pressure as cause of duodenal ileus, 384
Arteriosclerosis of extremities, 642
Arteriovenous fistula, subclavian, 564
— shunts between portal radicles and hepatic arterioles, 528
Arthritis in joint, consideration of, in choice of amputation site, 770
— traumatic, of spine compressing emerging nerves, 705
Arthrodesis of shoulder-joint, incision for, (*Fig.* 762) 805
Arthrodial joint, (*Fig.* 240) 252
Articular capsules of foot, 290
— cartilage, (*Figs.* 239, 240, 243, 244) 252, (*Fig.* 553) 580, (*Fig.* 682) 731
— — nutrition of, (*Fig.* 682) 732
— — synovial membrane covering, 730
— discs, (*Figs.* 246, 247) 254
— facets, lumbar, deficiency of, causing spondylolisthesis, (*Fig.* 655 A) 700
— menisci, 254

Articular processes of lumbar vertebrae, joints between, (*Figs.* 660, 661) 704
— — spine, (*Fig.* 119) 126
— — variations in direction of facets of, 695, 696
— surfaces, lubrication of, 730
— tropism, anomaly of, (*Fig.* 661) 705
Articulations of vertebral column, (*Fig.*119) 126
Artificial anus, 757
— limb, consideration of, in choice of amputation site, 769, 770
Ascites, production of, 527, 528
Aspiration pneumonia due to internal laryngeal nerve ligation, 22
Asthenic type of bodily habitus, (*Figs.* 456, 457) 473
Astragalo-scaphoid bone of Pirie, 230
Astragalus (*see also* Talus)
— accessory, (*Fig.* 214) 232
— secundarius, 231
Asymmetrical sacralization, (*Fig.* 654) 699
Atherosclerosis, aorto-iliac, 564
— gradual occlusion in, 533
Atlas, blood-supply of, (*Fig.* 230) 246
Atrial septal defect, 507
Atrium, opening of left superior vena cava, into, (*Fig.* 521) 540
Auditory canal, external, fistulous track ending in, (*Figs.* 357 C, 358) 365
— meatus, external branchial cleft in formation of, 363
— — — herpes of, 454
— — — nerve-supply of, (*Fig.* 130) 138
— — internal lesion of facial nerve at, (*Fig.* 435) 451
— nerve (8th), loss due to division of, 454
— tube, 180
— — in newborn, 130
Auerbach's plexus, (*Fig.* 584) 619
Auricle, development of, (*Fig.* 343) 354
Auricular glands, posterior, (*Fig.* 325) 326
— nerve, (*Fig.* 130) 137, 138, 139, 149, 151
— — great, (*Fig.* 130) 137, 138, 140, (*Fig.* 148) 158
— — posterior, 138, 148
— vein, posterior, (*Figs.* 303, 304) 301
Auricularis posterior muscle, 148
Auriculotemporal nerve, (*Fig.* 130) 137, 138, 139, 146, 150
— — paralysis (*Fig.* 434 C) 450
Autonomic innervation of iris, (*Fig.* 577) 611
— nerve supply to heart, (*Figs.* 579, 580) 615
— nervous system, (*Figs.* 159–165) 170–179
— — — abdominal, (*Figs.* 581–593) 618–631

826 INDEX

Autonomic nervous system, afferent side of, (*Fig.* 165) 178
— — — functions of, (*Figs.* 159, 160) 170
— — — peripheral, architecture of, (*Fig.* 161) 174
— — — plan of, 172
— — — reinnervation in, 646
— sensory nerves, abdominal, 618
— nerve-fibres, 178
— supply to bladder and colon, (*Figs.* 590–592) 625, 628
Avellis, syndrome of, 454
Axilla, accessory mammary tissue in, 373
— brachial plexus, branches in relaxation of, 468
— cold abscess of, at 724
— division of radial nerve in, sensory loss due to, 459
— relation of brachial plexus to, 160, 162
Axillary approach to sympathetic chain, (*Fig.* 596) 634
— artery, occlusion of, sudden, 553
— — relation of brachial plexus to, 160 (*Fig.* 151) 162, 163
— fascial 'tent', 34
— lymph-glands, (*Fig.* 27) 33, 35, 339
— — anterior, 30, (*Figs.* 27, 29) 33, 35, 339
— — apical, (*Figs.* 27, 30) 34, 35, 339
— — block dissection of, 34
— — central, (*Fig.* 27) 33, 35, 339
— — drainage area of, (*Fig.* 340) 346
— — lateral, (*Fig.* 27) 33, 35, 339
— — posterior, (*Fig.* 27) 33, 35, 339
— nerve, 161, 163, 457
— — compression by humeral head paralysing deltoid, 675
— — at shoulder-joint, (*Figs.* 618, 619) 660, 661
— sheath, (*Fig.* 196) 212
— tail of Spence, 30, (*Fig.* 29) 35
— — — cancer of, 33
— vein, (*Figs.* 27, 30) 31, 35 (*Fig.* 307) 303, 304, 305
Azygos continuation, 538, (*Fig.* 522 B) 540
— — entry of hepatic veins into right auricle in, 527
— lobe(s), lower, 45
— — of lung, (*Figs.* 36–38) 45–47
— — upper, 45
— system in communication with inferior vena cava, (*Fig.* 522 A) 540
— vein (*Fig.* 38) 46, 47, 197
— — development of (*Fig.* 520) 538
— — lobe of (*Figs.* 36–38) 45–47

Back, cold abscess in, 727
— deep muscles of, (*Figs.* 177–181) 189–194
— dermoids of, 427
— nerve-supply of, 165
— pain due to vertebral abnormalities, 127
— — low (*see* Low Back Pain)
— visible pulsation in, 520, 522
Backache due to lesion of recurrent nerve, 165
— — lumbar rib, 229
— lumbar (*see* Low Back Pain)
Balanic epispadias, 422
— type of hypospadias, (*Fig.* 408) 419
Ball-and-socket joint, (*Fig.* 245) 254
Ballooning of rectum, 585
Barber's hands, interdigital sinuses of, (*Fig.* 412) 423
Bartholinian glands, 200
Basilic vein, (*Fig.* 306) 304
— — median, (*Fig.* 306 B) 304
Basivertebral veins, (*Fig.* 322) 323
Battle's incision, (*Fig.* 706) 749
Berry, suspensory ligament of, 24
— — — recurrent nerve embedded in, 22, 24
Beyer's method of measuring girth of limbs, (*Fig.* 565) 596
Biceps insertion, bursae in relation to, 262
— long head of, 254
— reflex spasm of, 305
— rupture of long head of, 546
— synovial sheath of, 261, 262
— tendon injury from irregularities of tuberosity, 680
Bicipital groove, 675, 676
Bifid sternum associated with mediastinal dermoid, 428
— uvula, 359
Bifurcation of ureter, (*Fig.* 394) 400
Bile reflux in causation of pancreatitis, 495, 497
Bile-duct(s), (*Fig.* 69) 78–87
— accessory, (*Fig.* 382 B) 388
— common, (*Figs.* 69, 70) 78
— — congenital, cyst of (*Fig.* 382 D) 388
— — relation of pancreatic duct to, (*Fig.* 488) 494
— — vascular arrangements of, 87
— — venous plexus on, 87
— entrance of, into duodenum, 55, 56, 61
— extrahepatic, congenital atresia of, 86
— incisions giving access to, 745, (*Fig.* 709) 751, (*Fig.* 711) 753, 754
— mucus secretion by glands of, 86
— relations of, to arteries of liver, (*Figs.* 72, 73) 82
— structure of, 86

INDEX 827

Bile-duct(s), variations in, (*Figs.* 70, 71) 80
Biliary colic not the cause of shoulder-tip pain, 88
— fistula developing due to accessory bile-ducts, 85, 86
— passages, (*Figs.* 69–77) 78–89
Bimanual examination, per vaginam or per rectum, 587
Binding bands at wrist and ankle, (*Figs.* 287–291) 284–290
Bipartite bones of hand, (*Fig.* 220) 236
— patella, (*Fig.* 220) 238
Birth palsy, lower-arm type of, 458
— — upper-arm type of, 163, 456
Bitemporal hemianopia, 354
— — due to pituitary tumour, (*Fig.* 14) 16
Black eye, 3
Bladder abnormalities, (*Fig.* 395) 402
— in child compared with that of adult, (*Fig.* 128) 136
— congenital abnormalities of, 397
— development of, (*Fig.* 395) 402
— diverticulum of, (*Fig.* 395 C) 402
— — acquired, 446
— extroversion of, (*Figs.* 410, 411) 420
— fascial sheath of, (*Fig.* 207) 222, 223
— function, mechanism of, 629
— growth of prostatic adenoma into, (*Fig.* 91) 102, 104
— incisions giving access to, 745, 761, 762
— nerve-supply to (*Figs.* 590–592) 625
— — functions of, 628
— pain, presacral neurectomy for, 630
— puncture, (*Fig.* 696) 740
— rectal examination of, 585
— sphincters, 499
Blalock operation for Fallot's tetralogy, (*Fig.* 496) 509
Blindness in both eyes, 449
— unilateral, 449
Blood sinuses of cranium, 297
— — surrounding pituitary, (*Fig.* 8) 13
Blood-clot, removal of, from tonsillar fossa, (*Fig.* 24) 29
Blood-supply to adrenals, 95
— of bones, (*Figs.* 226–231) 242
— to breast, 31
— of colon, (*Fig.* 52) 61, 62–64, 599
— to gall-bladder and bile-ducts, 87
— of greater omentum, (*Figs.* 526, 527) 546
— gut, (*Figs.* 50–52) 61–64
— — diverticula in relation to, (*Figs.* 428, 429) 443
— — in relation to lymph drainage, 67
— intervertebral discs, 711
— jaw in relation to osteomyelitis, 575
— joints, 731

Blood-supply of kidney, (*Fig.* 82) 92, (*Figs.* 514–516) 531
— to lungs, (*Fig.* 40) 50
— parathyroid glands, 25
— of small gut, (*Fig.* 44) 57, (*Fig.* 51) 61, 62
— spinal cord, (*Figs.* 490–495) 499
— stomach, 61
— tendons, (*Fig.* 525) 545
— thymus gland, 134
— tonsil, (*Fig.* 23) 27
— ureter, (*Fig.* 517) 534
Blood-vessels of liver, (*Figs.* 509–513) 523–531, 558
— remains of, at umbilicus, (*Fig.* 41) 53, 392
— of thyroid gland, (*Figs.* 16, 17) 17
Bloodless fold of Treves, 71
Bodily habitus, (*Figs.* 454–462) 472
— — gall-bladder positions in relation to, (*Fig.* 462) 475
Bochdalek, foramen, 682, 683
Bockel-Langenbeck approach to wrist-joint, (*Fig.* 765) 807
Boeck's sarcoid, biopsy in diagnosis of, 338
Bone(s), (*Figs.* 209–234) 224–250
— abscess, acute, 583
— accessory, (*Figs.* 212–222) 229–240
— blood-supply of, (*Figs.* 226–231) 242
— cartilage, 580
— — pathological facts of, (*Fig.* 555) 582
— cavity, discharge from, 584
— cyst causing coxa vara, 476
— development of, (*Figs.* 232–234) 247
— disease, congenital, 582
— infection, 582
— — spread of, to joint, 266
— long (*see* Long Bone)
— maintaining arch of foot, 296
— membrane, 580, 582
— necrosis in infected terminal phalanx, 654
— pathological facts of, (*Fig.* 555) 581
— pathology of, in terms of anatomy, (*Figs.* 553–555) 580
— in tonsil, 29
— treatment of, in amputation stump, 772
— tumours, sites of, (*Fig.* 555) 584
Bony abnormalities of spine, 127
Bougie, false passage of, recognition of, per rectum, 585
Bow-knee, (*Fig.* 471 C) 480
Bow-leg, (*Fig.* 471 B) 480
Bowel (*see* Gut)
— wall, excessive contraction of, causing prolapse, 721
Boxer's muscle, 181
Brachial artery, injury to, causing ischaemia of forearm muscles, 324

828 INDEX

Brachial artery, occlusion of, collateral circulation in, 558
— — — gangrene following, 549
— — — sudden, 554
— — venae comites of, 304
— plexus, 157, (*Figs.* 150, 153) 160 (*Fig.* 196) 212
— — branches from, (*Fig.* 150) 160, 161
— — communication between phrenic nerve and, (*Fig.* 154) 164
— — compression by cervical rib, (*Fig.* 209) 225, 226
— — — first rib, 227
— — connexions of, with sympathetic, (*Fig.* 595) 634
— — injury to lowest trunk of, pupillary changes due to, 612
— — lesions of, (*Fig.* 438) 455, 457
— — plan of, (*Fig.* 150) 160
— — post- and pre-fixed, 164, 225, 226, 227
— — relation of head of humerus to, (*Fig.* 620) 661
— — relationships of, (*Fig.* 151) 161, 225
— — relaxation of nerves of, (*Fig.* 449) 467, 468
— — type of paralysis, whole, (*Fig.* 438, VIII) 458
Brachialis, reflex spasm of, 305
— splitting of, in exposure of humerus, (*Fig.* 778) 816
Brain abscess, danger of, in Fallot's tetralogy, 509
— cavities of, communication between subarachnoid space and, 9
— collateral mechanisms in, (*Fig.* 532) 552
— pressure effects on, due to pituitary tumour, 16
— puncture of ventricles of, (*Fig.* 690) 735
— surgical approach to, (*Figs.* 743–748) 786
Brain-stem, taste fibres to, 147
Branchial arches, (*Figs.* 354, 355) 361
— cleft, first, anomalies of, (*Fig.* 357) 363
— — — anomalous development of auricle at, (*Fig.* 343) 354
— — second, persistence of, 26
— cyst(s), (*Figs.* 354, 355) 361, 363
— — of first cleft, 365
— fistula(ae), (*Figs.* 354–358) 361, 362
— — or cyst associated with postfaucial diverticulum, 434
— sinus, 363
Breast(s), (*Figs.* 25–34) 30–41
— abscess due to lactiferous duct obstruction, (*Fig.* 33) 40
— architecture of, (*Fig.* 25) 30

Breast(s), cancer invading ligaments of Cooper, 31, (*Fig.* 34) 40
— — prognosis in, based on lymphatic drainage, 38
— — removal of lymph plexus on pectoralis major in, 345
— — retraction in relation to, (*Fig.* 34) 40
— — secondary invasion of skin in, (*Fig.* 28) 34
— — spread of, through internal mammary glands, 37
— — vertebral secondaries of, (*Fig.* 323) 324
— congenital errors of, (*Fig.* 368) 371
— development of, 371
— extent of, 30
— lymphatic drainage of, 30, (*Figs.* 27–31) 33–38, 339
— parenchyma, lymphatics of, (*Figs.* 29–31) 35–38
— supernumerary, 373, 374
— tissue, aberrant, cancer of, 374
Breathing, slow irregular, due to bilateral vagus nerve lesion, 454
Broad ligament(s), 717
— — of lung, 798
— — vestigial structures in, (*Fig.* 406) 417
Bronchial arteries, 51
— blood-vessels, 51
— and pulmonary circulations, anastomoses between, 51
— tree, (*Fig.* 39) 47–49
— — anomalies, 49
Bronchogenic carcinoma, pre-scalene gland biopsy in, 338
Bronchomediastinal lymphatic trunk, 336, 337, (*Fig.* 339) 345
Bronchus(i), lung buds of, 439, 440
— lymph drainage of, (*Fig.* 334) 337
— main left, (*Fig.* 39) 49
— — right, (*Fig.* 39) 47
— middle, glandular enlargement affecting, 44
— supernumerary, (*Fig.* 424 C) 437
Bryant's triangle, (*Fig.* 562) 594
Buccal pad of fat, 133
Buccinator glands, 327
— muscle, 148
Buccopharyngeal aponeurosis, (*Figs.* 194, 195) 210
Bucket-handle tear of meniscus, (*Fig.* 278) 279
Buerger's disease, 642
Bulbo-urethral glands, 200, 585
Bulbus cordis of fetal heart, 507
Bunion, 266
Burns, space of, 209

INDEX 829

Bursa(ae), 255, (*Figs.* 254–258) 261–266
— adventitious, 265
— around elbow, (*Fig.* 254) 262
— — knee-joint, (*Figs.* 257, 258) 264
— — the hip, (*Figs.* 255, 256) 262
— radial, (*Figs.* 249, 250) 257, (*Fig.* 287) 285
— ulnar, (*Figs.* 249, 250) 256, (*Fig.* 287) 285
Bursitis of prepatellar bursa, 265
— subdeltoid, 261
Buttock, cold abscess in, 726
— cutaneous nerve of, 166
By-pass shunt, use of, in aortic resection, (*Fig.* 495) 506

Caecal fossae, 67, (*Fig.* 60) 71
Caecocolic sphincter, 494
Caecostomy, incision for, 757
Caecum and ascending colon, resection of cancer of, (*Fig.* 569) 602
— cancer of, area of resection for, 67
— development of, (*Figs.* 371, 372, 374) 377, 380
— — appendix and, (*Fig.* 46) 59
— displaced, due to abnormal rotation, 381, 382
— mobile, congenital bands from, causing duodenal ileus, (*Fig.* 377) 384
— peritoneal relations of, 58
— tension gangrene and rupture of, 494
— volvulus, of, mesentery to ascending colon and, 77
Calcaneal angle, (*Fig.* 476) 485
— bursa, 266
— spurs, (*Fig.* 218) 231, 235
Calcaneocuboid joint, 292
Calcaneofibular ligament, (*Figs.* 283, 284) 281, 282
Calcaneonavicular ligament, inferior or plantar, 281, (*Fig.* 292) 291
Calcaneus, (*Fig.* 225 B) 242
— crush fracture of, reduction of, (*Fig.* 476) 485
— epiphysis on posterior surface of, 242
— os trigonum fused to, (*Fig.* 214 A) 233
— peroneal process of, 231
— secondary, (*Fig.* 212) 230
Calcification in supraspinatus tendon, (*Fig.* 638) 678
Calculus associated with hiatus hernia, 689
Calf muscles, postural activity of, 181
— — venous sinuses of, 312
— — pump, 313
Camper, fascia of, (*Figs.* 203, 204) 218
Canalis innominatus, (*Fig.* 141) 150
Cancellous exostosis, 582

Capitate bone, (*Fig.* 224 B) 241, 242
Capsular ligament of knee-joint, 667
— reflections and epiphyseal lines, (*Figs.* 259–265) 266–270
Capsule(s) of joint, (*Figs.* 553, 554) 580
— kidney, 93
— prostate, (*Fig.* 92) 103
— shoulder-joint, 660, 661
— — tearing of, 661, 662
— thyroid, (*Figs.* 20, 21) 23
— tonsil, 26, 28
Caput Medusae, 54 (*Fig.* 320) 321
Carcinoma, metastatic, of bone, (*Fig.* 555, 1) 583
Cardia, displacement of, into chest, (*Fig.* 645) 686
— mechanism at, preventing regurgitation, 491, 492
— obstruction at, due to achalasia, 492
Cardiac (*see also* Heart)
— accelerator nerves, 615, 799
— arrest, incision for dealing with (*Fig.* 497 A) 510
— branch(es) of cervical sympathetic ganglia, 153, (*Fig.* 145) 156, 157
— — recurrent nerve, 153
— — vagus, 153
— depressor nerves, 615
— ganglia, intrinsic, 615
— pain, 615
— — neurectomy for, (*Fig.* 758 B) 799
— — surgical treatment of, (*Fig.* 580) 616
— plexus(es), 176
— — superficial, 153
— — — and deep, (*Fig.* 579) 615
— sphincter, (*Fig.* 487) 490, 491
Cardinal veins, (*Figs.* 518–520) 536, 538, 540, (*Fig.* 524) 543
Cardio-inhibitory nerves, paralysis of, 454
Cardio-oesophageal junction, maintenance of position of, (*Fig.* 646) 686
Caroticotympanic nerves, superior and inferior, 149
Carotid aneurysm, diagnosis from cervical aortic arch, 516
—. artery(ies), common, 209
— — — anomaly affecting, 519
— — — danger of ligation of, 553
— — — occlusion of, collateral circulation in, 557
— — — relation of internal jugular veins to, 301
— —.— vagus nerve to, 151
— — digital control of, danger of, 614
— — external, plexus to, (*Fig.* 145) 156
— — interior, in relation to pituitary, (*Figs.* 10, 11) 13

830 INDEX

Carotid artery(ies), internal, plexus round, (*Fig.* 145) 155, 156
— — — relations of, (*Fig.* 143) 151
— — — — of tonsil to, 27
— — — relationships of, 149
— — left common, development of, 515
— — pressure on, by ossified stylohyoid ligament, 30
— bifurcation, branchial fistula and, (*Fig.* 356) 363
— — nerve plexus at, (*Fig.* 578) 614
— body, (*Fig.* 608) 650
— — tumour, 650
— sheath, 151, 153, 155, 159, 160, (*Fig.* 194) 209
— sinus plexus, (*Fig.* 578) 614
— system, 209, 210
Carotid-basilar anastomosis, 552
Carpal bones, accessory, (*Fig.* 220) 236
— — dislocation of, (*Figs.* 622, 623) 663
— ligament, transverse, (*Fig.* 250) 257 (*Fig.* 613) 655, 657, 658
— tunnel, 285
— — syndrome, (*Fig.* 288) 286, 470
Carpalia, (*Fig.* 224 A) 240, 241
Carpometacarpal joints, 567
Carpus, homologies of, (*Fig.* 224) 240, 242
'Carrying angle', (*Fig.* 476) 485
Cartilage(s), articular, (*Fig.* 682) 731
— bone(s), 580
— — pathological facts of, (*Fig.* 555) 582
— plates of intervertebral disc, (*Fig.* 666) 710
— in tonsil, 29
Cartilaginous intra-articular structures, (*Fig.* 246) 254
— joints, (*Figs.* 237, 238) 251
Causalgia complicating dislocated shoulder 661
— following sympathetic involvement in injury, 571
— ganglionectomy for, 634
Caval diverticulum, (*Fig.* 523 C) 543
— opening in diaphragm, (*Fig.* 184) 197
Cavernomatous transformations of portal veins, 529
Cavernous sinus(es), 13, (*Figs.* 134, 135) 142, 143
— — communication of anterior facial vein with, (*Fig.* 299) 299
Cellulitis, diagnosis from erysipelas, 587
Central hernia, 684
— lymphatics of tongue, (*Fig.* 329) 330
Cephalhaematoma, 4
Cephalhydrocele, traumatic, 3, 4
Cephalic gland, 34
— vein, (*Fig.* 306) 303, 304
— — median, (*Fig.* 306 B) 304

Cerebellopontine angle, incision giving access to, (*Fig.* 747) 789
Cerebellum, incision giving access to, (*Fig.* 747) 789
Cerebral arteries, compared with peripheral artery, (*Fig.* 609) 653
— compression due to middle meningeal haemorrhage, 613
Cerebrospinal fluid, (*Fig.* 6) 9
— — blockage of, in vertebral canal, 9
— — meninges and, (*Figs.* 3–6) 5–10
— ganglia, (*Fig.* 133 A) 141
— nerves of anal region, (*Fig.* 99) 110, 111
Cerebrum, incisions giving access to, (*Figs.* 743–746) 787
Cervical aortic arch, 516
— cardiac branches of vagus, 153
— — nerves, (*Fig.* 579) 615
— — — inferior, 153
— — — superior, 153
— cord, blood-supply of, 500
— — ischaemic lesions of, 503
— coxa vara, (*Fig.* 464 B) 476
— curve of vertebral column, (*Fig.* 116 B) 123, 134
— disc prolapse causing neuralgia, 229
— lymph-glands, anterior, (*Fig.* 325) 328
— — clearance of, sacrifice of jugulars in, 549
— — deep, 326
— — — anterior, 328
— — — circular chain of, (*Fig.* 325) 326, 328
— — — drainage area of, (*Fig.* 340) 346
— — — inferior, 328
— — — superior, 328
— — — vertical chain of, (*Figs.* 326, 327) 328
— — superficial, (*Fig.* 325) 328
— lymph-nodes, lateral, benign thyroid follicles in, 24
— — — malignant thyroid tissue in, 25
— nerve(s), anterior rami of, (*Fig.* 129) 137, 160
— — eighth, and cervical rib, 163, 225
— — — thoracic first combined, lesion of, (*Fig.* 438, VI) 457
— — fifth and sixth, loss due to division of, (*Fig.* 438, I–III) 455
— — fourth, (*Figs.* 131, 132) 139
— — in neck, (*Figs.* 147–149) 158
— — posterior rami of, (*Fig.* 129) 137
— — seventh, loss due to division of, (*Fig.* 438, IV) 457
— — supplying trunk, 164, 165
— — third, (*Fig.* 131) 139
— — with cutaneous branches, 137, 141
— plexus, (*Figs.* 147–149) 157, 158

INDEX 831

Cervical plexus, branches of, (*Fig.* 148) 158
— — communication of, with vagus, 152
— prevertebral abscess, (*Fig.* 677) 723
— rib, (*Fig.* 153) 163, (*Fig.* 209) 224
— sinus, (*Fig.* 355) 361
— spine, cold abscesses of, (*Fig.* 677) 723
— sympathectomy, nerve sprouting after, 646
— — contribution to carotid sinus plexus, (*Fig.* 578) 614
— — ganglion(ia), (*Fig.* 145) 156, 176, (*Fig.* 579) 615
— — — inferior, 153, (*Fig.* 145) 156, 157
— — — middle, 153, (*Fig.* 145) 156
— — — superior, 149, 152, 153, (*Fig.* 145) 156, 159, (*Fig.* 577) 611
— — nerve(s) to eye, paralysis of, 613
— — — results of division of, 466
— — nerve-trunk, (*Fig.* 145) 155
— transverse processes, 127
Cervicobrachial junction, pressure at, 226
Cervicofacial nerve, (*Fig.* 140) 148
Cervicothoracic junction, rudimentary ribs at, 224
— scoliosis causing brachial plexus compression, 227
Cervix uteri, transverse ligaments of, (*Fig.* 674), 717, 718, 719
— — vaginal examination of, 586
Cheek, deep fascia of, 208
— nerve-supply of, 140
Chemodectoma, 650
Chest, access to, (*Fig.* 497) 509
— cutaneous nerves of, 166
— wall, 41–42
Chiasma, partial and complete lesions of, (*Fig.* 433) 449
Chiasmatic sulcus, 13
Child(ren), anatomy of, (*Figs.* 120–128) 129–136
— haemorrhage from fractured vault in, 5
— height of aortic arch in, 41
— rectal examination in, 586
— spinal cord of, 128, 134
— subaponeurotic haematoma in, 3
— umbilical hernia of, 52
— vertebral column in, (*Fig.* 116 A) 123, 134
Choanoid muscle of Müller, 612
Chocolate cyst of hilum of ovary, 432
Choking due to internal laryngeal nerve ligation, 22
Cholecystectomy, common bile-duct after, 79
— drainage mandatory after, 85
— — of peritoneal cavity after, 389
Cholecystitis, 495
— associated with hiatus hernia, 689

Cholecystitis, shoulder-tip pain associated with, 88
Cholecystography, position of gallbladder in, (*Figs.* 76, 77) 87
Choledochoduodenal mechanism, (*Figs.* 488, 489) 494
Choledochus, migration of, (*Fig.* 417) 431
Cholelithiasis associated with hiatus hernia, 609
Cholinergic receptors of oesophagus, 492
Chondroma, solitary, (*Fig.* 555, 3) 583
Chorda tympani nerve, 146, 147
— — taste fibres in, 147, 148, 151
Choroid processes of lateral ventricles, 9
Chromaffin material, sites of, (*Fig.* 607) 648
— paraganglioma, (*Fig.* 607) 648
Chyle, loss of, from circulation causing death, 609, 610
Chylothorax, 609, 610
Ciliary body, 144
— ganglion, 141, (*Fig.* 136) 143, (*Fig.* 577) 611
— nerves, long, 145*n*
— — short, (*Fig.* 136) 144
Circle of Willis, (*Fig.* 522) 552
Circular chain of deep cervical lymphglands, (*Fig.* 325) 326, 328
— muscle of anal canal, 116
— — pyloric sphincter, 493
Circularis arteriosus, 9
— vasculosus, (*Fig.* 227) 244, (*Fig.* 682) 731, 732
Circumflex iliac vein, 308, 320
Cirrhosis of liver, venous hypertension in, 528
Cisterna chyli, 335, 336, (*Fig.* 336) 342
— — surgical injury to, 610
— interpeduncularis, 9
— magna, 9
— pontis, 9
Cisternal puncture, (*Fig.* 691) 737
Claudication, intermittent, 553, 555, 643
Clavicle, compression of nerve or artery between first rib and, 227
— dislocations of, (*Fig.* 617) 659
— fracture of, excessive pain after, 140
— ligaments of, (*Figs.* 267, 268) 270
— ossification of, (*Figs.* 232, 233) 247
— relation of brachial plexus to, 160, 161
— supraclavicular nerve in relation to, (*Fig.* 132) 140
— variations of, (*Fig.* 233) 247
— vein crossing, 303
Clavipectoral fascia, 34
Claw-hand, (*Fig.* 444) 462
— in Klumpke's paralysis, 458
— ulnar, (*Fig.* 442) 461

832 INDEX

Cleft membrane, 361
— palate, (*Fig.* 352) 358
— — and hare-lip, (*Figs.* 345–352) 355
Clicking knee, 578
Clinical tests, anatomical bases of, (*Figs.* 556–565) 587–597
Clinoid processes, erosion of, due to pituitary tumour, 16
Clitoris, dorsal nerve of, 200, (*Fig.* 741) 785
Cloaca, development of bladder from, (*Fig.* 395) 402, 445
— entodermal, development of rectum from, (*Fig.* 384) 392, (*Fig.* 387) 395
— extroversion of, 380, 381
Club-foot, 484
— congenital, 206
Coagulation of cerebrospinal fluid, 9
Coarctation of aorta, (*Fig.* 507) 520
Coccygeal nerves, 166
Coccygeus, 198
Coccyx, 123
— and sacrum, congenital absence of, 695, 696
Coeliac artery, 61, (*Fig.* 53) 64, 334, 335
— — compression by median arcuate ligament, 447
— — variations in site of origin of, 448
— axis, hepatic vein arising from, 524
— branch of vagus, (*Fig.* 586) 620
— ganglion, 176
— — chromaffin paraganglioma found at, (*Fig.* 607) 649
— group of pre-aortic glands, 66
— lymph-glands, 334
— plexus, 175, 176, 623
Cold abscesses of spine, (*Figs.* 677–679) 723
— — in spinal tuberculosis, 124
— local sensitivity to, causing Raynaud's spasm, 644
Colic angle, 376, 379
— artery(ies), (*Fig.* 52) 63, 67, 589, 599
— — left, division of, in cancer of pelvic colon or rectum, 605
— — middle, (*Fig.* 48) 60, (*Fig.* 52) 63
— — variations in, 599, 600, 602, 603
— veins, 64
Collar-stud abscess, (*Fig.* 611) 654
Collateral arrangements of liver, (*Figs.* 512, 513) 527, (*Fig.* 534) 558
— channels for circulation of lymph, 609
— — enlargement of, in cirrhosis, 529
— — of lymph-glands, 324
— circulation(s), (*Figs.* 528–534) 548–560
— — after ligation of vena cava, (*Figs.* 318, 320 B) 318
— — in coarctation of aorta, (*Fig.* 508) 521

Collateral circulation(s), portal obstruction, 529
— — of spinal cord, 502, 503, 505, 506
— ganglia, autonomic, 172, (*Fig.* 164) 175, 176
— ligament(s), (*Fig.* 542) 569
— — of elbow-joint, (*Fig.* 270) 272, 486
— — knee-joint, (*Fig.* 276) 276, 279
— — metacarpophalangeal and interphalangeal joints, (*Fig.* 273) 275
— — tibial, (*Figs.* 276, 279, 280) 277, 279
— — of wrist-joint, (*Fig.* 272) 274
— mechanisms in brain, (*Fig.* 532) 552
— — venous, (*Figs.* 529–531) 549
— nerve sproutings, (*Fig.* 606) 646
— pathways to lungs in Fallot's tetralogy, 509
Colles, fascia of, 199, (*Fig.* 205) 219, 220, 221
— — fluid extravasated under, 221
Colon, (*Figs.* 45–49) 57–61
— anastomosis of, division of mesentery in, (*Fig.* 567 B) 601
— ascending, and caecum, resection for cancer of, (*Fig.* 509) 602
— autonomic supply to, (*Fig.* 587) 622, 623, 628
— blood-supply of, 61 (*Fig.* 429) 443
— blood-vessels to, 599
— cancer of, anatomical principles underlying surgery of, (*Figs.* 567–576) 598–608
— — quarantining, 598
— — resection of, extent of, 598, 601
— — — typical, (*Figs.* 569–576) 602
— descending and pelvic, resection for cancer of, (*Fig.* 572) 604
— displaced, due to abnormal rotation, 381
— diverticula of, (*Fig.* 429) 443, 445
— — acquired, 442
— 'double-barrelled', (*Fig.* 65) 75
— incisions giving access to, 750, 754
— left, deficient collateral circulation of, 599
— lymph drainage of, (*Fig.* 54) 66
— lymph-glands of, 335
— mesentery(ies) of, (*Figs.* 48, 49) 60
— — to ascending or descending, (*Figs.* 67, 68) 76
— mobile proximal, 382
— pelvic and descending, resection for cancer of, (*Figs.* 572, 573) 604
— — mesocolon of, (*Fig.* 49) 60, 61
— — resection of, for cancer, 64
— peritoneal relations of, 58
— portal-systemic anastomosis behind, (*Fig.* 319) 321

INDEX 833

Colon, positioning of, by rotation of gut, 380
— right transverse, resection for cancer of hepatic flexure and, (*Fig.* 570) 602
— sphincters of, 490
— transverse, mesocolon of, (*Figs.* 48, 49) 60, 61
— — relation to duodenum, (*Fig.* 43) 56
— — and splenic flexure, resection for cancer of, (*Fig.* 571) 603
— venous drainage of, 64
Colonic anastomosis, blood-supply and, (*Fig.* 52) 63
— enlargement in Hirschsprung's disease, 630
— obstruction, rise in caecal tension in, 494
Colonic-rectal anastomosis after resection for cancer, 604, 608
Colostomy after operation for rectal cancer, 607, 608
— left inguinal, incision for, 755, 757
— sparing marginal artery in, (*Fig.* 567 A) 600
Common bile-duct, hepatic duct (*see* Bile-duct, Hepatic Duct, Common)
— channel, (*Fig.* 489) 495
Communicans(tes) cervicalis nerves, (*Fig.* 149) 160
— hypoglossi, (*Fig.* 149) 159
Compensatory regenerative hyperplasia of liver, 528
Compound dislocation of testis, 416
Compression fracture of spine causing disc prolapse, 712
Condyloid canal, veins of, 297
— joint, (*Fig.* 243) 253, 567
Congenital abnormalities of oesophagus, (*Figs.* 369, 370) 374
— — at umbilicus, 52
— — of urinary organs, (*Figs.* 389–397) 397–405
— anomalies of great vessels, (*Figs.* 498–508) 510–523
— atresia of extra-hepatic bile-ducts, 86
— — oesophagus, posterior approach to, 802
— bone disease, 582
— club-foot, 206
— defects of heart, (*Fig.* 496) 507
— deficiency in ganglion cells of colon, 630
— deformities of rectum and anus, (*Figs.* 384–388) 392–397
— diaphragmatic hernia, (*Figs.* 641, 642) 681
— dislocation of head of femur, (*Fig.* 467) 479

27

Congenital dislocation of hip, (*see* Hips Dislocation, Congenital)
— — patella, 667
— diverticulum, characteristics of, (*Fig.* 419) 433
— — of oesophagus, (*Figs.* 423, 424) 436
— errors, anatomy of, (*Figs.* 342–432) 353–448
— — of breast, (*Fig.* 368) 371
— hydrocele, (*Fig.* 400 B) 408
— inguinal hernia, 98, (*Fig.* 398 A) 407, 408
— oesophageal hiatal hernia, (*Fig.* 643) 685
— polycystic kidney, (*Fig.* 389) 397
— pulmonary stenosis, 507
— retraction of nipple, (*Fig.* 32) 38
— spondylolisthesis, (*Fig.* 655 A) 700
— talipes equinovarus, 484
— theory of causation of peritoneal bands, 73
— umbilical hernia, 52
— valves in urethra, 403, 404
Conjoint tendon (falx inguinalis), (*Fig.* 87) 98, 99, (*Fig.* 715) 757
Connective tissue, dense, of scalp, (*Fig.* 1) 1
— — loose, of scalp, 1, 2
Conoid ligament, (*Fig.* 268) 271
Constrictor muscle(s), inferior, 153
— — middle, plexuses on, 157
— — of pharynx, (*Fig.* 166) 179, 491
— — superior, in relation to tonsil, 27, 28
Contracture of scar in popliteal area, 567
Cooper, ligaments of, (*Fig.* 25) 31, 100
— — cancer invading, 31, (*Fig.* 34 A) 40
— — suture of inguinal ligament to, 759
Coraco-acromial ligament, 271
Coracobrachialis, paralysis of, 457
Coracoclavicular ligaments, (*Fig.* 268) 271
Coracohumeral ligament, (*Fig.* 269) 272, (*Figs.* 618, 619) 660, 661
Corneal reflex, loss of, 453
— ulcers, prevention of, in facial paralysis, 613
Corns due to hammer-toe, 484
Coronary ligament(s), (*Fig.* 379 B) 386
— — short and long, 279
— sinus, left superior vena cava and, (*Fig.* 521) 540
Corrugator cutis muscle, 116
Cortical lesion of facial nerve, (*Fig.* 435) 451
— — optic nerve, (*Fig.* 433) 448
— veins, swollen, 298
Cortisone cover in adrenalectomy, 432
Costal elements of lumbar vertebrae, 694, 697
Costalis, 192

Costocervical arteries, 500
Costochondral junction, prominence seen at, 42
Costoclavicular ligament, (*Fig.* 267) 271
Costocoracoid ligament, 271
Costophrenic sinus, 739
Costotransversectomy, 798
Cough, persistent, due to wax in ear, 139
Covered anus, (*Fig.* 385) 392, 397
Cowper's glands, 200, 585
Coxa valga, (*Fig.* 467) 478
— vara, (*Figs.* 464–466) 476
— — sign of, (*Fig.* 556 B) 588
Cranial fossa, posterior, incision giving access to, (*Fig.* 747) 789
— nerve(s) (*see also* Facial Nerve; Fifth Cranial Nerve, etc.)
— — autonomic fibres in, (*Fig.* 163) 175
— — loss due to division of, (*Figs.* 433–437) 448–455
— — in neck, (*Figs.* 140–144) 148–154
— — pain after tonsillectomy, 30
— — in relation to pituitary body, (*Fig.* 10) 13
— parasympathetic, 171, 175
— sympathetic nerve, (*Fig.* 145) 155
Craniectomy, 787, 789
Craniopharyngeal canal, 353
Craniopharyngioma, pressure on chiasma by, 15
Craniosacral outflow (*see* Parasympathetic Nervous System)
Craniotomy, osteoplastic, (*Figs.* 743–746) 787
Cranio-cleido-dysostosis, 582
Cranium, blood sinuses of, 297
— sensitive and insensitive structure of, 652
Creases of hand and fingers, 658
— interphalangeal, (*Fig.* 610) 654, 658
Creeping periostitis, 582
Cremaster muscle, 406
Cremasteric artery, anastomoses of, 406, (*Fig.* 401) 410
— fascia, 98, 405
Cricopharyngeal sphincter, (*Fig.* 487) 490, 491
Cricopharyngeus, 491
Cricothyroid ligament, 328
— muscle, nerve of, 19
— — — supply to, 152
Crista urethralis, 102
'Critical point' of Sudek, (*Fig.* 52) 63
Cross-bow cut of Cushing, (*Fig.* 747) **789**
Cruciate ligaments, 254, (*Fig.* 277) 277
— — of knee-joint, 667
Crura of diaphragm, 196, 197, 198
— inguinal ring, 97

Crural dislocation of testis, 416
— ectopia testis, 411
— sling, (*Fig.* 644) 686
— — repair of, in sliding hernia, (*Fig.* 648) 688, 689
Crusta petrosa, 574
Cryptorchidism, 409
Crypts of tonsil, 26, 27
Cubital vein, median, (*Fig.* 306 A) 304
Cubitus valgus and cubitus varus, (*Fig.* 478) 486
— — nerve compression in, 471
Cuboid bone, (*Fig.* 225 B) 242
— secondary, (*Fig.* 212) 230
Cuneiform bones, (*Fig.* 225 B) 242
Cushing, cross-bow cut of, (*Fig.* 747) **789**
Cutaneous branches of cervical plexus, (*Fig.* 148) 158
— — posterior rami of spinal nerves, 165
— intercostal nerves, (*Fig.* 155) 166
— nerves of forearm, 459, 460
— — lateral and anterior intercostal, (*Fig.* 155) 166
— — posterior, of thigh, 310
— — of trunk, (*Figs.* 155–158) 164–170
— nerve-supply of head and neck, (*Figs.* 129–132) 136–141
— root-areas, (*Figs.* 156–158) 167
Cyanosis due to Fallot's tetralogy, 508
Cyst(s), branchial, (*Figs.* 354, 355) 361, 363
— of common bile-duct, congenital, (*Fig.* 382 D) 388
— dermoid, (*see* Dermoid, Dermoid Cyst)
— enterogenous, of gut, (*Figs.* 426, 427) 440, 441
— fimbrial, 418
— solitary, of osteititis fibrosa, (*Fig.* 555, 5) 583
— thyroglossal, (*Fig.* 360) 366
— of urachus, (*Fig.* 396 C) 403
Cystic artery, 525
— — abnormalities of, (*Figs.* 72, 73) 83
— disease of organs associated with polycystic kidneys, 398
— duct, (*Figs.* 71–74) 78, 84
— — absence of, (*Fig.* 70 F) 81
— — variations in, (*Fig.* 70) 81
— lymph-gland, 64, 65
— tumour at umbilicus, 52, (*Fig.* 383 G) 390, 392
— vein, 87
Cystitis, presacral neurectomy for, 630
Cystocele, 720
Cystogastrocolic band, 76, (*Fig.* 380) 386

'Dancing fracture', 234
'Dangerous area' of face, (*Fig.* 300) 299
Dartos muscle of scrotum, 219

INDEX 835

Dawbarn's sign, 261, 589
Deafness due to auditory nerve lesion, 454
Deciduous teeth, extraction of, not followed by osteomyelitis, 575
Declination angle of femur, (*Fig. 463*) 475
Decompression of brain, 787, 789
Deep cervical glands, (*Fig. 22*) 24
— fascia of breast, (*Fig. 25*) 30, (*Fig. 30*) 36
— median vein of forearm, 304
Degenerative spondylolisthesis, (*Fig. 655 A*) 700
Deltoid, 201, 202
— bursa, incision giving access to, (*Fig. 760*) 803
— ligament, (*Figs. 281, 282*) 281, (*Fig. 292*) 291
— paralysis of, 204
— — by axillary nerve compression, 675
— — complicating dislocated shoulder, 661
— prominence of, in rupture of supraspinatus, (*Fig. 634*) 675
Deltopectoral lymph-glands, 339
— triangle, 303
Denervation of heart, (*Figs. 758, 759*) 799
— sympathetic, (*see* Sympathetic Denervation)
Denonvilliers, fascia and space of, (*Fig. 93*) 105
Dental formulae, (*Figs. 548, 549*) 574
— sac, 573
— shelf, (*Fig. 546*) 572
Dentine, 572
Dentition, first, (*Fig. 548*) 574
— second, (*Fig. 549*) 574
Depressors, fascia of, 209
Dermal sinus, congenital, 422
Dermoid(s) (*see also under specific parts*)
— cysts of face, sequestration, (*Fig. 353*) 359
— — nose, 360
— in line of embryonal concrescence, 426
— sacral, 424, 427
— sequestration, (*Figs. 414-416*) 424
— of skull, (*Fig. 415*) 426
Descendens cervicalis nerve, (*Fig. 149*) 160
— hypoglossi, 155, (*Fig. 149*) 159
Desegmentation of radicular arteries, (*Figs. 490, 491*) 499
Developmental defects, anatomy of (*Figs. 342-432*) 353-448
Dextrocardia, 523
Diacondylar fracture of humerus, 487
Diagonal conjugate, measurement of, per vaginam, 586
Diaphragm(s), (*Fig. 184*) 195
— of body, (*Figs. 182-187*) 194-200
— development of, (*Fig. 641*) 681

Diaphragm(s), eventration of, 684
— hernia, through dome of, 684
— incision of, in exploring upper abdomen, 794
— — sparing phrenic nerve, (*Fig. 649*) 691
— irritation of peritoneal surface of, causing shoulder-tip pain, 88, 89
— of lower aperture of thorax, (*Fig. 184*) 195
— mouth, (*Fig. 182*) 194
— nerve-supply of, 157
— openings in, (*Fig. 184*) 197
— orifices of, relations of, 347
— paralysis of, due to division of phrenic nerve, 466
— pelvic, (*Fig. 185*) 198, 224, 718
— 'pinch-cock' effect of, 492
— relation of 1st lumbar ganglion to crus of, (*Fig. 603*) 640
— — kidneys to, (*Figs. 79, 80*) 89
— relationships of, 196
— of upper aperture of thorax, (*Fig. 183*) 195
— urogenital, (*Figs. 186, 187*) 199, 718, 719
Diaphragma sellae, 6, 11
Diaphragmatic hernia, (*Figs. 641-649*) 681
— — central, 684
— — hiatal, (*Figs. 643-649*) 685
— — posterior, 683
— — posterolateral, (*Fig. 642*) 683, 684
— — retrosternal, (*Fig. 642*) 682, 684
— — route to, 792
— — traumatic, 684
— lymph-glands, (*Fig. 184*) 196, 335, 336
— respiration in child, 133
— veins in portal obstruction, 529
Diaphysial aclasia, 582
Diaphysis, 242, 246, 251
— of bone, (*Figs. 553, 554*) 580
— infections of, 583
Diarrhoea causing rectal prolapse, 721, 723
Diarthroses, (*Figs. 239-245*) 252
Diffuse bearing stump, 770
Digastric muscle, nerve to posterior belly of, 148, (*Fig. 142*) 150
Digital arteries supplying terminal phalanx, (*Fig. 611*) 653
— flexor sheaths, 657
— joints, (*Figs. 542-544*) 567
— mobility, factors limiting, 569, 570
— processes of palmar fascia, (*Figs. 198, 199*) 213
Digits, (*Figs. 542-544*) 567
Dilator pupillae muscle, (*Fig. 136*) 144
Dimpling of skin due to breast cancer, (*Fig. 34 A*) 40
Diploic plexus, 296
— veins, (*Fig. 298*) 296

836 INDEX

Diplopia due to pituitary tumour, 16
Disarticulation at upper limb joints, 779
Disc(s) articular, (*Figs.* 246, 247) 254
— prolapse causing neuralgia, 229
Discharges at umbilicus, 54
Discoid lateral meniscus, 578
Dislocation(s), common, (*Figs.* 617–628) 659–670
— of testis, 407, (*Fig.* 404) 415
— tissue, (*Figs.* 417, 418) 428
— of vertebrae, (*Fig.* 119) 126
Dissecting aneurysms of aorta, (*Figs.* 538, 539) 561
Distal lymph-glands of gut, (*Fig.* 54) 66
Diverticulitis, 445
Diverticulosis associated with hiatus hernia, 689
Diverticulum(a) (*see also under specific parts*) (*Figs.* 419–431) 433–447
— of bladder, (*Fig.* 395 C) 402, 445
— caval, (*Fig.* 523 C) 543
— characteristics of, (*Fig.* 419) 433
— congenital, diagnosed from acquired, (*Fig.* 419) 433
— duodenal, 56 (*Fig.* 382 C) 389
— gut, congenital, (*Figs.* 426, 427) 440
— Meckel's (*see* Meckel's Diverticulum)
— of oesophagus, (*Fig.* 423) 436
— pathological, characteristics of, (*Fig.* 419) 433
— of pharynx, 361
— Vaterine, (*Fig.* 430C–E) 443
Dorsal aorta(ae) embryonic, (*Figs.* 498–502) 510, 511, 512, 515
— — right, persistence of 8th segment of, (*Fig.* 501), 512, 518
— carpal ligament, 258
— mesentery, (*Fig.* 379 A) 386
— motor nucleus of vagus, (*Figs.* 581–583) 618
— nerve of penis, (*Figs.* 96, 98) 108
— — — or clitoris, (*Figs.* 741, 742) 785
— spaces of hand, (*Fig.* 612) 658
— subaponeurotic space, (*Fig.* 612) 658
— subcutaneous space, (*Fig.* 612) 658
— vein of penis, (*Fig.* 187) 200
— venous plexus of hand, 303, 304
Dorsalis scapulae nerve, 161, 456
Dorsiflexors of foot, paralysis of, gait of, (*Fig.* 551 C) 578
Dorsum of fingers, 658
'Double aortic arch', (*Figs.* 504, 505) 518
— channel', (*Fig.* 489) 495
— 'inferior vena cava, (*Fig.* 523 B) 543
— ureter, (*Fig.* 394) 401
— vision due to fourth nerve division, 450
'Double-barrelled' colon, (*Fig.* 65) 75

Douglas, pouch of, abscess in, (*Fig.* 698) 742
— — boundaries of, 742
— — examination of, 585, 587
— — floor of, 105
— — puncture of, (*Fig.* 698) 741
Drainage, defective, consequences of, to shoulder-joint, 571
Drainage-tube(s), incisions for, 744
— in pararectal incision, (*Fig.* 707) 750
Drop foot, (*Fig.* 551 C) 578
— — following operation in popliteal area, 567
Drop-wrist due to radial nerve palsy, (*Fig.* 439) 458
Drowsiness, persistent, due to pituitary tumour, 16
Ductus arteriosus, (*Fig.* 499) 512, 519
— — patent, (*Fig.* 506) 520
— — relation of, to coarctation of aorta (*Fig.* 507) 520
— deferens (*see* Vas Deferens)
— venosus, fibrotic process taking place in, at birth, 529
Duodenal atresia associated with annular pancreas, (*Fig.* 418) 431
— compression by abnormal bands due to errors of gut rotation, (*Fig.* 378) 384
— diverticulum, 56, (*Fig.* 382 C) 389
— entrance of bile-duct, 55
— fossa(ae), (*Figs.* 56–59) 67–71
— — inferior, 67, (*Fig.* 58) 69
— ileus, (*Figs.* 377, 378) 383
— — chronic episodic, 384
— — treatment of, (*Fig.* 378) 384
— obstruction, acute, of newborn, 384
— — due to pre-duodenal portal vein, 524
— perforation causing shoulder-tip pain, 89
— ulcer(s) associated with chronic ileus, 384
— — causing diverticula, 445
— — infection of gall-bladder from, 87
Duodenocolic isthmus, (*Fig.* 377) 376, 377, 381
Duodenojejunal flexure, 56, 490
— — congenital stenosis at, 387
— — intestinal rupture at, 566
— fossae, 67, (*Fig.* 57) 69
Duodenum, (*Fig.* 43) 55
— accessory pancreatic tissue or surrounding, (*Figs.* 417 B, 418) 428, 431
— blood-supply of, (*Fig.* 428 A) 443
— congenital obstruction of, (*Figs.* 380, 381) 386
— — stenosis of, (*Fig.* 381) 387

Duodenum, development of, 376
— displaced, due to abnormal rotation, (*Fig.* 376) 387
— diverticula of, (*Figs.* 428, 430) 443, 445
— entry of bile duct and pancreatic ducts into, (*Fig.* 488) 494
— — common bile-duct into, (*Fig.* 69) 78, 79
— incisions giving access to, 745
— portal vein lying anterior to, (*Fig.* 509 A) 523, 524
— relations, 55
— suspensory ligament of, 56
Duplications of alimentary tract, 442
Dupuytren's contracture, 214, 324
Dura mater, (*Fig.* 3) 5
— — dermoids of skull attached to, (*Fig.* 415) 426, 427
Dural relations of semilunar ganglion, (*Figs.* 134, 135) 142
— sac, 128
Dysmenorrhoea, primary, presacral neurectomy for, 630
Dysphagia due to oesophageal compression by ligamentum arteriosum, 519
— intermittent, due to oesophageal spasm, 493
— lusoria, 515
Dyspnoea due to sliding hernia, 687
Dystrophia adiposogenitalis, 354

Ear, chemodectoma in, 651
— external, nerve-supply of, (*Fig.* 130) 138
— extrinsic muscles of, origins of, 4
— herpes of, 138
— internal, nerve-supply to, (*Fig.* 141) 149, 152
— — pharyngeal pouch in formation of, 363
— oesophageal pain referred to, 492
Earache associated with gastric disorder, 139
Eburnation of tuberosity of humerus due to calcification, (*Fig.* 639 A) 680
Eck fistula, (*Fig.* 513) 529
Ectoderm between skin and neural tube, (*Fig.* 415 B, C) 427
Ectodermal surfaces, developmental fusion of, and dermoids, (*Fig.* 414) 424
— vestiges causing sequestration dermoids, 424, 428
Ectopia testis, 411
— — varieties of, 411
— vesicae, 53
Ectopic gestation, intraperitoneal rupture of, causing shoulder-tip pain, 89
— phaeochrome tissue, tumour arising from, 648

Ectopic thyroid, 367
— — tissue, 24
— ureter, 401
Efferents of deep cervical circular chain, 328
Effort thrombosis, (*Fig.* 307) 305
Eighth nerve, loss due to division of, 454
Ejaculation, mechanism of, 647
Ejaculatory ducts, (*Fig.* 91) 102
— — effects of prostatectomy on, 104
Elbow, anatomical angles of, (*Figs.* 477–479) 485
— bursae around, (*Fig.* 254) 262
— collateral ligaments of, (*Fig.* 270) 272, 486
— injury, Volkmann's ischaemic contracture following, 324
— median nerve compression at, 470
— optimum position for ankylosis of, (*Figs.* 481, 482) 488
— paralysis of extensors of, 457
— ulnar nerve compression at, 470
— veins at, (*Fig.* 306) 304
Elbow-joint, (*Fig.* 241) 253
— approach to, (*Figs.* 763, 764) 805
— puncture of, (*Fig.* 684) 733
Elephantiasis, Kondoléon operation for, (*Fig.* 566) 598
Eleventh cranial nerve (*see* Spinal Accessory Nerve)
Elmslie's operation for talipes equinovarus, 291
Emargination of patella, 238
Embryonal concrescence, line of, (*Fig.* 414) 425
Embryonic tail, persistence of, 422
Emissary veins, 296
— — of scalp, (*Fig.* 1) 2
Emphysema, advanced, compressing brachial plexus, 226
Empyema, chronic, causing brain abscess, 321
Enamel bud, (*Fig.* 546) 572
— dental, (*Fig.* 546) 572
Enarthrosis, (*Fig.* 245) 254
Encephalocele, 360, (*Fig.* 367 B) 371
Encephalopathy, hypertensive, cause of, 653
Encysted hydrocele of testis, 416
— inguinal hernia, (*Fig.* 398 D) 407
End-bearing stump, 770
Endometrial tissue, accessory, 432
Endometriomata, 432
Enophthalmos, 466
— in Horner's syndrome, 613
Enteritis in children causing prolapse of rectum, 721

838 INDEX

Entero-anastomosis in oesophagojejunal anastomosis, (*Fig.* 756) 798
Enterocystocele, (*Fig.* 383 D)
Enterogenous cysts of gut, (*Figs.* 426, 427) 440, 441
Enteromata, (*Fig.* 383 C) 392
Ephippial joint, (*Fig.* 244) 253
Epicranius muscle, (*Figs.* 1, 2) 1
Epididymis, development of, 405
— and vas, single, in duplication of testis, (*Fig.* 402) 412
Epididymitis, prevention of post-prostatectomy, 104
Epidural space, 7
Epigastric artery, inferior, (*Fig.* 87) 98, 99
— — — pubic branch of, (*Fig.* 90) 101
— bruit due to coeliac artery compression, 448
— vein, inferior, 308, 320
— — superficial, 306
Epigastrium, intercostal nerve supplying, 167
Epiphrenic diverticulum of oesophagus, (*Fig.* 424 C) 437
Epiphyseal blood-vessels, (*Fig.* 226) 243
— cartilage, 242, 243 (*Figs.* 553, 554) 581
— — displaced in separation of epiphysis, 582
— centres in development of vertebra, (*Figs.* 664, 665) 708
— coxa vara, (*Fig.* 464 A) 476
— line(s) and capsular reflections, (*Figs.* 259–265) 266–270
— — of femoral head in adult and child, (*Fig.* 465) 478
Epiphysitis, vertebral, (*Fig.* 671) 715
Epiphysis(es), 242, 246, 251, (*Fig.* 554) 580
— of clavicle, (*Fig.* 232) 247
— long bones, union of, 248, 251
— separation of, 242, 478, 582
— upper femoral, slipping of, (*Figs.* 465, 466) 476, 477
Epiploic arcade, normal and abnormal, (*Figs.* 526, 527) 546
— arteries, (*Fig.* 526) 546
Epispadias, (*Fig.* 410) 422
Epoophoron, (*Fig.* 406) 417
Equilibrium, loss of, due to auditory nerve lesion, 454
Erb's paralyses, 139, 163
— point, (*Fig.* 152) 163, (*Fig.* 438) 455
Erb-Duchenne paralysis, 455
Erysipelas, diagnosis from cellulitis, 587
Essential hypertension (*see* Hypertension, Essential)
Eventration of diaphragm, 684
Evolutionary theory of causation of peritoneal bands, 73

Ewing's tumour, (*Fig.* 555, 7) 583
Exomphalos, 52, 383
Exostosis(es), cancellous, 582
— multiple, 582
Exploratory abdominal incision, 749
Expression, loss of movements of, 453
— motor nerve for muscles of, 138
— muscles of, 148
Extensor(s) of arm and hand, paralysis of, 457
— carpi radialis longus and brevis, 258, 287
— — ulnaris, 258, 288
— communis digitorum, (*Fig.* 174) 187, 189, 258, 287, 288, 289
— digitorum brevis, 288
— — longus, 205, 283
— — — tendon-sheath of, (*Fig.* 251) 259
— hallucis longus, 283, 288, 289
— — — of foot, effects of flat-foot on, (*Figs.* 473, 474) 482, 483
— — — tendon-sheath of, (*Fig.* 251) 259
— indicis proprius, 258, 287, 288
— — — origin of, 274
— minimi digiti, 258, 288
— pollicis brevis, 258, 287
— — — origin of, 274
— — — stenosis of, 259
— — longus, 258, 287
— — — origin of, 274
— retinaculum of hand, 258, (*Fig.* 289) 286
— — superior, relations under, 348
— — of wrist, 665
External abdominal ring, dislocation of testis through, 415
— inguinal ring, testis at, 409
— nasal nerve, (*Fig.* 129) 136
Extraparietal inguinal hernia, (*Fig.* 399) 408
Extraperitoneal abscess causing supralevator fistula, (*Fig.* 115) 123
— compartments, right and left, 727
Extravaginal torsion of testis, 414
Extra-embryonic coelom, 376
Extremities, diseases of arteries of, 642
Extroversion of bladder, (*Figs.* 410, 411) 420
— cloaca, 380, 381

Face, 'dangerous area' of, (*Fig.* 300) 299
— deep sensibility from, nerve conveying, 451
— development of, (*Figs.* 345, 346) 355
— — anomalies of, (*Figs.* 347–353) 356
— imperfect fusion of processes of, (*Figs.* 347–352) 356, 357
— inclusions along fusion lines of, 356, (*Fig.* 353) 359

INDEX 839

Face, lines of fusion of, (*Fig.* 414) 425
— nerve-supply of, (*Fig.* 129) 138
— paralysis, partial, of upper part of, 451
Facial glands, (*Fig.* 325) 327, 328
— nerve, anastomosis operation on, 155
— — autonomic fibres in, 175
— — communication(s) between glossopharyngeal and, (*Fig.* 142) 150
— — — of, with fifth nerve, 141, 149
— — — laryngeal nerve with, 152
— — crushing of, in facial tic, 138
— — in infant, vulnerability of, (*Fig.* 123) 131
— — lesions, herpes of ear connected with, 138
— — loss due to division of, (*Figs.* 435, 436) 451
— — mandibular branch of, 149
— — in neck, (*Fig.* 140) 148
— — posterior auricular branch of, 138
— — in relation to parotid gland, (*Fig.* 436) 453
— — relationship of first branchial cleft fistula to, 365
— — and taste sensations, 147, 151
— — temporal branch of, 138
— paralysis due to facial nerve division, 451
— — nerve anastomosis for, 155
— — prevention of corneal ulcers in, 613
— tic, 138
— vein, anterior, (*Figs.* 299, 300) 298
— — common, 298, 300, (*Figs.* 303, 304) 301, 303
— — deep, (*Fig.* 299) 299
— — posterior, 298, (*Figs.* 303, 304) 301
Faecal obstruction due to peritoneal bands, 73
— soiling following anal canal surgery, 118
Faeces discharged at umbilicus, 52
Falciform ligament, (*Fig.* 379 B) 386
— — separating anterior intraperitoneal compartments, 729
— — process, 284
Fallot, tetralogy of, (*Fig.* 496) 508
— — right aortic arch associated with, 516
False capsule of prostate, (*Fig.* 92) 104
— — thyroid, (*Figs.* 20, 21) 23
— external piles, 112
Falx cerebelli, 6
— cerebri, 5
— — incision giving access to, (*Fig.* 743) 787
— inguinalis (conjoint tendon), (*Fig.* 87) 98, 99, (*Fig.* 715) 757
Fascia(ae), (*Figs.* 191-208) 206-224

Fascia(ae), anal, 106, 224
— around calf muscles, 313
— behind prostate, (*Fig.* 93) 104
— of Camper, (*Figs.* 203, 204) 218
— Colles, (*Fig.* 205) 220
— colli, (*Figs.* 191-196) 206-212
— — general investing layer of, (*Figs.* 192, 193) 206
— cribrosa, 101
— deep, dissection of, with skin, in amputations, 598
— — excision of, in Kondoléon operation, (*Fig.* 566) 597
— — importance of, in amputations, 771
— — lymph plexus on, 345
— of depressors, 209
— iliaca, (*Fig.* 88) 99
— lata, attachment of Scarpa's fascia to, (*Fig.* 204) 220
— lunata, (*Fig.* 95) 106, 109
— obturator, 106, 221
— palmar and plantar, (*Figs.* 197-199) 212
— parotideomasseteric, 208, 327
— pelvic, (*Figs.* 206-208) 221, 623
— of pelvic diaphragm, 224
— popliteus, (*Fig.* 275) 276
— pretracheal, (*Fig.* 192) 206, 209, 210
— prevertebral, (*Figs.* 192, 194-196) 206, 209, 210, 216
— renal, (*Figs.* 84, 85) 93
— of scarpa, (*Figs.* 203-205) 218
— supporting arches of foot, (*Fig.* 297) 295
— transversalis, 97, 98, (*Fig.* 88) 99, 405, (*Fig.* 399) 408
— urogenital, (*Fig.* 186) 199
Fascial bands of cervicovaginal border, 718
— relations of kidney, (*Figs.* 84, 85) 93
— — of prostate, (*Figs.* 92-94) 103-106
— spaces of hand, (*Figs.* 612-614) 654
Fat of hibernating gland, 134
— in ischiorectal fossa, (*Fig.* 95) 106
— pads in joints, 731
— subcutaneous, of child, 134
Fatty capsule of kidney, 93, 95
— tissue, loss of perianal and perirectal, causing prolapse, 721
Fauces, pillars of, 26
Faucial tonsil (*see* Tonsil)
Female, development of external genitalia in, 419
— drainage of pouch of Douglas in, (*Fig.* 698) 742
— external genitalia, anaesthesia of, (*Figs.* 741, 742) 785
— information gained by rectal examination in, 585

840 INDEX

Female pelvic floor, (*Fig.* 674) 718, 719
— urethra, prolapse of, 721
— vestigial structures in connexion with genital organs in, (*Fig.* 406) 417
Femoral artery, common, occlusion of, sudden, 553
— — — patency of, in atherosclerosis, 564, 566
— — exposure of, (*Fig.* 540) 565
— — occlusion of, collateral circulations in, 555
— — — gangrene following, 549
— — superficial, occlusion of, sudden, 553
— canal, (*Fig.* 89) 99, 100
— — incisions giving access to, (*Fig.* 717) 759, 760
— condyle, lateral, (*Fig.* 627) 668, 669
— dislocation of testis, (*Fig.* 404) 415
— ectopia testis, 411
— epiphysis, upper, slipping of, (*Figs.* 465, 466) 476, 477
— hernia, 97, (*Figs.* 88–90) 99
— — coverings of, 101
— — operations for, (*Fig.* 717) 759
— — obliquity in female, (*Fig.* 468) 479
— — ring(s), 100
— — Henry's suprapubic approach to, 760
— — septum, 101
— — sheath, (*Figs.* 88, 89) 99, 101
— — relations of, 347
— — thrombosis, deep, collateral channel in, 308, (*Fig.* 318) 318
— triangle, occlusion of femoral artery at apex of, 555
— — relations in, 349
— vein, (*Fig.* 309) 310, 312
— — communication between long saphenous and, 316
— — ligation of, (*Fig.* 317) 318
Femoro-iliac thrombophlebitis, treatment of, 611
Femoropopliteal graft, exposure of popliteal artery for, (*Fig.* 541) 566
Femur, amputation(s) through broad end of, 774
— — — shaft of, 775
— anatomical angle of lower end of, (*Figs.* 468–471) 479
— — — shaft of, 479
— — — upper end of, (*Figs.* 463–467) 475
— bending of shaft of, below great trochanter, (*Fig.* 464 C) 476
— bursae on great trochanter of, (*Fig.* 255) 262, 263
— congenital dislocation of head of, (*Fig.* 467) 479

Femur, dislocations of head of, 276
— displacement of, on tibia, 667
— epiphyseal line and capsular reflections of, (*Figs.* 262, 263) 268
— exposure of, (*Fig.* 779) 817
— measuring length of, (*Fig.* 561) 594
— ossification of, 249, 250
— rotation of, on tibia, (*Fig.* 190) 204
— sarcoma of lower end of, 249
Fetal spine, 128
Fetus, blood-supply to spinal cord in, (*Fig.* 490) 499
Fever, headache of, 652
Fibrocartilage(s), 251
— intervertebral, (*Fig.* 117) 123
Fibrochondroma of face, (*Fig.* 353) 359
Fibrosarcoma, periosteal, (*Fig.* 555, 2) 583
Fibrotic processes causing portal block, 529
Fibrous joints, (*Figs.* 235, 236) 250
— sheaths of uterine blood-vessels, 718, 719
— tendon sheaths of hand, 256
Fibula, epiphyseal line and capsular reflections of, (*Fig.* 261) 269
— exposure of, 818
— ligaments attached to lower end of, (*Fig.* 284) 281
— measuring length of, (*Fig.* 564) 596
— ossification of, 248
— spread of disease between ankle-joint and, 270
— stump of, 774
Fibular collateral ligament, (*Figs.* 276, 279) 276, 277
Fibulare, (*Fig.* 225 A) 241, 242
Fifth cranial nerve, (*Fig.* 129) 136
— — — alcohol injection of, (*Figs.* 736–738) 780, 781
— — — conveying deep sensibility from face, 451
— — — divisions of, 136, 137
— — — ganglia of, (*Figs.* 133–139) 141–148
— — — loss due to division of, (*Fig.* 434) 450
— — — motor root of, (*Fig.* 133) 142
Fimbrial cysts, 418
Finger(s) amputations, (*Figs.* 732–735) 776
— — tendon suture in, 771, 778
— attachments of palmar fascia to, (*Figs.* 198, 199) 214
— contracture of, in Volkmann's ischaemic contracture, 324
— dorsum of, 658
— fifth, small muscles of, 189
— incisions on, 764
— infections, (*Fig.* 610) 653

INDEX 841

Finger(s), little, amputation of, (*Fig.* 735) 778
— — tendon-sheath of, (*Figs.* 249, 250) 256
— — thecal whitlow of, incision for, (*Figs.* 723, 725) 767
— paralysis of extensors of, 457
— — flexors of, 457
— splinting of, in extension, 570
— tendon, long flexor, blood-supply to, (*Fig.* 525) 545
— tendon-sheaths of, (*Fig.* 249) 256
— trigger, 579
— webbed, (*Fig.* 413) 424
Finger-joint(s) dislocation of, 568
— level of, at back, (*Fig.* 616) 658
First cranial nerve, loss due to division of, 448
Fisher (Timbrell) approach to medial meniscus, (*Fig.* 774) 813
Fissure(s) in ano, 111
— of lungs, 42, 46
Fistula(ae) in ano, 111, (*Figs.* 110–115) 120–123
— — subcutaneous or submucous, 123
— branchial, (*Figs.* 354–358) 361, 362
— Eck, (*Fig.* 513) 529
— first branchial cleft, (*Figs.* 357, 358) 364
— lactiferous duct, (*Fig.* 33) 40
— pre-auricular, (*Figs.* 343, 344) 354
— rectal, (*Fig.* 386) 393
— thyroglossal, 367
— tracheo-oesophageal, (*Fig.* 370 B–E) 374
'Flame-shaped' haemorrhage in conjunctiva, 3
Flaps of amputation stump, (*Fig.* 728) 770, 771
Flat bones, blood-supply of, (*Fig.* 228) 242, 245
— muscles, division of, in extending McBurney's incision, 756
— — incisions dividing, 754
Flat-foot, 291, 293 (*Figs.* 472–474) 482
Flexed stump, 772
Flexion creases of palm, incisions in, 764
— of uterus, 719
Flexor(s) aspects, avoidance of incisions on, 764
— carpi radialis, 286
— — ulnaris, 286
— — — paralysis of, 457
— digitorum longus, (*Fig.* 171 B) 185, 188, (*Fig.* 282) 281, 289
— — profundus, (*Fig.* 171 A) 185, 188
— — — tendons, blood-supply to, 545
— — — involved in Volkmann's ischaemic contracture, 324

Flexor(s), digitorum sublimis, 188
— — — testing integrity of, (*Fig.* 167) 181
— hallucis brevis, sesamoids of, (*Fig.* 216) 234
— — longus, (*Fig.* 282) 281, 283, 289
— of hand and wrist, paralysis of, 457
— pollicis longus involved in Volkmann's ischaemic contracture, 324
— — — origin of, 273
— — — stenosis of, 259
— — — tendon, 285
— profundus tendons, (*Figs.* 198, 199) 213
— — origin of, 273
— retinaculum of foot, 289
— — hand, (*Fig.* 250) 257, (*Figs.* 289, 290) 284
— — — division of, (*Fig.* 288) 286
— — — relations under, 348
— tendons of fingers, stenosis of, 259
— — hand, (*Fig.* 615) 654, 657
— — — sheaths of, (*Figs.* 249, 250) 256
Fontanelle(s), (*Figs.* 120–121) 129
— anterior puncture of, 735
Foot, accessory bones of, (*Figs.* 212–219) 229n, 230
— arches of, (*Figs.* 295–297) 292–296, (*Figs.* 472–474) 482
— dorsiflexors, paralysis of, gait of, (*Fig.* 551 C) 578
— fascia of, 212
— homologies of, (*Fig.* 225) 241
— interossei of, (*Fig.* 172 B) 185
— inversion and eversion of, 205
— ligaments and arches of, (*Figs.* 292–297) 290–296
— lumbricals of, (*Fig.* 171 B) 185, 186
— paralysis of, due to tibial nerve lesion, 465
— sensory loss in, due to peroneal nerve lesion, (*Fig.* 448) 465
— sesamoids of, (*Figs.* 212, 216) 234
— stenosing tenovaginitis of, 259
— subtaloid, dislocation of, (*Fig.* 628) 669
— tendon-sheaths of, (*Figs.* 251–253) 259
Foot-drop due to peroneal nerve lesion, 465
— — sciatic nerve lesion, (*Fig.* 446) 464
Foramen(ina) of Bochdalek, 682, 683
— caecum, 360, (*Fig.* 360) 365
— — vein of, 296, 297
— epiploicum, 729
— — small gut in, 67, 68
— intervertebral, 126
— lacerum, veins of, 297
— of Morgagni, 682
— ovale, 150
— — relation of otic ganglion to, (*Fig.* 138) 146
— — veins of, 297

842 INDEX

Foramen(ina) traversing fifth lumbar vertebra, 697
— Vesalii, veins of, 297
— of Winslow, 729
Forearm(s) (*see also* Upper Limb)
— amputation through, 779
— flexion of, acute, 305
— interosseous membrane of, (*Fig.* 271) 273
— medial cutaneous nerve to, (*Fig.* 151) 161, 162
— median vein of, (*Fig.* 306 B) 304
— muscles, ischaemia of, due to brachial artery injury, 324
— position of, to maintain shoulder-joint abduction, (*Fig.* 545) 572
— red streaks on, in lymphangitis, 339
— space, infection of, (*Fig.* 615) 657
— veins of, (*Fig.* 306) 303, 304, 305
Foregut of embryo, (*Figs.* 371, 372) 375, 376
Foregut-midgut junction, congenital abnormalities of region of, (*Figs.* 379–382) 386
Foreign bodies in joints, 731
Fossa(ae) intersigmoidea, 67 (*Fig.* 61) 72,
— ovalis, 99, 306, 308
— peritoneal, (*Figs.* 55–61) 67–72
Fourth aortic arch, embryonic, (*Figs.* 498–504) 510, 512, 515, 516
— cranial nerve, loss due to division of, 450
— — — palsy due to pituitary tumour, 16
— thyroid vein, 19
— ventricle, apertures of, 9
— — blockage at aperture to, (*Fig.* 6) 10
— — incision giving access to, (*Fig.* 747) 789
— — tela choroidea of, 8
Fracture-compression of vertebra, localization of, 128
Fracture-dislocation of spine, localization of, 128
— vertebrae, (*Fig.* 119) 126, 659
Frenula of ileocaecal valve, 494
Fresher's leg, 556
Fröhlich's syndrome, 354
Froin's syndrome, 9
Froment's sign, (*Fig.* 170) 183
Frontal approach to brain, (*Fig.* 744) 787
— bone, fracture of orbital plate of, 3
— diploic vein, 296
— lobe(s), incisions giving access to, (*Figs.* 744, 745) 788
— — pressure on, by pituitary tumour, 16
— sinus, development of, in child, (*Fig.* 125) 132
Frontalis muscle, (*Fig.* 2) 2, 148

Frontonasal process of embryo, (*Fig.* 345) 355
Frozen hand, 571
— shoulder, 678
Functional impairment due to sympathetic involvement in injury, 571
Fundoplication in prevention of reflux, 686
Funicular inguinal hernia, (*Fig.* 398 B) 407
— process, 407
Funiculitis, (*Fig.* 658) 703
Funiculus, 706
Fused kidney, unilateral, (*Fig.* 393 B) 400

Galea aponeurotica, 1, 2
Gallaudet's fascia, 747
Gall-bladder, adhesions of, to duodenum, causing diverticula, (*Fig.* 430 B) 445
— anatomy of, (*Fig.* 74) 84
— cancer of, 87
— cystic artery supplying, (*Figs.* 72, 73) 83
— developmental abnormalities of, (*Fig.* 75) 84–86
— incisions giving access to, 745, 749, (*Fig.* 709) 751, 754
— lymphatics of, 87
— palpation of, 590
— paths of infection to, 87
— positions in relation to bodily habitus, (*Fig.* 462) 475
— right hepatic duct entering, (*Fig.* 71) 82
— structure of, 86
— vascular arrangements of, 87
— venous drainage of, 83
Gall-stones in common bile-duct, 79
Ganglion(a) of autonomic system, 156, (*Fig.* 161) 172, (*Fig.* 164) 176
— cerebrospinal, (*Fig.* 133 A) 141
— of fifth nerve, (*Figs.* 133–139) 141–148
— nodosum, (*Figs.* 582, 583) 618, 619
— — of vagus, 149, 152, 615
Ganglionectomy in denervation of limb, (*Figs.* 595, 596) 633
— to relieve tachycardia and cardiac pain, (*Fig.* 758) 799, 800
— remove cardiac pain, 617
Ganglionitis, (*Fig.* 658) 703
Gangrene due to arterial embolism or thrombophlebitis, 611
— following sudden occlusion of arteries, 553
— incidence of, following war injury to main vessels, 549
— ischaemic, amputation in presence of, (*Fig.* 731) 775
— of testis, 414
Gartner's duct, (*Fig.* 406) 418
Gask and Ross's approach in ganglionectomy, 617

INDEX 843

Gasserian ganglion (*see* Semilunar Ganglion)
Gastrectomy, accessory left hepatic artery complicating, 525, 558
— total, incision for, 755
— — sternum-splitting operation for, (*Fig.* 701) 747
— — transthoracic, 792, 794
Gastric artery(ies), (*Fig.* 754) 795
— — left, hepatic artery arising in, 525
— — right, 525, 558
— branches of vagus nerves, (*Figs.* 585, 586) 620
— contents, reflux of, due to sliding hernia, 687
— — — factors preventing, 686
— disorder, earache associated with, 139
— fundus, cancer of, approach to, 793
— lymph-glands, (*Fig.* 53) 65
— — inferior, (*Fig.* 53) 65
— — superior, (*Fig.* 53) 65
— mucosa in Meckel's diverticulum, 391
— pain due to sliding hernia, 687
— perforation causing shoulder-tip pain, 89
Gastrocnemius limp, 577
— popliteal artery entrapment by, (*Fig.* 432) 447
Gastroduodenal artery, 525, 560
— junction, congenital stenosis at, 387
Gastro-epiploic artery(ies), (*Figs.* 526, 527) 546
— — right, (*Fig.* 754) 795
Gastro-intestinal disorders, pyloric spasm and hypertrophy following, 493
Gastro-oesophageal reflux, factors preventing, 686
Geniculate artery, inferior, (*Fig.* 276) 277
— ganglion, 138, (*Fig.* 141) 150
— — taste fibres in, 147
— neuralgia, 451
Genioglossus muscle, 154
Geniohyoid muscle, nerve to, 155, (*Fig.* 149) 158, 159
Genital folds, lateral, excessive fusion of, 392, 394, 397
— organs, vestigial structures in connexion with, (*Figs.* 405, 406) 416
— swellings, (*Fig.* 407) 419
— tubercle, (*Fig.* 407) 419
Genitalia, external, development of, (*Fig.* 407) 419
Genitofemoral nerve, (*Fig.* 331) 333
Genito-mesenteric fold of Douglas Reid, 73
Genu valgum, (*Figs.* 468–470) 479
— varum, (*Fig.* 471 C) 480
Gerlach, valve of, 490

Germinal epithelium, 405
— ridge (Wolffian ridge), 95, 405
Giant diverticulum of gut, 441
— Meckel's diverticulum, 391
Giant-cell tumour, benign, (*Fig.* 555, 6) 583
Giddiness, rotary, due to auditory nerve lesion, 454
Gimbernat's ligament, 31
Ginglymus joint, (*Fig.* 241) 253
Giraldès, organ of, (*Fig.* 405) 416
Glenoid cavity, (*Fig.* 619) 660
— — of scapula, 254
— — temporal bone, 255
Globular processes of embryo, 356, 357
Glomerulus, (*Fig.* 389) 397
Glomic artery, 650
Glomus intravagale, (*Fig.* 608) 650
— jugulare, (*Fig.* 608) 650
— tympanicum, (*Fig.* 608) 650
Glossopharyngeal nerve, 28, 146, 148, (*Figs.* 141, 142) 149
— — autonomic fibres in, 175
— — branches of, (*Fig.* 142) 149, 150
— — contribution to carotid sinus plexus, (*Fig.* 578) 614
— — geniculate neuralgia and, 451
— — loss due to division of, 454
— — taste fibres in, 147, 151
— — tympanic branch of, (*Figs.* 141, 142) 149
Gluteus maximus, bursae under, (*Fig.* 255) 262
— — hernia under cover of, 692
— — limp, 576
— medius, bursa under, (*Fig.* 255) 263
— — limp, (*Fig.* 551 A) 576
— minimus, bursa under, (*Fig.* 255) 263
— muscles, postural activity of, 181
Goitre, suspensory ligament of Berry supporting, 24
Goodsall's law, (*Fig.* 112) 121
Great vessels, congenital anomalies of, (*Figs.* 498–508) 510–523
— — development of, (*Figs.* 498–504) 510
— — of upper mediastinum, exposure of, (*Fig.* 535) 560
Grey rami communicantes (*see* Rami Communicantes, Grey)
Gridiron incision, McBurney's, (*Figs.* 713–715) 755, 758
Gritti-Stokes amputation, 774
Groin, lymph-glands and cutaneous vessels of, (*Fig.* 204) 219
Gubernaculum testis, 405
Gut, (*Figs.* 43–54) 55–67
— blood-supply of, (*Figs.* 50–52) 61–64
— cancer, factor governing surgery for, 67

Gut, diverticula of, acquired, (*Figs.* 428–430) 442
— fixation of, excessive or deficient, 382, 383
— — to posterior abdominal wall, 380
— large (*see* Colon)
— lymph drainage of, (*Figs.* 53, 54) 64–67
— lymph-glands of, 335
— obliteration of, at attachment of vitello-intestinal duct, (*Fig.* 383 J) 390
— parasympathetic motor and sensory innervation of, (*Fig.* 584) 619
— primitive, (*Fig.* 46 A) 59, 61, 73
— — attachments of, (*Fig.* 379) 386
— rotation of, (*Figs.* 371–376) 375–383
— — errors in, (*Fig.* 376) 380, 384
— small, 56–57
— — anastomosis of, (*Fig.* 51) 62
— — blood-supply of, (*Fig.* 44) 57, (*Fig.* 51) 61, 62
— — development of, from pre-arterial segment of midgut, (*Fig.* 374) 379
— — displaced, due to abnormal rotation, 381
— — mesentery of, 57, (*Fig.* 49) 61
— sphincters of, (*Fig.* 487) 490
— sympathetic supply to, 623
Gynaecomastia, 373

H fistula, tracheo-oesophageal, (*Fig.* 370 E) 374
Habitual dislocation of shoulder, 661
Haemangioma of liver, 527
Haematoma ani, 112
— subaponeurotic, 3
— subdural, 298
Haemorrhage, severe, complicating surgery in portal obstruction, 529
Haemorrhagic pancreatitis, acute, pathology of, 80
Haemorrhoidal artery(ies), inferior, 64, (*Figs.* 98, 109) 599, 601
— — middle, 64, 599, 601
— — superior, 60, (*Fig.* 52) 63, 64, 599
— — — branches of, (*Fig.* 101) 112
— nerves, inferior, (*Figs.* 98, 99) 108, 110, (*Figs.* 741, 742) 785
— vein(s), middle and inferior, (*Fig.* 100) 111, 321
— — superior, (*Figs.* 100, 101) 111, 112, 321
— — thrombophlebitis of, 112
— venous plexus, external and internal, 116, 117
Haemorrhoids (*see* Piles)
Haller, vas aberrans of, (*Fig.* 405) 417
Hallux flexus, 483
— rigidus, (*Fig.* 474) 483

Hallux valgus, (*Fig.* 473) 482
Hamate bone, (*Fig.* 224 B) 241, 242
Hammer-toe, 483
Hand(s), accessory bones of, (*Fig.* 220) 236
— amputation, 779
— compartments of, 215
— development of, (*Fig.* 413) 424
— fascia of, (*Figs.* 197–199) 212
— fascial spaces of, (*Figs.* 612–614) 654
— homologies of, (*Fig.* 224) 240
— infections, (*Figs.* 610–616) 653
— — on dorsum of, incisions for opening, (*Fig.* 722) 766
— — treatment of, 764
— interdigital sinuses of barber's, (*Fig.* 412) 423
— interossei of, (*Fig.* 172 A) 185
— lumbricals of, (*Fig.* 171 A) 185, 186
— movements, coarse and fine, nerves responsible for, 460
— muscles, (*Figs.* 167–176) 181–189
— — intrinsic, (*Figs.* 168–170) 182
— — producing abduction and adduction, 182
— nerve-supply of, 186
— — anomalous, to muscles of, 462
— oedema, 569, 571
— optimum position of, (*Fig.* 445) 463
— paralysis due to median nerve lesion, 460
— — — radial nerve lesion, (*Fig.* 439) 458
— — — ulnar nerve lesion, (*Fig.* 442) 461
— — of intrinsic muscles of, 457
— sensory loss in, due to median nerve lesion, (*Fig.* 441) 460
— — — — radial nerve division, (*Fig.* 440) 459
— — — — ulnar nerve lesion, (*Fig.* 443) 461
— stenosing tenovaginitis of, 259
— tendon-sheaths of, (*Figs.* 249, 250) 256
Hare-lip and cleft palate, (*Figs.* 345–352) 355
— lower, (*Fig.* 349) 358
— types of upper, (*Fig.* 347) 359
Harris's method of injecting third division of fifth nerve, (*Fig.* 737) 781
Härtel's method of injecting semilunar ganglion, (*Fig.* 738) 781
Hartmann, pouch of, 84
— — adhesions between duodenum and, 445
Head of child, (*Figs.* 120–125) 129–132
— and neck, cutaneous nerve-supply of, (*Figs.* 129–132) 136–141
— — — route of blood to, in occlusion of innominate artery, 557
Headache, anatomy of, (*Fig.* 609) 651

Heart (*see also* Cardiac)
— anatomy of defects of (*Figs.* 496, 497) 506
— defects, acquired, (*Fig.* 497) 509
— — congenital, (*Fig.* 496) 507
— denervation of, (*Figs.* 758, 759) 799
— displacement due to sliding hernia, 687
— and great vessels, surgical anatomy of, (*Figs.* 496–506) 506–523
— incisions giving access to, (*Fig.* 497) 510
— inhibitory nerve to, 153
— intracranial drainage routes to, after excision of jugulars, 549
— lymphatic drainage of, 338
— muscle, ischaemia of, pain of, 615
— nerves of, accelerator, (*Fig.* 758 A) 799
— — autonomic, 171
— — pain-conveying, (*Fig.* 758 B) 799
— pain-conducting nerves to, attack on, (*Fig.* 580) 616
— slowing of, reflex, due to pressure on carotid sinus, 614
— transverse, 472
— vertical, 473
Heister, valve of, 86
Hemianopia, bitemporal, 354, 449
— homonymous crossed, 448
— — due to pituitary tumour, (*Fig.* 14) 16
Hemiazygos system in communication with inferior vena cava, (*Fig.* 522 A) 540
— — development of, (*Fig.* 520) 538
— vein, anomalies of, (*Fig.* 522 B) 542
— — associated with left superior vena cava, 540
Hemi-hepatectomy, (*Fig.* 512) 527
Hemiopic pupillary reaction, 448
Hemiplegia, accoucheur's position of hand in, 463
Hemivertebrae, congenital absence of one, (*Fig.* 651) 695, 696
— vertebral body represented by two, 695, 696
Henry's incision to expose humeral shaft, (*Figs.* 777, 778) 815
— — for exposure of femur, (*Fig.* 779) 818
— suprapubic approach to femoral rings, 760
Hepatectomy, partial, dealing with hepatic veins in, 527
Hepatic (*see also* Liver)
— aneurysm, ligation of hepatic artery in, 560
— artery, (*Figs.* 510, 511) 524, 526
— — abnormalities of, (*Figs.* 72, 73) 82, 83
— — anomalies, 524, 525, 558

Hepatic artery, common, aneurysm of, (*Fig.* 511) 525
— — ligation of, collateral circulation in, (*Fig.* 534) 558
— — surgical injury to, 558
— branches of vagus, (*Fig.* 585) 620
— duct(s), (*Figs.* 70, 73–74) 78
— — accessory right, (*Fig.* 70 E) 81
— — common, (*Figs.* 72, 74) 78
— — — variations in, (*Figs.* 70, 71) 81
— — variations in right, (*Fig.* 71) 82
— flexure, resection of cancer of, (*Fig.* 570) 602
— lymph-glands, (*Fig.* 53) 64, 65
— veins, 87
— — at upper hilum of liver, 526
— venous radicles, obstruction of, in cirrhosis of liver, 528
— — system, 526
Hepato-cardiac channel, (*Figs.* 519, 520) 540
Hepatocystic communications, persistent, (*Fig.* 75 D) 85
Hepatoma, hemi-hepatectomy for, 527
Hepatorenal pouch, (*Fig.* 83) 92
— — abscess in, 728
Hernia(ae), acquired, (*Figs.* 643–650) 684–693
— containing Meckel's diverticulum, 391
— diaphragmatic (*see* Diaphragmatic Hernia)
— diaphragmatica transversa, 683
— femoral (*see* Femoral Hernia)
— hiatal (*see* Hiatal Hernia)
— incisional, 743, 747
— inguinal (*see* Inguinal Hernia)
— internal, sites of, 67
— into fossa of Waldeyer, 70
— — ischiorectal fossa, (*Fig.* 95) 108
— Littre's, 391
— lumbar, 692
— obturator, (*Fig.* 650) 691
— pudendal, 692
— rare, (*Figs.* 641–650) 681–693
— scar, 743
— sciatic, 692
— sliding, of Allison, (*Figs.* 644–649) 685
— Spigelian, 691
— through dome of diaphragm, 684
— — pelvic diaphragm, 198
— umbilical, 52
— ventral, 743
Heron-Watson approach to wrist-joint, (*Fig.* 766) 807
Herpes on back of thigh, 706
— of ear, 138
— in facial nerve lesion, 454
— of supraclavicular nerves, 139

Hesselbach, triangle of, (*Fig.* 87) 99
Hiatal hernia, acquired, (*Figs.* 644–649) 685
— — of diaphragm, (*Figs.* 643–649) 685
— — sliding, (*Figs.* 644–649) 685
— — — effects of, (*Fig.* 645) 687
— — — mechanism of, (*Fig.* 645) 686
Hiatus hernia, earache associated with, 139
— — sliding, repair of, (*Figs.* 647, 648) 687
— oesophageal, (*Fig.* 644) 686
— sacralis, injection into, (*Fig.* 739) 783
— of Schwalbe, (*Fig.* 95) 107
Hibbs's operation for spinal tuberculosis, 126
Hibernating gland, 134
Hilar structures, arterial supply to, 51
Hilton's law, 255
— line, 109*n*
Hilum of liver, vessels at lower, (*Figs.* 509–511) 523
— — — upper, 526
— relations of kidneys at, (*Fig.* 82) 91
Hind-gut, 109
— of embryo, (*Figs.* 371, 372) 375, 376
Hinge joint, (*Fig.* 241) 253
Hip adductors, paralysis of, test for, 576
— bursae around, (*Figs.* 255, 256) 262
— dislocation, congenital, limp of, 576
— — — Trendelenburg's test for, (*Fig.* 556) 588
— flexion test, Thomas's, 589
— flexors, paralysis of, limp of, (*Fig.* 551 B) 577
— optimum position for ankylosis of, (*Fig.* 484) 488
— snapping, 578
Hip-joint, amputation at, 775
— dislocations at, 276 (*Fig.* 625) 666
— ligaments of, (*Fig.* 274) 275
— puncture of, (*Fig.* 686) 734
— subpsoas bursa communicating with, (*Fig.* 256) 263
— surgical approach to, (*Figs.* 767, 768) 808
Hirschsprung's disease, (*Fig.* 593) 630
His, angle of, 686, 687
— cervical sinus of, (*Fig.* 355) 361
Histamine, headache produced by, 652
Hoarseness due to injury to external laryngeal nerve, 20
Homologies of carpus and tarsus, (*Figs.* 224, 225) 240
Horizontal joint lines, (*Figs.* 475–479) 484
Horner's syndrome, 613
Horseshoe kidney, (*Figs.* 390–392) 399
Hour-glass dermoid of skull, (*Fig.* 415 G) 426

Housemaid's knee, 265
Houston, valve of, palpation of, 585
Humeral angle, lower, (*Fig.* 479) 487
— shaft, exposure of, (*Figs.* 777, 778) 815
Humero-ulnar and humeroradial joints, (*Fig.* 476) 485
Humerus, abduction of, limit to, (*Fig.* 188) 201
— degenerative changes spreading from supraspinatous to head of, (*Fig.* 639) 680
— dislocation of head of, (*Figs.* 618–620) 659
— epiphyseal lines and capsular reflections of, (*Fig.* 259) 266
— external rotation of, to prevent fixation at shoulder, 681
— fractures of lower end, 485, 487
— insertion of supraspinatus into great tuberosity of, (*Fig.* 629) 670
— intertubercular sulcus of, 262
— measuring length of, (*Fig.* 557) 592
— ossification of, 249
— rotation of, in abduction of shoulder, (*Fig.* 189) 202, 204
— surgical approach to, (*Figs.* 777, 778) 815
Hump-back due to disease or injury of vertebra, 125
Hunter's canal, occlusion of femoral artery in, 555
Huter's approach to hip-joint, (*Fig.* 767) 808
Hyaline cartilage, 251
Hydatid of Morgagni, (*Fig.* 406) 417, 418
— stalked, 417
Hydrencephalocele, (*Fig.* 367 C) 371
Hydrocele, (*Fig.* 400) 408
— of cord, (*Fig.* 400 D) 409
— drainage of, 743
— incision giving access to, (*Fig.* 716 A) 758
— tapping of, in anterior inversion of testis, 414
— of testis, encysted, 416
— types of, (*Fig.* 400) 408
Hydrocephalus, (*Fig.* 6) 9
— due to pituitary tumour, 16
— surgery for, 10
Hydronephrosis due to retention of urine in kidney, 499
— — retrocaval ureter, 544
— in pregnancy due to aberrant ovarian vein, 536
Hyoglossus muscle, 149, (*Fig.* 301) 300
— — relation of submaxillary ganglion to, (*Fig.* 139) 147
— relationship of lymph-glands to, 330
Hyoid arch, 361

INDEX 847

Hyoid bone, 209
— — relation of thyroglossal duct to, (*Figs.* 359 B, 360) 366
Hyperacusis due to facial nerve lesion, 453
Hyperalgesia, local, due to sympathetic involvement in injury, 571
Hyperhidrosis, ganglionectomy for, 634
Hyperparathyroidism, 26
Hypersthenic type of bodily habitus, (*Figs.* 454, 455) 472
Hypertension, chromaffin paraganglioma causing, 649, 650
— chronic, transient paralysis in, 653
— determination of popliteal blood-pressure in, 520
— due to coarctation of aorta, relief of, 522
— essential, (*Fig.* 588) 624
— headache of, 652
— with tachycardia, neurectomy for, (*Fig.* 758 A) 799
Hypertensive encephalopathy, cause of, 652
Hypertrophic pyloric stenosis, 493
Hypochondrium, incision giving access to, (*Fig.* 711) 753
Hypogastric artery(ies), occlusion of, collateral circulation in, 554
— — remains of obliterated, at umbilicus, (*Fig.* 41) 53
— lymph-glands, 334
— nerves, 624, 628
— plexus, inferior, (*Fig.* 164) 177, (*Fig.* 587) 622, 624
— plexus, superior (*see also* Presacral Nerve), (*Fig.* 164) 177
— vein, 321
Hypogastrium, nerve supplying, 167
Hypoglossal canal, veins of, 297
— nerve (12th), (*Fig.* 139) 147, 148, 154, (*Fig.* 149) 159
— — anastomosis of, to facial, 155
— — communication of, with vagus, 152
— — loss due to division of, 455
Hypoparathyroidism, post-thyroidectomy, 26
Hypophysis, developmental defects of, (*Fig.* 342) 353
Hypospadias, (*Figs.* 407–409) 419
Hyposthenic type of bodily habitus, (*Figs.* 460, 461) 475
Hypothalamus in relation to pituitary, 13
Hypothenar eminence, fascia of, 213
— muscles, 655
Hysterectomy, reactionary haemorrhage after, ligature of hypogastric arteries in, 554

Ileal membrane, Lane's, (*Fig.* 62) 74
Ileocaecal cyst, 441
— fold, 71
— fossa, 67, 71
— — superior, 71
— junction, (*Fig.* 487) 490, 494
— valve, 490, 494
— volvulus, 383
Ileocolic artery, (*Fig.* 52) 63, 67, 599
— fold, 71
— fossa, 67, 71
— vein, 64
Ileo-inguinal nerve compression, 471
Ileopectineal line, 100
Ileum, 56
— differences between jejunum and, (*Fig.* 44) 57
— displaced, due to abnormal rotation, 381
— diverticulum of, 57
— terminal, 57
Ileus complicating spinal fracture, 623
— duodenal, (*Figs.* 377, 378) 383
Iliac apophysis, ossification of, (*Fig.* 234) 249
— artery(ies), common, lymph-glands at bifurcation of, (*Fig.* 574) 606, 607
— — — occlusion of, collateral circulation in, 554
— — exposure of, (*Fig.* 540) 564
— — external, occlusion of, collateral circulation, in, 555
— — — sudden, 553
— — incision giving access to, (*Fig.* 716 B) 760, 761
— — internal (*see also* Hypogastric Artery), 599, 601
— — left common, bifurcation of, 72
— crest, articulation of 5th lumbar transverse process with, 127
— fossa, incision giving access to, (*Fig.* 707) 750
— — right, incision giving access to, (*Figs.* 713–715) 755
— — — pain in, due to obstructed flow of urine, 405
— lymph-glands, common, (*Fig.* 332) 333
— — external, (*Fig.* 331) 333
— — internal, 334, 604
— spine, anterior inferior, avulsion of, (*Fig.* 221) 237
— testis, 409
— vein, circumflex, 308, 320
— — common, 313
— — — anomalous position of confluence of, 543
— — — ligation of, (*Fig.* 317) 318
— — external, valve in, 313

848 INDEX

Iliococcygeus muscle, (*Fig.* 102) 114
Iliocostalis group of muscles, (*Figs.* 179, 180) 192
Iliofemoral ligament, (*Fig.* 274) 275
— muscles, 588
Iliohypogastric nerve, 167, 216, 757, 758
— — protection of, in hernial repair, 764
Iliolumbar ligament(s), 216
— — ossification of, (*Fig.* 653) 698
— — — causing painful back, 127
Iliopubic tract, 97
Iliotrochanteric muscles, 588
Ilio-inguinal nerve, 216, (*Fig.* 715) 757, 758
— — protection of, in hernial repair, 764
Ilium, articulation of transverse process of fifth lumbar vertebra with, (*Fig.* 653) 698
— blood-supply of, 245
— ossification of crest of, (*Fig.* 234) 249
Imperfect descent of testis, 412
Imperforate anus, 111, 392
Incisional hernia, 743, 747
Incisions, abdominal, anatomy of, (*Figs.* 699–717) 743–761
Index finger, amputation of, (*Fig.* 732) 776
Infancy, thymus gland in, 134
Infant, aortic arch anomaly in, 519
— hypertrophic pyloric stenosis in, 493
— newborn, spinal cord of, 128, 134
Infantile hydrocele, (*Fig.* 400 C) 409
— inguinal hernia, (*Fig.* 398 C) 407
— paralysis, muscle transplantation in, 181
— type of coarctation of aorta, (*Fig.* 508 A) 521
Infarction in metaphysis, 246
Inferior constrictor muscles, transverse and oblique, 434, 435
— extensor retinaculum of foot, (*Fig.* 290) 288
Inflammatory retraction of nipple, (*Fig.* 33) 40
— theory of causation of peritoneal bands, 73
Infraclavicular lymph-glands, 34, 339
Infrahyoid lymph-glands, 328
Inframammary incision, (*Fig.* 497) 509
Infrarenal anomalies of inferior vena cava, (*Fig.* 523) 540, 543
Infraspinatus, loss of function of, 672
— tendon, (*Fig.* 630) 670
Infratrochlear nerve, (*Fig.* 129) 136
Infra-orbital glands, 327
— nerve, (*Fig.* 129) 136
— — injection of, 782
— — paralysis, (*Fig.* 434 D) 450
Infra-umbilical incision, 745, 754

Infundibular type of pulmonary stenosis, 507
Infundibulum, fascia, 98
— of gall-bladder, (*Fig.* 74) 84
— pituitary body, 11
— relationship to optic chiasma, (*Figs.* 12, 13) 13
Inguinal canal, 97
— — exposure of, 758
— — opening of, to obtain access iliac vessels, 565
— colostomy, left, incision for, 755, 757
— — right, incision for, 757
— dislocation of testis, (*Fig.* 404) 415
— hernia, (*Fig.* 87) 97, 98
— — congenital, 98, (*Fig.* 398 A) 407, 408
— — direct, (*Fig.* 87) 98
— — following McBurney incision, (*Fig.* 715) 757
— — incisions giving access to, (*Fig.* 716 A) 758, 760
— — indirect, 98, (*Figs.* 398, 399) 407
— — — types of, (*Figs.* 398, 399) 407
— — recurrent, section of cord in, 411
— — strangulated, 98, 407
— ligament, (*Fig.* 87) 97, 98
— — occlusion of femoral artery below, collateral circulation in, 555
— — relationship of lymph-glands with, (*Fig.* 335) 340
— — suture to Cooper's ligament, 759
— lymph-glands, (*Fig.* 335) 340
— — drainage area of, (*Fig.* 340) 346
— — nerve injury causing painful scar, 764
— region, (*Figs.* 87–90) 96–101
— — anatomy of, (*Figs.* 87–90) 97
— rings, abdominal and subcutaneous, 97, 406
— testis, 409
Inhibitory nerves to gut, origin of, 172
Inion, 298
Injections into nerves, anatomy of, (*Figs.* 736–742) 780
Innominate artery, anomaly affecting, 519
— — development of, 515
— — exposure of, 564
— — occlusion of, collateral circulations in, 557
— — in relation to sternum, 41
— vein, obstruction to, collateral circulation for, (*Fig.* 529) 551
Inspiration causing movement of organs, 590
Interauricular septum, imperfect closure of, 507
Interbronchial lymph-glands, (*Fig.* 334) 336
Intercaval anastomoses, (*Fig.* 523 D) 543

INDEX 849

Intercavernous sinus(es), 6, 13
Interclavicular ligament, 209, (*Fig.* 267) 271
Intercolic membranes, (*Fig.* 65) 75
Intercostal artery(ies), anterior, 42
— — enlarged, in coarctation of aorta, 522
— — first aortic, (*Fig.* 499) 511, (*Figs.* 502, 503) 515
— — lateral branches of, 31, (*Fig.* 31) 36
— — section of, (*Figs.* 493, 495) 503, 506
— — supplying radicals, 500
— division in transthoracic operation, 791
— lymph-glands, 335, 336
— nerve(s), cold abscess following course of, (*Fig.* 679) 725
— — cutaneous, (*Fig.* 155) 166
— — injury causing painful scar, 764
— — removal of, in Smithwick's operation, 637
— — serving rectus muscle, (*Figs.* 709 B, 710) 752
— — supplying abdomen, 167
— — — breast, 33
— neuralgia following paravertebral alcohol injection, 618
— respiration, 133
— space, choice of, for ligation of internal mammary artery, 41
— vein(s), 31
— — superior, (*Figs.* 519, 520) 538
— vessels and nerves, relations of, 347
Intercostobrachial nerve, 166
— — pressure pain from, due to enlarged gland, 33
Interdigital sinuses of barber's hands, (*Fig.* 412) 423
Intermediate lymph-glands of gut, (*Fig.* 54) 66
Intermesenteric plexus, (*Fig.* 590) 627
Intermetatarseum, (*Fig.* 212) 230
Intermittent claudication, 553, 555, 643
— hydrocele, (*Fig.* 400 B) 408
Intermuscular enterogenous cyst of gut, (*Fig.* 427 B) 441
Internal abdominal ring, 97, 406
— capsule, lesion of facial nerve at, (*Fig.* 435) 451
— group of dislocated testes, (*Fig.* 404) 415
— oblique muscle, aponeurosis of origin of, (*Fig.* 200) 216
— — — nerve-supply of, 167
Interossei, (*Fig.* 172) 185
— action of, (*Fig.* 175) 188, 189
— nerve-supply of, 187
— test for, (*Fig.* 176) 189
Interosseous ligaments, 215, (*Figs.* 224 B, 236) 241, 242, 251
— of foot, 290

Interosseous and lumbrical muscles of hand, paralysis of, (*Fig.* 444) 463
— membrane of forearm, (*Fig.* 271) 273
— — leg, (*Fig.* 285) 283
— nerve, posterior, compression of, 471
Interparietal inguinal hernia, (*Fig.* 399) 408
Interphalangeal creases, (*Fig.* 610) 654, 658
— joints, 567, 569
— — flexure at, in Volkmann's ischaemic contracture, 324
— — ligaments of, 275
— — proximal and distal levels of, (*Fig.* 616) 659
— — sesamoids of, 235
Intersegmental arteries, embryonic, (*Figs.* 498, 499) 511, 512
Intersigmoid fossa, 67, (*Fig.* 61) 72
Interstitial inguinal hernia, (*Fig.* 399) 408
Inter-subcardinal anastomosis, (*Figs.* 519, 520) 538, 543
Intertarsophalangeal joints, ligaments of, 275
Intertracheobronchial lymph-glands, (*Fig.* 334) 336, 337
Intertransversales, nerve to, 159
Intertubercular sulcus, 675
— — of humerus, 262
Interureteric bar, (*Fig.* 395) 402, 446
Interventricular foramen, blockage of, (*Fig.* 6) 10
— septal defect in Fallot's tetralogy, 508
Intervertebral canal(s), boundaries of, 704
— — cold abscess in, 723
— — fourth and fifth lumbar nerves in, 706
— — pressure in, causing sciatica, 703
— disc (*see* Intervertebal Fibrocartilages)
— — anatomy of, (*Fig.* 666) 708
— — changes in aged, (*Fig.* 672) 716
— — degeneration narrowing foramen, 707
— — development of, (*Figs.* 664, 665) 708
— — function of, (*Figs.* 667, 668) 711
— — lesions, (*Figs.* 663–672) 707–716
— — — compression by, causing sciatica, 703
— — prolapse causing maternal obstetrical palsy, 715
— — — and herniation, 712
— — lesions causing low back pain, 695
— fibrocartilages, (*Fig.* 117) 123
— foramen(ina), effects of anomalies on, 705
— — 126
— — sizes of, 705
— sheath, compression of funiculus in, (*Fig.* 662) 707

850 INDEX

Intervertebral veins, 323
Intestinal lymphatic trunk, 335, 341, 342
— obstruction due to Meckel's diverticulum, 391
— — — remains of vitelline duct, 391
— — — volvulus, 382
— rupture following abdominal trauma, site of, 565
Intestine, large (*see* Colon)
— small (*see* Gut, small)
Intracranial blood sinuses, formation of, (*Fig.* 3) 5
— dermoid, (*Fig.* 415 F) 426
— pressure, increased, causing headache, 652
— — raising pressure of cerebrospinal fluid, 591
— spread of middle-ear disease in child, (*Fig.* 124) 132
— venous drainage after excision of jugulars, 549
Intramesenteric enterogenous cyst, (*Fig.* 427 D) 441
— inguinal hernia, (*Fig.* 399) 408
Intraparietal inguinal hernia, (*Fig.* 399) 408
Intraperitoneal compartments, posterior and anterior, (*Figs.* 681, 689) 727
Intrathoracic dermoid, (*Fig.* 416) 427
— stomach, 796
Intratonsillar cleft, 27
Intravaginal torsion of testis, 414
Intra-abdominal pressure, increased, causing prolapse of rectum, 722
Intra-articular ligaments, 254
— structures, (*Figs.* 246, 247) 254
Intrinsic muscles of hand, (*Figs.* 168–170) 182
Intussusception, diagnosis of, from rectal prolapse, 723
— due to Meckel's diverticulum, 391
— enlarged ileocaecal valve causing, 494
— mesentery to ascending colon and, 77
Inversion of testis, (*Fig.* 403) 413
Investing layer of dura mater, (*Fig.* 3) 5
Iris, autonomic innervation of, (*Fig.* 577) 611
— nerve supply to, (*Fig.* 136) 144
Irregular dislocations of hip, 667
Ischaemia of abdominal viscera due to coeliac artery compression, 447
Ischaemic contracture, Volkmann's, 324
— cord lesions following aortic surgery, 500, 503
— paralysis, acute, in anterior tibial compartment, (*Fig.* 533) 556
— — of peroneal nerve, 465

Ischaemic symptoms due to obstruction at origin of subclavian artery, 557
Ischiofemoral ligament, 276
Ischiopubic ramus, conjoined, 222
Ischiorectal abscess, (*Fig.* 95) 107, 110
— — causing sinus and fistula, (*Fig.* 114) 122
— fossa, (*Figs.* 95–98) 106–109, 284
— — cold abscess in, 726
— — contents of, 108
— — hernia into, (*Fig.* 95) 108
Isthmic type of coarctation of aorta, (*Fig.* 507 B) 520, 521
Ivory osteoma, 582

Jackson's membrane, (*Fig.* 66) 76
Jacobson's nerve, (*Fig.* 141) 149
Jaundice due to blocking of bile-duct, 86
Jaw incision behind angle of, 149
— osteomyelitis of, 575
— snapping, 579
Jejunum, 56
— accessory pancreatic tissue in, 428
— anastomosis of, with oesophagus, (*Figs.* 755, 756) 796
— differences between ileum and, (*Fig.* 44) 57
— diverticula of, in relation to blood-supply, (*Fig.* 428 B) 443
Jenkins's method of tapping lateral ventricle, (*Fig.* 690 B) 736
Joint(s), (*Figs.* 235–247) 250–255
— blood-supply of, 731
— capsule, metaphysis partially in, 243, 266
— development of, (*Fig.* 246) 254, 729
— function, restricted, in causalgia, 571
— lines, horizontal, (*Figs.* 475, 479) 484
— loose bodies in, 731
— movements, intricate, (*Figs.* 188–190) 201–206
— nerve-supply of, 255
— puncture of, (*Figs.* 683–689) 733
— 'snapping', 578
— spread of bone infection to, 266
— stiff, optimum attitudes for, (*Figs.* 480–486) 487
— surgical approach to, (*Figs.* 760–776) 803, 815
Jones's (Sir Robert) incision of knee-joint, (*Fig.* 771) 810, 812
Jugular foramen, ganglia in, 149, 151, 152
— — relations of, 349
— ganglion, 151 (*Figs.* 582, 583) 618, 619
— lymph trunk, 329, (*Fig.* 339) 345
— vein(s), anterior, 206, 209 (*Figs.* 304, 305) 302

Jugular vein(s), external, 206, 209 (*Figs. 303, 304*) 301, 302, 303
— — internal, 209, (*Fig. 302*) 299, 300, 303
— — — compression of, in Queckenstedt's test, 591
— — — relation of vagus nerve to, (*Fig. 143*) 151
— — — relationship with deep cervical glands, 329
— — ligation or excision of, collateral drainage after, 549
— — oblique, 303
— — posterior external, 303
— venous system, (*Figs. 302–305*) 300
Jugulodigastric gland, 28, 299, (*Fig. 327*) 329
Jugulo-subclavian junction, lymph-ducts entering, 329, 336–339
— — thoracic duct joins, (*Fig. 339 C*) 342
Juxta-epiphyseal strain, 242
— vessels of Lexer, (*Fig. 226*) 243

Keen's method of tapping lateral ventricle, (*Fig. 690 A*) 736
Kehr's sign, 89
Keloid formation in popliteal area, 566, 567
Keratitis, neuro-paralytic, section of sympathetic in neck for, 613
Kidney(s), (*see also* Renal), (*Figs. 78–86*) 89–96
— abscess, drainage of, Sherren's suggestion for, 761
— accessory, 400
— adrenal fused to, 94
— and adrenals, (*Figs. 78–86*) 89–96
— angle, 90, 761
— — danger of opening pleura at, (*Fig. 719*) 762
— blood-supply of, (*Fig. 82*) 92, (*Figs. 514–516*) 531
— of child in relation to peritoneum, (*Fig. 127*) 135
— congenital abnormalities of, 397–400
— — absence of one, (*Fig. 393 A*) 399
— — — obstructions to flow of urine from, (*Fig. 397*) 403
— development of, (*Fig. 389*) 397
— disease, unilateral, as cause of hypertension, (*Fig. 589*) 624
— double, associated with ectopic ureter, 402
— exposure of, by lumbar incision, 90
— horseshoe, (*Figs. 390–392*) 399
— incisions, 745, (*Figs. 718–720*) 761
— — giving access to, (*Figs. 711, 712*) 753, 754

Kidney(s) incisions, oblique, (*Figs. 718 B, 719*) 761
— — vertical, (*Fig. 720*) 763
— lymphatics of, 608
— movable (*see* Movable Kidney)
— nerve-supply of, 92
— palpation of, 590
— pelvic, (*Fig. 393 C*) 400
— portal-systemic anastomosis near, (*Fig. 319*) 321
— position of, 89
— relations of, (*Figs. 78–83*) 89–91, 93
— — adrenals to, (*Fig. 78*) 90, (*Figs. 83, 86*) 94, 95
— — to diaphragm, 196
— — at hilum, 347
— — lumbar rib to, (*Fig. 211*) 229
— removal of single, 400
— segmental resections of, 533
— segments of, conforming to arterial distribution, (*Figs. 514–576*) 531
— stone due to retrocaval ureter, 544
— transplantation, renal vessels in, 534
— unilateral fused, (*Fig. 393 B*) 400
Kienböck's disease, 665
Killian's dehiscence, 434
Klumpke's paralysis, 458
Knee, amputation at, 774
— clicking, 578
— compression of peroneal nerve at, 471
— optimum position for ankylosis of, (*Fig. 485*) 489
— snapping, 578
Knee-joint, approach to back of, 814
— bursae around, (*Figs. 257, 258*) 264
— dislocation of, 667
— excision of bone-ends forming, (*Figs. 769, 770*) 810, 811
— extensor mechanism of, (*Fig. 626*) 667
— fixation of popliteal artery to capsule of, 565
— injury in relation to age at, 673
— intra-articular manipulations of, (*Figs. 771, 772*) 810, 812
— ligaments of, (*Figs. 275–280*) 276
— loose bodies in, incisions for dealing with, 811, 814
— non-extensive intra-articular operations on, (*Figs. 773, 774*) 810, 813
— puncture of, (*Figs. 687, 688*) 734
— rotation at, (*Fig. 190*) 204
— surgical approach to, (*Figs. 769–774*) 810
Knock-knee, (*Figs. 468–470*) 479
— encouraging dislocation of patella, (*Fig. 626 C*) 669
Kobelt's tubes, (*Fig. 406*) 418

852 INDEX

Kocher's approach to hip-joint, (*Fig.* 768) 808, 809
— — shoulder-joint, (*Figs.* 761, 763) 804, 805, 806
— incision, (*Figs.* 709, 710) 751
— — of ankle-joint, (*Fig.* 775) 814
— — to expose fibula, 819
— — of knee-joint, (*Fig.* 769) 810, 811
— reduction of shoulder dislocation, (*Fig.* 619) 661
Kondoléon operation for lymphoedema, (*Fig.* 566) 597
Kümmell's disease of spine, 712
Kuntz, nerve of, (*Fig.* 596) 635
Kyphosis, adolescent, (*Fig.* 671) 715
Kyphotic bursa, 266
— due to disc lesions, 715
— — Kümmell's disease, 712
— — senile, (*Fig.* 668 B) 711, 716
— tuberculosis, localization of, 128

Labial sinuses, inferior, (*Fig.* 348) 358
Labium(a) majus(ora), hernia into, 692
— — swelling of, due to varicose veins, 311
Labour, rectal estimation of size of os uteri in, 586
Labourer's nerve, 187
Labrum glenoidale, 254
Lacertus fibrosus, 304
Lacrimal nerve, (*Fig.* 129) 136
Lactiferous duct(s), cancer invading, causing retraction of nipple, (*Fig.* 34 B) 40
— — fistula, (*Fig.* 33) 40
— — obstruction of, causing abscess and fistula, (*Fig.* 33) 40
Lacunae of Luschka, (*Fig.* 396 A) 403
Lacunar ligament, 100, 101
— — extension of, 31
Lambdoidal suture, Wormian bones in, 247
Lane's 'first and last kink', (*Fig.* 63) 74
— ileal membrane, (*Fig.* 62) 74
Langenbeck's approach to elbow-joint, (*Fig.* 764) 805, 806
Langer, foramen of, 30
Langley's ganglion, 141, (*Fig.* 139) 147
Lanz incision, 757
Larrey, space of, 682
Laryngeal nerve, external, 152
— — — in relation to thyroid, (*Fig.* 18) 19
— — inferior, 153
— — internal, 22, 152
— — non-recurrent, 22
— — recurrent (*see also* Recurrent Laryngeal Nerve), (*Fig.* 437) 454
— — superior, 152
Larynx of child, 133

Larynx, nerve-supply to, 152, 153
— paralysis and anaesthesia of, in vagus nerve lesion, 454
Latarjet, nerve of (*see also* Presacral Nerve), (*Fig.* 585) 620, (*Figs.* 590, 591) 625
Lateral aperture of fourth ventricle, 9, 10
— approach to brain, (*Fig.* 743) 787
— cutaneous nerve of thigh, compression of, 471
— ganglia, autonomic, 172, 175, 176, (*Fig.* 164) 177
— inversion of testis, (*Fig.* 403 D) 414
— J incision of ankle-joint, (*Fig.* 775) 814
— — knee-joint, (*Fig.* 769) 810, 811
— lobes of thyroid, (*Fig.* 16) 17
— transthoracic approach, (*Figs.* 750, 751) 791
— (transverse) sinus, 6, 297, 298
— ventricle(s), approach to, (*Fig.* 121) 130
— — choroid processes of, 9
— — puncture of, (*Fig.* 690) 735
Lateral-bearing stump, 770
Latum pulmonis, 798
Leg (*see also* Lower Limb)
— amputation, 770, 771
— — at site of election, (*Fig.* 730) 773
— interosseous membrane of, (*Fig.* 285) 283
— paralysis of, due to tibial nerve lesion, 465
— — in peroneal nerve lesion, 465
— — — sciatic nerve lesion, (*Fig.* 446) 464
— sensory loss in, due to peroneal nerve lesion, (*Fig.* 448) 465
— — — — sciatic nerve lesion, (*Fig.* 446) 464
— veins, thrombosis of, (*Figs.* 317, 318) 318
— venous system of, (*Figs.* 309–319) 306–320
Leontiasis, 582
Leptomeninges, 7
Leugart's pouch, 437
Levator ani, (*Fig.* 95) 107, (*Fig.* 102) 113, (*Fig.* 185) 198, 222, 224
— — fasciae of, 109, 110
— — separation of, in causation of prolapse of uterus, 720
— — supporting rectum, 721
— — — uterus, (*Fig.* 674) 718
— glandulae thyroideae, 17
— palpebrae superioris, sympathetic fibres to, 612, 613
— prostatae, 103
— scapulae, nerve to, 159
Lexer, juxta-epiphyseal vessels of, (*Fig.* 226) 243

Lid engorgement due to pituitary tumour, 16
Ligament(s), (*Figs.* 266–297) 270–296
— and arches of foot, (*Figs.* 292–297) 290–296
— disease of, causing low back pain, 695
— holding together lumbosacral joint, 693
— inability of, to withstand strain, 295*n*
— of Mackenrodt, 717, 719
— maintaining arch of foot, 290, 291, 292, 296
— tears of digital, 569
— traversing joints, 254
— of Treitz, 56
— uterus, (*Figs.* 673, 674) 717
Ligamenta flava, 251
Ligamentum arteriosum, 520
— — left, with right aortic arch, (*Fig.* 505) 518
— denticulata, (*Fig.* 5) 8
— flavum, thickening of, compressing fifth lumbar nerve, 704
— nuchae, 207
— patellae, 667
— teres, (*Fig.* 41) 53, 54, 254
Ligature of common hepatic artery, (*Fig.* 511) 525
— large veins, (*Figs.* 317, 318) 318
Limb(s) arteries further occluded by postoperative bedrest, 553
— denervation of, sympathetic, (*Figs.* 595–606) 633–648
— enlargements of spinal cord, (*Fig.* 161) 174
— ischaemia in, due to arterial embolism, 611
— long bones of, ossification of, 248
— measuring girth of, by Beyer's method, (*Fig.* 565) 595
— nerves conveying pain in, 178
— vessels, plexuses supplying, (*Fig.* 594) 632
Limp due to coxa vara, 477
— of infantile paralysis, (*Figs.* 551, 552) 576
Linea alba, incision through, 745
— — suture of, in lower abdominal incision, 747
— semilunaris, extending McBurney's incision through, (*Fig.* 714 B) 756
— — hernia of liver through, 691
— — through, 99
— — incision through, (*Fig.* 708) 751
— splendens, 8
Lingual glands, 330
— nerve(s), (*Fig.* 139) 147 (*Fig.* 142) 151
— — injection of, 783
— — taste sensation and, 147

Lingual thyroid, 367
— tonsils, (*Fig.* 324) 325
— vein, (*Fig.* 301) 300
Lingula, 49
Lingular segment of left lung, bronchus to, 49
Lip(s) cancer, gland removal in, 330
— — of lower, invading mandible, 332
— lymph drainage of, 330
Lipiodol injection in diagnosis of nuclear retropulsion, (*Fig.* 670) 714
Lipoma, axillary mammary tissue simulating, 373
Littre's hernia, 391
Liver (*see also* Hepatic)
— aneurysm within, ligation of hepatic artery in, 560
— arteries of, relations of bile-ducts to, (*Figs.* 72, 73) 82
— bare area of, portal-systemic anastomosis at, (*Fig.* 319) 321
— bile-ducts in, communicating direct to gall-bladder, (*Fig.* 75 D) 85
— blood-supply to, 523
— blood-vessels of, (*Figs.* 509–513) 523–531, 558
— cancer, secondary of, at umbilicus, 55
— caudate lobe of, hernia of, 691
— of child, 135
— cirrhosis of (*see* Cirrhosis of Liver)
— collateral arrangements in, (*Figs.* 512, 513) 527, (*Fig.* 534) 558
— cystic disease of, 398
— development of, (*Fig.* 379) 386, 387
— — causing pressure on midgut loop, 377, 378
— hilum of, blood vessels at, (*Figs.* 509–511) 523, 526
— incisions giving access to, 745, (*Fig.* 709) 751, 754
— metastases of breast cancer, 38
— necrosis due to ligature of hepatic artery, 558, 560
— puncture, (*Fig.* 694) 739
— relations of, to diaphragm, 196, 197
— — at hilum, 347
— sinusoids, 526, 528
— spaces in periphery of, (*Fig.* 680) 727
— tissue, accessory, 432
— vascular arrangements in, 526, 560
Lobe(s) of azygos vein, (*Figs.* 36–38) 45–47
— lung, left, (*Fig.* 35) 42, 47
— — right, (*Figs.* 35–38) 42, 44–47
Lobectomy, lower lobe, importance of relative position of middle lobe bronchus to, 48
Lockwood, tails of, 406
Loculation syndrome, 9

854 INDEX

Long arteries of ureter, (*Fig.* 517) 534
— bone(s), 242
— — after growth is complete, 581
— — blood-supply of, (*Fig.* 226) 243
— — constituent parts, before completion of growth, (*Figs.* 553, 554) 580
— — law of ossification of, 248
— — measurement of, (*Figs.* 557–564) 592
— — osteomyelitis of, 582
— — short, blood-supply of, (*Fig.* 227) 242, 244
— — surgical approach to, (*Figs.* 777–779) 815
— flexors of toes maintaining arch of foot, 295
— thoracic nerve of Bell, 161, 456
Longissimus group of muscles, (*Figs.* 179, 180) 191, 192
Longitudinal arch of foot, (*Figs.* 295–297) 292, 294
— — forming collateral circulation, (*Fig.* 528) 548
— ligament, anterior, of spine, (*Fig.* 118) 125
— — posterior, weakening of, in nuclear retropulsion, (*Fig.* 667 A) 712
— muscle of anal canal, (*Fig.* 105) 115, 117
— — pyloric sphincter, 493
— — spread of infection through, 121
— sinus (*see* Sagittal Sinus, Superior)
Longus capitis, nerve to, 159
— colli, nerves to, 159, 161
Loop inversion of testis, (*Fig.* 403 E) 414
Loose bodies in joints, 731
— — knee-joint, incisions for dealing with, 811, 814
Lotheissen operation, 759
Louis, angle of, as landmark to deeper structures, 41
Low back pain, (*Figs.* 651–657) 693–702
— — — classification of causes of, 694
— — — referred from viscera, 695
Lower arm type of birth palsy, 458
— extremity, lymphatic drainage of, (*Fig.* 335) 339
— limb(s) amputations, (*Figs.* 729–731) 772
— — measuring girth of, (*Fig.* 565 B) 597
— — — length of, 594
— — — long bones of, (*Figs.* 561–564) 594
— — perforating veins of, (*Figs.* 303, 313–315) 312, 313–318
— — pumping mechanism of, 570

Lower limb(s), sympathetic denervation of, (*Figs.* 600–606) 638
— — thrombosis of veins of, (*Figs.* 317, 318) 318
— — union of epiphyses in, 248
— — venous system of, (*Figs.* 309–319) 306–320
Lower-leg amputation, 770, 771
Ludloff's test, 587
Lumbar arteries supplying radicals, 500, 501
— curve of vertebral column, (*Fig.* 116 D) 123, 134
— ganglion(ia), 176
— — exposure of, (*Fig.* 603) 641
— — first, (*Figs.* 601, 602) 640, 641
— — recognition of, (*Figs.* 600–602) 638
— ganglionectomy, (*Fig.* 600) 639
— — intermittent claudication persisting after, 644
— hernia, lower, 692
— — upper, 692
— intervertebral foramina, sizes of, 126
— lymphatic trunks, 335, 341
— lymph-glands, (*Fig.* 333) 334
— manometer, use of, in Queckenstedt's test, 592
— nerve(s), emerging, 706
— — fifth, 693, 694
— — — compression of, by disc prolapse, 712, 713
— — — predisposed to sciatica, 706
— — — pressure on, in lumbosacral transverse articulation, 697, (*Fig.* 659) 704
— — first, 164
— — posterior root of, (*Fig.* 5) 9
— — foramina for, 126
— — fourth, 693, 694
— — predisposed to sciatica, 706
— — referred pain from in sacralization, 699
— psoas abscess following course of, 727
— supplying trunk, 164, 165, 166
— plexus, 218
— puncture, (*Figs.* 692, 693) 737
— — headache produced by, 652
— rib, (*Fig.* 211) 229
— spine, anatomical facts in, relating to sciatica, (*Figs.* 660–662) 704
— — cold abscesses of, 726
— — disc prolapse in, 712
— testis, 409
— transverse processes, 127
— veins, ascending, (*Fig.* 318) 320
— vertebra(ae), detachment of transverse processes of, 127

INDEX

Lumbar vertebra(ae), fifth, 694
— — — abnormalities of, 127
— — — anomalies of, (*Figs.* 653, 654) 695, 697, (*Fig.* 659) 704
— — — development of, 700
— — — sacralization of, (*Fig.* 654) 696, 698
— — first, rib articulating with, (*Fig.* 211) 229
— — joints between, (*Figs.* 660, 661) 704
— — slipping forward of, 700
'Lumbarization' of first sacral vertebra, 700
Lumbocostal arch(es) cold abscesses tracking through, (*Fig.* 678) 724
— — lateral, (*Fig.* 201) 216
— — medial, 218
— ligament, (*Fig.* 201) 216
Lumbodorsal fascia, (*Figs.* 200-202) 215
— — thoracic part of, 217
— triangle, cold abscess of, 727
Lumbosacral angle, 693
— — variations in, 700
— articular joint, anomaly in, (*Fig.* 661) 705
— articulation, 693
— cord, ischaemic lesions of, 500, 504
— deformities causing low back pain, 695
— — detailed consideration of, (*Figs.* 651-657) 696-702
— — general classification of, 695
— disc herniation of, 712
— joint, transverse, 127
— plexus, alterations in position of, due to sacralization, 700
— — compression of, causing sciatica, 703
— region of spine, anatomical details, 695
— **transverse** articulation, 697
— trunk, 693
— vertebrae, development of, 694
Lumbrical canals, (*Fig.* 613) 655, 657
— muscles, (*Fig.* 171) 184, 215, 654, 655, 656
— — action of, (*Fig.* 174) 187, 189
— — nerve-supply of, 186
— — sheaths, 655
Lunate bone, (*Fig.* 224 B) 241, 242
— — dislocation of, (*Figs.* 622, 623) 663, 664
Lung(s) abscesses, sites of, 49
— accessory lobes of, (*Figs.* 36-38) 45-47
— blood-supply of, (*Fig.* 40) 50
— and bronchial tree, (*Figs.* 35-40) 42-51
— cancer, biopsy in diagnosis of, 338
— collapse complicating transthoracic transdiaphragmatic approach, 792
— complete absence of, 51
— exposure of, 791

Lung(s), fissures of, 42, 46
— hilum, calcified glands near, 44
— infection after laparotomy, 49
— lymphatic drainage of, (*Fig.* 334) 337
— position of roots of, 41
— relations of, at hilum, 347
— segmental structure of, (*Fig.* 35) 42, 43
— segments of, (*Fig.* 35) 42-45, 47
— — localization of infection or growth to, 42
— surgery through intersegmental planes, 42
— surgical collapse of lower lobe of, 466
— tissue, ectopic, (*Fig.* 424 C) 437
Luschka, foramina of, 9. 10
— lacunae of, (*Fig.* 396 A) 403
— recurrent nerve of, (*Fig.* 155) 165
Luxatio erecta, 661
Lymph, drainage of, 324
— — colon and extent of cancer resection, 598
— — — left, and rectum, in relation to inferior mesenteric artery, 604
— plexus on deep fascia, 345
Lymph-ducts, great, (*Figs.* 336-339) 341-345
— — injury to, 609
— — principles governing surgery to, 610
— — right, 336, 337, 338, (*Fig.* 339 A) 345
Lymph-glands of abdomen, (*Figs.* 331-333) 333
— collateral channels of, 324
— diseased, causing oesophageal diverticulum, (*Fig.* 425) 437
— — draining adenoids, spinal accessory nerve and, (*Fig.* 144) 154
— — in femoral canal, (*Fig.* 89) 100
— of head and neck, (*Figs.* 325-327) 326
Lymphangiomatous mesenteric cyst, 441
Lymphangitis of forearm, 339
Lymphatic(s), (*Figs.* 324-340) 324-346
— in amputations, 597
— anatomy governing surgery of, (*Figs.* 566-576) 597-610
— channels of lower limb, 339
— drainage of breast, 30, (*Figs.* 27-31) 33-38, 339
— — stomach, (*Fig.* 53) 64-66
— — thymus gland, 134
— — tongue, 195, 327, 329, (*Figs.* 328-330) 330
— of gall-bladder, 87
— kidney, 608
— metastases of thyroid cancer, 25
— obstruction causing peau d'orange in breast cancer, (*Fig.* 34 C) 41
— of pectinate line, (*Fig.* 99) 110
— rectum, (*Figs.* 573, 574, 576) 605

Lymphatic(s), stasis in causation of 'white leg', 611
— of synovial membrane, 731
— system, formation of lymphocytes by, 609
— of thyroid, (*Fig.* 22) 24
— tissue of head and neck, (*Figs.* 324–330) 325–333
— of tonsil, 28
— watersheds of skin, (*Fig.* 340) 345
Lymphatic-portal communications, 321
Lymphocytes, formation of, by lymphatic system, 609
Lymphoedema, anatomical basis of surgical treatment of, (*Fig.* 566) 597
Lymphoid follicles of tonsil, 26
— tissue collections in alimentary tract, 59
— — pharyngeal, (*Fig.* 324) 325
— — in submaxillary salivary gland, 208, 327
Lympho-venous anastomosis, 597

McArdle's disease, 644
McBurney's gridiron incision, (*Figs* 713–715) 755, 758
— — — left, 755, 757
McGrae-Aitken incision of ankle-joint, (*Fig.* 776) 814, 815
McEvedy operation, (*Fig.* 717) 759
Mackenrodt, ligaments of, 223, 717, 719
Macrostoma, (*Fig.* 350 A) 358
Magendie, foramen of, 9, 10
Malassez, paradental debris of, (*Fig.* 550) 574, 575
Male, development of external genitalia in, 419
— drainage of pouch of Douglas in, 742
— information gained by rectal examination in, 584
— occurrence of female breasts in, 373
— sex organs, effects of sympathectomy on, 647
— vestigial structures in connexion with genital organs in, (*Fig.* 405) 416
Malignant secondary deposits causing ileus, 623
Mammary (*see also* Breast)
— abnormalities, congenital, 372
— artery, internal, 31, (*Fig.* 31) 36
— — internal, branches of, 42
— — — choice of site for ligation of, 41
— glands, internal, 34, 35, (*Fig.* 31) 36, 37
— — internal, spread of breast cancer through, 37
— line, 739
— lymph-glands, internal, 335
— vein, internal, 31

Mandible, lymphatic route of lip cancer into, 330
— mylohyoid line on, 194
— ossification of, 132, 147
— regenerative powers of, 582
— tooth extraction in, and osteomyelitis, 575
— vulnerability of, to cancer, (*Fig.* 330) 331
Mandibular arch, 361
— branch of facial nerve, 149
— nerve, (*Fig.* 129) 137, 141, 142, (*Fig.* 138) 146
— — paralysis, (*Fig.* 434 C) 451
— processes of embryo, (*Fig.* 345) 355, 356
— recesses, (*Fig.* 348) 358
Manubrium, junction of, with body of sternum, 41
— splitting of, to approach superior mediastinum, (*Fig.* 749) 790
— sterni, (*Fig.* 267) 271
Marginal artery, (*Fig.* 52) 63
— — of colon, (*Fig.* 567) 600
— lymphatics of tongue, 330
— vein, 64
Massive rectal prolapse, (*Fig.* 676) 723
Mastectomy, radical, prevention of bleeding in, 42
Mastication, muscles of, nerve-supply of, 141
— paralysis of muscles of, due to fifth nerve division, 451
Mastoid process in child, (*Figs.* 122, 123) 130, 131
— vein, 297
Mastoiditis in infant, 130
Maternal obstetrical palsy, 715
Maxillary antrum, development, in child, (*Fig.* 125) 132
— artery, external, 208, 327
— — — plexus round, 147
— — — in relation to tonsil, 27
— nerve, (*Fig.* 129) 136, 141, (*Fig.* 137) 145
— — paralysis, (*Fig.* 434 D) 451
— processes of embryo, (*Fig.* 345) 355, 356
— sinus, puncture of, (*Fig.* 697) 741
Mayo's incision in repair of umbilical hernia, (*Fig.* 42) 53
Mayo-Robson paramedian incision, (*Fig.* 704) 748
Meckel's cave, (*Figs.* 134, 135) 142
— diverticulum, 57, 224 (*Fig.* 383 B) 389
— — adenoid tumour associated with, (*Fig.* 383 A) 390
— — giant, 391
— — inflammation of, 390, 391
— — patent, (*Fig.* 383 A) 389

INDEX 857

Meckel's diverticulum, tumour of, 391
— — vestiges of, (*Fig.* 383) 390
— ganglion, 141, (*Fig.* 137) 145
Medial cutaneous nerve(s), (*Fig.* 151) 161, 162
— — — of forearm, 304, 305
— muscle-splitting incisions, (*Fig.* 716 A) 758
— patella ligament, 668, 669
Median abdominal incisions, (*Figs.* 700, 701) 745
— aperture of fourth ventricle, 9, 10
— nerve, (*Fig.* 151) 161, 162, 186, 187, 215, (*Fig.* 287) 285, 286
— — branch of, to thenar muscles, (*Fig.* 724) 767
— — combined lesions of ulnar and, (*Fig.* 444) 462
— — compression at wrist and elbow, 470
— — involved in dislocated shoulder, 661
— — loss due to division of, (*Fig.* 441) 460
— — pressure of lunate bone on, 663
— — relaxation, posture for, (*Fig.* 450) 468
— and ulnar nerves, combined lesion of, 457
— vein of forearm, (*Fig.* 306 B) 304
Mediastinal dermoids, 428
— lymph-glands, posterior, 335, 336
— — superior, 336
Mediastinum, approach to superior, (*Fig.* 749) 790
— cold abscess at, 724
— upper, exposure of great vessels of, (*Fig.* 535) 560
Medulla, incision giving access to, (*Fig.* 747) 789
— pupil-dilating centre in, 144
Megacolon (*see* Hirschsprung's disease)
Meissner's plexus, 619
Membrane(s), accessory peritoneal, (*Figs.* 62–66) 74–76
— bones, 580, 582
Meningeal artery, middle, (*Fig.* 138) 146
— branch, 165
— — of vagus, 152
— veins or sinuses, middle, 297
Meninges and cerebrospinal fluid, (*Figs.* 3–6) 5–10
Meningocele, (*Fig.* 364 A) 369, (*Fig.* 367 A) 371
— anterior sacral, 424
Meningomyelocele, (*Fig.* 364 B) 369
Meniscus(i), (*Figs.* 277–280) 278
— articular, 254
— attachments of, (*Fig.* 277) 278

Meniscus(i), bucket-handle tear of, (*Fig.* 278) 279
— discoid lateral, 578
— lateral, (*Fig.* 277) 278, 279
— medial, (*Fig.* 277) 277, 278
— — injury to, (*Fig.* 280) 279, 280
— — relation of tibial collateral ligament to, (*Fig.* 279) 279
— operations on, incisions for, (*Figs.* 771–774) 810, 812, 813
— re-formation of, 280
Menstrual bleeding from accessory endometrical tissue, 432
Mental dullness due to pituitary tumour, 16
— foramen, cancer of mouth and, (*Fig.* 330) 331
— nerve, (*Fig.* 129) 137
— — injection of, 783
— — paralysis, (*Fig.* 434 C) 450
Meralgia paraesthetica, 471
Mesenteric artery, haemorrhage from, due to remains of vitelline duct, 391
— — inferior, (*Fig.* 52) 61, 63, 64, 598, 599
— — — high ligation of, in cancer of left colon, (*Fig.* 573) 604
— — — relation of lymph-glands to, 334, 335
— — — removal of, in pelvic cancer, 64
— — superior, (*Fig.* 52) 61, 63, 64, (*Fig.* 59) 70, 599
— — — compression of, by median arcuate ligament, 448
— — — ensuring adequacy of, before colonic resection, 599
— — — hepatic artery arising in, 525
— — — relation of lymph-glands to, 334, 335
— — — supplying midgut, (*Figs.* 371, 372) 376
— cysts, (*Fig.* 427 D) 441
— — of urogenital origin, 441
— lymph-glands, inferior, 334, 335
— — superior, 334, 335
— plexus, inferior, (*Fig.* 164) 177, (*Fig.* 587) 623
— vein, inferior, (*Figs.* 56, 57) 68, 321
— — superior, 523
— — — implantation of, into vena cava, (*Fig.* 513) 530
— — — lack of collaterals for, 549
Mesenterico-parietal fossa of Waldeyer, 67, (*Fig.* 59) 69
Mesentery(ies) to ascending colon, (*Figs.* 67, 68) 76
— of colon, (*Figs.* 48, 49) 60
— division of, in colonic anastomosis, (*Fig.* 567 B) 601
— of gall-bladder, 86

858 INDEX

Mesentery(ies) of Meckel's diverticulum, 390, 391
— primitive pre-arterial and post-arterial, (*Figs.* 371–375) 377, 380
— roots of, nerve-supply to, 618
— of small gut, 57, (*Fig.* 49) 61
— ventral, (*Fig.* 379) 386
Meso-azygos, (*Fig.* 38) 46, 47
Mesoblast, paraxial bar of, (*Fig.* 246) 255
Mesocolic mesenteric cyst, 441
Mesocolojejunal membrane, (*Fig.* 64) 75
Mesocolon, 380
— transverse, (*Fig.* 48) 60, 380
Mesoderm, 427
Mesonephric arteries, persistent, 534
Mesosigmoid membrane, (*Fig.* 63) 74
Metacarpal ligament, transverse, 213, 214, 215
Metacarpophalangeal joint(s), (*Figs.* 542, 543) 567
— — dislocations of, (*Fig.* 624) 665
— — level of, (*Fig.* 616) 658
— — ligaments of, (*Fig.* 273) 275
— — related structures, (*Fig.* 544) 569
Metanephros, (*Fig.* 389) 397
Metaphysis, (*Figs.* 226, 227) 242, 243, (*Figs.* 553, 554) 581
— diseases affecting region of, (*Fig.* 555) 582, 583, 584
— infarction in, 246
— partially in joint capsule, 243, 266
Metastatic carcinoma of bone, (*Fig.* 555, 1) 583
Metatarsal arch of foot, dropping of, 293
— bones, attachment of tibialis posterior tendon to, (*Fig.* 296) 293
— fifth, fracture of, 234
— — os Vesalianum on, (*Fig.* 215) 233
— ligament, transverse, 215, 292
Metatarsalgia, 293
Metatarsophalangeal angle, (*Fig.* 474) 483
— joints, ligaments of, 275
— — sesamoids of, (*Fig.* 216), 234, 235
Metopic suture, 247
Microscopic anus, 394
Microstoma, (*Fig.* 350 B) 358
Middle meningeal veins or sinuses, 297
Middle-ear disease in infant, ease of intracranial spread of, (*Fig.* 124) 132
Midgut, communication of, with yolk-sac, 389
— of embryo, (*Figs.* 371, 372) 375, 376
— loop, malrotation of, 381, 382
— — non-rotation of, 381
— — reversed rotation of, (*Fig.* 376) 381
— — rotation of, (*Figs.* 372–375) 377

Midgut-foregut junction, congenital abnormalities of region of, (*Figs.* 379–382) 386
Mid-inguinal appendix, (*Fig.* 47) 60
Mid-palmar space, (*Figs.* 612–614) 654
— — drainage of pus in, 655
— — incisions giving access to, (*Fig.* 727) 767
Mid-Poupart appendix, (*Fig.* 47) 60
Migraine headache of, 652
'Milchleisten', (*Fig.* 368) 371
Miles's operation for cancer of rectum, (*Figs.* 575, 576) 607, 608
Milian's midline vertical division of sternum, 510
— sign, 587
Milk ducts, absence of, in breast, 373
— line, (*Fig.* 368) 372
Mitral stenosis, recurrent laryngeal nerve compression in, (*Fig.* 437) 454
— valve, obstruction at, 509
Mixed spinal nerves, 165
Mondor's disease, (*Fig.* 26) 32
Mongolism associated with congenital duodenal obstruction, 389
Monorchidism, 412
Monro, foramen of, blockage of, (*Fig.* 6) 10
— — closure of, by pituitary tumour, 16
Morgagni, columns of (anal columns), (*Fig.* 99) 110, 111
— foramen of, 682
— hydatid of, (*Fig.* 406) 417, 418
— valves of, (*Fig.* 105) 116
Morison (Rutherford) incision, (*Fig.* 711 B) 754
Morison's pouch, (*Fig.* 83) 92
— — abscess in, 728
Morton's disease, 293
Mouth, cancer of floor of, invading mandible, (*Fig.* 330) 331, 333
— dermoids of floor of, 428
— diaphragm of floor of, (*Fig.* 182) 194
— sphincter of, 490
Movable kidney, 95
— — palpation test for, 590
Movements, intricate, at shoulder, knee and foot, (*Figs.* 188–190) 201–206
Mucous membrane of anal region, 110, 111
— — gall-bladder and bile-ducts, 86
— — tendon-sheaths of foot, (*Figs.* 251–253) 259
— — hand, (*Figs.* 249, 250) 256
— tumours of rectum causing prolapse, 721
Müller, choanoid muscle of, 612
Multangulum majus and minus, (*Fig.* 224 B) 241, 242

Multifidus, 192
Multiple accessory organs, 432
— exostosis, 582
Murphy's sign of carpal dislocation, 663
— test, 591
Muscle(s), (*Figs.* 166–190) 179–206
— of anus, (*Figs.* 102–105) 113–116
— atrophy due to supracapsular, nerve compression, 471
— division of, 565
— incisions through, principles regarding, (*Fig.* 699) 744
— insertion of, into skull, 4
— power of, to withstand strain, 295
— supporting arches of foot, 295
— tendons arising in joint capsule, 254
— torus, 493
— transplantation and postural activity, 181
— trimming of, in fashioning stump, (*Fig.* 728) 771
— tunica media of arteries to, 561
Muscle-cutting incisions, (*Figs.* 709–711) 751
— — present status of, 754
Muscle-splitting incisions, (*Figs.* 713–717) 755
— — inferior, (*Figs.* 716, 717) 758
Muscular disease causing low back pain, 695
— effects of cervical rib, 226
Musculocutaneous nerve, (*Fig.* 151) 161, 162
Musculotendinous cuff of shoulder, (*Fig.* 630) 670
— — — injury to, (*Fig.* 631) 671, (*Fig.* 633) 673
— — — rim rent at, (*Fig.* 640) 680
Musician's nerve, 187
Myasthenia gravis, thymectomy for, 135
Myelocele, (*Fig.* 363) 369
Mylohyoid, (*Fig.* 182) 194

Nail-fold, infection of base of, treatment of, (*Fig.* 722) 766
Nasal nerves, 146
— processes of embryo, medial and lateral, (*Fig.* 345) 355
Nasmyth's membrane, (*Fig.* 547) 572
Nasociliary nerve, 143, 145*n*
Nasopalatine nerve, 146
Nasopharyngeal sphincter, 490, 491
Navicular bone, accessory, (*Figs.* 212, 213) 231
— — dislocation of, (*Fig.* 622) 663
— — of foot, (*Fig.* 225 B) 242
— — fracture of, 663

Navicular bone, of hand, (*Fig.* 224 B) 241, 242
— — — bipartite, (*Fig.* 220) 236
— tuberosity, relationship of os tibiale externum to, 231
Neck, access to, after splitting sternum, (*Fig.* 535) 561
— cold abscess at back of, 724
— deep fascia of, (*Figs.* 191–196) 206–212
— nerves in, cutaneous, 206
— nerve-supply of, (*Fig.* 129) 137, (*Fig.* 131) 139, (*Figs.* 140–154) 148–164
— parts of sacrospinalis reaching, (*Figs.* 179, 180) 192
— plexuses in, 157
— snapping, 579
— visceral compartment of, 210
— wounds, bleeding from, 206
Neighbourhood symptoms of pituitary tumours, (*Figs.* 14, 15) 15
Nélaton's line, (*Fig.* 563) 595
Neonatal death due to diaphragmatic hernia, 684
Nephrectomy causing lowering of blood-pressure, 624
— for renal artery stenosis, (*Fig.* 589 C) 625
Nephroptosis, 590
Nerve(s), (*Figs.* 129–165) 136–179
— anomalies due to sacralization of fifth lumbar process, 696, 700, 704
— approximation in stages, 467, 470
— compression effects of cervical rib, 226
— — results of, 470
— division, anatomical and physiological loss resulting from, (*Figs.* 433–448) 448–467
— entrapment, peripheral, 470
— grafting, 467
— injections, anatomy of, (*Figs.* 736–742) 780
— injury(ies), anatomy of, (*Figs.* 433–453) 448–471
— — surgical, causing painful scar, 763
— of Kuntz, (*Fig.* 596) 635
— regeneration, 646
— — prevention of, after denervation, (*Fig.* 604) 643
— — prevention of, in preganglionic section, 635
— relaxation of, (*Figs.* 449–453) 467
— root(s), 165
— — compression causing sciatica, 703
— — sprouting, collateral, (*Fig.* 606) 646
— — suture, approximation of ends for, 467
— — symptoms arising from asymmetrical sacralization, 699
— of synovial membrane, 731

860 INDEX

Nerve(s), treatment of, in amputation stump, 772
Nerve-block preliminary to sympathetic operation, 642
Nerve-root irritation by disc prolapse, 712
Nerve-supply of body, segmental, (*Fig.* 156) 167
— breast, 33
— to deep muscles of back, 190
— of ear, external, (*Fig.* 130) 138
— face, (*Fig.* 129) 138
— ischiorectal fossa, 108
— joint, 255
— kidney, 92
— neck, (*Fig.* 129) 137, (*Fig.* 131) 139, (*Figs.* 140-154) 148-164
— oesophagus, 492
— to pharyngeal constrictors, 180
— of scalp, 138
— to tongue, 154
Nervi erigentes, 175, 179, (*Fig.* 587) 622
— — functions of, regarding male sex organs, 647
Nervous system, autonomic (*see* Autonomic Nervous System)
— — central, puncture of, (*Figs.* 690-693) 735
Nervus cutaneus colli, 137 (*Fig.* 148) 158
— intermedius, 451, 454
— — taste fibres in, 147
Neural canal, (*Fig.* 415 A-C) 427
— groove and canal of embryo, (*Fig.* 361) 368
— tube, faulty fusion of, 423
Neuralgia from cervical rib, 227, 228
— — first rib, 228
— geniculate, 451
— intractable, alcohol injection of nerve in, 780
— reflex sciatic, 702
Neurectomy of presacral plexus, 629
— to relieve tachycardia and heart pain, (*Fig.* 758) 799, 800
Neurenteric canal, persistent, 127
Neuritis, primary sciatic, 702
— sciatic, due to compression, (*Fig.* 658) 707
Neurocentral synchondrosis, 694
Neurodocitis, 703
— sciatic, anatomical bases of, (*Figs.* 659-662) 704
Neurological damage due to aortic surgery, 499, 500, (*Figs.* 493-495) 503
Newborn infant, rectal examination in, 586
Ninth cranial nerve (*see* Glossopharyngeal Nerve)

Nipple(s), (*Fig.* 25) 30, 31
— congenital retraction of, (*Fig.* 32) 38
— inflammatory retraction of, (*Fig.* 33) 40
— retraction of, (*Figs.* 32-34 B) 38-41
— supernumerary, 373
Non-chromaffin paraganglioma, (*Fig.* 608) 650
Non-recurrent laryngeal nerve, 22
Nose, dermoid cysts of, 360
Notochord, (*Fig.* 362) 368
Nuclear expansion, (*Figs.* 667 B, 671) 711, 715
— retropulsion, (*Figs.* 667 A, 669, 670) 711, 712
Nucleus ambiguus of vagus, (*Figs.* 581-583) 618
— pulposus, (*Fig.* 666) 708
Nutrient artery, (*Figs.* 226-228, 231) 243, 245, 246
— foramina of limb bones, 249
Nutritiae (*Fig.* 226) 243

Oblique aponeurosis, external, 747
— cord, (*Fig.* 271) 273
— fascia, external, incisional hernia through, 747
— inguinal hernia associated with ectopia testis, 412
— muscle(s) external, (*Figs.* 204, 205) 220, 405, (*Fig.* 399) 408
— — external and internal, division of, 564, 565
— — internal, (*Fig.* 399) 405, 408
— popliteal ligament, (*Fig.* 275) 276
— vein of Marshall, (*Fig.* 520) 538
Obstetric injury causing prolapse of uterus, 720
Obstetrical palsy, maternal, 715
Obturator artery, abnormal, (*Fig.* 90) 101
— fascia, 106, 221
— foramen, (*Fig.* 90) 101, 221
— — hernia of peritoneum through, (*Fig.* 650) 691
— hernia, (*Fig.* 650) 691
— internus, (*Figs.* 95, 96) 106, 107, 221, 222, 223
— — tendon in dislocation of hip, (*Fig.* 625) 667
— nerve, 224
— — compression, 471
— test for pelvic appendicitis, 591
— type of dislocation of hip, 666
— vessels and nerves, relations of, 347
Occipital approach to brain, (*Fig.* 746) 788
— artery, sternomastoid branch of, 154
— diploic vein, 296
— glands, (*Fig.* 325) 326

INDEX 861

Occipital lobe, incision giving access to, (*Fig.* 746) 788
— nerve, great, 137, 138
— — — pressure of occipital glands on, 326
— — lesser (small), (*Fig.* 130) 137, 138, (*Fig.* 148) 158
— — least (third), 138
— sinus, 6
Occipitalis muscle, (*Fig.* 2) 2, 143
Occipito-atlantoid ligament, posterior, puncture through, (*Fig.* 691) 737
Occipitofrontalis muscle (*see* Epicranius Muscle)
Oculomotor nerve (3rd), 143
— — autonomic fibres in, 175
— — compression of, causing fixed dilated pupil, 613
— — loss due to division of, 449
Oddi, sphincter of, (*Fig.* 489 A) 495
Odditis, 497
Odontomes, (*Fig.* 550) 575
Oedema of brain causing hypertensive encephalopathy, 653
— following strain, narrowing, of foramen, 707
Oesophageal diverticula, production of, 436, 493
— hiatus, 492, 620, 686, 687
— — hernia, congenital, (*Fig.* 643) 685
— — stretching of, causing submammary pain, 687
— lesions, transthoracic route to, 792
— manometry, 686
— opening in diaphragm, (*Fig.* 184) 197
— orifice of diaphragm, relations of, 347
— plexus, 176
— sphincter, inferior, 492
— — lower, 686, 687
— — superior, 491
— ulceration and structure due to sliding hernia, 687
— varices, 197, 321
— — complicating cirrhosis of liver, 529
Oesophagitis due to sliding hernia, 687
Oesophago-gastrectomy, incision for, 755
Oesophagogastric anastomosis, (*Figs.* 752–756) 794
— — high, 792, 793
— junction, 491
Oesophagojejunal anastomosis, (*Figs.* 755, 756) 796
Oesophagus, atresia of, (*Fig.* 370 A) 374
— blood-supply of, (*Fig.* 752) 794
— cancer of lower, approach to, 792, 793
— congenital abnormalities, (*Figs.* 369, 370) 374
— — atresia of, posterior approach to, 802

Oesophagus, development of, (*Fig.* 369) 374
— diffuse spasm of, 493
— diverticula of, (*Figs.* 423–425) 436
— exposure of, 791
— mobilization of, 795
— nerve-supply of, 492
— portal-systemic anastomosis at lower, (*Fig.* 319) 321
— separation of upper from lower, (*Figs.* 423 C, 424 A, B) 437
— and trachea, developmental anomalies of, (*Figs.* 423, 424) 437
— traumatic rupture of, site of, 565
— vascular ring encircling, (*Figs.* 504, 505) 518
Old age, atrophy of intervertebral discs in, (*Fig.* 117) 124
Olfactory groove, incision giving access to, (*Fig.* 745) 788
— nerve (2nd), loss due to division of, 448
— pits, (*Fig.* 345) 355
Ollier's approach to shoulder-joint, (*Fig.* 760) 803
Omentum, greater, blood-supply to, (*Figs.* 526, 527) 546
— in infancy and childhood, 135
— lesser, (*Fig.* 379 B) 386
— — control of blood-vessels in border of, 525
— — vagus nerve in, 620
— mobilization of, from greater curvature of stomach, (*Figs.* 526, 527) 546, 547
Omohyoid, 209, 210
— muscle, nerve supplying, 159, 160
Omphalocele, 376
Omphalomesenteric duct (*see* Vitello-intestinal Duct)
Opponens, action of, 182
Opposite-sided test for appendicitis, 591
Ophthalmic artery, sympathetic plexus around, 143, 144
— nerve, (*Fig.* 129) 136, 141, 143
— — paralysis, (*Fig.* 434) 451
— — sympathetic fibres in, 612
— veins, 297
Optic chiasma, incision giving access to, (*Fig.* 745) 788
— — pressure on, by adamantinoma, 354
— — — pituitary tumour, (*Fig.* 14) 14, 15
— — relationship of infundibulum, (*Figs.* 12, 13) 13
— — superior relation of, 15
— — variations in position of, (*Fig.* 13) 14
— nerve (2nd), 144
— — complete lesion of, (*Fig.* 433) 449

862 INDEX

Optic nerve, incision giving access to, (*Fig.* 745) 788
— — loss due to division of, (*Fig.* 433) 448
— tract(s) lesions, (*Fig.* 433) 448
— — retinal fibres in, 15
Optimum attitudes for nerve relaxation, (*Figs.* 449–451) 467
— — stiff joints, (*Figs.* 480–486) 487
— position of hand, (*Fig.* 445) 463
Orbicular ligament, (*Fig.* 270) 273
— — of radial head, (*Fig.* 621) 662
Orbicularis oris, 490
Orbit, arterial anastomosis in, 553
— ciliary ganglion in, 143
— cyst at outer angle of, (*Fig.* 353) 360
— haemorrhage into, 3
Orbital ciliary body, 650
— fissure, superior, relations of, 349
— muscle of Müller, paralysis of, 466
— nerve, 146
— plate of frontal bone, fracture of, 3
Organ of Giraldès, (*Fig.* 405) 416
Os acetabuli, (*Figs.* 221, 234) 237, 249
— calcis (see Calcaneal; Calcaneum)
— centrale, (*Fig.* 220) 236
— — of foot, (*Fig.* 225 A) 242
— — hand, (*Fig.* 224 A) 241
— innominatum, ossification of, (*Fig.* 234) 249
— intercuneiforme, (*Fig.* 212) 230
— intermedium of foot, (*Fig.* 225 A) 241, 242
— — hand, (*Fig.* 224 A) 240, 241
— paracuneiforme of Cameron and Carlier, (*Fig.* 212) 231
— para-trapezium, (*Fig.* 220) 236
— radiale externum, (*Fig.* 220) 236
— styloideum, (*Fig.* 220) 236
— subtibiale, 231
— sustenaculum proprium, 231
— tibiale externum, (*Figs.* 212, 213) 230, 231
— triangulare, (*Fig.* 220) 236
— trigonum, (*Figs.* 212, 214) 230, 232, 242
— ulnare externum, (*Fig.* 220) 236
— uncinatum, 231
— Vesalianum carpi, (*Fig.* 220) 236
— — tarsi, (*Figs.* 212, 215) 230, 233
Ossicle(s) separate, at end of spinous process, 697
— X-ray demonstration of, 229, 230
Ossification, (*Figs.* 232–234) 247
— of iliolumbar ligament, (*Fig.* 653) 698
— law of, in long bones of limbs, 248
— of sutural joints, 250
Osteitis fibrosa, solitary cyst of, (*Fig.* 555, 5) 583

Osteoarthritis, (*Fig.* 682) 729
— cervical, causing neuralgia, 229
— due to faulty position at ankle joint, 485
Osteoarthritic spurs and osteophytes narrowing intervertebral foramen, (*Fig.* 662) 707
Osteogenic sarcoma, (*Fig.* 555, 4) 583
Osteoma, ivory, 582
Osteomyelitis, acute, (*Fig.* 555, 8) 582
— — pyogenic, 582
— chronic, 582, 583
— of jaw, 575
Osteophytes from intervertebral joint, (*Fig.* 662) 707
Osteoplastic craniotomy, (*Figs.* 743–746) 787
— flaps of skull, (*Figs.* 743–746) 787
— — — blood-supply of, 787, 788, 789
— — — periosteum, 4
Osteoporosis following causalgia, 571
— of spine, senile, (*Fig.* 672) 716
Otic ganglion, 141, (*Fig.* 138) 146, (*Fig.* 141) 149
Outflow block of hepatic veins, 527
Ovarian cyst diagnosed from fimbrial cyst, 418
— — pseudomucinous, causing pseudomyxoma peritonei, 445
— tissue in broad ligament, 432
— vein, right and right ureter, association of, 536
Ovaries, prolapsed, palpable per rectum, 586

Pacchionian bodies, 7
Pain in abducting or adducting arm, 677, 678
— autonomic transmission of sensations of visceral, 178
— cardiac (see Cardiac Pain)
— due to obturator hernia, 692
— radiating to ear after tonsillectomy, 30
— referred from oesophagus, 492
— — to shoulder-tip, 88
— in rupture of supraspinatus, 674, (*Fig.* 635) 675
Painful scars, 763
Palatal part of nasopharyngeal sphincter, 491
Palate, cleft (see Cleft Palate)
— hard, bony ridge in, (*Fig.* 221) 240
— normal, (*Fig.* 351) 358
— paralysis of, due to vagus nerve lesion, 454
Palatine artery, ascending, in relation to tonsil, 27
— nerves, 146
— processes, sutures of, (*Fig.* 223) 240

INDEX 863

Palatine tonsil (see Tonsil)
Palatoglossal folds, 26
Palatoglossus muscle, 154
Palatopharyngeal folds, 26
Palatopharyngeus muscle, 180
Palmar fascia, density of, 569
— — pathological contracture of, 214
— — relation of skin to, 654
— incisions, anatomy of, (Figs. 721–726) 764–769
— ligament(s), (Figs. 542, 543) 568, 569
— — in dislocation of metacarpophalangeal joint, (Fig. 624) 665
— — of metacarpophalangeal and interphalangeal joints, (Fig. 273) 275
— and plantar fasciae, (Figs. 197–199) 212
— spaces, incisions of, (Figs. 726, 727) 767
Palmaris longus tendon, 213, 286
Palpation of anorectal ring, (Fig. 108) 117
Pancreas, annular, (Figs. 417 D, 418) 428
— cystic disease of, 398, 399
— development of, (Fig. 417 A, B) 431
— groove in, containing bile-duct, 79
— incision giving access to, 745, 754
— regurgitation of bile into, 80
— relation to duodenum, (Fig. 43) 55
— suspension of transverse colon from, (Fig. 48) 60
Pancreatic duct(s), (Figs. 69, 74) 78
— — anatomy of, (Fig. 488) 494
— — entrance of, into duodenum, 55
— — obstruction in pancreatitis, acute, 495
— — variations in terminations of, 80
— ferments, reflux of, into gall-bladder, 495
— tissue, accessory, (Figs. 417, 418) 428
— — — in Meckel's diverticulum, 390
Pancreatico-duodenal artery, posterior-superior, 87
Pancreatico-lienal lymph-glands, (Fig. 53) 65, 66
Pancreatitis, acute haemorrhagic, pathology of, 80
— anatomy of, 495
— postoperative, due to trauma, 495
Papilla duodeni, (Fig. 69) 78, 79
— — stone blocking, 80
— of Vater (see Vater, Papilla of)
Papillary thyroid tissue in lymph-node, 25
Papillomata at umbilicus, 54, 55
Para-aortic lymph-glands, (Fig. 333) 335, 341, 608
Paracardiac lymph-glands, 65
Paracolic appendix, (Fig. 47) 59
Paradental debris of Malassey, (Fig. 550) 574, 575
Paradidymis, (Fig. 405) 416

Paraduodenal fossa, (Fig. 56) 67, 68
Paraesthesiae due to painful scar, 763
Paraganglioma, chromaffin, (Fig. 607) 648
— non-chromaffin, (Fig. 608) 650
Paralysis, transient, in chronic hypertension, 653
Paralytic ileus, postoperative, 172
Paramedian abdominal incision, (Figs. 702–705) 747
Parapatellar incision, 811
Pararectal incision, (Figs. 706–708) 749
Parasympathetic fibres to constrictor pupillae of iris, (Fig. 577) 611
— innervation of bladder and colon, (Fig. 592) 628, 629
— nerve(s), functions of, in male sex organs, 647
— — — to heart, 615
— nervous system, (Fig. 161) 174, 175
— — — functions of, (Fig. 159) 170
— — — origin of, (Fig. 163) 175
— — — surgery on, 610, 611
— supply to abdominal viscera, (Figs. 581–587) 618
Paratenon carrying blood to tendons, (Fig. 525) 545
Parathyroid arteries, 25
— gland, 25
— — surgical significance of, 26
Paratracheal lymph-glands, 329
Paravertebral alcohol injection, 617
— space, lumbar, chromaffin paraganglioma in, (Fig. 607) 649
— — in thorax, chromaffin paraganglioma found, (Fig. 607) 649
Paraxial bar of mesoblast, (Fig. 246) 255
Paresis or paralysis due to pituitary tumour, 16
Parietal cell vagotomy, 621
— emissary vein, 297
— layer of pelvic fascia, (Figs. 206, 208) 221, 224
— lobe, incision giving access to, (Fig. 746) 788
— lymph-glands of abdomen, (Figs. 331–333) 333
— — thorax, 335
— spider, (Fig. 298) 296
Parona's space, (Fig. 615) 657
Paronychial infections of hand, incisions for opening, (Fig. 722) 766
Parotid gland, facial nerve in relation to, (Fig. 436) 453
— — nerve-supply to, 146, (Fig. 140) 148
— — secretory nerve-fibres to, 150
— — veins of, (Fig. 303) 301
— investment, 208
— lymphatic glands, (Fig. 325) 327

864 INDEX

Parotid tumours, enucleation of, sparing facial nerve, (*Fig.* 436) 453
Parotideomasseteric fascia, 208, 327
Parovarian cysts of urogenital origin, 441
Parovarium, (*Fig.* 406) 417
Pars anterior, 11
— interarticularis, defect in, causing spondylolisthesis, (*Figs.* 655 B, 656) 700, 702
— intermedia, 11, 12
Passavant, ridge of, 491
Patella, 276
— bipartite or tripartite, (*Fig.* 222) 238
— cubiti, 238
— dislocation of, (*Figs.* 626, 627) 667
— ossification of, unusual, (*Fig.* 222) 238
Patella-displacing approach to knee-joint, (*Fig.* 772) 810, 812
Patella-splitting approach to knee-joint, (*Fig.* 771) 810, 812
Patellar ligament, 276
— — medial, 668, 669
— tendon, lateral attachment of, 669
Patent ductus arteriosus, (*Fig.* 506) 520
— Meckel's diverticulum, (*Fig.* 383 A) 389
— urachus, 52, (*Fig.* 396 B) 403
Pathological spondylolisthesis, (*Fig.* 655 B) 700
Payr's membrane, 75
Peau d'orange in breast cancer, (*Fig.* 34 C) 41
Pecten band, 119
Pectinate line, (*Figs.* 99–101) 109–113, 115
— — abscess opening at, (*Figs.* 112, 114) 121, 123
— — carcinoma at, 110
— — piles in relation to, (*Fig.* 100) 110, 111, 112
Pectoralis major, lymph plexus on, removal of in breast cancer, 345
— — in relation to breast, (*Fig.* 25) 30, (*Fig.* 30) 35
— minor, relation of brachial plexus to, 160
Pelvic abscesses, 742
— appendix, (*Fig.* 47) 60
— bleeding, control of, by ligature of hypogastric arteries, 554
— cancer, colonic resection for, 64
— colon (*see* Colon, Pelvic)
— — antagonistic roles of sympathetic and parasympathetic in, 628
— — blood-supply to, 599, 601
— diaphragm, (*Fig.* 102) 113, (*Fig.* 185) 198, 224, 718
— fascia, (*Figs.* 206–208) 221, 623
— floor, female, (*Fig.* 674) 718, 719
— kidney, (*Fig.* 393 C) 400

Pelvic mass causing sciatica, 707
— mesocolon, (*Fig.* 49) 60, 61
— — fossa intersigmoidea in attachment of, (*Fig.* 61) 72
— metastases of breast cancer, 38
— peritonitis, small gut affected by, 57
— viscera, pain from, referred to low back, 695
— — parasympathetic supply to, (*Fig.* 587) 622
Pelvirectal abscess causing supralevator fistula, (*Fig.* 115) 123
Pelvis, abnormality of, in extroversion of bladder, (*Fig.* 411) 420
— arrangement of structures on wall of, (*Fig.* 208) 223
— incisions giving access to, 750, 754
— in infancy and childhood, (*Fig.* 128) 136
— part of small gut lying in, 57
— sympathetic supply to, 624
Penile dislocation of testis, (*Fig.* 404) 416
— epispadias, 422
— type of hypospadias, (*Fig.* 409) 419
Penis, dorsal nerve of, (*Figs.* 96, 98) 108
— gutter on, in extroversion of bladder and epispadias, 420, 421, 422
— muscle and fascia covering of, 219, 220, 221
— vein of, 104
Penopubic epispadias, 422
Peptic ulcer of Meckel's diverticulum, 391
— ulceration associated with hiatus hernia, 689
Perforating branches of internal mammary artery, 42
— cutaneous branches of internal mammary artery, 31, 36
— veins, ankle, (*Fig.* 310) 307, 310, 316
— — direct and indirect, (*Figs.* 314 A, 315) 313
— — of leg, (*Figs.* 309, 313–315) 312, 313–318
— — — test for competence of, (*Fig.* 316) 317
Perforation of diverticulum of appendix, 445
Perianal vein, rupture of, 112
Periarterial plexuses, 623
— — of limb vessels, (*Fig.* 594) 632
— sympathectomy, (*Fig.* 594) 631
Periarticular fluids, stagnation of, due to trauma and/or disuse, 571, 572
Pericardium, puncture of, 739
Perichondrium of articular cartilage, 732
Pericranium, (*Fig.* 1) 1, 4
Perineal anaesthesia, (*Fig.* 742) 785
— artery, (*Fig.* 98) 109
— dislocation of testis, (*Fig.* 404) 416

Perineal ectopia testis, 411
— nerve, (*Figs.* 741, 742) 785
— pouch, deep, 199
— prostatectomy, 106
Perineoscrotal type of hypospadias, (*Fig.* 409) 419
Perinephric fat, lymph-glands of, 608
Perineum, dermoids of, 427
— development of, (*Fig.* 387) 395
— extravasation of fluid in, 221
— laceration of, causation of prolapse of uterus, 720
— nerve-supply of, (*Fig.* 741) 784
— shotgun, (*Fig.* 388) 396
Perineus, deep transverse, 199
Periodontal membrane, (*Fig.* 547) 574
Periosteal blood-vessels, (*Fig.* 226) 243, 245, 246
— fibrosarcoma, (*Fig.* 555, 2) 583
— layer of dura mater, (*Fig.* 3) 5
Periosteum, (*Figs.* 553, 554) 581
— bone-forming function of, 581, 584
— of scalp (*see* Pericranium)
Periostitis, creeping, 582
Peripheral autonomic system, (*Fig.* 167) 172
— mixed nerve injury causing painful scar, 763
— nerve(s) entrapment, 470
— — ischaemia of, (*Fig.* 493) 504
— — oxygenation of, when nutrient vessels are occluded, 567
— vascular disease, (*Figs.* 594–606) 631–648
Perirenal fat, absence of, in child, (*Fig.* 127) 135
Peristalsis, renal lesions interfering with, 92
Peritoneal bands, accessory, (*Figs.* 62–68) 73–78
— — accessory, theories of causation of, 73, 386
— — due to persistence of ventral mesentery, (*Fig.* 380) 386
— cavity, multiple accessory spleens in, 432
— — puncture of, 739
— fossae, (*Figs.* 55–61) 67–72
— metastases of breast cancer, 38
— recess, 739
— relations of colon, 58
— — duodenum, (*Fig.* 43) 56
— surface of diaphragm, shoulder-tip pain due to irritation of, 88, 89
Peritoneum, ease of stripping, 761
— lesser sac of, (*Fig.* 55) 67
— parietal, nerve-supply to, 618
— prolapse of, in rectal prolapse, (*Fig.* 676) 722, 723

Peritoneum, relationship in child to kidneys, (*Fig.* 127) 135
— — of ureter to, 534
Peritonitis, appendicitis resulting in, 60
— pelvic, small gut affected by, 57
Peritracheobronchial lymph-glands, (*Fig.* 334) 336
Peri-urethral glands, 419
Perivascular spaces of brain, (*Fig.* 4) 7
Peroneal nerve, deep, (*Fig.* 285) 283
— — injury to, in operation in popliteal area, 567
— — ischaemic palsy of, 465
— — at knee, compression of, 471
— — loss due to division of, (*Fig.* 448) 465
— — relation of, to fibula, 818, 819
— — relaxation, posture for, (*Fig.* 451) 468
— process of os calcis, 231
— retinaculum(a) of foot, (*Fig.* 291) 289
— — stenosis of, 259
— sesamoid, (*Fig.* 212) 234
— vein, 312, 316
Peroneus(i) longus and brevis, 289
— — sheath for, (*Fig.* 253) 260
— — sesamoid in, (*Fig.* 212) 234
— — slipping, 579
— — tendon, (*Fig.* 294) 292
— — — supporting arch of foot, (*Fig.* 295) 293
— and movements of foot, 205
— tertius, 283, 288, 289
Pes anserinus, 148
— cavus, 295
Petit, triangle of, cold abscess of, 727
— — hernia at, 692
Petrosal nerve, great deep, 142, (*Fig.* 37) 145
— — — superficial, 142, (*Fig.* 37) 145
— — lesser superficial, 146
— — small superficial, 146, (*Fig.* 141) 150
— sinus, inferior, (*Fig.* 302) 300
— — superior, 6 (*Fig.* 135) 143
Petrous bone, lesion of facial nerve in below offshoot to stapedius, (*Fig.* 435) 453
— ganglion, 149
Peyer's patches, 335
Phaeochromocytoma, 648, 649, 650
— securing adrenal vein in, 802
Phalangeal spurs, (*Fig.* 219) 231, 236
Phalanx(ges), first and second, incisions of, (*Fig.* 723) 766
— terminal, incisions of, (*Figs.* 721–723) 764
Pharyngeal aponeurosis, 180
— branch of vagus, 152

866 INDEX

Pharyngeal canal, 146
— constrictors, (Fig. 166) 179, 491
— dimple, (Fig. 421) 434
— diverticulum, lateral, 26
— — production of, 491
— part of nasopharyngeal sphincter, 491
— pressure diverticulum, deep, (Figs. 421, 422) 434
— nerves, 146, (Fig. 142) 150
— plexus, (Fig. 142) 150, 152, 157
— — branch from cervical sympathetic to, (Fig. 145) 156
— — of nerves, 180
— — veins, 181
— tonsils (see Adenoids)
— venous plexus, 157
Pharyngobasilar fascia, 180
Pharynx, anaesthesia of, due to glossopharyngeal nerve lesion, 454
— diverticulum(a) of, 361 (Figs. 420-422) 433
— lymphoid tissue of, 59
— sphincters of, 491
Phimosis, extreme, 404
Phlebitis commencing in soleal sinuses, 312
— of vein of breast, (Fig. 26) 32
Phrenic arteries, inferior, collateral circulation to liver through, (Fig. 534 B) 558, 560
— exairesis, 467
— nerve, 158, 216
— — accessory, (Fig. 154) 164
— — avulsion of, 164, 467
— — communication between brachial plexus and, (Fig. 154) 164
— — division of, causing paralysis of diaphragm, 466
— — intradiaphragmatic distribution of, (Fig. 649) 690
— — pain referred to shoulder tip, 88
— — protection of, in repair of hiatus hernia, (Fig. 649) 689
— plexus, 176
Phreno-oesophageal membrane, (Fig. 646) 686
Pia mater, (Fig. 4) 7
Piles, (Figs. 100, 101) 111
— external, 112
— false external, 112
— injection of, 110
— internal, 112
— interoexternal, 112, 117
— position of, (Fig. 101) 112
— removal of, anatomical considerations, (Fig. 106) 117, 119
— sentinel, 111
— strangulated, (Figs. 105, 106) 117
— thrombotic, 112

Pilonidal sinuses, sacrococcygeal, 423
Pin-point meatus, 404
Pinna, developmental anomalies of, (Figs. 343, 344) 354
— nerve-supply of, (Fig. 130) 138
— sensory loss to, in fifth nerve paralysis (Fig. 434 B) 450
Pirie, astragalo-scaphoid bone of, 230
Piriformis, 221, 223
— hernia escaping at border of, 692
Pirogoff's amputation, 772
Pisiform bone, 242, 286
— — bipartite, (Fig. 220) 236
'Pistoning' of amputation stump, 774
Pituitary body, developmental defects of, (Fig. 342) 353
— — enlarged, (Figs. 14, 15) 15
— — normal, (Figs. 7-13) 11-15
— — relationships of, (Figs. 8-10) 12
— — vascular relationships of, (Fig. 11) 13
— fossa, 11
— — expansion of, by tumour, (Fig. 15) 16
— — removal of floor of, (Fig. 748) 790
— gland, routes giving access to, (Fig. 745) 788, (Fig. 748) 790
— tumour, approach to, (Fig. 748) 790
— — causing optic nerve lesion, 449
— — symptoms of, (Figs. 14, 15) 15
— — visual defects due to, (Fig. 14) 14, 15
Pivot joint, (Fig. 242) 253
Plantar aponeurosis, 289
— — maintaining arch of foot, (Fig. 297) 295
— fascia, digital processes of, 215
— — fibrosis of, 214
— ligament, long, (Fig. 294) 292
— — short, (Fig. 294) 292
— and palmar fasciae, (Figs. 197-199) 212
Platt's law, 625
Platysma, 148, 149, 194, 206
Pleura, danger of opening, in kidney incision, (Fig. 719) 762
— puncture of, during preganglion denervation of arm, 637
— tear of, prevention of pneumothorax due to, 747
Pleural cavity, approach to, 791
— — divided by meso-azygos, 46
— — left, stomach brought into, 796
— — puncture of, 738
— relationship with oesophagus, 795
— surface of diaphragm, shoulder-tip pain due to irritation of, 89
Pleurohilar arteries and veins, 51
Pleuroperitoneal hiatus, 682, 683
Plexitis, (Fig. 658) 707

INDEX 867

Plexuses on anterior rami, 157, 165
— scalenus medius, (*Fig.* 146) 157
Plica semilunaris, 26, 27
— triangularis, 26, 27
Pneumonia, liability of children to, 133
Pneumothorax, tension, due to pleural tear, prevention of, 747
Poirier's gland involved in rectal cancer, 606
Polycystic kidney, congenital, (*Fig.* 389) 397
Polymastia, 373
Polyorchidism, (*Fig.* 402) 412
Polythelia, 373
Pons, taste fibres to, 147
Popliteal artery, 565
— — atherosclerotic, patency of, 566
— — at bifurcation, occlusion of, sudden, 553
— — entrapment, (*Fig.* 432) 447
— — occlusion of, collateral circulation in, 555
— — — gangrene following, 549
— — — sudden, 553
— — surgical approach to, (*Fig.* 541) 566
— blood-pressure in coarctation of aorta, 520
— fossa, short saphenous vein in, 311
— ligament, oblique, (*Fig.* 275) 276
— lymph-glands, 340
— thrombosis in young, 565
— tributaries, varicosities of, 311
— vein, 310, 312
Popliteus, 205
— — (*Fig.* 275) 276
— tendon of, bursa under, (*Fig.* 257) 264
— — at knee-joint, 254
Portal bed block, surgery for, (*Fig.* 513) 529
— block, extrahepatic, 528, 529
— — intrahepatic, 528, 529
— hypertension, factors causing, 528
— — ligature of hepatic artery, invalid in, 526
— obstruction, (*Fig.* 513) 528
— — collateral circulations in, (*Fig.* 319) 320
— shunts, (*Fig.* 513) 529
— vein(s), 306, 523, 528
— — anomalies of, (*Fig.* 509) 523
— — cavernomatous transformations of, 529
— — communicating at umbilicus with systemic veins, 54
— — congenital stricture of, (*Fig.* 509 C) 523
— — development of, 523
— — implantation of, into inferior vena cava, (*Fig.* 513) 529, 543

Portal vein(s), lack of collaterals for, 546
— venous radicle, 526
— — system, 526, 528
— — thrombosis causing portal block, 529
Portal-lymphatic communications, 321
Portal-systemic communications, (*Fig.* 100) 111, 197, (*Figs.* 319–321) 321
Porter's shoulder, 265
— tip hand, 456
Portio minor, 142
Postcentral vertebral venous plexus, 320, 323
Postdeglutition coughing due to internal laryngeal nerve ligation, 22
Posterior approach in denervation of heart, (*Fig.* 759) 801
— arch vein, (*Figs.* 310, 311) 307, 316
— clinoid processes, (*Fig.* 8) 12
— cord lesion, paralysis due to, (*Fig.* 438, V) 457
— dislocations of hip, high and low, (*Fig.* 625) 667
— hernia, 683
— lobe of pituitary, (*Fig.* 7) 11, 12
— rhizotomy, (*Fig.* 580) 616
— root ganglion compression causing sciatica, 703
— temporal diploic vein, 296
— triangle, 207, 208, 212, 302, 303
Posterolateral hernia, (*Fig.* 642) 683, 684
Posteromedial vein of thigh, (*Fig.* 311) 307, 311
Postfaucial diverticulum of pharynx, 434
Postganglionic autonomic fibres to heart, 615
— fibres of autonomic system, (*Figs.* 159–161) 171, 172
— section in denervation of limb, (*Figs.* 595, 597) 633, 635
Postprandial pain due to coeliac artery compression, 448
Postural activity, 181
— defects causing low back pain, 695
Posture, relaxation of nerves by, (*Figs.* 449–451) 467
Pott's fracture of ankle, 485
— operation for Fallot's tetralogy, 509
Poupart's ligament, 98
Pre-aortic lymph-glands, (*Fig.* 333) 334, 342
— — coeliac group of, 66
Pre-auricular fistulae, (*Figs.* 343, 344) 354
— gland, (*Fig.* 325) 326
Preganglionic fibres of autonomic system, (*Figs.* 159–161) 171, 172
— — — — to heart, 615
— section in denervation of limb, (*Figs.* 597–603) 635

868 INDEX

Pregnancy, enlarged aberrant ovarian vein in, compressing ureter, 536
— vulval vaginal veins in, 311
Prelaminar vertebral venous plexus, 320, 323
Prelaryngeal lymph-glands, (*Fig.* 22) 24, 328
Premaxilla, 358
Prepatellar bursa, (*Fig.* 258) 265
'Prerectal' space, (*Fig.* 93) 105
— nerve or plexus (superior hypogastric plexus), (*Figs.* 585–587) 620, 622, 624, (*Figs.* 590, 591) 625
— — neurectomy of, 629
— plexus, 177
Pre-scalene lymph-gland biopsy, 338
Pre-tracheobronchial lymph-glands, (*Fig.* 334) 336, 337
Pre-ureteric left inferior vena cava, 543
Pressure diverticula, deep pharyngeal, (*Figs.* 421, 422) 434
Pretracheal fascia, (*Figs.* 192, 194) 206, 209, 210
— — supplying false capsule to thyroid, 23
— lymph-glands, (*Fig.* 22) 24, 328
Prevertebral abscess, costotransversectomy for, 798
— cold abscess, 723
— fascia, (*Figs.* 192, 194–196) 206, 209, 210, 216
— muscles, 155
Primary diverticula of gut, (*Figs.* 428–430 A) 443
Principal plane of Rex, (*Fig.* 512) 527
Pringle's manœuvre, 525
Procaine nerve-block, paradoxical response to, 643
Processus vaginalis, 96, 406
— — diverticula of, complicating indirect inguinal hernia, 407, 408
— — failure of, to close, 407
— — fluid in (*see* Hydrocele)
Proctodeal membrane, persistence of, 394
Proctodeum, 109, 421
Profunda artery, anomalous origin of, 310
— vein, 304
— — collateral circulation through, (*Fig.* 317) 318
Profundus tendon, 285
— — sheath for, (*Fig.* 249) 256, (*Fig.* 287) 285
Prolapse, (*Figs.* 673–676) 716–723
— of disc (*see* Intervertebral Disc Prolapse)
— female urethra, 721
— rectum, (*Fig.* 676) 721
— uterus and vagina, (*Figs.* 673–675) 717

Promontoric appendix, (*Fig.* 47) 60
Pronator teres, paralysis of, 457
Proparietal inguinal hernia, (*Fig.* 399) **408**
Properitoneal inguinal hernia, (*Fig.* 399) 408
Proptosis due to pituitary tumour, 16
Prostate, (*Figs.* 91–94) 102–106
— adenoma of, (*Fig.* 91) 102
— capsules of, (*Fig.* 92) 103
— — compared to those of thyroid, (*Fig.* 21) 23
— enucleation of, (*Fig.* 21) 23, 104
— fasciae behind, (*Fig.* 93) 104
— fascial sheath of, (*Fig.* 207) 222, 223
— lobes of, (*Fig.* 91) 102
— rectal examination of, 585
— surfaces and relations of, 103
Prostatectomy, perineal, 106
— suprapubic, 104
Prostatic calculi, recognition of, per rectum, 585
— carcinoma, vertebral secondaries of, 321
— tumours, upward growth of, 23, 102, 104
— urethra (*see* Urethra, Prostatic)
— veins, 104
Prostato-perineal fascia, (*Fig.* 93) 105
Prosthesis, replacement of aortic aneurysm by, 561
Proust, retroprostatic space of, (*Fig.* 93) 105
Proximal lymph-glands of gut, (*Fig.* 54) 66
Pseudo-cysts of pancreas, 497
Pseudo-duplication of testis, 412
Pseudo-short saphenous veins, 311
Pseudomyxoma peritonei, 445
Psoas fascia, opening of, in approach to sympathetic chain, (*Fig.* 603) 642
— major, 218
— — test for, 218
— muscle, 127
— sheath, (*Figs.* 200, 202) 217
— — cold abscesses in, 218, 725, 726
— test, 587
Pterygoid canal, nerve of, 142, (*Fig.* 137) 145, 146
— muscle, internal, (*Fig.* 138) 146
— plexus, (*Fig.* 299) 299
Pterygopalatine fossa, (*Fig.* 137) 145
Ptosis, 449, 458, 466
Pubic dislocation of testis, (*Fig.* 404) 416
— symphysis, (*Fig.* 238) 251
— type of dislocation of hip, 666
Pubis, anchoring of rectum to, (*Figs.* 103, 104) 114
— pilonidal sinus at, 423
— transverse ligament of, 200

Pubococcygeal line, 394
Pubococcygeus muscle, (*Fig.* 102) 114
Pubofemoral ligament, (*Fig.* 274) 276
Pubopenile ectopia testis, 411
Puboprostatic ligaments, 103
Puborectalis muscle, (*Figs.* 102–104) 114, 115, 117
— sling, (*Fig.* 644 C) 686
Pudendal artery, internal, (*Figs.* 96–98) 108, 109, 200
— canal, (*Fig.* 742) 785
— — relations of, 348
— hernia, 692
— nerve(s), (*Figs.* 96–98) 108, 625, 628
— — block, (*Fig.* 742) 785
— — injection of, (*Figs.* 741, 742) 784
— plexus, 200
— vein(s), external, 308
— — external, incompetence of, 311
— — internal, enlarged tributaries of, 311
— venous plexus, 104
Pulmonary agenesis, 51
— artery(ies), development of, 510, 519
— — left, (*Fig.* 40 B) 50
— — right, (*Fig.* 40 A) 50
— — stenosis or ligation of, 51
— and bronchial circulations, anastomoses between, 51
— embolism, prevention of, by venous ligation, (*Figs.* 317, 318) 318
— glomus bodies, 650
— plexus, 176
— stenosis, congenital, 507
— — in Fallot's tetralogy, 508
— valve, defective, 507
— vein(s), inferior, (*Fig.* 40) 51
— — joining portal, (*Fig.* 509 B) 523
— — superior, (*Fig.* 40) 51
— vessels, (*Fig.* 40) 50
Pulp space infections, incisions for, (*Fig.* 721) 764
— of tooth, (*Figs.* 546, 547) 573
Pulsation, visible, in coarctation of aorta, 520, 522
Pulsion diverticulum, pharyngeal, (*Figs.* 421, 422) 434, 435
Punctures (*see also under specific parts*)
— anatomy of, (*Figs.* 683–698) 733–743
Pupil, Argyll Robertson, 145
— contraction of, 466
— — in whole brachial plexus lesion, 458
— dilated, due to oculomotor nerve division, 449
— fixed dilated, indicating side of lesion in cerebral compression, 613
Pupillary changes due to brachial plexus injury, 612
— — — cervical cord injury, 612

Pupillary constriction, 144
— dilatation, 144
— reflexes, loss of, 449
Pyelogram of normal and horseshoe kidney, (*Fig.* 392) 399
— polycystic kidney, 398
Pyelonephritis in pregnancy due to aberrant ovarian vein, 536
Pyloric antrum, vagus nerves ending at, 620
— sphincter, (*Fig.* 487) 490, 493
— stenosis, diagnosis from congenital duodenal obstruction, 387
— — hypertrophic, 493
Pylorus, 493
Pyramidal lobe of thyroid, 17, 366
— tract, pressure on, by pituitary tumour, 16

Quadratus labii inferioris muscle, paralysis of, 149
— lumborum, 127, (*Figs.* 200–202) 216
— — cold abscess on, 725, 726
— — hernia at border of, 692
— plantae, 292
Quadriceps, imperfect development of, 238
— limp, (*Fig.* 552) 577
— line of pull of, and dislocation of knee, (*Fig.* 626) 667
— muscle, postural activity of, 181
— tendon of, 276
— — degeneration of, with age, 673
Queckenstedt's test, 9
— — for spinal block, 591
Quinsy, 28
— location of commencement of, 27

Rachischisis, (*Fig.* 363) 369
Radial artery, incision for ligature of, 817
— bursa, (*Figs.* 249, 250) 257, (*Fig.* 287) 285, 657
— — infection in, incision for, (*Figs.* 723, 724) 767
— collateral ligament, (*Figs.* 270, 272) 272, 274
— flexors of wrist, paralysis of, 457
— nerve, 161, 163, 457
— — injury causing painful scar, 764
— — loss due to division of, (*Figs.* 439, 440) 458
— — paralysis, 457
— — relaxation, posture for, 468
— — sparing of, in exposure of humerus and radius, (*Fig.* 778) 816, 817
— — transplantation, (*Fig.* 452) 468
— and ulnar styloids, determination of relative levels of, (*Fig.* 560) 593
Radiale (*Fig.* 224 A) 240, 241

870 INDEX

Radicular artery(ies), anterior, 501
— — great, (*Fig.* 491) 501, 502, (*Fig.* 495) 506
— — lower thoracic, 506
— spinal arteries, (*Figs.* 490–492, 494, 495) 499–503, 506
Radiculitis, (*Fig.* 658) 703
Radio-ulnar joint, superior, (*Fig.* 242) 253
Radiography, position of gall-bladder in, (*Figs.* 76, 77) 87
Radiohumeral joint, dislocation of, (*Fig.* 621) 662
Radiology demonstrating ossicles of foot and hand, 229, 230
Radius, diagnosis of fracture of, (*Fig.* 560) 593
— dislocation of head of, (*Fig.* 621) 662
— epiphysial lines and capsular reflections of, (*Fig.* 260) 267
— exposure of, 817
— measuring length of, (*Fig.* 558) 593
— ossification of, 249
Rami, anterior, in brachial plexus, 160
— — of spinal nerves, 157, (*Fig.* 155) 164, 165, 166
— communicantes, grey, 156, 159, 172, 175
— — white, 156, 172, 175, 179, 622, 624
— — — sympathetic supply to heart through, 615
— posterior, of spinal nerves, 165
Ramstedt operation, 493
Ranine vein, (*Fig.* 301) 300
Ranula, diagnosis from dermoid, 428
Rathke's pouch, 353
— — congenital cysts of, 15
— folds of, (*Fig.* 384) 392
Raynaud's disease, 642
— — ganglionectomy for, 634
— — results of sympathetic denervation in, 644
— phenomenon in hands after operation for hypertension, 647
Reaction of degeneration in facial nerve injury, 453
Receptaculum chyli (*see* Cisterna Chyli)
Rectal agenesis, 392
— angle, 106
— arteries, superior and middle, 601
— biopsy, total, 119
— continence, preservation of, 118
— estimation of size of os uteri in labour, 586
— examination (P.R.) information gained by, in female, 585
— — — — male, 584
— sinus(es), 111

Rectal spasm, chronic, causing colonic enlargement, 630
— stalks, 601, 721
— and vaginal examination, 584
— — — combined, 587
Recto-urethral fistula, (*Fig.* 386 B) 393, 446
Recto-urethralis muscle of Roux, (*Fig.* 94) 106, 116, 721
Recto-uterine fold, 717
— pouch (*see* Douglas, Pouch of)
Rectocele, 720
Rectovaginal fistula, (*Fig.* 386 C) 393
— pouch, vaginal examination of, 586
— septum, accessory endometrial tissue in, 432
— — examination of, 587
Rectovesical pouch (*see* Douglas, Pouch of)
— fistula, (*Fig.* 386 A) 393
— septum, (*Fig.* 384) 392
Rectovestibular fistula, 393
Rectum, anchoring of, to pubis, (*Figs.* 103, 104) 114
— antagonistic roles of sympathetic and parasympathetic in, 628
— anterior resection of, 608
— ballooning of, 585
— blood-supply of, 61, 599, 601
— carcinoma of, 110
— — causing ballooning, 585
— — extension of, via lymphatics, (*Fig.* 574) 606
— — resection of, (*Figs.* 573–576) 605
— congenital deformities of anus and, (*Figs.* 384–388) 392–397
— deformities of, (*Figs.* 385, 386) 392
— development of, (*Fig.* 384) 392, (*Fig.* 387) 395
— excision of, protection of vesical nerves in, 623
— fasciae between prostate and, (*Fig.* 93) 104
— fascial sheath of, 222, 223
— high blind termination of, (*Fig.* 385) 393
— lateral ligaments of, 601
— line dividing anus from, 394
— lymphatics of, (*Figs.* 573, 574, 576) 605
— palpation of kidney per, 400
— peritoneal relations of, (*Fig.* 45) 58
— portal-systemic anastomosis in lower, (*Fig.* 100) 111, 197, (*Figs.* 319–321) 320
— prolapse of, 586 (*Fig.* 676) 721
— resection of, 601
— supports of, 721
Rectus abdominis, extending McBurney's incision through, 757

INDEX 871

Rectus abdominis, incisions through, (*Fig.* 699 B) 744, (*Figs.* 702–704) 747, 748
— — — — principles of, 754
— — nerves in, 167
— — nerve-supply to, (*Fig.* 699 B) 744, (*Fig.* 703) 748, (*Figs.* 708–712) 751, 752
— capitis lateralis and anterior, nerves to, 159
— femoris, sesamoid of, (*Fig.* 221) 237
— oculi, paralysis of external, 451
— sheath, cold abscess in, 726
— — significance of transversely running fibres of, (*Fig.* 42) 53
Rectus-displacing incisions, (*Figs.* 705, 707) 749, 750
Recurrent chain, glands of, (*Fig.* 22) 24
— dislocation of patella, (*Fig.* 627) 667, 669
— — shoulder, 661
— laryngeal nerve in relation to inferior thyroid artery, (*Fig.* 18) 18
— — — varying relation to thyroid, (*Fig.* 19) 19, 20
— nerve (of Luschka), 153, (*Fig.* 155) 165
Referred pain (*see* Pain Referred)
— — oesophageal, 492
— — due to sciatic nerve compression, 702
Reflex acute arterial spasm due to vascular insult, 611
— sciatic neuralgia, 702
Regeneration after denervation, prevention of, (*Fig.* 604) 643
Regular dislocations of hip, 667
Reid's base line, (*Fig.* 690) 736
— (Douglas), genitomesenteric fold of, 73
Relations, important, (*Fig.* 341) 347–349
Relaxation of nerves, (*Figs.* 449–453) 467
Renal artery(ies), (*Fig.* 82) 92
— — aberrant, 534
— — anastomosis of splenic artery to, 533, (*Fig.* 589 B) 625
— — divisions of, (*Fig.* 515) 531
— — stenosis causing hypertension, (*Fig.* 589) 624
— collar, venous, 543
— fascia, (*Figs.* 84, 85) 93, 216
— pedicle, venous anomalies in region of, 543
— pelvis, junction of, with ureter, 499
— — shape of, in horseshoe kidney, (*Fig.* 392) 399
— plexus. 176
— vein(s), 534
— — anastomosis of, to splenic vein, (*Fig.* 513) 530
— — left, 543

Renal vessels in kidney transplantation, 534
Respiration of child, 133
Respiratory disease causing tracheoceles, 439, 440
Rete testis, appendages of, (*Fig.* 405) 417
Retinaculum(a) of foot, flexor, 289
— — peroneal, (*Fig.* 291) 289
— — superior and inferior extensor, (*Fig.* 290) 288
— of hand, extensor, 258, (*Fig.* 289) 286
— — flexor, (*Fig.* 250) 257, (*Figs.* 289, 290) 284
— — — division of, (*Fig.* 288) 286
— uteri, 223, 717
Retinal fibres in optic chiasma, arrangement of, 15
— vein, lack of collateral for, 549
— vessels, sympathetic fibres to, 612
Retinitis pigmentosa, 613
'Retraction' in breast pathology, (*Figs.* 32–34) 38–41
— of nipple, (*Figs.* 32–34 B) 38–41
Retro-aortic lymph-glands, (*Fig.* 333) 335
Retro-ureteric branch of renal artery, (*Fig.* 82) 92
Retrocaval ureter, (*Fig.* 524) 543
Retrocolic appendix, (*Fig.* 47) 59
— fossa, 67, (*Fig.* 60) 72
'Retrograde menstruation' causing endometriomata, 432
Retroparietal inguinal hernia, (*Fig.* 399) 408
Retropharyngeal abscess, (*Fig.* 195) 210
— — acute, (*Fig.* 677) 724
— cold abscess, (*Fig.* 677) 723
— lymph-glands, (*Figs.* 194, 195) 210, 328
Retroprostatic space of Proust, (*Fig.* 93) 105
Retrosternal hernia, (*Fig.* 642) 682, 684
— pain due to oesophageal spasm, 493
Retroversion of uterus, 719
Rex, principal plane of, (*Fig.* 512) 527
Rhizotomy, posterior, (*Fig.* 580) 616
Rhomboid fossa of clavicle, (*Fig.* 233) 248
— ligament, (*Fig.* 267) 271
Ribs, accessory, (*Figs.* 209–211) 224
— blood-supply of, (*Fig.* 231) 242, 246
— cervical, (*Fig.* 153) 163, (*Fig.* 209) 224
— first, anterior relations of neck of, (*Fig.* 153) 163
— — cervical rib and, (*Fig.* 209) 225
— — compression of brachial plexus by, (*Fig.* 153) 163, 227
— — congenital abnormalities of, 227
— lumbar, (*Fig.* 211) 229
— removal in transthoracic approach to abdomen, (*Fig.* 751) 793
— — — operations, (*Figs.* 750, 751) 791

Ribs, resection in denervation of heart, (*Fig.* 759) 801
— — Smithwick's denervation operation, (*Fig.* 598) 637
— — transthoracic approach to abdomen, (*Fig.* 751) 794
— second, identification of, 41
— — joined to first rib, 228
— twelfth, hernia escaping under, 692
— — relations of kidneys to, (*Figs.* 80, 81) 89, 91
Rickety knock-knee, (*Fig.* 470) 480
Ridge of Passavant, 491
Right lymph-duct, 336, 337, 338, (*Fig.* 339 A) 345
Rim rents of supraspinatus, (*Fig.* 640) 680
Rima glottidis, growth of, 133
Roscoe Graham manœuvre in oesophagojejunal anastomosis, (*Fig.* 756 B) 796
Rotation errors of gut, (*Fig.* 376) 380, 384
— of gut, (*Figs.* 371–376) 375–383
Rotatores, 192
Round ligaments, 717
Roux Y anastomosis for duodenal obstruction due to annular pancreas, 432
— recto-urethralis muscle of, (*Fig.* 94) 106, 721
Rovsing's operation for polycystic kidneys, 398
— test, 591

Sacculations of colon, 58
Sacral articular facets, superior, variation in direction of, 596
— curve of vertebral column, (*Fig.* 116) 123, 134
— ganglia, 176
— lymph-glands, 334, 606
— meningocele, anterior, 424
— nerve(s), 166
— — first, compression of, by disc prolapse, 712, 713
— — injection of, (*Fig.* 739) 783
— — roots giving off nervi erigentes, (*Fig.* 587) 622
— parasite, 423
— parasympathetic, 171, 174, 175
— plexus, 221, 223
— vertebra, first, lumbarization of, 700
Sacralization of fifth lumbar vertebra, 127, (*Fig.* 654) 696, 698, 704
Sacrococcygeal region, congenital defects in, 423
— root-areas, (*Fig.* 158) 170
Sacro-iliac joint diseases causing sciatica, 707
Sacrosciatic foramina, 221, 283

Sacrospinalis, (*Fig.* 200) 216
— group of muscles, (*Figs.* 177–180) 189, 190
— muscle, postural activity of, 181
— — relation of kidneys to, (*Fig.* 81) 90
Sacrospinous ligament, 198, (*Fig.* 286) 284
Sacrotuberous ligament, (*Fig.* 286) 283
Sacrum, 123
— anomalies of, 696, 700
— articulation of transverse process of fifth lumbar vertebra with, 697, (*Fig.* 659) 704
— attachment of aponeurosis of origin of sacrospinalis, (*Fig.* 178) 190
— and coccyx, congenital absence of, 695, 696
— — — defects in region of, 422
— development of, 694
— fusion of transverse process of fifth lumbar vertebra with, (*Fig.* 654) 698
— kidney in hollow of, 400
— ossification of, 248
— teratoma of, 423
Saddle emboli of aortic bifurcation, 553
— joint, (*Fig.* 244) 253
'Safety-valve' haematoma, 3
Sagittal sinus, inferior, 6
— — superior, 6, 297, 298
— — — approach to, (*Fig.* 121) 130
— — — injury to, 298
Saint's triad, 689
Salivary glands, fascial sheath of, (*Fig.* 193) 207
Saphenofemoral valve, test for competence of, (*Fig.* 316) 317
Saphenopopliteal valve, test for competence of, (*Fig.* 316) 318
Saphenous nerve, 307, 310
— — compression in thigh, 471
— — injury causing painful scar, 764
— opening, 99, 306
— vein(s), accessory, 308
— — long, (*Figs.* 309–312) 306, 309, 315, 316
— — — incompetence of, 311
— — — test for varicosities of, 587
— — pseudo-short, 311, 315
— — short (small), (*Fig.* 309) 306, 308, 310, 315, 316
— venous system, hypertension in, causing varicosities, 313
Sappey, subareolar lymph plexus of, 35
Sarcoma of long bones, sites of, 249
— osteogenic, (*Fig.* 555, 4) 583
— torus palatinus diagnosed as, 240
Sartorius muscle, postural activity of, 181
Scalenus anterior, 216
— — nerves to, 159, 161

Scalenus anterior syndrome, (*Fig.* 210) 226
— maximus muscle, plexuses on, (*Fig.* 146) 157
— medius, falciform process of tendon of insertion of, (*Fig.* 210) 227
— — nerves to, 159, 161
— posterior, nerve to, 161
Scalp, (*Figs.* 1, 2) 1–4
— dangerous area of, 3
— dermoids, (*Fig.* 415) 426
— layers of, (*Figs.* 1, 2) 1
— nerve-supply of, 138
— skin, relationship to epicranial aponeurosis, 654
— swelling due to escape of cerebrospinal fluid, 3
— wounds, danger of infection from, 297
Scaphoid, accessory, 231
Scapula, blood-supply of, (*Fig.* 228) 245
— development of, 248
— displacement of, in spinal accessory nerve lesion, 455
— movements of, 201, 202
— — by serratus anterior, 181
— winging of, 204
Scapular ligaments, transverse, 272
— notch, 272
Scar(s) hernia, 743
— painful, 763
Scarpa, fascia of, (*Figs.* 203–205) 218
— triangle, occlusion of femoral artery at apex of, 555
Scheuermann's disease, (*Fig.* 671) 715
Schmorl's nodes, (*Fig.* 671) 715
Schwalbe, hiatus of, (*Fig.* 95) 107
Sciatica, (*Figs.* 658–662) 702
— due to nuclear retropulsion, 712, 713, 714, 715
— — pressure on fifth lumbar nerve, 698, (*Fig.* 659) 704
— — — lumbar nerves, 127
— sensory or motor signs associated with, 703
Sciatic hernia, 692
— nerve, (*Fig.* 658) 703
— — compression by causes outside spine, (*Fig.* 658) 703, 707
— — — with referred pain, 702
— — great, injection of, (*Fig.* 740) 784
— — loss due to division of, (*Figs.* 446, 447) 464
— — relaxation, posture for, (*Fig.* 451) 468
— — suture, functional results of, in tibial and peroneal nerve lesions, 465
— neuralgia, reflex, 702

Sciatic neuritis, primary, 702
— neurodocitis, anatomical bases of, (*Figs.* 659–662) 704
Scissors gait due to bilateral coxa vara, 477
Scoliosis due to asymmetrical sacralization, 699
— — coxa vara, 477
— — disc prolapse, (*Fig.* 669) 712, 714
— — hemivertebra, (*Fig.* 651) 696
— — vertebral abnormality, 127
Scrotal arteries supplying testis, 411
— dimpling in torsion of testis, 415
— testis, 409
Scrotum, dartos muscle of, 219
— descent of testis into, 405
— muscle and fascia covering, 219, 220, 221
Sebaceous cyst, diagnosis from sequestration dermoid, 425
Second cranial nerve (*see* Optic Nerve)
Secondary diverticula of gut, (*Fig.* 430) 445
Segmental arteries of spinal cord in fetus, (*Figs.* 490, 491) 499
— nerve-supply of body, (*Fig.* 156) 167
— — rectus abdominis, (*Fig.* 699 B) 744
Segments of lungs, (*Fig.* 35) 42–45, 47
— — bronchi to, (*Fig.* 39) 48, 49
Sella turcica, 11
— — changes in, due to pituitary tumour, (*Fig.* 15) 16
— — removal of floor of, (*Fig.* 748) 790
Sellaris joint, (*Fig.* 244) 253
Semilunar bone (*see* Lunate Bone)
— cartilages (*see* Meniscus)
— ganglion, (*Figs.* 133–135) 141
— — alcohol injection into, (*Fig.* 738) 780, 781
— — dural relations of, (*Figs.* 134, 135) 142
— — removal of, taste loss after, 147
Semimembranosus, 205
— bursa, 264, 265
— ligaments of, (*Fig.* 275) 276
— tendon, (*Fig.* 257) 264, (*Fig.* 275) 276, 279
Seminal vesicles, rectal examination of, 585
Semispinalis capitis, (*Figs.* 180, 181) 192, 193
— group of muscles, 192, 193
Senile kyphosis, (*Fig.* 668 B) 711, 716
— osteoporosis of spine, (*Fig.* 672) 716
Sensory loss due to combined lesion of ulnar and median nerves, 457
— — — fifth nerve division, (*Fig.* 434) 450, 451
— nerve(s) from heart, 615
— — injury causing painful scar, 763
— — nucleus of vagus, (*Fig.* 581) 618

874 INDEX

Sentinel pile, 111, 113
Separation of epiphysis, 242
Septum transversum, 681
Sequestration dermoid(s), (*Figs.* 414–416) 424
— — of face, (*Fig.* 353) 359
Sequestrum, 584
Serratus anterior, 181, 201, 202
— — paralysis, test for, 181
— paralysis of, 204
— posterior, 217
Sesamoid bones, 230
— at finger joint, 569
— of foot, (*Figs.* 212, 216) 234
— fracture of, 235
— of rectus femoris, (*Fig.* 221) 237
Sesamum peronaeum, 231
Seventh cranial nerve (see Facial Nerve)
Sex, difficulty in determining, in perineoscrotal hypospadias, 420
— organs, male, effects of sympathectomy on, 647
Sexual efficiency, impaired, following sympathectomy above diaphragm, 648
Sherren's suggestion on draining kidney abscess, 761
Short long bones, infections of, 583
— muscles maintaining arch of foot, 295
Shotgun perineum, (*Fig.* 388) 396
Shoulder(s), abduction at, (*Figs.* 188, 189) 201, 681
— bursae around, 261, 265
— compression of supracapsular nerve at, 471
— dislocation of, 201
— — examination for ruptured supraspinatus in, 675
— — habitual or recurrent, 661
— — rupture of supraspinatus complicating, (*Fig.* 633 B) 673, 674, 675
— mobility, restriction of, by arm position, 571
— musculotendinous cuff of, (*Fig.* 630) 670, 671, (*Fig.* 633) 673
— optimum position for ankylosis of, (*Fig.* 480) 488
Shoulder-girdle, movement of, 202
— sagging, leading to brachial nerve compression, 227
Shoulder-hand syndrome, 571
Shoulder-joint abduction, position of forearms to maintain, (*Fig.* 545) 572
— bursae communicating with, 261
— capsule, exposure of, 804
— communicating with subdeltoid bursa, (*Fig.* 631) 671, (*Fig.* 634) 675
— consequences of defective drainage in, 571

Shoulder-joint, dislocations at (*Figs.* 618–620) 659
— — nerve lesions complicating, 661
— involved in rim rent, (*Fig.* 640) 680
— ligament accessory to, (*Fig.* 269) 272
— movement, (*Figs.* 188, 189) 201, 202
— puncture of, (*Fig.* 683) 733
— supraspinatus tendon lesions and, 678
— surgical approach to, (*Figs.* 760–762) 803
Shoulder-tip pain, 88
Shunt(s), left to right, in atrial septal defect, 507
— portal, (*Fig.* 513) 529
— resection of aortic aneurysm, using, (*Fig.* 537) 561
Sibson's fascia, (*Fig.* 184) 195
Sigmoid artery(ies), (*Fig.* 52) 72, 599, 600
— colon, diverticula of, 445
— sinus, 297
Sinus(es) bleeding, 297
— blood, of cranium, 297
— pocularis, enlargement of, 446
Sinusoids of liver, 526, 528
Sinu-vertebral nerve, 165
Situs inversus, 523, 543
Sixth cranial nerve, loss due to division of, 451
— — — palsy due to pituitary tumour, 16
Skene's ducts, 418
Skin of anal region, 110, 111
— breast, lymphatics of, (*Fig.* 28) 34
— — retraction of, due to cancer invading ligaments of Cooper, (*Fig.* 34) 40
— lymphatic watersheds of, (*Fig.* 340) 345
— oedema in peau d'orange, (*Fig.* 34 C) 41
— of scalp, (*Fig.* 1) 1
— segmental nerve supply of, (*Fig.* 157) 168
— tags at anus, 112
Skin-flaps in operations on breast, 32
Skoog's ganglion, (*Fig.* 605) 644
Skull, adamantinomata of, results of, 353
— bone, defective, causing encephalocele, 371
— dermoids of, (*Fig.* 415) 426
— development of vault of, and dermoids, (*Fig.* 415) 427
— fracture of base of, haemorrhage from, 5
— — sinus bleeding due to, 297
— — of vault of, in children, 3, 4
— — — haemorrhage from, in children, 5
— obstruction to cerebrospinal fluid in, (*Fig.* 6) 10
— ossification of, 247
— sutural joints of, (*Fig.* 235) 250

Skull, vault of, lacking regenerative power, 582
— veins of, (*Fig.* 298) 296
Sliding hernia (*see* Hiatal Hernia, Sliding)
— — of Allison, (*Figs.* 644–649) 685
Sling position of shoulder restricting shoulder mobility, 571
Slipping peroneus longus, 579
Small gut anastomosis, blood-supply and, (*Fig.* 51) 62
Smell sensations due to pituitary tumour, 16
Smithwick approach to denervation of heart, (*Fig.* 759) 801
— — in ganglionectomy, 617
— denervation of lower limb, (*Fig.* 603) 641
— — upper limb, (*Figs.* 597–599) 635
— transthoracic sympathectomy, bone removed in, (*Fig.* 750) 791
Smith-Petersen approach to hip-joint, (*Fig.* 767) 808
'Snapping' joints, 578
Sojius glands, 33
Soleus muscle, thrombosis in venous sinuses of, 318
— veins in, 312
Soleal venous sinuses, 312, 316
Solitary chondroma, (*Fig.* 555, 3) 583
— cyst of osteitis fibrosa, (*Fig.* 555, 5) 583
Somatic afferent and efferent fibres of vagus, (*Fig.* 583) 619
— pain fibres, 178
Spasm of oesophagus, diffuse, 493
Spastic paresis due to sagittal sinus injury, 298
Spermatic cord, 97, 98
— — incision giving access to, (*Fig.* 716 A) 758
— — relations in, (*Fig.* 341) 349
— — relationship to fasciae of Scarpa and Colles, (*Fig.* 204) 221
— — torsion of, 414
— fascia, external, 747
— — — and internal, 98, 99, 405
Spermatoceles, anatomical basis of, (*Fig.* 405) 416
Spence, axillary tail of, 30, 33, (*Fig.* 29) 35
Sphenoid bone, 11
Sphenoidal air sinus, descent of pituitary fossa into, due to tumour, (*Fig.* 15) 16
Sphenomandibular ligament, (*Fig.* 266) 270
Sphenopalatine foramen, 146
— ganglion, 141, (*Fig.* 137) 145
Sphenoparietal sinus, (*Figs.* 134, 135) 143
Sphincters, (*Figs.* 487–489) 490–499
— ani (*see* Anal Sphincters)

INDEX 875

Sphincters, ani externus, (*Fig.* 105) 115, 117, (*Fig.* 108) 119, 491
— — internus, (*Fig.* 105) 116, 117, (*Fig.* 108) 119, 491
— — re-orientation of, (*Fig.* 108) 119
— of gut, (*Fig.* 487) 490
— Oddi, (*Fig.* 489 A) 495
— oris, 490
— urethrae membranaceae, 199, 499
— of urinary tract, 499
— vesicae, 199, 499
— — pressure of prostatic adenoma on, 102
Sphincteric action of ileocaecal junction, 494
— control, preservation of, 118
Sphincterotomy, internal, 119
Spigelian hernia, 691
Spina bifida, 127, (*Figs.* 361–366) 368
— — anterior, (*Fig.* 366) 370, 424
— — defective fusion of vertebral arches causing, (*Fig.* 652) 697
— — occulta, (*Fig.* 365) 370
— — — at sacrum, 423
— — at sacrum, 423
Spinal accessory nerve (11th), 148, (*Fig.* 144) 153, 180, 618
— — — anastomosis of, to facial, 155
— — — injury to, 326
— — — joins vagus, 152, 153
— — — loss due to division of, 455
— anaesthesia, fall in blood pressure due to, 172
— artery(ies), anterior, enlarged, in coarctation of aorta, 522
— — desegmentation of, (*Fig.* 491) 499
— — segmentation of, in fetus, (*Fig.* 490) 499
— block, Queckenstedt's test for, 591
— column (*see* Vertebral Column)
— — compression by non-disc lesions in, causing sciatica, 703
— — development of, (*Fig.* 362) 368
— cord, 128
— — blood-supply of, (*Figs.* 490–495) 499
— — ciliospinal centre in, (*Fig.* 136) 144
— — collateral circulation of, 502, 503, 505, 506
— — compression causing low back pain, 695
— — development of, (*Figs.* 361, 362) 368
— — dural tube of, 6
— — injury or disease relation of most prominent vertebral spine in, 128
— — lesion between 4th cervical and 2nd thoracic segments, 140
— — pressure on, by dermoid, 427
— — limb enlargements of, (*Fig.* 161) 174

Spinal cord, reflex mechanism in, causing sciatica, 702
— — upper, incision giving access to, (*Fig.* 747) 789
— dura, 6
— localization, 128
— nerves, anterior rami of, 157, (*Fig.* 155) 165, 166
— — arrangement of, (*Fig.* 155) 165
— — compression by dural sheath causing neuralgia, 229
— — foramina for, 126
— — localization of function of, 455
— — loss due to division of, (*Figs.* 438–448) 455–467
— — mixed, 165, 174
— — posterior rami of, 165
— nerve-roots, anterior, accessory ganglia in, (*Fig.* 605) 645
— subarachnoid space, tapping of, 737
— tumour, Queckenstedt's test for, 591, 592
Spinalis group of muscles, (*Fig.* 179) 191, 192
Spine(s), cold abscesses of, (*Figs.* 677–679) 723
— extensors, paralysis of, 578
— fracture of, ileus complicating, 623
— lumbosacral region of, 693
— senile osteoporosis of, (*Fig.* 672) 716
— tuberculosis of (*see* Tuberculosis of Spine)
— of vertebrae, localization of spinal segments by, 128
Spinous processes, anomalies of, 695, 696
— — development of, 697
Splanchnic branches of sympathetic trunk, 175
— nerves, 92, 176, 623
— — excision of, (*Fig.* 588) 624
— — exposure of, 791
— — functions of, 623
Splanchnicectomy of White and Smithwick, (*Fig.* 588) 624
Splanchnicus ima nerves, 92
Spleen(s), accessory, 432
— cystic disease of, 398, 399
— enlarged, puncture of, (*Fig.* 695) 740
— incisions giving access to, (*Fig.* 709) 751, (*Figs.* 711, 712) 753, 754
— multiple accessory, in peritoneal cavity, 432
— palpation of, 590
Splenectomy rendered ineffective by accessory spleens, 432
— transthoracic route to, 792, 794
Splenic appendix, (*Fig.* 47) 59

Splenic artery, anastomosis of, to renal artery, 533 (*Fig.* 589 B) 625
— — occlusion of, collateral circulation in, 558
— enlargement due to portal obstruction, 529
— flexure, 380
— — blood-supply to, 599
— — resection for cancer of, (*Fig.* 571) 603
— rupture causing shoulder-tip pain, 89
— vein, 523
— — anastomosis of, to renal vein, (*Fig.* 513) 530
— — puncture for, 740
Splenius muscle, 193
Spondylitis, tuberculous, pus in psoas sheath in, 218
Spondylolisthesis, (*Figs.* 655–657) 700
— causes of, (*Fig.* 655) 700
— clinical features of, (*Figs.* 656, 657) 702
Spondylolytic spondylolisthesis, (*Fig.* 655 B) 700
Spondylosis deformans, (*Fig.* 668 A) 711, 716
— osteoarthritica, 715, 716
Spring ligament, 281, (*Fig.* 292) 291
— — attachments and relations of, (*Fig.* 293) 291
Spur(s), calcaneal, (*Fig.* 218) 231, 235
— from articular facet narrowing foramen, (*Fig.* 662) 707
— phalangeal, (*Fig.* 219) 231, 236
Stalked hydatid, 417
Stapedius, paralysis of, 453
Stellate ganglion, removal of, 613
Stenosing tenovaginitis, 259
Step cut incision, (*Fig.* 497 C) 510
Sterility following prostatectomy, 104
Sternebrae, 248
Sternoclavicular joint movement, 201, 202
Sternohyoid, 209
— nerve supplying, 160
Sternomastoid(s), 209
— cold abscess at posterior border of, 724
— fascial sheath of, (*Fig.* 192) 207
— nerve-supply of, (*Fig.* 144) 153, 159
— paralysis of, 455
— relations of jugular veins with, (*Fig.* 305) 302, 303
Sternothyroid, 209
— nerve supplying, 160
Sternum, bifid, associated with mediastinal dermoid, 428
— dermoid over, (*Fig.* 416) 427
— division of, in gaining access to heart, (*Fig.* 497) 510
— as landmark to deeper structures, 41

Sternum, ossification of, 248
— splitting of, in exposure of great vessels, (*Fig.* 535) 560
— swelling over centre of, 167
Sternum-splitting approach to superior mediastinum, (*Fig.* 749) 790
Sternum-splitting operation, (*Fig.* 701) 747
Sthenic type of bodily habitus, (*Figs.* 458, 459) 473
Stiff joints, optimum attitudes for, (*Figs.* 480–486) 487
Stiles's modification of McBurney's incision, 756
Stohr, gland of, 327, 330
Stomach, accessory pancreatic tissue in, 428
— blood-supply of, 61
— development of, 376
— incisions giving access to, 745, 754
— lesions, transthoracic route to, 792
— lymph drainage of, (*Fig.* 53) 64–66
— — territories of, (*Fig.* 53) 66
— mobilization of, (*Fig.* 754) 795
— sphincters of, (*Fig.* 487) 490, 493
Stomodeum of embryo, 355, 356
Straight sinus, 6
Strangulated femoral hernia, 101
— inguinal hernia, 98, 407
— pile, (*Figs.* 105, 106) 117
Strap-hanger's oedema, 305
Stretch strains on popliteal artery, 565
Stylohyoid ligament, ossification of, 29
— nerve to, 148
Styloids, radial and ulnar, determination of relative levels of, (*Fig.* 560) 593
Stylomandibular ligament, 208
Stylomastoid foramen, (*Fig.* 140) 148
— — lesion of facial nerve at, (*Fig.* 435) 453
Stylopharyngeus muscle, 149, 180
— nerve from glossopharyngeal nerve to, 148, (*Fig.* 142) 150
Subacromial bursa (*see* Subdeltoid Bursa)
Subaponeurotic space of scalp, 3
Subarachnoid space, 9
— — testing for increased pressure in, 591, 592
Subareolar lymph plexus of Sappey, 35
Subcaecal fossa, 67, (*Fig.* 60) 72
Subcardinal veins, (*Figs.* 518–520) 536, 540, (*Fig.* 524) 543
Subcervical glands of Albarran, 102
Subclavian, anastomosis of to pulmonary artery, (*Fig.* 496) 509
— aneurysm, 226, 564
— artery(ies), (*Fig.* 196) 212
— — aberrant right, (*Fig.* 501) 512, 515
— — compression by cervical rib, 225, 226

Subclavian artery(ies), development of, (*Figs.* 498–500) 512
— — exposure of, 564
— — fixation of, and scalene syndrome, 227
— — obstruction at origin of, effects of, 557
— — occlusion of third part of, collateral circulation in, 557
— — plexus to, (*Fig.* 145) 157
— — relation of brachial plexus to, 160
— — supplying radicals, 500, 503
— — groove of first rib, 225
— lymph trunk (*see also* Jugulo-subclavian Junction), (*Fig.* 339) 345
— steal syndrome, 557
— vein, (*Figs.* 302, 304) 301
— — damage to, in phrenic avulsion, 164
Subclavicular dislocation of humerus, 661
Subclavius muscle, (*Fig.* 267) 271
— — nerve to, (*Fig.* 152) 161, 163
— — — communication of, with phrenic nerve, (*Fig.* 154) 164
— relation of axillary vein to, (*Fig.* 307) 305
Subconjunctival haemorrhage diagnosed from 'flame-shaped' haemorrhage, 3
Subcoracoid dislocation of humerus, 661
Subcortical regions, incision giving access to, (*Fig.* 743) 787
Subcutaneous dermoid of skull, (*Fig.* 415 E) 426
— fat of child, 134
— (external) inguinal ring, 97, 406
— whitlow, 653
Subdeltoid bursa, 261
— — anatomy of, (*Figs.* 636, 637) 676
— — communicating with shoulder-joint, (*Fig.* 631) 671, (*Fig.* 634) 675
— — effects of lesions of supraspinatus tendon on, 678
— — examination of supraspinatus tendon through, 676
— — involvement of, in upper arm injuries, 678
— bursa test, 589
— bursitis, 679
Subdural haematoma, 298
— space, 7
Subglenoid dislocation of humerus, 661
Subgluteal bursae, (*Fig.* 255) 262
Sub-infraspinatus bursa, 261
Sublimis tendons, 285
— — sheath for, (*Fig.* 249) 256, (*Fig.* 287) 285
Sublingual artery, 195
— gland, 147, 194
Submammary pain, 687

Submaxillary ganglion, 141, (*Fig.* 139) 147
— gland, (*Fig.* 139) 147, 149
— lymph-glands, 194, (*Fig.* 325) 327
— — relationship with salivary gland, (*Fig.* 193) 207, 327
— salivary gland, 194, (*Fig.* 193) 207
— — — excision of, 208
— — — relation with lymph-glands, (*Fig.* 193) 207, 327
Submental lymph-glands, 194, (*Fig.* 325) 327, 328, (*Fig.* 328) 330
— triangle, 194, 327
Submucosal enterogenous cyst of gut, (*Fig.* 427 A) 441
Suboccipital decompression, 789
— exploration of skull, (*Fig.* 747) 789
Subperitoneal enterogenous cyst, (*Fig.* 427 C) 442
— lymph-plexus, secondaries from breast cancer in, 38
Subphrenic abscess, (*Figs.* 680, 681) 727
Subpleural structures, arterial supply to, 51
Subpsoas bursa, (*Fig.* 256) 263
Subpyloric lymph-glands, (*Fig.* 53) 64, 65
Subscapular bursa, 261
— nerves, 161
— vein, (*Fig.* 27) 33
Subscapularis tendon, (*Fig.* 630) 670
Subserous enterogenous cyst of gut, 441
Subspinous dislocation of humerus, 661
Substernal pain due to sliding hernia, 687
Subsuperior bronchus, 49
Subtaloid dislocation of foot, (*Fig.* 628) 669
Subtemporal decompression, 787
Subtrigonal glands, 102
Suctorial pad, 133
Sudek, 'critical point' of, (*Fig.* 52) 64
Superficial group of dislocated testis, (*Fig.* 404) 415
— inguinal dislocation of testis, (*Fig.* 404) 416
— — ectopia testis, 411
— — hernia, (*Fig.* 399) 408
Superior extensor retinaculum of foot, 288
— ganglion on glossopharyngeal nerve, 149
— inversion of testis, (*Fig.* 403 B) 414
Supernumerary bronchus, 49
Suppurative pneumonitis, sites of, 49
Supracardinal veins (lateral sympathetic line veins), (*Figs.* 518–520) 536, 538, 540, (*Fig.* 544) 543
Supraclavicular lymph-glands, 34
— nerves, 137, (*Figs.* 131, 132) 139
— — descending, (*Fig.* 148) 158, 164, 166, 209
Supracondylar fracture of humerus, 487

Supradiaphragmatic vagotomy, (*Fig.* 757) 798
Supraduodenal artery of Wilkie, (*Fig.* 50) 61
Supralevator fistula due to pelvirectal abscess, (*Fig.* 115) 123
Supramalleolar amputation, (*Fig.* 729) 773
Supramandibular glands, 327
Supra-omohyoid gland, (*Figs.* 327, 328) 329
Supra-orbital nerve, (*Fig.* 129) 136, 138
— — injection of, 782
Suprapatellar bursa, (*Fig.* 258) 264
— pouch, puncture of, (*Fig.* 687) 734
— — separation of, in exposing femur, 818
Suprapleural membrane, (*Fig.* 183) 195
Suprapubic prostatectomy, 104
Suprarenal anomalies of inferior vena cava, (*Fig.* 522) 540
Suprascapular nerve, (*Fig.* 152) 161, 163, 201, 672
— — compression of, at shoulder, 471
Suprasellar region, incision giving access to, (*Fig.* 745) 788
Supraspinous fossa, 670, 671
Supraspinatus, 201
— anatomy of, (*Figs.* 629–631) 670
— function of, 672
— lesions, (*Figs.* 629–635) 670–676
— nerve-supply of, 672
— rim rent of, (*Fig.* 640) 680
— rupture of, (*Figs.* 631, 633, 634) 671, 672
— — examination for, (*Figs.* 634, 635) 675
— sprain of tendon of exertion of, 590
— tendinitis of, 678
— tendon, (*Figs.* 630, 631) 670
— — calcification in, (*Fig.* 638) 678
— — effects of lesions of, on subdeltoid bursa, (*Fig.* 638) 678
— — degeneration of, with age, 673, 678
— — examination for point of tenderness in insertion of, (*Fig.* 635) 675
— — exploration of insertion of, 676
— — relationship of shoulder-joint and subdeltoid bursa to, (*Fig.* 636) 676
— wasting of, (*Fig.* 632) 672, 675
Suprasternal space, 209, 302
Suprategmental space, (*Fig.* 95) 107
Supratonsillar recess, 27
Supratrochlear lymph-gland, 339
— nerve, (*Fig.* 129) 136, 138
Supra-umbilical incision, 745, 754
— median incision converted to right angled incision, (*Fig.* 711) 753
Sural nerve, large, relation to short saphenous vein, 310, 311
Surgery, neurological complications of, 499, 500, (*Figs.* 493–495) 503

Surgery, vascular pattern in relation to, (*Figs.* 490–545) 499–572
Surgical approach, anatomy of, (*Figs.* 743–799) 786 786–819
— procedures, anatomy of, (*Figs.* 683–742) 733–786
Suspensory ligament of duodenum, 56
Sutura harmonia, (*Fig.* 235 C) 251
— serrata, (*Fig.* 235 A) 251
— squamosa, (*Fig.* 235 B) 251
Sutural joints, (*Fig.* 235) 250
— membrane, 4
Suture(s), (*Fig.* 235) 250
— lines of scalp, 4
Swallowing, mechanism of, 491
Sweating, excessive, following sympathetic denervation, 647
Swenson's operation in Hirschsprung's disease, (*Fig.* 593) 630
Sylvian system, 298
Syme's amputation, 770, 772
Sympathectomy for essential hypertension, (*Fig.* 588) 624
— nerve sprouting after, (*Fig.* 606) 646
— periarterial, (*Fig.* 594) 631
— physiological derangements following, 647
— results of, on male sex organs, 648
— transthoracic, (*Fig.* 750) 791
Symphysis absent in extroversion of bladder, (*Fig.* 411) 420
Sympathetic activity, vasoconstrictor, causing Raynaud's spasm, 644
— cardiac denervation, 799
— denervation of limbs, (*Figs.* 595–606) 633–648
— — — failure of, 642
— — — prevention of regeneration after, (*Fig.* 604) 643
— fibres to brachial plexus, 164
— — dilator pupillae of iris, (*Fig.* 577) 611
— — innervation of anal region, (*Fig.* 99) 110
— — bladder and colon, (*Figs.* 590–592) 625, 628, 629
— involvement in injury, 570
Sympathetic line veins, (*Figs.* 518–520) 536, 538, 540, (*Fig.* 524) 543
— nerves, functions of, in male sex organs, 647
— — to gut, irritation of, 623
— — iris, (*Fig.* 136) 144
— — supply to abdominal viscera, 623
— — — heart, (*Fig.* 579) 615
— nervous system, (*Fig.* 161) 174
— — — anatomy governing surgery of, (*Figs.* 577–608) 610–651
— — — functions of, (*Fig.* 160) 170
— — — origin of, (*Fig.* 162) 174

Sympathetic, operations on, prognosis in, (*Figs.* 604–606) 642
— pathways, alternative, (*Fig.* 605) 644
— plexuses, (*Fig.* 164) 176
— root to ciliary ganglion, 145
— surgery, preoperative tests of benefit of, 610
Sympathetico-parasympathetic imbalance of gut, 623
Symphysis menti, dermoid behind, 428
— pubis, (*Fig.* 238) 251
Synapses of autonomic system, 172
Synchondrosis, (*Fig.* 237) 251
Syndactylism, (*Fig.* 413) 424
Syndesmoses, (*Fig.* 236) 251
Synostosis, 250
Synovial cells, 730
— fluid, 252, 729
— joints, (*Figs.* 239–245) 252
— membrane, 252, 729
— reflection, 731
— sheath(s) of biceps, 261, 262
— — flexors of hand, (*Fig.* 615) 657
— — hand, (*Figs.* 249, 250) 256
— villi, 730
Syphilis of bone, 583, 584
Syringomyelocele, (*Fig.* 364 C) 369
Systemic-portal communications, (*Fig.* 100) 111, 197, (*Figs.* 319–321) 321

Tachycardia due to bilateral vagus nerve lesion, 454
— neurectomy for, (*Fig.* 758 A) 799
Taeniae coli, 57
Tail(s) of Lockwood, 406
— persistence of embryonic, 422
Tailor's ankle, 265
Talipes equinovarus, 206
— — congenital, 291, 484
Talocalcaneonavicular joint, 291
Talofibular ligament, anterior, (*Figs.* 283, 284) 281, 282
— — posterior, (*Figs.* 283, 284) 281, 282
Talonavicular capsule, (*Fig.* 293) 291
Talus, (*Fig.* 225 B) 242
— accessory, (*Fig.* 214) 232
— descent of, in flat-foot, 291, 293
— lateral tubercle of, 242
— process from middle of upper surface of, 231
— trochlear process of talus, (*Fig.* 217) 235
Tarsal bones, attachment of tibialis posterior tendon to, (*Fig.* 296) 293
— tunnel syndrome, 471
Tarsalia, (*Fig.* 225 A) 242
Tarsometatarsal joints, amputation at, 772
— — of great toe, 253
Tarsus, homologies of, (*Fig.* 225) 241, 242

880 INDEX

Taste fibres paralysed in facial nerve lesion, 453
— nerve of, 141, 147
— pathways for, 147, 151
Taussig-Blalock shunt, (*Fig.* 496) 508, 509
Teeth, (*Figs.* 545–550) 572
— of child, 133
— constituent parts of, (*Fig.* 546) 572
— development of, (*Fig.* 546) 572
— extraction, osteomyelitis of jaw in relation to, 575
— socket, (*Fig.* 547) 574
Tegmentum, (*Fig.* 95) 107
Tela choroideae of ventricles, 8
Telford's denervation of upper limb, (*Fig.* 597) 635
Temporal bone, cartilage between squamous and petrous parts of, in child, (*Fig.* 124) 131
— fascia, 4
— lobe, incisions giving access to, (*Figs.* 743, 744) 787
— — pressure on, by pituitary tumour, 16
— muscle, 4
— nerve, 138
— region of scalp, layers of, 4
Temporofacial nerve, (*Fig.* 140) 148
Temporomandibular joint, (*Fig.* 247) 255
— — accessory ligament of, (*Fig.* 266) 270
— — snapping, 579
Tendinitis of supraspinatus, 678
Tendo Achillis, rupture of, 546
— — sheath for, (*Fig.* 252) 260
Tendon(s), blood-supply of, (*Fig.* 525) 545
— function, restricted, in causalgia, 571
— graft, blood-supply to, from adhesions, 546
— rupture of, 546
— supporting arches of foot, (*Figs.* 295, 296) 293
Tendon-sheath(s), (*Figs.* 248–253) 256–260
— and bursae, (*Figs.* 248–258) 255–266
— of finger, incision of infected, 766
Tenosynovitis of little finger, 256, 257, 258
Tenovaginitis, stenosing, 259
Tension gangrene of caecum, 494
Tensor palati muscle, 146, 150
— tympani, 146
Tenth cranial nerve (*see* Vagus Nerve)
Tentorium cerebelli, 6, 789
— — blockage at opening of, 10
Teratoma of sacrum, 423
— tridermal, of mediastinum, 428
Teres minor tendon, (*Fig.* 630) 670
Terminal ganglia, autonomic, 172, 175, 177
— phalanx, result of infection in, 654
Testicular artery, anastomoses of, (*Fig.* 401) 410

Testicular artery, ligature of, 411
Testis, blood-supply to, (*Fig.* 401) 410
— 'bringing down', practicability of, 409
— concealment of, malignant potential of, 412
— congenital abnormalities of, (*Figs.* 398–404) 405–416
— descent of, 96, 405
— — chronology of, 406
— development of, 405
— — faulty, abnormalities resulting from, (*Figs.* 398–403) 407
— dislocation of, 407, (*Fig.* 404) 415
— duplication of, with single epididymis and vas, (*Fig.* 402) 412
— encysted hydrocele of, 416
— imperfect descent of, 412
— — fixation of, leading to torsion, 414, 415
— incision giving access to, (*Fig.* 716 A) 758
— incomplete descent of, (*Fig.* 401) 409
— — — hernia associated with, 408
— inversion of, (*Fig.* 403) 413
— normal position of, (*Fig.* 403 A) 413
— torsion of, 412, 414
— — in polyorchidism, 412
— undescended, 406
Tests, anatomical bases of clinical (*Figs.* 556–565) 587–597
Tetralogy of Fallot (*see* Fallot, Tetralogy of)
Thecal whitlow, 654
— — of thumb or little finger, incisions for, (*Figs.* 723–725) 767
Thenar eminence, fascia of, 213
— space, (*Figs.* 612–614) 655, 656
— — incisions giving access to, (*Fig.* 726) 767
Thigh amputation, 770, 771
— cold abscess in, 727
— compression of saphenous nerve in, 471
— leg prosthesis, 775
— lymph-glands at root of, (*Fig.* 335) 340
— place of fifth lumbar nerve in innervation of, 706
— venous system of, (*Fig.* 311) 307, 316
— cranial nerve, (*see* Oculomotor Nerve)
— nerve palsy due to pituitary tumour, 16
— ventricle, pituitary gland and, (*Fig.* 7) 11
— — pressure on, by pituitary tumour, 16
— — tela choroidea of, 8
Thomas's hip flexion test, 589
Thomson's ligament, 97
Thomson-Walker's incision for exposing terminal ureter and bladder, 761

INDEX 881

Thoracic aortic aneurysm, exposure of and resection of, (*Fig.* 537) 561
— approach to hiatus hernia, 688, (*Fig.* 649) 690
— artery, lateral, 31
— cage, unequal rib growth causing prominence in, 42
— cardiac nerves, (*Fig.* 579) 615
— cord, ischaemic lesions of, 500, 503, 504
— curve of vertebral column, (*Fig.* 116) 123, 134
— duct, (*Figs.* 336–339) 341, 609
— — anomalies of, (*Fig.* 338) 343
— — course of, (*Fig.* 337) 342
— — injury to, effects of, 609
— — ligation of, 609
— — lymph trunk entering, 329
— — passage of, through diaphragm, (*Fig.* 184) 197
— — relationship of, with oesophagus, 795
— — tributaries of, 343
— ganglia, 176
— nerve(s) twelfth, lateral cutaneous branch of, division of, 761
— — anatomy of, (*Fig.* 155) 166
— — anterior rami to, 164, (*Fig.* 155) 166
— — cold abscess following course of, (*Fig.* 679) 725, 726
— — first, in brachial plexus, 160, 161, 166
— — — and cervical eighth, combined lesion of, 457
— — — rib, (*Fig.* 153) 163
— — lesion of, 458
— — medial and lateral anterior, 161
— — in neck, (*Fig.* 150) 160, 161, (*Fig.* 153) 164
— — second, 139
— — supplying kidney, 92
— — trunk, 164, 165
— — twelfth, 216
— posterior nerve-roots, section of upper five, (*Fig.* 580) 616
— respiration, 133
— spine, cold abscesses of, (*Figs.* 678, 679) 724
— sympathetic ganglia, removal of upper, for tachycardia and cardiac pain, (*Fig.* 758) 799, 800
— — upper, alcohol injection of, 617
— transverse processes, 127
— vein, lateral, (*Fig.* 27) 33, (*Fig.* 308) 306
Thoraco-abdominal exposure of right lobe of liver, 527
Thoracodorsal nerve, 161
Thoracolumbar outflow (*see* Sympathetic Nervous System)

Thoraco-epigastric vein, (*Fig.* 308) 306, 320
Thoracotomy, protection of nerves during, 764
Thorax of child, (*Fig.* 126) 133
— dermoids of, (*Fig.* 416) 427
— diaphragms of, (*Figs.* 183, 184) 195
— exposure of, (*Fig.* 497) 509
— lymph-glands of, (*Fig.* 334) 335
— sympathetic plexuses in, 176
— upper, nerve supply of skin of, 139
Thrombo-endarterectomy, 564
— exposure of popliteal for, (*Fig.* 541) 566
Thrombophlebitis causing reflex vasoconstriction, 611
— of haemorrhoidal vein, 112
Thrombosis of axillary vein, primary, (*Fig.* 307) 305
— secondary, due to popliteal artery entrapment, 447
— of veins of lower limb, (*Figs.* 317, 318) 318
Thrombotic pile, 112
Through-thigh amputation, 775
— — weight bearing in, 770
Thumb amputation, 779
— small muscles of, (*Figs.* 168–170) 182, 189
— tendon-sheath of, (*Fig.* 249) 257, 258, 259
— thecal whitlow of, incision for, (*Figs.* 723, 724) 767
Thumb-joint, 253
Thymus gland, 134
— — approach to, (*Fig.* 749) 791
Thyrohyoid arch, 361
— membrane, 152
— muscle, nerve to, 155, (*Fig.* 149) 158, 159
— nerve, 155
Thyroid artery(ies), accessory, 19
— — inferior, (*Figs.* 16, 17) 17
— — — plexus to, (*Fig.* 145) 157
— — superior, (*Figs.* 16, 17) 17
— cartilage, (*Fig.* 359) 366
— gland, (*Figs.* 16–22) 17–25
— — absence of lobe of, 367
— — accessory or ectopic, 367
— — anomalies, 367
— — blood-vessels of, (*Figs.* 16, 17) 17, 19
— — capsules of, (*Figs.* 20, 21) 23
— — connexion of thymus to, 134, 135
— — developmental errors of, (*Figs.* 359, 360) 365
— — fascial sheath of, 209
— — lingual, 367
— — lymphatics of, (*Fig.* 22) 24
— — nerves related to, (*Figs.* 18, 19) 19

Thyroid isthmus, 17
— scanning, 367
— tissue, accessory, 428
— — ectopic, 24, 367
— vein, fourth, 19
— — inferior, (*Fig.* 17) 19
— — middle, (*Fig.* 17) 19
— — superior, (*Fig.* 17) 19
Thyroidea ima artery, 19
Thyroidectomy, avoidance of parathyroids in, 26
— removal of true capsule with thyroid in, 23, 24
— vulnerability of nerves to injury in, 20, 22
Thyroglossal cysts, (*Fig.* 360) 366
— duct, (*Fig.* 359) 365
— — anomalies of, (*Fig.* 360) 366
— — carcinoma of, 367
— fistulae, 367
Thyrothymic ligament, 134
Tibia, curved, causing bow-leg, 480
— displacement of, on femur, 667
— epiphyseal line and capsular reflections of, (*Fig.* 264) 269
— exposure of, 818
— measuring length of, (*Fig.* 564) 596
— ossification of, 249
— relations of upper surface of, 348
— rotation of, in club-foot, 484
— sarcoma of upper end of, 249
Tibial artery(ies), anterior, occlusion of, (*Fig.* 533) 555
— — anterior and posterior, 565
— — collateral ligament, (*Figs.* 276, 279, 280) 277, 279, 668
— lymph-gland, anterior, 340
— nerve, anterior and posterior, compression of, at ankle, 471
— — loss due to division of, 465
— — nutrient arteries of, 465
— — relaxation, posture for, (*Fig.* 451) 468
— tuberosity, attachment of patellar tendon to, 276
— vein, 312
— — anterior, (*Fig.* 309) 307
— — posterior, (*Figs.* 309, 313) 312, 316
Tibiale, (*Fig.* 225 A) 241, 242
Tibialis anterior, 205, 283, 288
— — tendon-sheath of, (*Fig.* 251) 259
— posterior, 205, (*Figs.* 281, 282) 281, 283, 289, 291
— — relationship of os tibiale externum to, 231
— — tendon supporting arch of foot, (*Fig.* 296) 293
Tibiofibular mortice, (*Fig.* 628) 669, 670

Tibiofibular syndesmosis, (*Fig.* 236) 251
Tilting table prosthesis, 775
Tissue dislocation, (*Figs.* 417, 418) 428
Toe(s), amputations of, 772
— fifth, small muscles of, 189
— great, deviation of, in hallux valgus, (*Fig.* 473) 482
— — retention of, in amputation, 772
— — sesamoids of, (*Fig.* 216) 234, 235
— — small muscles of, 189
Tongue (*see also* Lingual)
— anaesthesia due to glossopharyngeal nerve lesion, 454
— cancer, metastases from, 195, 332
— — removal of lymph-glands in, 327, 331
— lymph drainage of, 195, 327, 329, (*Figs.* 328–330) 330
— main lymph-gland of, (*Figs.* 327, 328) 329, 330
— nerve-supply to, 154
— paralysis of, due to hypoglossal nerve lesion, 455
— taste sensations from, 147, 151
— veins of, (*Fig.* 301) 300
Tonsil, (*Figs.* 23, 24) 26–30, (*Fig.* 324) 325
— blood-supply of, (*Fig.* 23) 27
— lymphatics of, 28
— main lymph-gland of, 325, (*Fig.* 327) 329
— nerves of, 28
— pharyngeal (*see* Adenoids)
— special features of practical importance, (*Fig.* 24) 28–30
Tonsillar arteries, (*Fig.* 23) 27
— fossa, 26
— — bleeding from, after removal of tonsil, (*Fig.* 24) 29
— gland, 28, 299
— nerves, (*Fig.* 142) 151
Tonsillectomy, prevention of haemorrhage after, (*Fig.* 24) 29
Torcular Herophili, 298
Torkildsen's operation for hydrocephalus, 10
Torsion of testis, 414
Torus palatinus, (*Fig.* 221) 240
Tourniquet test, (*Fig.* 316) 316
Trachea, bifurcation of, landmark to, 41
— development of, (*Fig.* 369) 374
— — and structure of, 437, 438
— diverticula of, 437, 438
— and oesophagus, developmental anomalies of, (*Figs.* 423, 424) 437
— vascular ring encircling, (*Figs.* 504, 505) 518
Tracheal compression by innominate or left common carotid artery, 519

INDEX 883

Trachealis muscle, 439
Tracheobronchial fistula, posterior approach to, 802
Tracheoceles, 437, 438
Tracheo-oesophageal fistulae, (*Fig.* 370) 374, (*Figs.* 423 D, 424 B) 437
Traction diverticulum of oesophagus, (*Fig.* 425) 437
Tractus arteriosus anterior, (*Figs.* 491, 492, 494, 495) 502, 503, 506
— solitarius, (*Figs.* 581–583) 619
Tragus, swelling in front of, 326
Transplantation, relaxation of nerves by, 467, 468
Transthoracic procedures, posterior, 798
Transverse arches of foot, 292, 293
— carpal ligament, (*Fig.* 250) 257, (*Fig.* 613) 655, 657, 658
— colic sphincter, 491
— heart, 472
— incision dividing both recti, 754
— (lateral) sinus, 6
— ligament(s) of cervix, 223, (*Fig.* 674) 717, 718, 719
— — deep, of palm, (*Fig.* 543) 569
— — of knee-joint, (*Fig.* 277) 279
— — pubis, 200
— lumbosacral joint, 127
— mesocolon, (*Fig.* 48) 60
— metatarsal ligament, 292
— process(es) of 5th lumbar vertebra, anomalies of, (*Figs.* 653, 654) 695, 697
— — spine, 127
— scapular ligaments, 272
— sinus, (*Fig.* 302) 300
Transdiaphragmatic approach to upper abdomen, (*Fig.* 751) 792
Transfrontal approach to brain, (*Fig.* 745) 788, 790
Transillumination of colic arteries, 602
Transmetatarsal amputation, (*Fig.* 731) 775
Transrectal incision, inferior, 754
— — middle, (*Figs.* 711, 712) 753
— — superior, (*Figs.* 709, 710) 751
Trans-sphenoidal operation, (*Fig.* 748) 790
Transthoracic approach(es), (*Figs.* 749–759) 790–803
— — lateral, (*Figs.* 750, 751) 791
— route to upper abdomen, (*Fig.* 751) 792
— sympathectomy, (*Fig.* 750) 791
Transtrochanteric amputation, 775
Transversus abdominis, 97, 98, 405, (*Fig.* 399) 408
— — aponeurosis of origin of, (*Figs.* 200, 201) 216
— — division of, 564, 565

Transversus abdominis, nerve-supply of, 167
— spinalis, 261
— — group of muscles, (*Fig.* 177) 189, 192
Trapezius, 201, 202
— fascial sheath of, (*Fig.* 192) 207
— nerve-supply of, 153, 159
— paralysis of, 204, 455
Trapezoid ligament, (*Fig.* 268) 271
Traumatic cause of dislocation of testis, 415
— cephalhydrocele, 3, 4
— disease of cartilage bone, 582
— dislocation of patella, 667
— spondylolisthesis, (*Fig.* 655 B) 700
Treitz, ligament of, 56
Trendelenburg operation for varicose veins, (*Fig.* 312) 308, 310, 317, 588
— test for congenital hip dislocation, (*Fig.* 556) 588
— — varicose veins, 587
Treves, bloodless fold of, 71
Triangular ligament, (*Fig.* 186) 199, 222
— — bile-duct remnants in, 85
Triceps insertion, bursae in relation to, (*Fig.* 254) 262
— loose bone in tendon on, 238
Tridermal teratoma of mediastinum, 428
Trigeminal artery, 552
— nerve (*see* Fifth Cranial Nerve)
— neuralgia, alcohol injection for, (*Figs.* 736–738) 780
Trigger finger, 259, 579
Tripartite patella, (*Fig.* 220) 238
Triquetrum, (*Fig.* 224 B) 241
— bipartite, (*Fig.* 220) 236
Trochanter(s), great, relative heights of upper borders of, (*Figs.* 562, 563) 594
— raising of, in coxa vara, 477
Trochlear nerve (4th), loss due to division of, 450
— process of talus, (*Fig.* 217) 231, 235
Trochoid joint, (*Fig.* 242) 253
Trophic changes in hand due to median nerve lesion, 461
— ulcers in foot due to sciatic nerve lesion, 465
Truncal vagotomy, 621
Truncus arteriosus, 515
Trunk, cutaneous nerves to, (*Figs.* 155–158) 164–170
Tuberculosis of adenoid glands, 326
— salivary gland, 208
— spine, cold abscesses in, 124, 723
— — Hibbs's operation for, 126
— vertebra, 583
Tuberculous kyphosis, localization of, 128

884 INDEX

Tuberculous osteomyelitis affecting membrane bone, 582
— spondylitis, pus in psoas sheath in, 218
Tuberosity of humerus, degenerative changes spreading from supraspinatus to, (*Fig.* 639) 680
Tubules, failure of fusion of, (*Fig.* 389) 397
Tumours in fusion lines of face, (*Fig.* 353) 359
Tunica media of arteries to muscles, 561
— vaginalis testis, 97, 407
— — — fluid in, 408
— — — incision giving access to, (*Fig.* 716 A) 758
— — — puncture of, 743
Tuning-fork of larynx, 153
Twelfth cranial nerve (*see* Hypoglossal Nerve)
Tympanic antrum in child, 130
— branch of glossopharyngeal nerve, (*Fig.* 141) 149
— membrane, nerve-supply of, 138
— plexus, (*Fig.* 141) 149
Typhoid fever, Peyer's patches in, 335

'Ulcer bearing area' of leg, 316
Ullman's sign, (*Fig.* 656 C) 701
Ulna, epiphyseal line and capsular reflections of, (*Fig.* 261) 267
— exposure of, 817
— failure of fusion of upper epiphysis of, 238
— measuring length of, (*Fig.* 559) 593
— ossification of, 249
Ulnar bursa, (*Figs.* 249, 250) 256, (*Fig.* 287) 285, 657
— — infection in, incision for, (*Figs.* 723, 724) 767
— claw-hand, (*Fig.* 442) 461
— collateral ligament, (*Figs.* 270, 272) 273, 274
— and median nerves, combined lesion of, 457
— nerve, (*Fig.* 151) 161, 162, 186, 187
— — combined lesions of median and, (*Fig.* 444) 462
— — compression at wrist and elbow, 470
— — loss due to division of, (*Figs.* 442, 443) 461
— — relaxation, posture for, 468
— — transplantation, (*Fig.* 453) 469
Ulnare, (*Fig.* 224 A) 240, 241
Umbilical concretions or stones, 54
— cord, hernia of, 52
— — midgut loop in, (*Figs.* 371, 372) 376, 377, 379, 380
— — — — after birth, 383
— hernia, 52

Umbilical hernia, acquired, (*Fig.* 42) 53
— — of adults, (*Fig.* 42) 53
— — children, 52
— — diagnosis of exomphalos from, 383
— — physiological, (*Figs.* 371, 372, 374) 376, 377, 383
— region, intercostal nerve supplying, 167
— ring, lax, causing non-rotation of midgut loop, 381
— tumour, raspberry-red, 52, 392
— vein, fibrotic process taking place in, at birth, 529
— — left, pressure from, on midgut loop, (*Fig.* 372) 377
— — remains of, at umbilicus, (*Fig.* 41) 53
Umbilicus, (*Figs.* 41, 42) 52-55
— acquired abnormalities at, (*Fig.* 42) 53
— congenital abnormalities at, 52
— cyst at, 52, (*Fig.* 383 G) 390
— discharges at, 54
— imperfect, in extroversion of bladder, (*Fig.* 410) 420
— level of, 52
— new growths at, 54
— pilonidal sinus at, 423
— portal-systemic anastomoses around, (*Figs.* 319-321) 321
— spread of cancer at, 346
— veins around, in portal obstruction, 529
— weeping, 53
'Umbrella ring', 115, 116
Uncinate fits due to pituitary tumour, 16
Undescended testis, 406
Upper arm type of birth palsy, 456
— extremity, lymphatic drainage of, 338
— limb amputations, (*Figs.* 732-735) 776
— — defective drainage in, problems of, 567
— — disarticulation at joints of, 779
— — extensor nerves of, 457
— — measuring girth of, (*Fig.* 565 A) 597
— — — long bones of, (*Figs.* 557-560) 592
— — medial cutaneous nerve to, (*Fig.* 151) 161, 162
— — nerve-supply of, 157
— — neuralgia, ganglionectomy for, 634
— — pumping mechanism of, 570
— — rotation to prevent fixation at shoulder, 681
— — sympathetic denervation of, (*Figs.* 595-599) 633
— — union of epiphyses in, 248
— — veins of, (*Figs.* 306, 307) 303
— — whole brachial plexus palsy of, 458
Urachus, abnormalities of, (*Fig.* 396) 402
— congenital abnormalities of, 397

INDEX 885

Urachus, cysts of, (*Fig.* 396 C) 403
— patent, 52, (*Fig.* 396 B) 403
— persistence of connexion between bladder and, 52, (*Fig.* 396 B) 403
Ureter(s), abnormalities of, (*Fig.* 394) 400
— bifurcation of, (*Fig.* 394) 400
— blood-supply of, (*Fig.* 517) 534
— congenital abnormalities of, 397, (*Fig.* 394) 400
— — narrowing of, (*Fig.* 397) 403, 404
— development of, (*Fig.* 389) 397
— ectopic, 401
— incisions giving access to, (*Fig.* 716 B) 760, 761, 762
— junction of renal pelvis with, 499
— left, surgeon's guide to, 60 (*Fig.* 61) 72
— position of, in horseshoe kidney, (*Fig.* 391) 399
— retrocaval, (*Fig.* 524) 543
— right and right ovarian vein, association of, 536
— vaginal examination of, 586
Ureteric incisions, 745
— — horizontal, 764
Uretero-intestinal anastomosis, division of ureter in, 536
Urethra, abnormal development of, in hypospadias, (*Figs.* 408, 409) 419
— anterior, diverticula of, (*Fig.* 431) 447
— congenital valves in, (*Fig.* 397) 403, 404
— fascial sheath of female, 223
— forming gutter in epispadias, 422
— membranous, diverticula of, (*Fig.* 431) 446
— prolapse of female, 721
— prostatic, diverticula of, (*Fig.* 431) 446
— — prominence in floor of, (*Fig.* 91) 102
— — removal of, with prostate, 104
— vaginal examination of, 586
Urethral diverticula, (*Fig.* 431) 446
— meatus, internal, obstruction at, (*Fig.* 397) 403
Urinary bladder, puncture of, (*Fig.* 696) 740
— obstruction causing diverticula of bladder, 446
— organs, congenital abnormalities of, (*Figs.* 389–397) 397–405
— outflow, congenital obstruction of, 397
— tract, sphincters of, 499
Urine, congenital causes of obstruction to, (*Fig.* 397) 403
— desire to pass, due to prostatic enlargement, 103
— discharged at umbilicus, 52, 403
Urogenital diaphragm, (*Figs.* 92–94) 103, (*Figs.* 186, 187) 199, 718
— — fusion of Colles fascia with, 221

Urogenital diaphragm, inferior fascia of, 222
— — superior layer of, 222
— fasciae, (*Fig.* 186) 199
Urorectal septum, 392, (*Figs.* 387, 388) 395, 396
Uterine arteries, fibrous sheaths of, 719
— tube (*see* Fallopian tube)
Uterosacral ligaments, (*Fig.* 673) 717, 718
Uterus, change in position of, causes of, 719
— — — facilitating prolapse, (*Fig.* 675) 719, 720
— ligaments of, (*Figs.* 673, 674) 717
— retroversion of, facilitating prolapse, (*Fig.* 675) 719, 720
— supports of, 718
— typical position of, 719
— and vagina, prolapse of, (*Figs.* 673–675) 717
Utriculus prostaticus, enlargement of, 446
Uvula, bifid, 359
— vesicae, 102

Vagina, fascial sheath of, 223
— nerve-supply of, 784
— palpation of kidney per, 400
— prolapse of uterus on, (*Figs.* 673–675) 717
Vaginal arteries, fibrous sheaths of, 719
— examination (P.V.), information gained by, 586
— — of rectum, 586
— hydrocele, (*Fig.* 400 A) 408
— inguinal hernia, (*Fig.* 398 A) 407
— prolapse preceding uterine prolapse, 721
— wall, cysts of, 418
— — prolapse of anterior, 720
— — — posterior, 720
Vagotomy, 611
— parietal cell, 621
— selective, 621
— super-selective, 621
— supradiaphragmatic, (*Fig.* 757) 798
— truncal, 621
Vagus(i), abdominal course of, (*Figs.* 585, 586) 620
— anatomical arrangement of, over lower oesophagus (*Fig.* 737) 798
— nerve (10th) 148, 149, (*Fig.* 143) 151–153, 179, 209, (*Figs.* 581–586) 618
— — auricular branch of, (*Fig.* 130) 137, 138, 139, 149, 151, 454
— — autonomic fibres in, 175
— — changes in, in achalasia of oesophagus, 492
— — contribution to carotid sinus plexus, (*Fig.* 578) 614

886 INDEX

Vagus(i) nerve, functions of, 621
— — loss due to division of, (*Fig.* 437) 454
— — passage of, through diaphragm, (*Fig.* 184) 197, 620
— — supplying oesophagus, 492
— parasympathetic efferent and afferent fibres of, (*Fig.* 582) 618
— — supply to heart via, 615
— pharyngeal branch of, 180
— recurrent branch of (*see* Laryngeal Nerve, Recurrent)
Valve(s) of Gerlach, 490
— lymphatic channels, 341
— in thoraco-epigastric vein, 306
— venous, 321
Valvular heart abnormalities, congenital, 523
— obstructions in urethra, (*Fig.* 397) 403, 404
— type of pulmonary stenosis, 507
Varicose saphenous veins, (*Fig.* 312) 309, 311, 313, 315
— ulcers, genesis of, 313
— veins, accessory saphenous, 308
— — genesis of, 313
— — oesophageal, 197, 321
— — tourniquet test for, (*Fig.* 316) 316
— — Trendelenburg operation for, (*Fig.* 312) 308, 310, 317
— — — test for, 587
— — vulval, in pregnancy, 311
Vas aberrans of Haller, (*Fig.* 405) 417
— deferens, artery to, (*Fig.* 401) 410
— — congenital absence of, 405
— — rectal examination of, 585
Vasa recta, (*Fig.* 567) 600
— — of small gut, (*Fig.* 51) 62
— vasorum, (*Fig.* 538) 562
Vascular approach, (*Figs.* 535–541) 560–567
— arrangements in liver, 526
— disease, peripheral, (*Figs.* 594–606) 631–648
— effects of cervical rib, 226
— insult, reflex acute arterial spasm due to, 611
— pattern in relation to surgery, (*Figs.* 490–545) 499–572
— remnants at umbilicus, (*Fig.* 41) 53
— ring in thorax, persistence of, (*Fig.* 504) 518
Vasoconstriction, reflex, due to thrombophlebitis, 611
Vasoconstrictive drugs causing intermittent claudication, 644
Vasoconstrictor nerves to retinal vessels, paralysis of, 613
Vasomotor nerves, origin of, 171

Vasospastic conditions, sympathetic denervation in, 642
Vastus medialis, 669
Vater, ampulla of, (*Figs.* 69, 74) 78
— — diverticulum of, (*Fig.* 430 C–E) 443
— papilla of, 494
— — stenosis at, (*Fig.* 489 B) 497
Vaterine diverticulum, (*Fig.* 430 C–E) 443
Veins, (*Figs.* 298–323) 296–324
— emissary, 296
— lymphatics draining directly with, 321
— of thyroid gland, (*Fig.* 17) 19
— with and without valves, 321
Vena azygos, 320
— cava(ae), anomalies of, (*Figs.* 518–524) 536–545
— — hepatic veins entering, 527
— — inferior, 313
— — — absence of (*see* Azygos Continuation)
— — — anastomoses of portal vein to, (*Fig.* 513) 530, 543
— — — anomalies of infrarenal, (*Fig.* 523) 540, 543
— — — — suprarenal, (*Fig.* 522) 540
— — — development of, (*Figs.* 519, 520) 538, 540, 543
— — — implantation of mesenteric vein into, (*Fig.* 513) 530
— — — left-sided, (*Fig.* 523 A) 542, 543
— — — ligation of, (*Fig.* 317, 318) 318
— — — occlusion of, 306
— — — portal vein emptying into, 523
— — — suprarenal, lack of collaterals for, 549
— — pressure on, from horseshoe kidney, 399
— — superior, absence of right, (*Fig.* 521 E) 540, 543
— — — anastomosis between left and right, (*Fig.* 521 B) 540
— — — lack of collaterals for, 549
— — — obstruction of, above azygos collateral circulation for, (*Fig.* 530) 551
— — — — involving azygos, collateral circulation for, (*Fig.* 531) 551
— — — occlusion of, 306
— — — persistent left, (*Fig.* 521) 538
— caval obstruction, inferior, (*Fig.* 320 B) 322
— — opening in diaphragm, (*Fig.* 184) 197
— comes nervi hypoglossi, 300
Venae comites of lingual artery, (*Fig.* 301) 300
— — in portal obstruction, 529
— hemiazygos, inferior, 320

Venous back pressure in 'white leg', 611
— collateral circulation after ligation of vena cava, (*Figs.* 318, 320 B) 318
— — mechanisms, (*Figs.* 529–531) 549
— development, (*Figs.* 518–520) 536
— drainage of breast, (*Fig.* 26) 31
— — colon, 64
— — gall-bladder, 83, 87
— hypertension due to phlebitis in soleal sinuses, 312
— — in leg, 310, 311, 316
— — transmission of, in saphenous vein, 313
— infarction of colon, postoperative, 64
— ligation, prevention of pulmonary embolism by, (*Figs.* 317, 318) 318
— plexus(es) around funiculus, 706, 707
— — of vertebral bodies, (*Fig.* 322) 323
— renal collar, 543
— sinuses in dura mater, (*Fig.* 3) 5, 6
— system of lower limb, (*Figs.* 309–318) 306–320
— thrombosis of lower limbs, (*Figs.* 317, 318) 318
Ventral aortae, embryonic, (*Fig.* 498) 510
— hernia, 743
— mesentery, (*Fig.* 379) 386
— — persistence of, (*Fig.* 380) 386
Ventricle, lateral, puncture of, (*Fig.* 690) 736
Ventricular hydrocephalus, (*Fig.* 6) 10
— hypertrophy, right, 507
— — — in Fallot's tetralogy, 508, 509
Ventriculo-auriculostomy for hydrocephalus, 10
Ventriculocaval anastomosis for hydrocephalus, 10
Ventriculocisternostomy for hydrocephalus, 10
Ventriculography in hydrocephalus, 10
Version of uterus, 719
Vertebra(ae), abnormalities of, 127
— accessory, in whole or part, 127
— blood-supply of, (*Figs.* 229, 230) 242, 245
— collapse of diseased, (*Fig.* 118) 124
— development of typical, (*Figs.* 663–665) 708
— dislocations of, 659
— forming sacrum, 248
— fusing of bodies of, 695, 696
— lumbosacral, development of, 694
— represented by shapeless mass of bone, 695, 696
— sacralization of fifth lumbar, 127
— transverse processes of, 127
— tuberculosis of, 583
Vertebral arch(es), defects in development of, (*Fig.* 652) 695, 697

Vertebral arch(es), dermoids superficial and deep to, 427
— — failure of, to fuse, (*Fig.* 364) 369
— — development of, (*Fig.* 362) 368, (*Fig.* 663) 708
— — incomplete, 127
— artery(ies), exposure of, 564
— — supplying radicals, 500
— body, defects in development of, 695
— — development of, (*Fig.* 362) 368, (*Figs.* 663–665) 708
— column, (*Figs.* 116–119) 123–128
— — abnormalities of bone in, 127
— — articulations of, (*Fig.* 119) 126
— — assessment of skeletal maturity of, 249
— — bearing and transmission of weight by, (*Fig.* 118) 124
— — in child, (*Fig.* 116 A) 123, 134
— — curves of, (*Fig.* 116) 123, 134
— — extension of, in treatment of collapsed vertebra, (*Fig.* 118) 125
— — movements of, 128
— disease causing low back pain, 695
— epiphysitis, (*Fig.* 671) 715
— fracture with callus narrowing foramen, 707
— metastases of breast cancer, (*Fig.* 323) 324
— — from prostatic carcinoma, 321
— system of veins, (*Fig.* 322) 321
— venous plexuses, external and internal, (*Fig.* 322) 323
Vertical chain of deep cervical lymph-glands, (*Figs.* 326, 327) 328
— heart, 473
Verumontanum, 102
Vesical nerves, injury to, in excision of rectum, 623
Vestibular glands, greater, 200
Vestigial fold, 538
— glands of anus, 111
— structures in connexion with genital organs, (*Figs.* 405, 406) 416
Vibrating tools causing Raynaud's spasm, 644
Vidian canal, nerve of, 142, 145
Vinculum brevis and longus, (*Fig.* 525) 546
Virchow-Robin space, 8
Viscera, high, in hypersthenic type, (*Fig.* 454) 472
— low, in asthenic type, (*Fig.* 457) 473
Visceral arches, (*Figs.* 354, 355) 361
— clefts, (*Figs.* 354, 355) 361
— lymph-glands of abdomen, (*Fig.* 334) 335, 336
— pain, transmission of, 178
— layer of pelvic fascia, (*Figs.* 206, 207) 222

INDEX

Visceral motor nucleus of vagus, (*Fig.* 581) 618
— pelvic fascia supplying false capsule to prostate, 23
— pouches, (*Fig.* 354) 361
Viscero-sensory nerve-fibres, (*Fig.* 165) 178
— parasympathetic fibres to heart, 615
Visual defects due to pressure of pituitary tumour, (*Fig.* 14) 14, 15, 16
Vitelline artery, remains of, at umbilicus, (*Fig.* 41) 53, (*Fig.* 383 F) 390, 392
— veins, anastomosis of, 523
— vessels, remnant of, (*Fig.* 383 F) 390
Vitello-intestinal duct, 377
— — artery of, (*Fig.* 41) 53
— — persistent abnormalities due to, 52, 57, (*Fig.* 383) 389–392
Vocal cord(s), effect on, of injury to external laryngeal nerve, 20
— — palsy due to recurrent nerve injury, 22
— — — — — laryngeal nerve compression, (*Fig.* 437) 454, 455
— — tensor muscle to, 153
Volar accessory ligaments, 215
— arch, superficial, 215
— carpal ligament, (*Fig.* 289) 286
Volkmann's incision of knee-joint, (*Fig.* 772) 810, 812
— ischaemic contracture, 324
Voluntary motor nucleus of vagus, (*Fig.* 581) 618
Volvulus of caecum, mesentery to ascending colon and, 77
— due to abnormal rotation, 382, 383
— neonatorum, 382
Vomiting due to appendicitis, 60
Vulval varicose veins in pregnancy, 311

Waldeyer's fascia (*see* Pelvic Fascia)
— fossa of, 67, (*Fig.* 59) 69
— lymphatic ring, (*Fig.* 324) 325
Wallerian degeneration affecting vagus, 492
Warts at umbilicus, 54
Wax in ear, cough associated with, 139
Weaver's bottom, 262, 266
Webbed fingers, (*Fig.* 413) 424
Wedge deformity of spine, treatment of, (*Fig.* 118) 125
Weeping umbilicus, 53
Weight bearing, considerations of, in planning amputation, 770
— — and transmission by vertebral column, (*Fig.* 118) 124
White bile, 86
— leg, factors causing swelling in, 611
— line, 113, 117
— rami communicantes (*see* Rami Communicantes, White)

Whitlow, subcutaneous, 653
— thecal, 654
— — of thumb or little finger, incisions for, (*Figs.* 723–725) 767
— of terminal phalanx, incisions for opening, (*Figs.* 721, 723) 765
Whooping cough causing diaphragmatic hernia, 684
Wilkie, supraduodenal artery of, (*Fig.* 50) 61
Willis, circle of, 9, (*Fig.* 532) 552
Winged scapula, 204
Winging of scapula test for serratus anterior, 181
Winslow, foramen of, (*Fig.* 55) 67, 68, 729
Wolffian body, epididymis developed from, 405
— duct(s), (*Fig.* 389) 397
— — structures developed from, (*Fig.* 395) 402, 405, 416, 417
— ridge (germinal ridge), 95, 405
Wormian bones, 247
Wrist, binding bands at, (*Figs.* 287–289) 284
— fixation in full extension causing adhesions of tendons to sheaths, 570
— fracture at, restoration of horizontal joint lines of, (*Fig.* 475) 484, 485
— median nerve compression at, 470
— optimum position for ankylosis of, (*Fig.* 483) 488
— paralysis of extensors of, 457
— relations of, 348
— ulnar nerve compression at, 470
Wrist-joint, (*Fig.* 243) 253
— creases marking level of, 658
— position of hand for splinting, (*Fig.* 445) 463
— puncture of, (*Fig.* 685) 734
— surgical approach to, (*Figs.* 765, 766) 807

X-ray appearance of lobe of azygos vein, (*Fig.* 38) 47
— — spondylolisthesis, (*Figs.* 656, 657) 702
— detection of adamantinoma, 354
Xanthochromia, 9
Xiphisternal junction, position of, 41
Xiphisternum, removal of, in midline incision, (*Fig.* 701) 745

Y, anastomosis in, oesophagojejunal, (*Fig.* 755 B) 796

Zuckerkandl, organ of, chromaffin paraganglioma found at, (*Fig.* 607) 649
Zygomatic nerve, 137
Zygomaticofacial nerve, (*Fig.* 129) 137
Zygomaticotemporal nerve, (*Fig.* 129) 137, 138